Tietz's Applied
Laboratory Medicine

Second Edition

THE WILEY BICENTENNIAL—KNOWLEDGE FOR GENERATIONS

$\mathcal{E}$ach generation has its unique needs and aspirations. When Charles Wiley first opened his small printing shop in lower Manhattan in 1807, it was a generation of boundless potential searching for an identity. And we were there, helping to define a new American literary tradition. Over half a century later, in the midst of the Second Industrial Revolution, it was a generation focused on building the future. Once again, we were there, supplying the critical scientific, technical, and engineering knowledge that helped frame the world. Throughout the 20th Century, and into the new millennium, nations began to reach out beyond their own borders and a new international community was born. Wiley was there, expanding its operations around the world to enable a global exchange of ideas, opinions, and know-how.

For 200 years, Wiley has been an integral part of each generation's journey, enabling the flow of information and understanding necessary to meet their needs and fulfill their aspirations. Today, bold new technologies are changing the way we live and learn. Wiley will be there, providing you the must-have knowledge you need to imagine new worlds, new possibilities, and new opportunities.

Generations come and go, but you can always count on Wiley to provide you the knowledge you need, when and where you need it!

WILLIAM J. PESCE
PRESIDENT AND CHIEF EXECUTIVE OFFICER

PETER BOOTH WILEY
CHAIRMAN OF THE BOARD

Tietz's Applied Laboratory Medicine

Second Edition

Mitchell G. Scott
Washington University School of Medicine

Ann M. Gronowski
Washington University School of Medicine

Charles S. Eby
Washington University School of Medicine

BICENTENNIAL
1807
WILEY
2007
BICENTENNIAL

WILEY-INTERSCIENCE
A JOHN WILEY & SONS, INC., PUBLICATION

For general information on our other products and services or for technical support, please contact our Customer Care Department within the United States at (800) 762-2974, outside the United States at (317) 572-3993 or fax (317) 572-4002.

Wiley also publishes its books in a variety of electronic formats. Some content that appears in print may not be available in electronic formats. For more information about Wiley products, visit our web site at www.wiley.com.

Library of Congress Cataloging-in-Publication Data is available.

ISBN-13 978-0-471-71457-6
ISBN-10 0-471-71457-6

10 9 8 7 6 5 4 3 2

Contents

Preface   xi
Contributors   xiii

Part One   Cardiac Disease

**Case 1. A 45-Year-Old Man
with Substantial
Chest Pain**   3
Fred S. Apple

**Case 2. A 48-Year-Old Cocaine User
with Chest Pain**   11
Fred S. Apple and Ramona Evans

Part Two   Pulmonary Diseases

**Case 3. Shortness of Breath with
Productive Cough**   19
Nausherwan K. Burki

**Case 4. Genotype–Phenotype
Correlations in Cystic
Fibrosis**   25
*Latisha Love-Gregory,
Barbara Zehnbauer,
and Dennis Dietzen*

Part Three   Renal Disease

**Case 5. Man with Hypertension
and Fever**   33
C. Darrell Jennings

**Case 6. Oliguria with Metabolic Acidosis
after Renal Transplantation**   41
C. Darrell Jennings

**Case 7. A Woman with Uremia,
Pulmonary Infiltration,
and Hemoptysis**   49
C. Darrell Jennings

**Case 8. Young Man with Edema and
Decreased Urine Output**   55
H. William Schnaper

**Case 9. A New Doctor for a Man with
Diabetes and Hypertension**   65
Michael E. Hull

Case 10. A Pain in the Back   75
*Kevin J. Martin and
Esther A. González*

**Case 11. Refractory Hyponatremia
with Lung Cancer**   79
Manish J. Gandhi

Part Four   Liver Diseases

**Case 12. Adolescent Female with
Tremor, Depression,
and Hepatitis**   91
Steven I. Shedlofsky

v

Case 13. Adult Male with New-Onset Ascites   99
Steven I. Shedlofsky

Case 14. An Unexpected Finding   105
Nathan C. Walk

Case 15. I Did It Just Once—A 37-Year-Old Man with Hepatitis C   111
Alvaro Koch and Luis R. Peña

Case 16. Obese Woman with Persistently Abnormal Liver Enzymes   121
Iliana Bouneva

Part Five   Thyroid Diseases

Case 17. The Irritable Wife   131
William E. Winter

Case 18. The Fatigued Attorney   139
Kenneth B. Ain

Case 19. The Reluctant Chef   143
Kenneth B. Ain

Part Six   Adrenocortical Diseases

Case 20. Child with Rapid Growth and Precocious Sexual Maturation   149
Phyllis W. Speiser

Case 21. Weight Gain, Infertility, and Hypertension   155
William E. Winter

Case 22. The Tired Teenager   167
William E. Winter

Case 23. The Hypertensive Accountant   175
Michael Stowasser and Richard D. Gordon

Case 24. *Don't* "Take Two Aspirin and Call Me in the Morning"   183
Jacqueline E. Payton

Case 25. Unpleasant Spells   189
Les G. K. Q. Burke and Ravinder J. Singh

Part Seven   Diabetes

Case 26. Recent Weight Loss and Polyuria in a 52-Year-Old Man   199
Anders H. Berg and David B. Sacks

Case 27. An Unconscious Diabetic Male   205
Anders H. Berg and David B. Sacks

Case 28. A Diabetic Woman's "Episode"   211
Anders H. Berg and David B. Sacks

Part Eight   Calcium and Parathyroid Hormone (PTH)

Case 29. Bad to the Bone   219
Chelsea A. Sheppard and Corinne R. Fantz

Case 30. A Middle-Aged Woman with Colle's Fracture   225
Catherine A. Hammett-Stabler

Case 31. **A 10-Year-Old Boy with Pain-Induced Seizures** 233
Lorin M. Henrich, Alan D. Rogol, and David E. Bruns

Part Nine   Miscellaneous Endocrine Diseases

Case 32. **Laboratory Tests Ignored** 243
Oren Zinder

Case 33. **Hot Flashes and Abdominal Pain** 249
Jennifer Snyder

Part Ten   Genetically Inherited Disorders

Case 34. **Feed a Cold** 257
Dennis Dietzen

Case 35. **Acute Neonatal Ammonia Intoxication** 263
Dennis Dietzen

Case 36. **Not Just a Picky Eater** 269
Douglas F. Stiekle and Richard E. Lutz

Case 37. **The "Fussy" Neonate** 275
Patricia M. Jones and Dinesh Rakheja

Case 38. **The "Sleepy" Neonate** 281
Dinesh Rakheja and Patricia M. Jones

Case 39. **A Happy but Developmentally Delayed 5-Year-Old Boy** 287
Alison E. Presley and David E. Bruns

Case 40. **The Asymptomatic Iron Man** 293
Elise Krejci

Part Eleven   Infectious Diseases

Case 41. **Tired, Hot, and Lumpy** 301
J. Stacey Klutts

Case 42. **A Rash on the Soles of the Feet** 305
Robyn M. Atkinson

Case 43. **When Life Gives You Lemons** 311
Robert S. Liao

Case 44. **The Wheezing Woodsman** 315
Paula Revell

Case 45. **Not Just Heartburn** 319
Ariel Goldschmidt

Case 46. **The Dangers of Yardwork** 329
Nathan A. Ledeboer

Part Twelve   Nonhematologic Malignancies

Case 47. **An Important Finding on Routine Screening** 337
Joan K. Riley

Case 48. **Increasing Abdominal Girth** 343
Nicholas P. Taylor and Randall K. Gibb

Case 49. **To Screen or Not to Screen?** 349
Da-elene van der Merwe and Eleftherios P. Diamandis

**Case 50. A Male with Confusing
hCG Results**   355
Kingshuk Das

Case 51. Size Greater than Dates 363
*Randall K. Gibb and
Nicholas P. Taylor*

Part Thirteen   Hematologic Malignancies

**Case 52. A Man with Anemia and
Lymphocytosis**   371
*Sylva Bem, Robert E. Hutchison,
and Naif Z. Abraham, Jr.*

**Case 53. A Teenager with Pneumonia,
Leukopenia, and Ecchymoses**   379
Anna Hallsdordottir

**Case 54. A Middle-Aged Man with
Chronic Foot Ulcer**   387
Brian Watson

**Case 55. A Man with Progressive Effort
Intolerance and Splenomegaly** 393
*Mrinal M. Patnaik and
Ayalew Tefferi*

**Case 56. A Man with Splenic Vein
Thrombosis and
Polycythemia**   401
Karen Austin

Part Fourteen   Benign Hematologic
Disorders

Case 57. A Child with Pneumonia   411
John A. Koepke

**Case 58. A Man with a Tender Toe
and Anemia**   419
John Koepke

**Case 59. A Woman with Fatigue
and Pallor**   425
*Naif Z. Abraham, Jr. and
Robert E. Hutchison*

**Case 60. Pulseless Leg 9 Days after
a Myocardial Infarction**   435
Majed Refaai

**Case 61. Young Girl with a Bloody
Knee Effusion**   443
Danielle Stueber

**Case 62. A Young Man with
Chest Pain Following
a Knee Injury**   453
Ganesh C. Kudva

**Case 63. A Young Woman with
Postpartum Cerebral Venous
Thrombosis and Abnormal
Coagulation Tests**   459
Hans-Joachim Reimers

**Case 64. A Baby with Petechiae
and Bruises**   465
Lori Luchtman-Jones

**Case 65. Evaluation of a Reference
Range Outlier**   475
Charles Eby

**Case 66. A Woman with Abdominal
Pain and Thrombocytopenia**   485
Ji Lu

**Case 67. Sudden Jaundice and
Painful Fingers**   491
Arnel Urbiztondo

**Case 68. The Good in "Bad"
Fish Tacos**   497
Kimberley G. Crone

Case 69. The Jaundiced Mother   503
Nathan Walk

Part Fifteen   Porphyrias

Case 70. **Young Woman with Recurrent Abdominal Pain**   513
Steven I. Shedlofsky

Case 71. **A 9-Year-Old Boy with Skin Lesions and Headaches**   523
David Bruns and Audrey K. Bennett

Part Sixteen   Pharmacogenomics

Case 72. **Personalized Medicine for a Renal Transplant Patient**   533
Paul J. Jannetto

Case 73. **Personalized Medicine for Pain Management**   539
Paul J. Jannetto and Nancy C. Bratanow

Case 74. **A Man with Colitis and Pancytopenia**   543
Alison Woodworth

Case 75. **A 46-Year-Old Female with a Painful, Swollen Right Calf**   551
Syamal Bhattacharya, Bradley D. Freeman, and Barbara A. Zehnbauer

Part Seventeen   Toxicology

Case 76. **A Case of Mixed Club Drugs Abuse**   557
Susan B. Gock, Run-Zhang Shi, Jeffery M. Jentzen, and Steven H. Wong

Case 77. **A 43-Year-Old Male with Chronic Pain**   561
Run-Zhang Shi, Susan B. Gock, Jeffrey M. Jentzen, and Steven H. Wong

Case 78. **Metabolic Acidosis of Unknown Origin Among Burn Patients**   567
Deborah Chute and David Bruns

Part Eighteen   Lipid Disorders

Case 79. **The Family Reunion Party**   575
Veronica Luzzi

Case 80. **A 5-Year-Old Boy with Yellow-Orange Tonsils: Hypoalphalipoproteinemia**   581
Raffick A. R. Bowen and Alan T. Remaley

Case 81. **Worsening Diarrhea in a 5-Year-Old Girl**   585
Masako Udewa and Alan T. Remaley

Case 82. **A 4-Year-Old Girl with Yellow Xanthomas and Arthritis**   589
Robert D. Shamburek and Alan T. Remaley

Part Nineteen   Autoimmune Diseases

Case 83. **Woman with Morning Stiffness and Tender, Swollen Joints**   595
Liron Caplan and Sterling G. West

Case 84. **Woman with a Rash and Lower Extremity Pain**   601
Liron Caplan and Sterling G. West

Case 85. Woman with Diarrhea and Anemia 609
Nikola Baumann

Case 89. Is That Really the Calcium Value? 635
Mitchell G. Scott

Part Twenty   Analytical Errors

Case 86. Where's My Baby? 617
Jennifer A. Egan and David G. Grenache

Case 87. Elevated Concentrations, but Not Elevated Enough 623
Ann M. Gronowski

Case 88. I Want To Go Home! 629
Mitchell G. Scott

Part Twenty-One   Miscellaneous

Case 90. A Man with Fever and Acute Polyarthritis 643
William Eugene Davis

Case 91. Middle-Aged Alcoholic with Jaundice and Ascites 649
Luis R. Peña and Alvaro Koch

Case 92. Where Did the Red Cells Go? 658
Arnel Urbiztondo

Index 665

Contributors

Naif Z. Abraham, Jr., M.D., Ph.D. Staff Pathologist, Veterans Affairs Medical Center; Assistant Professor, State University of New York, Upstate Medical University, Syracuse, NY
Case 52, A Man with Anemia and Lymphocytosis; Case 59, A Woman with Fatigue and Pallor

Kenneth B. Ain, M.D. Assistant Professor of Medicine, Division of Endocrinology and Metabolism, Department of Medicine, University of Kentucky Medical Center; Veterans Administration Medical Center, Lexington, KY
Case 18, The Fatigued Attorney; Case 19, The Reluctant Chef

Fred S. Apple, Ph.D. Professor, Department of Laboratory Medicine and Pathology, University of Minnesota School of Medicine; Medical Director of Clinical Chemistry and Toxicology Laboratories, Hennepin County Medical Center, Minneapolis, MN
Case 1, A 45-Year-Old Man with Substantial Chest Pain; Case 2, A 48-year-old Cocaine User With Chest Pain

Robyn Atkinson, Ph.D. Director of Bacteriology, New York State Department of Health, Wadsworth Center, Albany, NY
Case 42, A Rash on the Soles of the Feet

Karen Austin, M.D. Resident, Department of Medicine, Washington University School of Medicine, St. Louis, MO
Case 56, A Man with Splenic Vein Thrombosis and Polycythemia

Nikola Baumann, Ph.D. Director of Clinical Laboratories, Assistant Professor of Pathology, University of Illinois Medical Center, Chicago, IL
Case 85, A Woman with Diarrhea and Anemia

Sylva Bem, M.D. Staff Pathologist, Veterans Affairs Medical Center, Assistant Professor, State University of New York, Upstate Medical University, Syracuse, NY
Case 52, A Man with Anemia and Lymphocytosis

Anders H. Berg Department of Pathology, Harvard Medical School, Boston, MA
Case 26, Recent Weight Loss and Polyuria in a 52-Year-Old Man; Case 27, An Unconscious Diabetic Male; Case 28, A Diabetic Woman's "Episode"

Syamal Bhattacharya Medical Student, University of Tennessee, Memphis, TN
Case 75, A 46-Year-Old Female with a Painful, Swollen Right Calf

Iliana Bouneva, M.D. University of Kentucky, Department of Gastroenterology, Lexington, KY
Case 16, Obese Woman with Persistently Abnormal Liver Enzymes

Raffick A. R. Bowen, Ph.D. Department of Laboratory Medicine, National Institutes of Health, Bethesda, MD
Case 80, A 5 Year-old Boy with Yellow-orange Tonsils: Hypoalphalipoproteinemia

Nancy Bratanow, M.D.   Midwest Comprehensive Pain Care Center, Milwaukee, WI
Case 73, Personalized Medicine for Pain Management

David E. Bruns, M.D.   Professor, Department of Pathology, University of Virginia Medical Center, Charlottesville, VA
Case 31, 10-Year-Old Boy with Pain-Induced Seizures; Case 39, A Happy, But Developmentally Delayed, 5-Year-Old Boy; Case 71, 9-Year-old with Hyperpigmentation and Stomach Aches; Case 78, Metabolic Acidosis of Unknown Origin Among Burn Patients

Les G.K.Q. Burke, M.D.   Department of Laboratory Medicine and Pathology, Mayo Clinic, Rochester, MN
Case 25, Unpleasant Spells

Nausherwan K. Burki, M.D.   Professor of Medicine, Division of Pulmonary and Critical Care Medicine, University of Connecticut Health Centre, Farmington, CT
Case 3, Shortness of Breath with Productive Cough

Liron Caplan, M.D.   University of Colorado at Denver and Health Science Center, Denver, CO
Case 83, Woman with Morning Stiffness and Tender, Swollen Joints; Case 84, Woman with a Rash and Lower Extremity Pain

Deborah Chute, M.D.   Resident, Department of Pathology, University of Virginia Medical Center, Charlottesville, VA.
Case 78, Metabolic Acidosis of Unknown Origin Among Burn Patients

Kimberly Crone, M.D.   Resident, Department of Pathology and Immunology, Division of Laboratory Medicine, Washington University School of Medicine, St. Louis, MO
Case 68, The Good in "Bad" Fish Tacos

Kingshuk Das, M.D.   Resident, Department of Pathology and Immunology, Division of Laboratory Medicine, Washington University School of Medicine, St. Louis, MO
Case 50, A Male with Confusing hCG Results

William Davis, M.D.   Program Director of Internal Medicine Residency, Ochsner Clinical Foundation and Clinical Associate Professor of Medicine, Tulane University, New Orleans, LA
Case 90, A Man with Fever and Acute Polyarthritis

Eleftherios Diamandis, M.D., Ph.D.   Head, Section of Clinical Biochemistry, Department of Pathology and Laboratory Medicine, Mount Sinai Hospital, Professor and Head, Division of Clinical Biochemistry, Department of Laboratory Medicine and Pathobiology, University of Toronto, Ontario, Canada
Case 49, To Screen or Not to Screen

Dennis Dietzen, Ph.D.   Assistant Professor of Pediatrics and Pathology, Washington University School of Medicine, St. Louis, Missouri, Assistant Director, Clinical Chemistry and Metabolic Genetics Laboratories, St. Louis Children's Hospital, St. Louis, MO
Case 4, Genotype-Phenotype Correlations in Cystic Fibrosis; Case 34, Feed a Cold; Case 35, Acute Neonatal Ammonia Intoxication

Charles Eby, M.D.   Associate Professor of Pathology and Immunology, Division of Laboratory Medicine, Washington University School of Medicine, St. Louis, MO
Case 65, Evaluation of a Reference Range Outlier

Jennifer A. Egan, M.D.   Resident, Department of Pathology and Laboratory Medicine, University of North Carolina School of Medicine, Chapel Hill, NC
Case 86, Where's My Baby?

Ramona Evans, M.D.   Resident in Pathology, University of Minnesota, Department of Laboratory Medicine and Pathology, Minneapolis, MN
Case 2, A 48-Year-Old Cocaine User With Chest Pain

Corinne Fantz, Ph.D.   Assistant Professor, Core Labs, Emory University, Crawford Long Hospital, Department of Pathology and Laboratory Medicine, Atlanta, GA
Case 29, Bad to the Bone

Bradley D. Freeman, M.D.   Associate Professor of Surgery, Washington University School of Medicine, St. Louis, MO
Case 75, A 46-Year-Old Female with a Painful, Swollen Right Calf

Manish J. Gandhi, M.D.   Resident in Department of Pathology and Immunology, Division of Laboratory Medicine, Washington University School of Medicine, St. Louis, MO
Case 11, Refractory Hyponatremia with Lung Cancer

Randall K. Gibb, M.D.   Assistant Professor of Obstetrics and Gynecology, Washington University School of Medicine, St. Louis, MO
Case 48, Increasing Abdominal Girth; Case 51, Size Greater than Dates

Susan B. Gock   Technical Director, Milwaukee County Medical Examiners Office, Medical College of Wisconsin, Milwaukee, WI
Case 76, Case of Mixed Club Drugs Abuse; Case 77, A 43-Year-Old Male with Chronic Pain

Ariel Goldschmidt, M.D.   Resident in Laboratory Medicine, Department of Pathology and Immunology, Washington University School of Medicine, St. Louis, MO
Case 45, Not Just Heartburn

Esther A. González, M.D.   Associate Professor of Internal Medicine, Division of Nephrology, St. Louis University, St. Louis, MO
Case 10, A Pain in the Back

Richard Gordon, MBBS, FRACP, Ph.D., M.D.   Professor and Co-Director, Endocrine Hypertension Research Centre, University of Queensland School of Medicine, Princess Alexandra Hospital, Brisbane, Australia
Case 23, The Hypertensive Accountant

David Grenache, Ph.D.   Assistant Professor, Department of Pathology and Laboratory Medicine, University of North Carolina School of Medicine, Chapel Hill, Chapel Hill, NC
Case 86, Where's My Baby?

Ann M. Gronowski, Ph.D.   Associate Professor of Pathology and Immunology, Division of Laboratory Medicine, Washington University School of Medicine, Associate Medical Co-Director of Clinical Chemistry, Barnes-Jewish Hospital, St. Louis, MO
Case 87, Elevated Concentrations, but Not Elevated Enough

Anna Halldórsdóttir, M.D.   Resident in Department of Pathology and Immunology, Division of Laboratory Medicine, Washington University School of Medicine, St. Louis, MO
Case 53, A Teenager with Pneumonia, Leukopenia, and Ecchymoses

Catherine Hammett-Stabler, Ph.D.   Associate Professor of Pathology and Laboratory Medicine, University of North Carolina, Chapel Hill, NC
Case 30, A Middle-Aged Woman with Colle's Fracture

Lorin M. Henrich, Ph.D.   Postdoctoral Fellow in Clinical Chemistry, Department of Pathology, University of Virginia Medical Center, Charlottesville, VA
Case 31, 10-Year-Old Boy with Pain-Induced Seizures

Michael Hull, M.D.   Resident in Department of Pathology and Immunology, Division of Laboratory Medicine, Washington University School of Medicine, St. Louis, MO
Case 9, A New Doctor for a Man With Diabetes and Hypertension

Robert T. Hutchison, M.D.   Professor of Pathology, State University of New York, Upstate Medical University, Syracuse, NY
Case 52, A Man with Anemia and Lymphocytosis; Case 59, A Woman with Fatigue and Pallor

Paul Jannetto, Ph.D.   Assistant Professor of Pathology, Medical College of Wisconsin, Milwaukee, WI
Case 72, Personalized Medicine for A Renal Transplant Patient; Case 73, Personalized Medicine for Pain Management

C. Darrell Jennings, M.D.   Associate Professor, Department of Pathology and Laboratory Medicine; Director of Immunopathology, University of Kentucky College of Medicine; Associate Director of Clinical Laboratories, University of Kentucky Medical Center, Lexington, KY
Case 5, Man with Hypertension and Fever; Case 6, Oliguria with Metabolic Acidosis After Renal Transplantation; Case 7, A Woman with Uremia, Pulmonary Infiltration, and Hemoptysis

Jeffrey M. Jentzen, M.D.   Professor of Pathology, Medical College of Wisconsin, Milwaukee, WI
Case 76, Case of Mixed Club Drugs Abuse; Case 77, A 43-Year-Old Male with Chronic Pain

Patricia M. Jones, Ph.D.   Children's Medical Center, Dallas, TX
Case 37, The "Fussy" Neonate; Case 38, The "Sleepy" Neonate

J. Stacey Klutts, M.D., Ph.D.   Resident in Department of Pathology and Immunology, Division of Laboratory Medicine, Washington University School of Medicine, St. Louis, MO
Case 41, Tired, Hot, and Lumpy

Alvaro Koch, M.D.   Assistant Professor of Medicine, Medical Director, Liver Transplantation Program, Division of Digestive Diseases and Nutrition, University of Kentucky, Lexington, KY
Case 15, "I Just Did It Once"—A 37 Year-Old Man with Hepatitis C; Case 91, Middle-aged Alcoholic with Jaundice and Ascites

John A. Koepke, Ph.D.   Professor Emeritus, Duke University Medical Center, Durham, NC
Case 57, A Child with Pneumonia; Case 58, A Man with a Tender Toe and Anemia

Elise Krejci, M.D. Resident in Laboratory Medicine, Department of Pathology and Immunology, Washington University School of Medicine, St Louis, MO
Case 40, The Asymptomatic Iron Man

Ganesh C. Kudva, M.D. Division of Hematology and Oncology, St. Louis University School of Medicine, St. Louis, MO
Case 62, A Young Man with Chest Pain Following a Knee Injury

Nathan Ledeboer, Ph.D. Postdoctoral Fellow, Medical and Public Health Microbiology, Department of Pathology and Immunology, Division of Laboratory Medicine, Washington University School of Medicine, St. Louis, MO
Case 46, The Dangers of Yard Work

Robert Liao, Ph.D. Assistant Professor, Department of Pathology and Molecular Medicine and Director of Clinical Microbiology, Queens University Hospital, Kingston, Ontario, Canada
Case 43, When Life Gives You Lemons

Latisha Love-Gregory, Ph.D. Postdoctoral Fellow in Clinical Chemistry, Department of Pathology and Immunology, Division of Laboratory Medicine, Washington University School of Medicine, St. Louis, MO
Case 4, Genotype-Phenotype Correlations in Cystic Fibrosis (CF)

Lu Ji, M.D. Resident in the Department of Pathology and Immunology, Washington University School of Medicine, St. Louis, MO
Case 66, A Woman with Abdominal Pain and Thrombocytopenia

Lori Luchtman-Jones, M.D. Assistant Professor of Pediatrics, Division of Hematology and Oncology, Washington University School of Medicine, St. Louis, MO
Case 64, A Baby with Petechiae and Bruises

Veronica Luzzi, Ph.D. Research Associate Professor of Medicine, Department of Internal Medicine, Division of Lipid Research, Washington University School of Medicine, St. Louis, MO
Case 79, The Family Reunion Party

Richard E. Lutz, M.D. Department of Pathology and Microbiology, University of Nebraska Medical Center, Omaha, NE
Case 36, Not Just a Picky Eater

Kevin J. Martin, M.B., B.Ch. Professor of Internal Medicine, Director, Division of Nephrology, St. Louis University Health Science Center, St. Louis, MO
Case 10, A Pain in the Back

Mrinal M. Patnaik, M.D. Postdoctoral Fellow, Department of Hematology, Mayo Clinic, Rochester, MN
Case 55, A Man with Progressive Effort Intolerance and Splenomegaly

Jacqueline Payton, M.D., Ph.D. Resident in Department of Pathology and Immunology, Division of Laboratory Medicine, Washington University School of Medicine, St. Louis, MO
Case 24, Don't "Take Two Aspirin and Call Me in the Morning"

Luis R. Peña, M.D., F.A.C.G. Assistant Professor of Medicine, Director, Gastroenterology Fellowship Program, Division of Digestive Diseases and Nutrition, University of Kentucky Medical Center, Lexington, KY
Case 15, "I Just Did It Once "— A 37 Year-Old Man with Hepatitis C

Alison E. Presley, M.D. Transfusion Medicine Fellow, University of Virginia Health Systems, Department of Pathology, Charlottesville, VA
Case 39, A Happy, But Developmentally Delayed, 5-Year-Old Boy

Dinesh Rakheja Department of Pathology, University of Texas Southwestern Medical Center, Dallas, TX
Case 37, The "Fussy" Neonate; Case 38, The "Sleepy" Neonate

Majed Refaai, M.D. Resident in Department of Pathology and Immunology, Division of Laboratory Medicine, Washington University School of Medicine, St. Louis, MO
Case 60, Pulseless Leg Nine Days After a Myocardial Infarction

Hans-Jochim Reimers, M.D., Ph.D. St. Louis University, Department of Hematology and Oncology, St. Louis, MO 63110
Case 64, Acquired Venous Thromboembolism

Alan T. Remaley, Ph.D., M.D. National Institutes of Health, Department of Laboratory Medicine, Bethesda, MD
Case 80, A 5-Year-old Boy with Enlarged Yellow-orange Tonsils: Hypoalphalipoproteinemia; Case 81, Worsening Diarrhea in a 5-Year-old Girl; Case 82, A 4-Year-Old Girl with Yellow Xanthomas and Arthritis

Paula Revell, Ph.D. Postdoctoral Fellow, Medical and Public Health Microbiology, Department of Pathology and Immunology, Division of Laboratory Medicine, Washington University School of Medicine, St. Louis, MO
Case 44, The Wheezing Woodsman

Joan Riley, Ph.D. Postdoctoral Fellow in Clinical Chemistry, Department of Pathology and Immunology, Division of Laboratory Medicine, Washington University School of Medicine, St. Louis, MO
Case 47, An Important Finding on Routine Screening

Alan D. Rogol, M.D. Department of Pathology, University of Virginia Medical Center, Charlottesville, VA
Case 31, A 10-Year-Old Boy with Pain-Induced Seizures

David B. Sacks, M.B., ChB. Associate Professor of Pathology, Harvard Medical School, Boston, MA
Case 26, Recent Weight Loss and Polyuria in a 52-Year-Old Man; Case 27, An Unconscious Diabetic Male; Case 28, A Diabetic Woman's "Episode"

H. William Schnaper, M.D. Associate Professor, Department of Pediatrics, George Washington University; Department of Nephrology, Children's National Medical Center, Washington, DC
Case 8, Young Man with Edema and Decreased Urine

Mitchell G. Scott, Ph.D. Professor of Pathology and Immunology, Division of Laboratory Medicine, Washington University School of Medicine, Medical Co-Director of Clinical Chemistry, Barnes-Jewish Hospital, St. Louis, MO
Case 88, I Want to Go Home!; Case 89, Is that really the Calcium Value?

Robert D. Shamburek, M.D. National Institutes of Health, Department of Laboratory Medicine, Bethesda, MD
Case 82, A 4-Year-Old Girl with Yellow Xanthomas and Arthritis

Steven I. Shedlovsky, M.D.   Associate Professor, Department of Medicine and Graduate Center for Toxicology, University of Kentucky College of Medicine, Staff Gastroenterologist, Veterans Administration Hospital and University of Kentucky Medical Center, Lexington, KY
Case 12, Adolescent Female with Tremor, Depression, and Hepatitis (Wilson's Disease); Case 13, Adult Male with New Onset Ascites; Case 70, Young Woman with Recurrent Abdominal Pain

Chelsea Sheppard, M.D.   Clinical Fellow, Core Labs, Emory University, Crawford Long Hospital, Department of Pathology and Laboratory Medicine, Atlanta, GA
Case 29, Bad to the Bone

Run-Zhang Shi, Ph.D.   Department of Pathology, Medical College of Wisconsin, Milwaukee, WI
Case 76, Use of "Club Drugs" by a 24-Year-old Female

Ravinder Singh, Ph.D.   Department of Laboratory Medicine and Pathology, Mayo Clinic, Rochester, MN
Case 25, Unpleasant Spells

Jennifer Snyder   Department of Pathology and Laboratory Medicine, University of North Carolina School of Medicine, Chapel Hill, NC
Case 33, Hot Flashes and Abdominal Pain

Phyllis Speiser, M.D.   Associate Professor, Pediatric Endocrinology, Schneider Children's Hospital, New Hyde Park, NY
Case 20, Child with Rapid Growth and Precocious Sexual Maturation

Douglas F. Stickle, Ph.D.   Technical Director of Clinical Chemistry, Assistant Professor, Department of Pathology and Microbiology, University of Nebraska Medical Center, Omaha, NE
Case 36, Not Just a Picky Eater

Michael Stowasser, MBBS, FRACP, Ph.D.   Associate Professor and Co-Director, Endocrine Hypertension Research Centre, University of Queensland School of Medicine, Princess Alexandra Hospital, Brisbane, Australia
Case 23, The Hypertensive Accountant

Danielle Stueber, M.D.   Research Technologist, Department of Medicine, Washington University School of Medicine, St. Louis, MO
Case 61, Young Girl with a Bloody Knee Effusion

Nicholas Taylor, M.D.   Clinical Fellow, Department of Obstetrics & Gynecology, Washington University School of Medicine, St. Louis, MO
Case 48, Increasing Abdominal Girth; Case 51, Size Greater than Dates

Ayalew Tefferi, M.D.   Department of Hematology, Mayo Clinic, Rochester, MN
Case 55, A Man with Progressive Effort Intolerance and Splenomegaly

Masako Ueda, M.D.   Department of Laboratory Medicine, National Institutes of Health, Bethesda, MD
Case 81, Worsening Diarrhea in a 5-Year-Old Girl

Arnel Urbiztondo, M.D.   Transfusion Medicine Fellow, Department of Pathology and Immunology, Division of Laboratory Medicine, Washington University School of Medicine, St. Louis, MO
Case 67, Sudden Jaundice and Painful Fingers; Case 92, Where Did the Red Cells Go?

Da-olone van der Merwe, M.D.   Department of Pathology and Laboratory Medicine, Mount Sinai Hospital, Toronto, Ontario, Canada
Case 49, To Screen or Not to Screen

Nathan Walk, M.D.   Resident in Department of Pathology and Immunology, Division of Laboratory Medicine, Washington University School of Medicine, St. Louis, MO
Case 14, An Unexpected Finding. . .; Case 69, The Jaundiced Mother

Brian Watson, M.D., Ph.D.   Resident in Department of Pathology and Immunology, Division of Laboratory Medicine, Washington University School of Medicine, St. Louis, MO
Case 54, A Middle-Aged Man with Chronic Foot Ulcer

Sterling G. West, M.D.   Professor of Rheumatology/Allergy and Clinical Immunology, University of Colorado at Denver and Health Science Center, Denver, CO
Case 83, Woman with Morning Stiffness and Tender, Swollen Joints; Case 84, Woman with a Rash and Lower Extremity Pain

William E. Winter, M.D.   Professor, Department of Pathology, University of Florida, Gainesville, FL
Case 17, The Irritable Wife; Case 21, Weight Gain, Infertility, and Hypertension; Case 22, The Tired Teenager

Steven Wong, Ph.D.   Professor, Department of Pathology, Medical College of Wisconsin, Milwaukee, WI
Case 76, Case of Mixed Club Drugs Abuse; Case 77, A 43-Year-Old Male with Chronic Pain

Alison Woodworth, Ph.D.   Postdoctoral Fellow in Clinical Chemistry, Department of Pathology and Immunology, Division of Laboratory Medicine, Washington University School of Medicine, St. Louis, MO
Case 74, A Man with Colitis and Pancytopenia

Barbara Zehnbauer, Ph.D.   Clinical Professor in the Departments of Pathology and Immunology, and Pediatrics, Director, Molecular Core Laboratory, Site-man Cancer Center, Washington University School of Medicine, St. Louis, MO
Case 4, Genotype-Phenotype Correlations in Cystic Fibrosis (CF); Case 75, A 46-Year-Old Female with a Painful, Swollen Right Calf

Oren Zinder, Ph.D.   Professor, Department of Clinical Biochemistry, Rambam Medical Center, Haifa, Israel
Case 32, Laboratoy Tests Ignored

Part One

Cardiac Disease

Cases of cardiac risk with myocardial infarction and with cocaine abuse are
presented and discussed in Cases 1 and 2 [both edited by MGS (editors' names
are listed on title page in book Frontmatter)], respectively.

Tietz's Applied Laboratory Medicine, Second Edition. Edited by Mitchell G. Scott, Ann M. Gronowski, and
Charles S. Eby
Copyright © 2007 John Wiley & Sons, Inc.

Case 1

A 45-Year-Old Man with Substantial Chest Pain

Fred S. Apple

History of Current Presentation

The subject is a 45-year-old African-American male who presents with a chief complaint of "substantial chest pain" that radiated through his right arm and back. The pain awoke him from his sleep at approximately 3:30 am and was described as constant and as "8 out of 10." He also complained of nausea and shortness of breath. Over the past 2–3 months he stated that he had experienced similar symptoms that radiated through both arms. One month prior to admission, he visited his primary care internist, during which time his electrocardiogram (EKG) and x-rays were normal. A stress test was scheduled but the appointment was missed. On the morning of presentation, the patient took 1 aspirin (325 mg) within 30 minutes of awakening. The subject presents to the emergency department 1 hour [0430 h (4:30 am)] after onset of acute chest pain.

He had a past medical history of hypertension and takes both antihypertensive medication and aspirin daily. He is a smoker (20 years), and occasional drinker, and his father had a fatal myocardial infarction (MI) at the age of 72. At physical examination, temperature, pulse, and respiration were normal, blood pressure 200/40, O_2 saturation (pulse oximetry) 92% on room air and 99% after receiving 100% oxygen. He was alert, awake, and oriented in moderate discomfort. His lungs were clear to auscultation bilaterally with no rales or wheezes. Heart rate and rhythm were regular without murmurs. Chest x-ray showed borderline cardiomegaly, without infiltrates.

At presentation, routine chemistries, CBC, and cardiac biomarkers were within normal limits. The EKG at presentation shows poor R-wave progression anteriorly, with an ST depression in lead III. Consultation with the attending cardiologist following a similar EKG repeated at 1 hour after presentation ruled out MI. The patient was managed medically with nitroglycerin sublingually ($\times 3$ doses), which improved his discomfort to the point where he was pain-free. His blood pressure improved (decreased) following medication. He was also given multiple doses of morphine sulfate for his right arm pain.

Given the history and current presentation, the patient was admitted to the cardiac short-stay unit, and monitored. He was given nitrogycerine and low-molecular-weight

Tietz's Applied Laboratory Medicine, Second Edition. Edited by Mitchell G. Scott, Ann M. Gronowski, and Charles S. Eby
Copyright © 2007 John Wiley & Sons, Inc.

heparin (LMWH, enoxaparin). Repeat cardiac biomarkers were ordered for 4 and 8 hours after presentation. Four hours following presentation, the EKG showed inverted T waves, now with new Q waves in the anterior leads. Repeat measurements of biomarkers at 0845 h (8:45 am) showed elevated values for total CK, CKMB, and condiac troponin T(cTnT).

Day Reference Intervals	Time, h	Total CK U/L 60–300	CKMB, μg/L ≤7.0	cTnT, μg/L <0.01	EKG
1	0430	40	1.5	<0.01	ST depression
	0845	405	88	3.2	Q wave
	0930	—	—	—	Stent placement
	1445	4850	950	31.5	—
2	0600	3225	505	24.2	—
	1800	1258	245	18.1	—

The diagnosis of an evolving acute MI was made and the patient was immediately taken to the cardiac catheterization lab and a glycoprotein IIB IIIA inhibitor [ReoPro (abciximab)] was started. In the catherization lab (0930 h), the patient's 100% occluded left anterior descending (LAD) coronary artery was opened by angioplasty and a stent was placed, with successful reperfusion. His chest pain was relieved following the procedure, without recurrence. There were no signs of any congestive heart failure issues. His echocardiographic (echo) study showed an ejection fraction of 48%.

In the hospital, the patient tolerated progressive ambulation without difficulty. He was discharged on day 4, on multiple medications, and scheduled for cardiac rehabilitation, medication assessment, and outpatient follow-up. Presently use of biomarkers such as cardiac troponin, BNP (B-type natriurtic peptide), or hsCRP are not routinely used for follow-up in post-MI patients for risk assessment, unless clinically indicated.

Definition of the Disease

Acute myocardial infarction (AMI) is defined as an imbalance between myocardial oxygen supply and demand resulting in injury and eventual death of myocytes. It is now thought that the migration of stem cells has the potential to replace at least some damaged myocytes. When the blood supply to the heart is interrupted, "gross necrosis" of the myocardium results. Necrosis is most often associated with a thrombotic occlusion superimposed on coronary atherosclerosis. The process of plaque rupture and thrombosis is one of the ways in which coronary atherosclerosis progresses and that we currently recognize only the more severe of these events. Total loss of coronary blood flow in a major coronary artery results in a clinical syndrome known as *ST-segment elevation AMI* (STEMI). Partial loss of coronary perfusion can also lead to necrosis as well, is generally less severe, and is known as *non-ST-elevation myocardial infarction* (NSTEMI). Other events of still lesser severity may be missed entirely and can range from stable to unstable angina.

Presenting Symptoms

The clinical history remains of substantial value in establishing a diagnosis. A prodromal history of angina can be found in 40–50% of patients with AMI; approximately one-third have symptoms 1–4 weeks before hospitalization. In the remaining two-thirds, symptoms predate admission by a week or less, and one-third of these patients will have had symptoms for 24 hours or less.

The pain of AMI is variable in intensity; in most patients it is severe but rarely intolerable. The pain may be prolonged, up to 30 minutes. The discomfort is described as constricting, crushing, oppressing, or compressing; often the patient complains of something sitting on or squeezing the chest. Although usually described as a squeezing, choking, viselike, or heavy pain, it may also be characterized as a stabbing, knifelike, boring, or burning discomfort. The pain is usually retrosternal in location, spreading frequently to both sides of the chest, often favoring the left side and radiating down the left arm. In some instances, the pain of AMI may begin in the epigastrium and simulate a variety of abdominal disorders, which often causes MI to be misdiagnosed as indigestion. In other patients, the discomfort radiates to the shoulders, upper extremities, neck, and jaw. Older individuals, diabetics, and women often present without the typical pain. For example, less than 50% of those over age 80 who present with AMI will have chest discomfort. Sometimes, these patients will present with shortness of breath, fatigue, or even confusion. The pain of AMI may have disappeared by the time physicians first encounter the patient (or the patient reaches the hospital), or it may persist for a few hours.

Diagnostic Criteria

Previously, the diagnosis of AMI established by the World Health Organization in 1986 required at least two of the following criteria: a history of chest pain, evolutionary changes on the ECG, and/or serial elevations of cardiac markers. However, it was rare for a diagnosis of AMI to be made in the absence of biochemical evidence. A 2000 European Society of Cardiology/American College of Cardiology (ESC/ACC) consensus conference has codified the role of biomarkers, specifically cardiac troponin I or T, by advocating that the diagnosis be based on biomarkers of cardiac damage in the appropriate clinical situation.[1-5] The criteria for diagnosis of an acute and established AMI are described in Table 1.1. The guidelines recognize the reality that neither the clinical presentation nor the ECG has adequate sensitivity and specificity for myocardial necrosis. This guideline does not suggest that all elevations of these biomarkers should elicit a diagnosis of AMI;

Table 1.1   Diagnosis of Myocardial Infarction

Acute MI: Either one of the following criteria satisfies the diagnosis for an acute, evolving, or recent MI:
1. Typical rise and gradual fall (cardiac troponin) or more rapid rise and fall (CK-MB) of biochemical markers of myocardial necrosis with at least one of the following:
   a. Ischemic symptoms
   b. Development of pathological Q waves on ECG
   c. ECG changes indicative of ischemia (ST-segment elevation or depression)
   d. Coronary artery intervention (e.g., coronary angioplasty)
2. Pathological findings of an acute MI.

Established MI: Any one of the following criteria satisfies the diagnosis for established MI:
1. Development of new pathologic Q waves on serial ECGs. The patient may or may not remember previous symptoms. Biochemical markers of myocardial necrosis may have normalized, depending on the length of time that has passed since the infarct developed.
2. Pathological findings of a healed or healing MI.

Table 1.2   ESC/ACC Recommendations for Use of Cardiac Biomarkers for Detection of Myocardial Injury and Myocardial Infarction

Increases in biomarkers of cardiac injury are indicative of injury to the myocardium, but not an ischemic mechanism of injury.

Cardiac troponins (I or T) are preferred markers for diagnosis of myocardial injury.

Increases in cardiac marker proteins reflect irreversible injury.

Improved quality control of troponin assays is essential.

Myocardial infarction is present when there is cardiac damage, as detected by marker proteins (an increase above the 99th percentile of the normal range) in a clinical setting consistent with myocardial ischemia.

For patients with an ischemic mechanism of injury, prognosis is related to the extent of troponin increases.

If an ischemic mechanism is unlikely, other etiologies for cardiac injury should be pursued.

Samples must be obtained at least 6–9 hours after the symptoms begin.

After PCI and CABG, the significance of marker elevations and patient care should be individualized.

only those associated with the appropriate clinical and/or ECG findings.[6,7] When elevations that are not caused by an acute ischemia event, the clinician is obligated to search for another etiology for the elevation. The criteria suggested for use with these biomarkers by the Biochemistry Panel of the ESC/ACC Committee is listed in Table 1.2.

The use of these new criteria has led to the NSTEMI diagnosis. The initial ECG used to have a sensitivity of about 50% for AMI. As the diagnosis of NSTEMI is made with greater and greater sensitivity, the frequency of STEMI among all AMI has decreased. Serial ECG tracings are helpful for STEMI but not for what now makes up almost 70% of AMIs, those with NSTEMI. The classic ECG changes of an STEMI are ST-segment elevation, which often evolves to the development of Q waves without intervention. Most NSTEMIs present with either ST segment depression, with or without T-wave changes; T-wave changes alone; or occasionally in the absence of any ECG findings. Those with ST-segment change have a substantially worse prognosis. There are many other clinical aspects that might suggest AMI as the etiology of a given biomarker elevation. For example, the finding of significant coronary obstructive lesions, especially in a pattern suggestive of recent plaque rupture, is highly suggestive. At times, a positive stress test with or without imaging may be necessary to help make the diagnosis. However, if the clinical situation is not suggestive, other sources for cardiac injury should be sought.

The term *acute coronary syndrome* (ACS) is increasingly used in the literature and encompasses all patients who present with unstable ischemic heart disease. If they have STE, they are called *STEMI*. If they do not have STE but have biochemical criteria for cardiac injury, they are called *NSTEMI*, few of whom develop ECG Q waves. Those who have unstable ischemia and do not manifest cardiac necrosis markers are designated patients with unstable angina (UA). Most of these syndromes occur in response to an acute event in the coronary artery when circulation to a region of the heart is obstructed. If the obstruction is high-grade and persists, then necrosis usually ensues. Since necrosis is known to take some time to develop, it is apparent that opening the blocked coronary artery in a timely fashion can often prevent death of myocardial tissue.

Pathogenesis

The major cause of ACS is atherosclerosis, which contributes to significant narrowing of the artery lumen and a propensity for plaque disruption and thrombus formation.

Myocardial ischemia and subsequent infarction usually begin in the endocardium and spread toward the epicardium. The extent of myocardial injury reflects (1) extent of the occlusion, (2) duration of the imbalance between coronary supply and substrate availability, and (3) the metabolic needs of the tissue. Irreversible cardiac injury consistently occurs in animals when complete occlusion is present for at least 15–20 minutes. Most of the damage occurs within the first 2–3 hours. Restoration of flow within the first 60–90 minutes evokes maximal salvage of tissue, but the benefits of reperfusion up to 4–6 hours are sufficient to be associated with increased survival. The percentage of tissue at risk that undergoes necrosis (infarct size) is highly variable and difficult to predict.

In most cases, the left ventricle is affected by AMI. However, with right coronary and/or circumflex occlusions, the right ventricle can also be involved. Coronary thrombi will undergo spontaneous lysis, even if untreated, in about 50% of cases within 10 days. However, for patients with STEMI, opening the vessel earlier with clot-dissolving agents (thrombolysis) and/or percutaneous intervention (PCI) can often save myocardium and lives. Consequently, percutaneous intervention with stenting is the preferred therapy for STEMI. However, many hospitals cannot or do not offer urgent PCI 24 hours a day, 365 days per year. Thus clot-dissolving medications still play a major role in the treatment of these patients. It is now apparent that urgent invasive revascularization also benefits those with NSTEMI. We now know that many treatments, such as newer anticoagulant, antiplatelet, and antiinflammatory agents in conjunction with coronary revascularization, save lives in this group.

Precipitating Factors

In many patients with AMI, no precipitating factor can be identified. Studies have noted the following patient activities at the onset of AMI: modest, heavy, or usual physical exertion, surgical procedure, rest, and sleep. If and when these activities trigger an infarction, the window of risk is often brief, usually only an hour or two. The severe exertion that preceded an infarction was often performed at times when the patient was fatigued or emotionally stressed.

There are causes of infarction other than acute atherothrombotic coronary occlusion. Prolonged vasospasm can induce infarction, and spontaneous dissections are becoming more commonly appreciated, especially in pregnant females. Other conditions can also cause the death of cardiomyocytes and lead to a biochemical signal of myocyte damage, but should not be confused with myocardial infarction. These include (1) trauma that may precipitate myocardial contusion; (2) toxic reactions to chemotherapy agents, such as Adriamycin, or myocardial depressant substances released with sepsis; (3) heat-induced injury after cardioversion; (4) increases in wall stress with impairment of subendocardial perfusion caused by severe hypo- or hypertension; and/or (5) injury caused by catecholamine release in patients with acute neurological catastrophes. Pulmonary embolism is another common cause of biomarker increase.

Anatomy of an MI

On gross pathological examination, AMI can be divided into subendocardial (nontransmural) infarctions and transmural infarctions. The pathological changes correlate poorly with clinical, ECG, and biochemical markers of necrosis. In experimental infarction, the earliest ultrastructural changes in cardiac muscle following occlusion of a coronary artery noted within 20 minutes by electron microscopy, consist of a reduction in the size and number of glycogen granules, intracellular edema, and swelling and distortion of the transverse tubular system, the sarcoplasmic reticulum, and the mitochondria. These early changes are partially reversible. Changes after 60 minutes of occlusion include myocardial cell swelling and mitochondrial abnormalities. After 20 minutes to 2 hours of ischemia, changes in some cells become irreversible, with a progression of these alterations, including enlarged mitochondria with few cristae and clumping, and thinning and disorientation of myofibrils. Cells irreversibly damaged by ischemia are usually swollen, with an enlarged sarcoplasmic reticulum. Defects in the plasma membrane may appear.

In some infarcts a pattern of wavy myocardial fibers may be seen by light microscopy 1– 3 hours after onset, especially at the periphery. After 8 hours, edema of the interstitium becomes evident, as do increased fatty deposits in the muscle fibers. By 24 hours there is clumping of the cytoplasm and loss of cross-striations, with appearance of irregular cross-bands in the involved myocardial fibers. During the first 3 days, the interstitial tissue becomes edematous. On about day 4 after infarction, removal of necrotic fibers by macrophages begins, again commencing at the periphery. By day 8, the necrotic muscle fibers have become dissolved; by about 10 days the number of polymorphonuclear leukocytes is reduced, and granulation tissue first appears at the periphery. Removal of necrotic muscle cells continues until weeks 4–6 following infarction. By the sixth week, the infarcted area has usually been converted into a firm connective tissue scar with interspersed intact muscle fibers. Gross alterations of the myocardium are difficult to identify until at least 6–12 hours following the onset of necrosis. By 18–36 hours after onset of the infarct, the myocardium is tan or reddish purple (because of trapped erythrocytes). These changes persist for approximately 48 hours; the infarct then turns gray and fine yellow lines. Eight to 10 days following infarction, the thickness of the cardiac wall in the area of the infarct is reduced as necrotic muscle is removed by mononuclear cells. Over the next 2–3 months, the infarcted area gradually acquires a gelatinous, gray appearance, eventually converting into a shrunken, thin, firm scar that whitens and firms progressively with time.

Prognosis

The prognosis of patients with ischemia but without necrosis is far better, and there are no differences thus far described that distinguish medical from invasive therapies. A major determinant of mortality and morbidity is the amount of myocardial damage. With STEMI, most of it is acute whereas with NSTEMI, it may evolve because of repetitive events over many months. Thus interrupting the process improves survival.

STE and NSTE infarctions have distinctly different short-term prognoses. STEMI is associated with a higher early and in-hospital mortality. It is said that mortality associated by STEMI can occur up to 6 months postevent, but the vast majority (at least two-thirds) occurs during the first 30 or 40 days. It is this process that coronary recanalization seems to benefit. NSTEMI is associated with a lower acute mortality and complication rates but a longer period of vulnerability to reinfarction and death. As a result, 1–2-year survival rates are similar to those for transmural infarction. This is why intervention has been so effective in this group.

In today's environment of preventive and evidence-based medicine, the use of cTnI or cTnT measured once at presentation and again at 12–24 hours in patients with ischemia will allow clinicians to use markers as both exclusionary and prognostic indicators.[8-12] The results will assist in determining who is more at risk for AMI and death, and thereby determine who may benefit from early medical or surgical intervention. An evaluation of the majority of risk stratification studies shows that approximately 30% of all UA and NSTEMI patients present with an increased cardiac troponin level. Of these, approximately 30% (or 9–10% overall) have an adverse short-term (30–40 days) and long-term (1–2 years) prognosis. Identifying patients at greater risk for cardiac events allows them to be treated more aggressively, with proven beneficial outcomes. Clinical performance of cardiac troponin assays have been shown to be strongly dependent on the analytical sensitivity and precision of measured concentrations around the 99th percentile reference limit.[13-16] Several studies have now documented that assays with lower limits of detection are able to identify more ACS patients with poor prognosis who may be candidates for early invasive procedures. There are now data that such patients benefit from the use of low-molecular-weight heparin, IIB/IIIA platelet antagonists, and an early invasive strategy. General population screening of hospitalized patients with cTnI or cTnT is not recommended.

References

1. ALPERT, J. S, THYGESEN, K., ANTMAN, E. ET AL.: Myocardial infarction redefined—a consensus document of The Joint European Society of Cardiology/American College of Cardiology Committee for the redefinition of myocardial infarction. *J. Am. Coll. Cardiol.* *36*:959–69, 2000.

2. APPLE, F. S., WU, A. H. B., AND JAFFE, A. S.: European Society of Cardiology and American College of Cardiology guidelines for redefinition of myocardial infarction: How to use existing assays clinically and for clinical trials. *Am. Heart J. 144*:981–6, 2002.

3. BRAUNWALD, E., ANTMAN, E. M., BEASLEY, J. W. ET AL.: American College of Cardiology/American Heart Association Task Force on practice guidelines (Committee on the Management of Patients with Unstable Angina). ACC/AHA guideline update for the management of patients with unstable angina and non-ST-segment elevation myocardial infarction—2002: summary article: A report of the American College of Cardiology/American Heart Association Task Force on Practice Guidelines (Committee on the Management of Patients with Unstable Angina). *Circulation 106*:1893–2000, 2002.

4. LUEPKER, R. V., APPLE, F. S., CHRISTENSON, R. H. ET AL.: Case definitions for acute coronary heart disease in epidemiology and clinical research studies. *Circulation 108*:2543–9, 2003.

5. NEWBY, L. K., ALPERT, J. S., OHMAN, E. M. ET AL.: Changing the diagnosis of acute myocardial infarction: implications for practice and clinical investigations. *Am. Heart J. 144*:957–80, 2002.

6. APPLE, F. S.: Tissue specificity of cardiac troponin I, cardiac troponin T, and creatine kinase MB. *Clin. Chim. Acta 284*:151–9, 1999.

7. JAFFE, A. S., RAVKILDE, J., ROBERTS, R. ET AL.: It's time for a change to a troponin standard. *Circulation 102*:1216–20, 2000.

8. BERTRAND, M. E., SIMONS, M. L., FOX, K. A. A. ET AL.: Management of acute coronary syndromes: Acute coronary syndromes without persistent ST-segment elevation. *Eur. Heart J. 21*:1406–32, 2000.

9. HAMM, C. W., HEESCHEN, C., GOLDMANN, B. ET AL.: Benefit of ABCIXIMAB in patients with refractory unstable angina in relation to serum troponin T levels. *N. Engl. J. Med. 340*:1623–9, 1999.

10. HEIDENREICH, P. A., ALLOGGIAMENTO, T., MELSOP, K. ET AL.: The prognostic value of troponin in patients with non-ST elevation acute coronary syndromes: A meta analysis. *J. Am. Coll. Cardiol. 38*:478–85, 2001.

11. MORROW, D. A., CANNON, C. P., RIFAI, N. ET AL.: Ability of minor elevations of troponins I and T to predict benefit from an early invasive strategy in patients with unstable angina and non-ST elevation myocardial infarction. *JAMA 286*:2405–12, 2001.

12. VENGE, P., LAGERQUIST, B., DIDERHOLM, E. ET AL.: On behalf of the FRISC II study group. Clinical performance of three cardiac troponin assays in patients with unstable coronary artery disease (a FRISC II substudy). *Am. J. Cardiol. 89*:1035–41, 2002.

13. APPLE, F. S., QUIST, H. E., DOYLE, P. J. ET AL.: Plasma 99th percentile reference limits for cardiac troponin and creatine kinase MB mass for use with European Society of Cardiology/American College of Cardiology consensus recommendations. *Clin. Chem. 49*:1331–6, 2003.

14. APPLE, F. S., PARVIN, C. A., BUECHLER, K. F., CHRISTENSON, R. H., WU, A. H. B., AND JAFFE, A. S.: Validation of the 99th percentile cutoff independent of assay imprecision (%CV) for cardiac troponin

monitoring for ruling out myocardial infarction. *Clin. Chem.* *51*:2198–200, 2005.

15. LIN, J. C., APPLE, F. S., MURAKAMI, M. M. ET AL.: Rates of positive cardiac troponin I and creatine kinase MB among patients hospitalized for suspected acute coronary syndromes. *Clin. Chem.* *50*:333–8, 2004.

16. PANTEGHINI, M., GERHARDT, W., APPLE, F. S. ET AL.: Quality specifications for cardiac troponin assays. *Clin. Chem. Lab. Med.* *39*:174–8, 2001.

Case 2

A 48-Year-Old Cocaine User with Chest Pain

Fred S. Apple and Ramona Evans

Case Presentation

A 48-year-old male presented to the emergency department with constant, "squeezing," left sided and substernal chest pain following a night of partying with friends that included ingestion of alcohol and crack cocaine. He stated that the pain started acutely around 0230 h (2:30 am) while he was sleeping and was temporarily relieved following the ingestion of two nitroglycerin tablets at home. He was not short of breath or diaphoretic. The pain did not radiate, was nonpleuritic, and was not associated with exertion but was similar in character to the chest pain he experienced when admitted last month for a myocardial infarction. Improvement, but not resolution, of the pain was noted by the patient following administration of an aspirin, nitroglycerin, and metoprolol.

His past medical history is significant for a non-ST-segment elevation myocardial infarction suffered last month following the ingestion of crack cocaine. Cardiac catheterization at that time revealed essentially normal coronary arteries that required no intervention. An echocardiogram completed 2 months prior to this presentation revealed a normal ejection fraction, mild left ventricular hypertrophy, and no wall motion abnormalities.

His medical history is also noteworthy for a diagnosis of small cell lung carcinoma that was treated with radiation and chemotherapy 7 years ago. He had metastasis involving his brain with multiple strokes and transient ischemic attacks secondary to whole-brain radiation in 1998. He has only mild residual deficits secondary to these multiple strokes. Additionally, he has hypertension and a history of substance abuse.

His current medications include lisinopril, metoprolol, and atorvastatin.

On physical examination, his blood pressure was 170–200 systolic and 90–104 diastolic with a heart rate in the 60s and a respiration rate 20. His oxygen saturation was 98%; temperature, 97.3°F; and he appeared to be in mild distress. Diminished breath sounds were found on auscultation of the bilateral upper lobes of his lungs, while the remainder of his lung and cardiovascular examination was unremarkable. No neck vein distention or lower extremity edema was seen and his abdomen was benign. Neurologic examination was normal.

Tietz's Applied Laboratory Medicine, Second Edition. Edited by Mitchell G. Scott, Ann M. Gronowski, and Charles S. Eby

An EKG demonstrated a normal sinus rhythm. An echocardiogram completed the following morning demonstrated a normal left ventricular ejection fraction, no wall motion abnormalities, mild left ventricular hypertrophy, left atrial enlargement, a small pericardial effusion, and insufficiency of the aortic, mitral, and tricuspid valves.

Laboratory tests included a cTnI, total creatine kinase (CK) and CKMB and the calculated percent relative index (CKMB/total CK × 100). Additional tests included a basic chemistry profile and a complete blood count. Laboratory data were as follows:

Time, h Reference Interval	cTnI ≤0.3 ng/mL	CK Total 60–300 IU/L	CKMB ≤7.0 ng/mL	Relative CKMB Index >3% = MI
0330	0.2			
0420	0.9	190	12.5	6.6%
0520	1.6			
0100	3.6			
0615	3.7			
2015	3.1			
0100	2.6			
0615	2.3			

The final diagnosis was non-ST-segment elevation myocardial infarction secondary to cocaine abuse.

Definition of the Disease

Data from 1999 estimates that 25 million Americans have tried cocaine at least once and that 1.5 million people were active users during the data collection period.[1] Cocaine is noted to be the most frequent drug used in patients who present to the emergency department and is listed by medical examiners as the most common cause of drug-related deaths.[2-5] The risk of myocardial infarction increases to 24 times that of baseline in the first hour following cocaine use, and the risk of nonfatal myocardial infarction is 7 times greater in cocaine users versus nonusers.

Acute myocardial infarction is defined as an imbalance between oxygen supply and demand that results in injury and necrosis of the myocytes.[6] The European Society of Cardiology and the American College of Cardiology outline the diagnosis of acute, evolving or recent myocardial infarction to include either (1) a characteristic rise and fall of the biochemical markers cardiac troponin I or T and CKMB within 24 hours of the onset of ischemic symptoms, pathological Q waves on ECG, ECG changes consistent with ischemia (i.e., ST-segment elevation) and coronary artery intervention (angioplasty); or (2) pathological findings of an AMI.

Differential Diagnosis

The most important diagnostic decision to make in the setting of chest pain following cocaine use is to determine whether the patient has actually sustained acute myocardial damage that requires prompt medical and surgical management. It is estimated that only 6% of persons who present to the emergency department with chest pain after the ingestion of cocaine will actually have an acute myocardial infarction. This small percentage of persons likely to have myocardial ischemia together with the fact that distinguishing chest wall and skeletal pain from acute myocardial ischemia is challenging because three of the main criteria for a diagnosis of AMI are similar in both settings.

Frequently the patient's presentation is atypical for myocardial infarction, the electrocardiogram demonstrates nonspecific abnormalities, and the serum markers CK and CKMB, which lack specificity for cardiac muscle, are elevated. Also, although it is widely recognized that myocardial infarction can occur after use of cocaine, the specific risk and risk factors that portend acute myocardial damage following use of cocaine are not well characterized. Approximately one-half of patients with myocardial infarction will not have the classic risk factors associated with AMI such as older age and previous CAD history.

An electrocardiogram following cocaine use without myocardial infarction can demonstrate PR, QRS, and QT interval prolongation, elevation of ST segments, and pathologic Q waves. In contrast, 90% of patients with myocardial infarction following cocaine use have changes seen on the electrocardiogram that include ST-segment elevation, T-wave inversions, and Q waves. The use of echocardiography is often helpful in this setting to demonstrate new wall motion abnormalities.

The biochemical markers cardaiac troponin I (cTnI) or T (cTnT), total creatine kinase (CK), and CKMB are crucial in diagnosing AMI in these patients.[6-10] Total CK and CKMB levels rise to twice the reference range within 6 hours of myocardial necrosis and peak at approximately 24 hours, but these markers lack the specificity necessary to distinguish cardiac muscle necrosis from the skeletal muscle necrosis that is often seen in persons who have recently used cocaine. Serum CK and CKMB elevations seen are often thought to be secondary to skeletal muscle damage because of trauma or rhabdomyolysis, and the chest pain experienced by these patients may be a result of a transient coronary vasospasm without necrosis of the myocytes. A calculation of the percent relative index of the CKMB to total CK will usually be above 3% if actual myocardial necrosis has occurred and <3% if the elevation of these biochemical markers is due instead to skeletal muscle damage.

It is now widely recognized that cTnI or cTnT are the most specific markers for myocardial injury. The cardiac troponins are the serum markers of choice to differentiate myocardial infarction from skeletal muscle damage. Cardiac troponin I or T are contractile proteins of the myofibril, and thus the presence of these proteins in serum is consistent and specific for damage to myocardial tissue. Cardiac troponins are elevated within 4–6 hours of injury, peak at 12–36 hours, and remain elevated for 4–10 days. A characteristic rise or fall of cTnI or cTnT in the correct clinical setting should be seen in order to diagnose acute myocardial ischemia. The rise–fall pattern distinguishes AMI from other disorders that may lead to an elevation in cardiac troponins but are not related to myocardial infarction. Serial cardiac troponin levels taken over at least a 8–12-hour period is a conservative and reasonable diagnostic approach to evaluate a suspected infarction in high risk or suspicious patients.

In summary, the symptomatic presentation, electrocardiogram, and biochemical markers can be strikingly similar in patients with cocaine-related chest wall pain or acute myocardial infarction. The diagnosis of AMI depends on the use of cardiac troponins I or T and echocardiography to distinguish the two entities in this challenging patient population.

Pathogenesis

The etiology of acute myocardial infarction secondary to cocaine use is thought to be caused by an imbalance of the increased demand placed on the cardiovascular system by an elevation in heart rate and blood pressure versus the decreased delivery of oxygen secondary to coronary artery spasm. The decreased oxygen delivery via the coronary arteries has also been theorized by some to be exacerbated by enhanced atherosclerosis, increased platelet aggregation, and thrombus formation within the coronary arteries after cocaine ingestion. The incidence of myocardial infarction following cocaine use is not related to and cannot be predicted by the route, frequency, or dose of cocaine ingested. An elevated heart rate and increased systolic and diastolic blood pressures are known effects of cocaine ingestion secondary to blockage of the reuptake of norepinephrine into the preganglionic neurons with resultant elevation in the concentration of norepinephrine at the postganglionic neuron receptors. The coronary vasoconstriction is mediated by stimulation of the α-adrenergic receptors on the coronary vessels. Vasoconstriction of the arteries is further exacerbated by the cocaine-stimulated production of endothelin by endothelial cells and inhibition of the production of nitric oxide. Endothelin is a potent vasoconstrictor, while nitric oxide is a potent vasodilator, and the alteration of their production disallows a compensatory response to the α-adrenergic vasoconstriction. Vasoconstriction of the coronary arteries may disrupt susceptible atherosclerotic plaques in addition to causing the release of von Willebrand factor from the endothelium.

In one controlled cocaine administration trial, a significant elevation (40% at its peak) of von Willebrand factor was demonstrated which lasted for 30–240 minutes. This same study showed a transient erythrocytosis that was hypothesized to allow for maintenance of tissue oxygenation during vasoconstriction. The elevation of von Willebrand factor with the concomitant erythrocytosis were postulated as potential factors that lead to the elevated risk of platelet aggregation and thrombus formation.

Although cocaine is a known toxin to myocardial tissue, this toxicity is thought to only play a minor role in the damage to the tissue, and the main pathological disorder is due mainly to an imbalance of demand and delivery of oxygen to the myocytes.

Treatment

Administration of nitroglycerin, oxygen, aspirin, and oral calcium antagonists are first-line agents in these patients. Aspirin, as in non-cocaine-related myocardial infarction, should be administered to inhibit platelet aggregation. Percutaneous coronary angioplasty is indicated to evaluate the severity of a suspected underlying stenosis. Benzodiazepines can be administered to reduce the heart rate and systemic hypertension and may also decrease the direct toxicity of cocaine to the myocardium. The treatment of cocaine-induced myocardial infarction is complicated by the fact that thrombolytics may be contraindicated if the patient has had a seizure, intracranial hemorrhage, or severe hypertension.

Coronary vasospasm is best treated with nitrates, and either calcium channel blockers or α-blockers instead of the more commonly used β-blockers in non-cocaine-induced myocardial infarction. Unopposed α-receptor stimulation may intensify coronary vasospasm if β-blockers are administered and hence should be either avoided altogether or given with great caution. However, the administration of labetalol, which is both an α- and β-receptor blocker, may be used as it can reverse the systemic hypertension without exacerbating the α-adrenergic induced vasoconstriction.

References

1. WEBER, J., SHOFER, F., LARKIN, G., KALARIA, A. S., AND HOLLANDER, J. E.: Validation of a brief observation period for patients with cocaine-associated chest pain. *N. Engl. J. Med. 348*:510–17, 2003.

2. SIEGEL, A., SHOLAR, M., MENDELSON, J. ET AL:. Cocaine-induced erythrocytosis and increase in von Willebrand factor: Evidence for drug-related blood doping and prothrombotic effects. *Arch. Intern. Med. 159*:1925–9, 1999.

3. HOLLANDER, J. E., LEVITT, M. A., YOUNG, G. P., BRIGLIA, E., WETLI, C. V., AND GAWAD, Y.: Clinical investigations—acute ischemic heart disease, the effects of recent cocaine use on the specificity of cardiac markers for diagnosis of acute myocardial infarction. *Am. Heart J. 135*:245–52, 1998.

4. KLONER, R. AND REZKALLA, S.: Cocaine and the heart. *N. Engl. J. Med. 348*:487–8, 2003.

5. LANGE, R. AND HILLIS, L. Cardiovascular complications and cocaine use. *N. Engl. J. Med. 345*:351–8, 2001.

6. APPLE, F. S. AND JAFFE, A. S.: Cardiac function. In: *Tietz' Textbook of Clinical Chemistry and Molecular Diagnostics*, 4th ed., C. BURTIS, E. ASHWOOD, and D. E. BRUNS, eds., Saunders, Philadelphia, 2005, pp. 1619–70.

7. KONTOS, M., ANDERSON, F., ORNATO, J., TATUM, J. L., AND JESSE, R. L.: Utility of troponin I in patients with cocaine-associated chest pain. *Acad. Emerg. Med. 9*:1007–13, 2002.

8. LIVINGSTON, J., MABIE, B., AND RAMANATHAN, J.: Crack cocaine, myocardial infarction, and troponin I levels at the time of cesarean delivery. *Anesth. Analg. 91*:913–15, 2000.

9. MCLAURIN, M., APPLE, F., HENRY, T. D., AND SHARKEY, S. W.: Cardiac troponin I and T concentrations in patients with cocaine-associated chest pain. *Ann. Clin. Biochem. 33*:183–6, 1996.

10. LIN, J., APPLE, F., MURAKAMI, M. M., AND LUEPKER, R. V.: Rates of positive cardiac troponin I and creatine kinase MB mass among patients hospitalized for suspected acute coronary syndromes. *Clin. Chem. 50*:333–8, 2004.

Part Two

Pulmonary Diseases

Cases of chronic obstructive pulmonary disease (COPD) and cystic fibrosis are presented in Cases 3 and 4, respectively (both edited by MGS).

Tietz's Applied Laboratory Medicine, Second Edition. Edited by Mitchell G. Scott, Ann M. Gronowski, and Charles S. Eby
Copyright © 2007 John Wiley & Sons, Inc.

Case 3

Shortness of Breath with Productive Cough

Nausherwan K. Burki

A 61-year-old man was admitted to the hospital for treatment of increasing shortness of breath, cough, and sputum production. The patient had neither a family history of pulmonary disease nor a known contact with anyone with tuberculosis. He started smoking cigarettes at the age of 17 and since then had smoked one pack per day. He had been drinking about one or two cans of beer per week.

He gave a history of having developed a noticeable cough during the past 10–15 years. This cough had been present daily and had been productive of small amounts of sputum (approximately one tablespoon per day). Sputum production had occurred mainly in the morning. It was usually white but at times had been yellowish green. The patient also gave a history of shortness of breath on exertion that he first noticed about 5–7 years ago. This shortness of breath had steadily progressed until, in the month before admission, he was unable to walk one block or to go up one flight of stairs without pausing to catch his breath.

His current illness started about 3 days prior to admission when he developed increased frequency and intensity of coughing spells and increased production of sputum that became greenish yellow. He was febrile; his shortness of breath had increased; and he had developed some swelling of his feet and ankles that was particularly noticeable in the evening.

The patient's general health had otherwise been fair, and he had no history of allergies. He gave no history of eczema or childhood asthma. He had been hospitalized 4 times during the last 5 years with acute exacerbations of shortness of breath, cough, and increased sputum production. On each occasion, he was treated and discharged from the hospital after about one week; the last admission was approximately 4 months ago. His current medications consisted of inhaled bronchodilators (ipratropium and metaproterenol) as well as the diuretic furosemide taken as oral tablets.

On physical examination, the patient was alert, cooperative, and short of breath at rest; he had some central cyanosis but showed no pallor, jaundice, or lymphadenopathy. The oral temperature was 100.4°F (38°C).

The pulse rate was 110 per minute and regular. The blood pressure in the left arm with the patient in the supine position was 120/76 mm Hg. Jugular venous pressure was

Tietz's Applied Laboratory Medicine, Second Edition. Edited by Mitchell G. Scott, Ann M. Gronowski, and Charles S. Eby

elevated to the angle of the jaw, with normal pulsations. The first heart sound was normal, whereas the second heart sound and pulmonic component were accentuated; no murmurs or rubs were heard.

The patient was short of breath at rest and was coughing. The respiratory rate was 20/min, and the patient was using accessory muscles. Hyperresonance to percussion was noted over both lung fields. Auscultation revealed reduced breath sounds over the bases with expiratory rhonchi over both bases. The abdomen was scaphoid, soft; no palpable mass was observed, nor was tenderness elicited. His extremities showed peripheral cyanosis and bilateral 1+ ankle edema. There was no finger clubbing.

The chest radiograph showed low, flat diaphragms and a narrow heart. The right diaphragm dome level was below the sixth rib interspace anteriorly; this finding is a strong indication of airways obstruction. Hyperlucent lung fields (i.e., areas of lung parenchyma with decreased density) were observed; these findings were suggestive of emphysema.

The electrocardiogram (ECG) was consistent with a diagnosis of cor pulmonale: tall P waves (>2.5 mV) indicated right atrial hypertrophy, and right axis deviation suggested right ventricular hypertrophy.

Results of laboratory tests were as follows:

Analyte	Value, Conventional Units	Reference Interval, Conventional Units	Value, SI Units	Reference Interval, SI Units
Sodium (S)	138 mmol/L	136–145	Same	
Potassium (S)	3.2 mmol/L	3.8–5.1	Same	
Chloride (S)	100 mmol/L	98–108	Same	
Bicarbonate (S)	44 mmol/L	23–31	Same	
Urea nitrogen (S)	10 mg/dL	8–21	3.6 mmol urea/L	2.9–7.5
Creatinine (S)	0.8 mg/dL	0.8–1.4	71 μmo/L	71–124
Arterial Blood Gases				
1. FI O$_2$, 21%				
pO_2 (aB)	46 mm Hg	83–108	6.1 kPa	11.1–14.4
pCO_2 (aB)	56 mm Hg	35–45	7.5 kPa	4.7–6.0
pH (aB)	7.27	7.35–7.45	Same	
2. FI O$_2$, 24%				
pO_2 (aB)	50 mm Hg	83–108	6.7 kPa	11.1–14.4
pCO_2 (aB)	62 mm Hg	35–45	8.3 kPa	4.7–6.0
pH (aB)	7.26	7.35–7.45	Same	
3. After 6 h of FI O$_2$, 24%				
pO_2 (aB)	52 mm Hg	83–108	6.9 kPa	11.1–14.4
pCO_2 (aB)	54 mm Hg	35–45	7.2 kPa	4.7–6.0
pH (aB)	7.30	7.35–7.45	Same	
Hemoglobin	17.1 g/dL	14–18	10.61 mmol/L	8.69–11.17
Hematocrit	54%	40–54	0.54	0.40–0.54
Leukocyte count (B)	15.3×10^3/μL	4.8–10.8	15.3×10^9/L	4.8–10.8
Differential count (B)				
Band forms	14%	5–10	0.14	0.05–0.10
Polymorphonuclear neutrophils	64%	41–71	0.64	0.41–0.71

Analyte	Value, Conventional Units	Reference Interval, Conventional Units	Value, SI Units	Reference Interval, SI Units
Lymphocytes	17%	24–44	0.17	0.24–0.44
Monocytes	3%	3–7	0.03	0.03–0.07
Eosinophils	2%	1–3	0.02	0.01–0.03

Pulmonary Function Tests

	Actual	% Predicted
Total lung capacity (TLC)	7.20 L	132%
Residual volume (RV)	3.90 L	173%
Functional residual capacity (FRC)	5.20 L	182%
Forced vital capacity (FVC)	3.30 L	76%
Forced expired volume in 1 s (FEV$_1$)	1.12 L	23%
FEV$_1$/FVC ratio	34%	>75%
Carbon monoxide diffusing capacity (D$_L$CO)	17 mL/min/mm Hg	65%

Comments

An elevated hematocrit suggested polycythemia that was likely caused by the chronic hypoxemia. The total leukocyte count was increased, with a "left shift" (increased band forms and polymorphonuclear neutrophils) suggesting a pulmonary infection.

Decreased serum potassium was probably related to the use of the diuretic drug furosemide.

The sputum revealed many Gram-negative coccobacilli, suggesting that the patient had a bronchitis caused by *Haemophilus influenzae*. In patients with chronic bronchitis and emphysema, *H. influenzae* is the most common infecting organism that causes acute exacerbations. This interpretation was supported by the fact that the patient had an elevated leukocyte count.

Pulmonary function tests and a reduced FEV$_1$/FVC ratio were evidence of severe airways obstruction. The total lung capacity (TLC) was increased above the normal range, indicating that there was a significant amount of emphysema. Diagnosis of emphysema was further supported by the reduced carbon monoxide diffusing capacity (D$_L$CO).

Increased airway resistance leads to nonuniform distribution of ventilation in the lungs (since the increase in airway resistance in different lung segments is nonuniform). Because there is also loss of the alveolocapillary bed in emphysema, gas exchange is affected and hypoxemia occurs. As chronic bronchitis and emphysema progress in the patient, alveolar hypoventilation occurs. The reason for this is not clearly understood but is believed to be a combination of the increased mechanical abnormalities hindering ventilation, an alteration in ventilatory pattern, and a reduction in central respiratory drive.

Chronic bronchitis and emphysema may cause cor pulmonale (right ventricular hypertrophy or failure secondary to lung disease) by several mechanisms: hypoxemia is a strong stimulus to pulmonary vasoconstriction; similarly, hypercapnia, by increasing H$^+$ concentration (i.e., by decreasing pH), is also a strong stimulus for pulmonary vasoconstriction. The combination of hypoxemia and hypercapnia thus increases pulmonary vascular resistance and raises pulmonary artery pressure. In addition, emphysema causes destruction of the pulmonary vascular bed, thus reducing the effective capacitance of the system. Finally, prolonged vasoconstriction causes structural alterations in pulmonary arteriolar smooth muscle and narrowing of the arteries. The resulting increase in pulmonary artery pressure increases the afterload on the right ventricle and leads to right ventricular hypertrophy and failure.

The arterial pO_2 and pCO_2 on room air (FI O_2, 21%) indicated severe hypoxemia and alveolar hypoventilation. Elevated pCO_2 and reduced pH suggested that the cause was an acute exacerbation of chronic hypercapnia. The patient's elevated serum bicarbonate is an appropriate renal compensatory response to this chronic respiratory acidosis. When the patient was placed on 24% oxygen, the pO_2 rose, but so did the pCO_2, and there was a slight decrease in pH. This change was presumably due to a reduction in the hypoxic drive, secondary to the rise in pO_2, and resulted in the further reduction in alveolar ventilation, causing the rise in pCO_2. After six hours on 24% oxygen, the patient's pO_2 was not significantly changed, but the pCO_2 decreased—a change that indicated improved alveolar ventilation.

The patient's shortness of breath and cough gradually improved with antibiotic treatment, and after 2 days he was afebrile with arterial blood gases on FI O_2, 24%, as follows: pO_2, 56 mm Hg (7.5 kPa); pCO_2, 48 mm Hg (6.4 kPa); and pH, 7.36. His ankle swelling had disappeared.

The patient was readmitted to the hospital 6 months later with another acute exacerbation but, unfortunately, did not survive this episode.

Discussion

Chronic bronchitis usually results from chronic cigarette smoke exposure. The mucous glands of the airway enlarge and increase in number; the mucous membranes become inflamed from prolonged irritation. These processes are first noted in the small (>2-mm-diameter) airways but ultimately affect the entire bronchial tree. Thus, narrowed airways increase resistance to airflow.

Emphysema is defined as dilation and destruction of the gas-exchanging portions of the lung. This effect again is most commonly a result of cigarette smoking. The destruction of lung tissue causes a loss of elastic recoil (an increase in lung compliance), which then hinders expiration and causes narrowing of the airways and increased airway resistance.

Cough is one of the cardinal symptoms of disease of the pulmonary airways (the bronchi); it is due to stimulation of the irritant receptors in the airways. Therefore, any condition resulting in inflammation of the airways is likely to cause cough.

Sputum production implies increased secretions in the airways or alveoli. Bronchial inflammation with increased number and size of mucous glands results in increased sputum production in chronic bronchitis; this sputum is usually white/yellow; when infection occurs the sputum increases in quantity and changes in color to yellow/green. Since the patient described above had a history of chronic cough and sputum production over a period of 10–15 years, it is likely that he had chronic bronchitis at presentation. Indeed, chronic bronchitis is defined as present when a patient has a history of cough for the previous 2 years with daily sputum production for at least 3 months in each year. Another possibility to be considered is bronchiectasis; however, the quantity of sputum is usually much greater (a cupful per day or more) in bronchiectasis, and other symptoms and signs are present.

The presence of expiratory rhonchi confirms the airway narrowing. Hyperresonance to percussion and decreased breath sounds are suggestive of the presence of *emphysema*. The 44-pack-year history (=packs smoked per day × years smoked) of cigarette smoking is very significant, since smoking is the major cause of chronic bronchitis as well as of emphysema. Note that there is no history of exposure to dusts or fumes.

Dyspnea or shortness of breath, present in a large variety of pulmonary disorders, is one of the most common symptoms of cardiopulmonary disease. In most cases, dyspnea is first noted on exertion; if dyspnea progresses, the patient may become short of breath on lying down (orthopnea). In very severe cases, dyspnea is present even at rest. The mechanism of production of this symptom is unknown; for further discussion, please see review.[1]

Edema, the swelling of the feet and ankles, indicates salt and water retention. This situation may occur with heart, renal, or liver failure; other causes include severe hypo-albuminemia or secondary hyperaldosteronism or both. In the present case, the elevated jugulovenous pressure indicates right-sided heart failure, and the accentuated pulmonic component of the second heart sound indicates pulmonary hypertension. Since there is no clinical evidence of left-sided heart failure, the right-sided heart failure must be attributed to pulmonary hypertension secondary to lung disease, namely, *cor pulmonale*. This condition is associated with hypertrophy of the right ventricle. The presence of central cyanosis is suggestive of hypoxemia.

Treatment

The treatment of chronic obstructive pulmonary disease (COPD) due to chronic bronchitis and emphysema is both preventive and therapeutic. The most essential aspect of preventive treatment is cessation of exposure to cigarette smoke; patients are very strongly encouraged to avoid all cigarette smoke, although successful cessation occurs in less than 25% of patients, due to the addictive effect of nicotine. Therapeutic treatment consists of measures to improve airway function, prevent or treat pulmonary infections and treat cor pulmonale. Bronchodilator drugs, such as β agonists and parasympatholytics are useful in most patients with COPD. Pulmonary infections cause exacerbations of COPD and are commonly due to *Haemophilus influenzae* or *Streptococcus pneumoniae* and appropriate antibiotics are given to treat exacerbations. Cor pulmonale occurs in patients in respiratory failure and treatment is with supplemental oxygen provided for at least 14 hours per day, and the use of diuretic drugs.

In selected patients with end-stage COPD, lung transplantation or lung volume reduction surgery (LVRS) may be considered. When successful, either procedure can result in improvement in dyspnea and lung function.

Reference

1. BURKI, N. K.: Dyspnea. *Lung 165*:269–77, 1987.

Additional Reading

PAUWELS, R. A., BUIST, A. S., CALVERLEY, P. M. A. ET AL.: Global strategy for the diagnosis, management, and prevention of COPD: GOLD workshop summary. *Am. J. Respir. Crit. Care Med. 163*:1256–76, 2001.

HOGG, J. C.: Pathophysiology of airflow limitation in chronic obstructive pulmonary disease. *Lancet 21*:364:709–21, 2004.

BURKI, N. K. AND KRUMPELMAN, J. L.: Correlation of pulmonary function with the chest roentgenogram in chronic airway obstruction. *Am. Rev. Respir. Dis. 121*:217–23, 1980.

FLETCHER, C. AND PETO, R.: The natural history of chronic airflow obstruction. *Br. Med. J. 1*:1645–8, 1977.

THOMPSON, A. B., DAUGHTON, D., ROBBINS, R. A. ET AL.: Intraluminal airway inflammation in chronic bronchitis: Characterization and correlation with clinical parameters. *Am. Rev. Respir. Dis. 140*:1526–37, 1989.

NATHAN, S. D.: Lung transplantation: disease-specific considerations for referral. *Chest 127*:1006–16, 2005.

MILLER, BERGER, R. L., MALTHANER, R. A. ET AL.: Lung volume reduction surgery vs. medical treatment for patients with advanced emphysema. *Chest 127*:1166–77, 2005.

Case 4

Genotype–Phenotype Correlations in Cystic Fibrosis

Latisha Love-Gregory, Barbara Zehnbauer, and Dennis Dietzen

Case A

A 9-month-old Caucasian female was referred to the department of pediatric pulmonary medicine for evaluation of a chronic cough, wheezing, rhinorrhea, loose stools, and poor weight gain despite a ravenous appetite. Born at 38 weeks' gestation, the patient had an uneventful neonatal course. Several weeks prior, the patient exhibited worsening signs of wheezing, which the grandmother mentioned had persisted since early in life. In addition, the baby was beginning to show signs of decreased activity and intermittent difficulty sleeping. There was no history of known respiratory infections.

Physical exam revealed a somnolent child with no respiratory distress. However, she had mild signs of tachypnea, respiratory rate of 48 beats/min (20–35 bpm), temperature 36.2°C, heart rate of 136 (80–130 bpm), and weight 6.425 kg (<3rd percentile for age) and height 65.5 cm (~10th percentile for age). The nasopharyngeal mucosa was mildly inflamed, but no polyps were observed. The lungs had few coarse bronchi, but good air exchange. The abdomen was soft, not tender, and nondistended with normal bowel sounds.

The family history revealed that a paternal cousin and a maternal second cousin were diagnosed with cystic fibrosis. There was no known family history of recurrent pneumonitis or recurrent pancreatitis in either of these relatives. Laboratory tests included a BMP and CBC (the tabular list below). A sweat chloride test from an outside hospital revealed an elevated result of 123 mmol/L. A repeat quantitative sweat test again showed elevated electrolytes:

Analyte	Value, Conventional Units	Reference Interval, Conventional Units	Value, SI Units	Reference Interval, SI Units
Sodium	139 mmol/L	135–145	Same	
Potassium	4.2 mmol/L	4.2	Same	
Chloride	107 mmol/L	97–110	Same	
Total CO_2	21 mmol/L	20–28		

Tietz's Applied Laboratory Medicine, Second Edition. Edited by Mitchell G. Scott, Ann M. Gronowski, and Charles S. Eby

Analyte	Value, Conventional Units	Reference Interval, Conventional Units	Value, SI Units	Reference Interval, SI Units
BUN	4 mg/dL	9–18	1.4 mmol/L	3.2–6.4
Creatinine	0.3 mg/dL	0.1–0.5	26.5 mmol/L	8.84–44.2
Glucose (random)	89 mg/dL	65–199	4.9 mmol/L	3.6–11
Chloride (sweat)	111 mmol/L	0–40	Same	
Sodium (sweat)	78 mmol/L		Same	

The child's liver enzymes and albumin values were normal. Chest x-rays revealed mildly increased peribronchial markings with no infiltrates or atelectasis. The WBC was 13,600 (3.8–9.8 × 10^3/μL) with 61% segmented neutrophils, 32% lymphocytes, 1% eosinophils, a hemoglobin of 13.7 (13.8–17.2 g/dL), and a hematocrit of 39.3 (40.7–50.3%). The platelet count was 317,000 (140–440 × 10^3/μL).

The chronic respiratory and GI symptoms plus the laboratory results for this young patient were consistent with cystic fibrosis. To support the diagnosis, mutational analysis of the *CFTR* gene revealed that the patient was homozygous for the common delta F508 mutation. With these results in mind, the clinicians initiated antibiotic therapy for possible pneumonitis, conventional chest physiotherapy and Ultrase (Axcan Scandipharm Inc., Birmingham, AL) for the pancreatic insufficiency.

Case B

A 13-year-old Caucasian male presented to the clinic with a past medical history remarkable for asthma and pneumonia that required hospitalization on several occasions. The patient complained of a chronic cough, which affected his daily activities along with chronic sputum production and failure to thrive. He developed shortness of breath during minimal exercise activities. No hemoptysis was noted. GI evaluation indicated voluminous stools once a day and loose at times. Pancreatic insufficiency was not suspected.

On physical exam the short-stature 13-year-old ranked below the 3rd percentile for height and weight. He had a normal temperature at the time of exam with a heart rate of 72 bpm, respiratory rate of 20 (16–25 bpm), and blood pressure of 106/72 mm Hg. Also, clubbing of the extremities was evident. Although the patient was not in acute respiratory distress or wheezing, pulmonary exam revealed crackling sounds bilaterally. The abdomen was soft and supple, no hepatosplenomegaly noted.

To explore possible causes for the pulmonary involvement, allergy testing was performed. Skin testing was positive for *Aspergillosis* and *Alternaria*, two environmental fungi. Previous laboratory data from an outside facility revealed an elevated sweat chloride of 95 mmol/L (0–40 mmol/L), and a chest x-ray showed infiltration and mild bronchiectasis of the right upper lobe in addition to hyperinflation of both upper lobes with possible air trapping. His sweat chloride on the day of presentation was 99 mmol/L and sodium of 90 mmol/L. Hepatic enzymes tests were normal, ALP 192 (130–550 IU/L), AST 36 (10–40 IU/L), and ALT 18 (10–15 IU/L). Pulmonary function tests were consistent with air trapping, confirming the radiographic findings. Other laboratory findings are shown below.

Analyte	Value, Conventional Units	Reference Interval, Conventional Units	Value, SI Units	Reference Interval, SI Units
Sodium	140 mmol/L	135–145	Same	
Potassium	3.6 mmol/L	3.6–4.9	Same	
Chloride	103 mmol/L	97–110	Same	
Total CO_2	26 mmol/L	20–28	Same	
BUN	11 mg/dL	9–18	3.9 mmol/L	3.2–6.4
Creatinine	0.5 mg/dL	0.1–0.5	44.2 mmol/L	8.8–44.2
Glucose (random)	89 mg/dL	65–199	4.9 mmol/L	3.6–11
Chloride (sweat)	99 mmol/L	0–40	Same	Same
Sodium (sweat)	90 mmol/L			

The patient had no known family history of cystic fibrosis or other pulmonary diseases. However, the chronic respiratory symptoms, in addition to the abnormal sweat tests, were consistent with cystic fibrosis. Molecular diagnostic testing revealed that the patient was compound heterozygous for the common delta F508 allele and the 2789 + 5 G > A mutation. The plan of treatment included a course of antibiotics, along with albuterol, chest physiotherapy therapy, and dietary supplementation with ADEKS (Axcan Pharma, Birmingham, AL) fat-soluble vitamin tablets.

Definition of the Disease

Cystic fibrosis (CF) is a lethal multisystem disease caused by abnormal chloride ion transport. Andersen originally described cystic fibrosis in 1938 in a pediatric population with severe pancreatic insufficiency. Inherited as an autosomal recessive disease, the major cause of morbidity and mortality is complications related to decline in pulmonary function. As a result of damage to the distal airways and submucosal glands caused by thick secretions, patients are at risk for developing microbial infections with pathogens such as *Staphylococcus aureus*, *Pseudomonas aeruginosa*, and *Hemophilus influenza*. In addition, ~85–90% of all CF patients have exocrine pancreatic insufficiency. Approximately 13% of CF patients develop diabetes mellitus; 10%, meconium ileus; and approximately 5% suffer from severe liver disease. In addition, 99% of males with CF are infertile due to congenital bilateral absence of the vas deferens (CBAVD).[1]

One in 2500 Caucasians are affected with CF (1 in 25 are heterozygous carriers of a CF mutation) while the occurrence of this disease in other populations is less frequent. In African-Americans, the prevalence of CF is at 1 in 15,000, and in Asian Americans about 1 in 31,000.[1] The reported median survival for CF patients is currently 33 years. However, this age is continuing to increase as a result of improved diagnostic criteria and treatment options.

Differential Diagnosis[1]

As described in the cases presented here, some phenotypic features consistent with CF include chronic cough, sputum production, digital clubbing, bronchiectasis, and hyperinflation as seen on chest x-ray. In addition, pancreatic insufficiency and failure to thrive are also common characteristics of the disease. In most cases, the diagnosis of CF involves elevated Na^+ and Cl^- sweat concentrations as measured by quantitative pilocarpine iontophoresis. Elevated sweat tests can be seen in patients with other disorders such as fucosidosis, glycogen storage disease type 1 mucopolysaccharidosis, hypothyroidism, celiac disease, malnutrition, and asthma. These diseases are clinically distinguishable from CF, and an elevated sweat test (>60 mmol/L) is usually sufficient for CF diagnosis. However, atypical CF cases have been described in which the sweat chloride values were below 60 mmol/L.[2] The sensitivity of sweat chloride determined by quantitative pilocarpine iontophoresis using a cutoff of 60 mmol/L is ~98% with a specificity of ~83%. One drawback of sweat analysis is that a minimum weight of sweat collected (75 mg) is required to ensure accurate results and this requires good technical skills.

If exocrine pancreatic deficiency is the sole clinical symptom in the presence of a normal sweat test, the symptoms may be due to pancreatitis or distal abdominal obstruction syndrome. In the two cases presented here, case 1 is an example of a classic CF presentation in which there is an elevated sweat test and family history supported by the identification of known gene mutations. Case 2 is more representative of an intermediate phenotype with a later onset. Two percent of CF patients have an atypical presentation with a borderline sweat test (<60 mmol/L) and have pancreatic sufficiency.[1] In these cases, the utility of molecular diagnostic testing is evident.[3,4]

Pathogenesis

Cystic fibrosis manifests as an exocrine pancreatic disease that leads to abnormal functioning of the lungs, GI, and reproductive tracts. The inability of the airways to secrete Cl^- normally in CF patients is due to mutations in the gene for the cystic fibrosis transmembrane conductance regulator (*CFTR*). CFTR functions as a protein kinase A regulated chloride channel at the apical surface of epithelial cells. Phosphorylation by other proteins is also thought to occur. Not only is there damage to the submucosal glands, which express CFTR; the decrease or loss in CFTR activity results in the formation of thick mucinous secretions that can obstruct the pancreatic ducts, reducing the secretion of pancreatic enzymes. In males, deficient CFTR activity can obstruct the vas deferens in prepubertal males, resulting in infertility. There are two theories that attempt to explain the underlying pathophysiology of CF. The "low-volume model" suggests that the deficient activity of the CFTR Cl^- channel results in increased Na^+ absorption and uptake of Cl^- through alternative pathways, resulting in an increased potential difference across the transepithelial membrane and consequently, reduced airway–surface liquid volume. The "high-salt model" proposes that the CFTR channel is the major pathway for ion absorption. Thus the loss of CFTR activity results in excess airway–surface liquid NaCl concentrations, which lead to the thick mucus produced by CF patients. Nonetheless, both theories support reduced mucociliary clearance and eventual increased susceptibility of patients to bacterial infection.

The 1480 amino acid CFTR protein is encoded by a 180-kilobase (kb) gene (CFTR) on chromosome 7q. More than 1000 disease-associated mutations have been identified. The most common of these is the delta F508 allele (deletion of phenylalanine (F) codon at amino acid position 508). Fifty percent of Caucasian CF patients are homozygous for the delta F508 mutation (allele frequency of 0.7), which results in complete loss of CFTR activity in the homozygous state. These are the patients that present with a more severe phenotype and the disease occurs extremely early in life as described here in case A. Case B carries one delta F508 allele, but the second mutation ($2789 + 5G > T$) produces a splice variant that leads to abnormal mRNA expression and low levels of normal transcripts. This compound heterozygous combination has been associated with a milder phenotype, as described for the patient in case B.[2] Most CF mutations result in full-length CFTR proteins that have diminished CFTR activity because these alleles are either misfolded and prematurely degraded (type II), have abnormal nucleotide binding (type III), have reduced chloride conductance (type IV), or as a result of splicing variants, become unstable at the cell surface resulting in accelerated turnover of CFTR (type VI). Less than 10% of CF mutations are caused by type I mutations that result in prematurely truncated proteins.

In 2001, the American College of Medical Genetics (ACMG) published guidelines for genotyping 25 common CFTR mutations. These recommendations were established in conjunction with the American College of Obstetricians and Gynecologists (ACOG) for CF carrier detection. The mutations in the panel have allele frequencies $\geq 0.1\%$ in the general U.S. population.[3] The panel includes the following mutations:

delta F508	N1303K	A455E	1078delT
delta I507	R553X	R560T	$711 + 1G > T$
G542X	$621 + 1G > T$	R1162X	$1898 + 1G > A$
G551D	R117H	G85E	2184delA
W1282X	1717-1G > A	R334W	R347P
$3849 + 10kbC > T$	$2789 + 5G > A$	3659delC	I148T
$3120 + 1G > A$			

The carrier frequency for CF in non-Hispanic Caucasians and Ashkenazi Jewish is ~ 1 in 25. This panel of mutations has a $\sim 97\%$ sensitivity of detection for CF mutations in the Ashkenazi, 80% in non-Hispanic Caucasians, 69% in African-Americans, and 57% in Hispanic Americans. An additional set of reflex tests are recommended if patients are positive for the R117H mutation. R117H is associated with classic CF only when it is present in a cis configuration with a "5T" polymorphism (present in at least 1% of the general population) in intron 8 of the CFTR gene. 5T is a thymidine tract with 5 repeat T nucleotides. In addition, when R117H is on the same chromosome as a 7T or 9T thymidine repeat in intron 8, a variant of CF is present that results in infertility in otherwise healthy males. Recently, studies suggesting that I148T must occur on the same chromosome as a 3199delG mutation in order to confer a pathogenic role. This led to changes in ACMG's recommendations that this mutation be tested for when I148T is found.[4] More studies are needed to validate these findings, but these examples point out the complexity of genotyping for CF. It is also important to note that, depending on the methodology used for DNA genotyping, benign variants such as I506V, I507V, and I508V may lead to false-positive results, rendering an incorrect genotype for delta F508, for example. Nonetheless, the identification of such a substantial number of disease causing mutations has increased the understanding of genotype–phenotype correlations, subsequently improving the sensitivity and specificity of current CFTR mutation screening.

According to a report by Wilfond and Gollust, seven states have newborn screening programs that now include CF as mandated by legislative or executive actions.[5] The screening for CF is based on measuring immunoreactive trypsinogen (IRT) on newborn blood spots. An elevated IRT is significant for increased risk of cystic fibrosis.[6] Integrating molecular diagnostic test results with the clinical features and other laboratory findings is paramount to developing the most effective treatment plans for patients.

Treatment

Currently, there is no cure for cystic fibrosis. Treatment is specific to the patients' clinical presentation and needs. The overall goal of treatment is to maintain near-normal pulmonary function. This may require antibiotics, special exercises using a percussion vest for draining sputum, and albuterol nebulizers. Diet therapy, which emphasizes the replacement of deficient pancreatic enzymes and fat-soluble vitamins, is recommended. A DNase known as *Pulmozyme* (dornase alfa) (Genentech, South San Francisco, CA) is also used to reduce the viscosity of the mucous secretions, improving lung function. The induction of normal CFTR function using mutation-specific pharmacologic agents is also being investigated.[7] The aim of these studies is to use drugs that can correct the disrupted molecular mechanism caused by the different mutations or augment the activity of the mutated CFTR protein. Gene therapy trials are also under way. The first clinical trials were performed in 1993. Several viral and nonviral delivery systems have been utilized. In addition, a vector system consisting of compacted nanoparticles of single CFTR expression plasmids administered intranasally has shown promise in efficient gene transfer.

References

1. ROSENSTEIN, B. J. AND CUTTING, G. R.: The diagnosis of cystic fibrosis: A consensus statement. Cystic Fibrosis Foundation Consensus Panel. *J. Pediatr. 132*:589–95, 1998.
2. DUGUEPEROUX, I. AND DE BRAEKELEER, M.: The CFTR 3849 + 10kbC → T and 2789+5G → A alleles are associated with a mild CF phenotype. *Eur. Respir. J. 25*:468–73, 2005.
3. GRODY, W. W., CUTTING, G. R., KLINGER, K. W., RICHARDS, C. S., WATSON, M. S., AND DESNICK, R. J. (Subcommittee on Cystic Fibrosis Screening, Accreditation of Genetic Services Committee, ACMG): Laboratory standards and guidelines for population-based cystic fibrosis carrier screening. *Genet. Med. 3*:149–54, 2001.
4. MONAGHAN, K. G., HIGHSMITH, W. E., AMOS, J. ET AL.: Genotype-phenotype correlation and frequency of the 3199del6 cystic fibrosis mutation among I148T carriers: results from a collaborative study. *Genet. Med. 6*:421–5, 2004.
5. WILFOND, B. S. AND GOLLUST, S. E.: Policy issues for expanding newborn screening programs: The cystic fibrosis newborn screening experience in the United States. *J. Pediatr. 146*:668–74, 2005.
6. OGINO, S., FLODMAN, P., WILSON, R. B., GOLD, B., AND GRODY, W. W.: Risk calculations for cystic fibrosis in neonatal screening by immunoreactive trypsinogen and CFTR mutation tests. *Genet. Med. 7*:317–27, 2005.
7. KEREM, E.: Pharmacological induction of CFTR function in patients with cystic fibrosis: mutation-specific therapy. *Pediatr. Pulmonol. 40*:183–96, 2005.

Additional Reading

Tietz Textbook of Clinical Chemistry, 2nd. ed., C. A. BURTIS, AND E. R. ASHWOOD, eds., Saunders, Philadelphia, 1999, pp. 1314–16.
WELSCH, M. J., TSUI, L.-C., BOAT, T. F., AND BEAUDET, A. L.: In *The Metabolic and Molecular Basis of Inherited Disease*, 7th ed., Vol. 3, C. R. SCRIVER, A. L. BEAUDET, W. S. SLY, AND D. VALLE, eds., McGraw-Hill, New York, 1995, pp. 3799–876.

Part Three

Renal Disease

Acute and chronic renal failure are reported in Cases 5 and 9, respectively
(both edited by (MGS); Cases 6, 7, 8, and 11 (all edited by MGS) present cases
of renal transplant cyclosporin toxicity, glomerular nephritis, nephrotic
syndrome, and syndrome of inappropriate secretion of antidiuretic hormone
(SIADH), respectively; and a case of renal osteodystrophy is presented in
Case 10 (edited by AMG).

Tietz's Applied Laboratory Medicine, Second Edition. Edited by Mitchell G. Scott, Ann M. Gronowski, and
Charles S. Eby
Copyright © 2007 John Wiley & Sons, Inc.

Case 5

Man with Hypertension and Fever

C. Darrell Jennings

A 75-year-old man with longstanding hypertension developed a fever and upper respiratory illness 2 weeks prior to admission. The fever ranged between 103 and 104°F (39.4 and 40.0°C), and there were no localized pulmonary findings or productive cough. This illness did not respond to a cephalosporin, and thus amantadine was begun one week prior to admission. Four days prior to admission the patient's family stopped all medications, including his antihypertensive drugs, because they felt he was having a reaction to the medicine.

At 3:00 am the morning of admission, the patient awoke with severe dyspnea without chest pain. On arrival at the community hospital emergency room, a chest film revealed pulmonary edema. Vital signs were pulse, 140 bpm; temperature, 103°F (39.4°C); and blood pressure, 210/110 mm Hg. The patient was treated with intravenous furosemide and intravenous nitroglycerin. The blood pressure decreased modestly but then fell precipitously to a systolic pressure of 50 mm Hg. Dopamine, bicarbonate, and normal saline were started and the systolic pressure returned to the 100–110 mm Hg range. Laboratory values obtained at the community hospital were as follows:

Analyte	Value, Conventional Units	Reference Interval, Conventional Units	Value, SI Units	Reference Interval, SI Units
Sodium	138 mmol/L	136–145	Same	
Potassium	4.2 mmol/L	3.8–5.1	Same	
Chloride	101 mmol/L	98–108	Same	
CO$_2$, total	32 mmol/L	23–31	Same	
Urea nitrogen	9 mg/dL	8–21	3.2 mmol	2.9–7.5
Creatinine	1.7 mg/dL	0.8–1.4	150 μmol/L	71–124
Urea nitrogen/ creatinine ratio	5 : 1	12–20 : 1	20.2 : 1	48.5–80.8 : 1
Bilirubin, total	0.9 mg/dL	0.2–1.1	15 μmol/L	3–19
ALT	92 U/L	13–40	1.53 μkat/L	0.22–0.67
AST	107 U/L	19–48	1.78 μkat/L	0.32–0.80

Tietz's Applied Laboratory Medicine, Second Edition. Edited by Mitchell G. Scott, Ann M. Gronowski, and Charles S. Eby
Copyright © 2007 John Wiley & Sons, Inc.

Analyte	Value, Conventional Units	Reference Interval, Conventional Units	Value, SI Units	Reference Interval, SI Units
CK	479 U/L	38–174	7.98 μkat/L	0.63–2.90
LDH	433 U/L	110–210	7.2 μkat/L	1.83–3.50
ALP	91 U/L	56–119	1.5 μkat/L	0.9–1.98
Hemoglobin	14 g/dL	14–18	8.69 mmol/L	8.69–11.17
Hematocrit	42%	40–54	0.42	0.40–0.54
Platelet count	$85 \times 10^3/\mu L$	150–450	$85 \times 10^9/L$	150–450

The patient was transferred by air ambulance to a tertiary care hospital. Physical examination suggested pulmonary consolidation, and a chest x-ray examination confirmed right upper lobe pneumonia. No focal neurological deficits were found. A test for hemosiderin pigment in urine was requested in view of the decrease in hemoglobin and hematocrit compared with values obtained at the community hospital; in the absence of frank hemorrhage, the admitting physician considered the possibility of a hemolytic process.

Three hours after admission and stabilization, the following laboratory results were obtained:

Analyte	Value, Conventional Units	Reference Interval, Conventional Units	Value, SI Units	Reference Interval, SI Units
Urea nitrogen	12 mg/dL	8–21	4.3 mmol urea/L	2.9–7.5
Creatinine	1.4 mg/dL	0.8–1.4	124 μmol/L	71–124
Urea nitrogen/ creatinine ratio	9 : 1	12–20 : 1	36.4 : 1	48.5–80.8 : 1
Sodium	136 mmol/L	136–145	Same	
Potassium	3.3 mmol/L	3.8–5.1	Same	
pH	7.43	7.35–7.45	Same	
pCO_2	39 mm Hg	35–48	5.2 kPa	4.7–6.4
pO_2 (on 30% FI O_2)	116 mm Hg	83–108	15.5 kPa	11.1–14.4
Hemoglobin	13.1 g/dL	14–18	8.13 mmol/L	8.69–11.17
Hematocrit	39%	40–54	0.39	0.40–0.54
Urinalysis	Within normal limits; negative for hemosiderin			

About 8 hours later, the following additional laboratory data were obtained:

Analyte	Value, Conventional Units	Reference Interval, Conventional Units	Value, SI Units	Reference Interval, SI Units
Hemoglobin	12.9 g/dL	14–18	8.01 mmol/L	8.69–11.17
Hematocrit	38%	40–54	0.38	0.40–0.54
Platelet count	$67 \times 10^3/\mu L$	150–450	$67 \times 10^9/L$	150–450
Prothrombin time	12.2 s	11.5–13.5	Same	

Analyte	Value, Conventional Units	Reference Interval, Conventional Units	Value, SI Units	Reference Interval, SI Units
Partial thromboplastin time (PTT)	28.6 s	23.1–33.3	Same	
Protein, total	5.5 g/dL	6.2–7.8	55 g/L	62–78
Albumin	2.8 g/dL	3.4–4.8	28 g/L	34–48
Amylase	111 U/L	21–150	1.85 μkat/L	0.35–2.50

These data appeared to rule out pancreatitis or a coagulation disorder. Although hemoglobin and hematocrit appeared to have stabilized, thrombocytopenia persisted, and hemolytic anemia remained a possibility. By the second day, however, the patient had virtually no urine output. The following table shows his laboratory results for days 2 and 3:

Analyte	Second Day, am	Second Day, pm	Third Day, am
Urea nitrogen	22 mg/dL (7.9 mmol/L)	35 mg/dL (12.5 mmol/L)	42 mg/dL (15.0 mmol/L)
Creatinine	2.1 mg/dL (186 μmol/L)	3.6 mg/dL (318 μmol/L)	4.4 mg/dL (389 μmol/L)
Hemoglobin	11.6 g/dL (7.20 mmol/L)	10.5 g/dL (6.52 mmol/L)	10.6 g/dL (6.58 mmol/L)
Hematocrit	34% (0.34)	31% (0.31)	31% (0.31)
Platelet count	54 × 10³/μL (54 × 10⁹/L)	51 × 10³/μL (51 × 10⁹/L)	51 × 10³/μL (51 × 10⁹/L)
Magnesium	1.6 mg/dL (0.66 mmol/L)		
Peripheral blood smear	Unremarkable		Unremarkable
Coagulation studies		Within normal limits	
Reticulocyte count, corrected			1.8%
Urinalysis		Within normal limits	Leukocytes, 1–5/ hpf; erythrocytes, 5–10/hpf; renal tubular epithelial cells, 1–5/hpf
Sodium, urine			44 mmol/L
Osmolality, urine			258 mOsm/kg

Rapid rise in serum levels of urea nitrogen and creatinine and developing stability of hemoglobin, hematocrit, and thrombocyte values, together with barely elevated reticulocyte count, turned attention away from the hematological findings and focused it on acute renal failure.

Several consulting physicians, including a clinical pathologist, were called to see the patient. One consultant raised the question of thrombotic thrombocytopenic purpura (TTP) and the possibility of plasma exchange. A second consultant thought that acute renal failure secondary to acute tubular necrosis (ATN) was more likely and that anemia and thrombocytopenia were probably due to marrow suppression secondary to the infectious process. The pathologist also felt that TTP was unlikely and thus recommended against plasma exchange.

The morning of the next day, the fourth hospital day, the following laboratory studies indicated relatively stable hematological findings and a further increase in serum urea nitrogen and creatinine:

Analyte	Value, Conventional Units	Reference Interval, Conventional Units	Value, SI Units	Reference Interval, SI Units
Urea nitrogen	66 mg/dL	8–21	23.6 mmol urea/L	2.9–7.5
Creatinine	7.0 mg/dL	0.8–1.4	619 μmol/L	71–124
Urea nitrogen/ creatinine ratio (calculated)	9 : 1	12–20 : 1	36.4 : 1	48.5–80.8 : 1
Hemoglobin	10.2 g/dL	14–18	6.33 mmol/L	8.69–11.17
Hematocrit	29%	40–54	0.29	0.40–0.54
Platelet count	$67 \times 10^3/\mu L$	150–450	$67 \times 10^9/L$	150–450

Dialysis was started, and laboratory results reported on the fifth day were as follows:

Analyte	Value, Conventional Units	Reference Interval, Conventional Units	Value, SI Units	Reference Interval, SI Units
Hemoglobin	10.2 g/dL	14–18	6.33 mmol/L	8.69–11.17
Hematocrit	29%	40–54	0.29	0.40–0.54
Platelet count	$94 \times 10^3/\mu L$	150–450	$94 \times 10^9/L$	150–450
Bilirubin, total	0.6 mg/dL	0.2–1.1	10 μmol/L	3–19
Haptoglobin	Within normal limits			

Over the next several days the hematological picture improved spontaneously; hemoglobin rose to 12 g/dL (7.45 mmol/L), hematocrit to 36% (0.36), and platelet count to $191 \times 10^3/\mu L$ ($191 \times 10^9/\mu L$). Serum electrolytes, acid–base values, and urea nitrogen, determined during this period of hemodialysis, stabilized. A disintegrinlike and metalloproteinase domain with thrombospondin Motifs–13 (ADAMTS-13) enzyme level performed by a reference laboratory was normal, ruling out TTP. The patient remained in acute renal failure until the 22nd hospital day when urine output increased to 500–1000 mL/d. Renal biopsy performed on the 22nd hospital day showed regenerating tubules consistent with improving ATN. By the 27th hospital day, urine output was >1500 mL/day, and serum urea nitrogen and creatinine were decreasing without further dialysis. When serum potassium fell to 3.1 mmol/L, oral potassium supplementation was initiated. After an uneventful diuretic phase, the patient was discharged with only medications for his hypertension.

Differential Diagnosis

The case presented above poses the problem of a febrile illness, anemia, and thrombocytopenia evolving into acute renal failure. The combination caused serious consideration to be given to a diagnosis of thrombotic thrombocytopenic purpura (TTP). TTP is treated by plasma exchange (plasmapheresis), a procedure in which whole blood is removed and separated into plasma and cellular components with return of the cellular components to the patient but replacement of the plasma with donor plasma. Plasma exchange is automated in a continuous-flow device that requires extracorporeal circulation and anticoagulation. The risks of plasma exchange for this patient were bleeding due to anticoagulation, infection from the extracorporeal circulation, and most important, infection and adverse reactions from the large amount of donor plasma that would be required. Critical examination of the patient's physical status and laboratory data, as well as the relative rarity of TTP, led to a choice of hemodialysis as an immediate treatment. During dialysis, spontaneous improvement in the cytopenic state, normal levels of ADAMTS-13, together with recovery from anuria and the findings of the renal biopsy, resolved the diagnostic question in favor of ATN.

Thrombotic Thrombocytopenic Purpura (TTP)[1–3]

The clinical features of TTP have been reviewed in the case records of the Massachusetts General Hospital.[4] Originally described by Moschowitz in 1925, thrombotic thrombocytopenic purpura (TTP) consists of five classic findings: (1) neurologic deficit, (2) renal dysfunction, (3) fever, (4) thrombocytopenia, and (5) microangiopathic hemolytic anemia (also see the case presented in Case 67 of this book).

Since the previous edition of this book, the pathogenesis of TTP has been elucidated.[1] The fundamental defect is a deficiency in the activity of ADAMTS-13, a plasma metalloproteinase that cleaves ultra-high-molecular-weight (UHMW) multimers of von Willebrand factor normally produced by endothelial cells. These UHMW multimers initiate platelet aggregation and subsequent microthrombi. While rare inherited deficiencies of ADAMTS-13 have been described, most patients have acquired disease secondary to development of an inhibitory antibody. The recognition of the important role of ADAMTS-13 has allowed development of a useful but lengthy and not emergently available laboratory test that also helps differentiating TTP from hemolytic uremic syndrome.[2,3] Patients with both congenital and acquired TTP have ADAMTS-13 activity levels less than 5–10% of normal. However, the lack of routine availability of the assay requires initial treatment to be based on clinical and other laboratory features.[3]

Hemolytic uremic syndrome (HUS), seen predominantly in children, has overlapping clinical features and a similar pathophysiological process that instead initiates with endothelial injury but also consists of microvascular hyaline thrombi. It is frequently preceded by a febrile illness. It has been associated with 0157:H7 strain of *Escherichia coli* where a shigellalike endothelial toxin is crucial. Like TTP, DIC is not present. But unlike TTP, the findings are typically confined to the kidney and ADAMTS-13 values are not below 5–10% of normal.[3] HUS does not respond to plasmapheresis, whereas, TTP responds effectively to plasmapheresis. Presumably, exchange removes UHMW VWF multimers and ADAMTS-13 inhibitors, while the infused plasma replaces deficient enzyme activity.[1,2,3]

This case presents some of the features of TTP or HUS, but lacks certain critical laboratory and clinical findings. TTP is predominantly a disease of the third and fourth decades with only 18% of patients being over age 50.[4] It does, however, occasionally occur in older individuals.[5] Thrombocytopenia with a mean platelet count of $20{,}500/\mu L$ $(20.5 \times 10^9/L)$ is present in 83–93% of patients with TTP–HUS.[4] The drop in platelet count accompanies the formation of microthrombi, the central pathophysiological event. This patient's platelet count remained stable around $52 \times 10^3/\mu L$ $(52 \times 10^9/L)$, while renal function deteriorated. Subsequently, the platelet count rose dramatically as renal function further declined. This pattern is contrary to our current understanding of the pathophysiological mechanism of TTP.

The patient reported above lacked several key findings of TTP: (1) there was no evidence of intravascular hemolysis, since total serum bilirubin and haptoglobin levels were normal, urine hemosiderin was negative, and serum LDH was only mildly elevated despite coexisting pulmonary disease; (2) schistocytes (the hallmark of microangiopathic processes[4]) were not seen on blood smears; and (3) the low reticulocyte count suggested an inadequate bone marrow response as a probable cause of the anemia and thrombocytopenia. Failure to find laboratory evidence of hemolysis or evidence of a microangiopathic process in the peripheral blood smear placed the diagnosis of TTP in serious doubt. Finally, the renal dysfunction seen in 76–88% of the patients with TTP differs in several important aspects from this patient's findings. TTP or HUS are typically associated with an abnormal urine sediment, hematuria, and moderate proteinuria. This patient's urinalysis was unremarkable initially, despite increasing serum urea nitrogen and creatinine levels. When urinalysis results became abnormal, the urine contained renal tubular epithelial cells, a finding more suggestive of acute tubular injury. In addition, the patient's clinical course, characterized by anuria and daily doubling of urea nitrogen and creatinine values, is unusual in TTP or HUS; only 11% of patients present with acute renal failure[4] and even fewer with anuric renal failure.[6]

Although the combination of fever, anemia, thrombocytopenia, and renal failure in this patient initially suggested TTP, the diagnosis could not be sustained when the laboratory findings were critically examined. The subsequent normal ADAMTS-13 further excluded TTP. Because the anemia and thrombocytopenia were self-limited and could be explained as a secondary effect of bone marrow suppression by the pulmonary infection and drug therapy, the major question remaining was the etiology of anuric acute renal failure.

Prerenal Azotemia

Prerenal azotemia[7] is caused by diminished renal function due to poor renal perfusion. In prerenal azotemia there is relative preservation of tubular concentration function. Consequently, renal tubules respond to the decreased glomerular filtration rate (GF) with sodium and water retention and concentration of the urine.[7] The result is a urine sodium typically <20 mmol/L and an elevated urine osmolality, creatinine, and specific gravity; most characteristic is a fractional excretion (see next paragraph) of sodium $<1\%$.[7]

Fractional excretion (FE) for sodium is determined from an assay of sodium and creatinine on the same urine and serum specimens. The value is calculated as the sodium clearance divided by the creatinine clearance in an equation simplified by the cancellation of units and flow rate, thus:

$$FE\ (\text{sodium})\% = \frac{\text{creatinine (S), mg/dL} \times \text{sodium (U), mmol/L}}{\text{creatinine (U), mg/dL} \times \text{sodium (S), mmol/L}} \times 100.$$

In *acute renal failure* due to intrinsic renal disease, there is loss of tubular function. This loss results in a glomerular filtrate that is little altered by the tubules. Thus, urine may be isosthenuric (specific gravity of urine similar to that of unmodified glomerular filtrate, 1.010 ± 0.002), urine sodium >20 mmol/L, and the fractional excretion of sodium greater than 3%.[7] This patient's urine osmolality, urine sodium, and specific gravity are all typical of intrinsic renal disease and not prerenal azotemia.

Serum findings may also help differentiate prerenal azotemia from intrinsic renal disease. With the reduced GFR of prerenal azotemia, intact tubules will allow reabsorption of urea without creatinine (creatinine is only minimally absorbed by the tubules). Additionally, tubules secrete creatinine but not urea from the blood to the glomerular filtrate, increasing the net excretion of creatinine but not urea. The result is that serum urea concentrations will climb faster than creatinine levels so that the urea nitrogen/creatinine ratio will rise above 20 : 1. In ATN, the tubule does not exclude creatinine, and a normal or a low ratio is maintained. This patient's ratio remained very close to 10 : 1 throughout the period of renal dysfunction, favoring the diagnosis of intrinsic renal disease.

The most common cause of acute reversible oliguric renal failure is ATN. The renal tubules are particularly vulnerable to ischemic injury because they have a very high metabolic rate and also because their blood supply comes from the portal circulation via the efferent arteriole. The portal supply is less oxygenated and under less pressure than a direct arterial supply is. Also, because of their resorptive and concentrating functions, the renal tubular epithelial cells are vulnerable to toxins such as heavy metals and some drugs. Toxic injury and ischemic injury are therefore the two most common causes of ATN.

In this patient there was a well-documented episode of sudden hypotension following the treatment of the patient's hypertensive crisis. Renal function was only very mildly compromised until this event. Subsequently, the patient was anuric with daily doubling of creatinine and urea nitrogen values, a situation indicative of almost complete cessation of renal function. This is a classic picture of ATN secondary to a single ischemic event—in this case, hypotension.

Treatment

Once injured, the renal tubular epithelial cells require 3–4 weeks to regenerate. During this time the patient must be supported with dialysis as well as fluid and electrolyte management. The most common cause of morbidity is infection. Once regeneration occurs, the patient enters a diuretic phase. The patient must be monitored because there may be wasting of electrolytes such as potassium and sodium. Many patients, such as this one, experience complete recovery of renal function with good supportive care.

References

1. MOAKE, J. L.: Von Willebrand factor, ADAMTS-13, and thrombotic thrombocytopenic purpura. *Semin. Hematol.* *41*:4–14, 2004.
2. KREMER-HOVINGA, J. A., STUDT, J. D., AND LAMMLE, B.: The Von Willebrand factor-cleaving protease (ADAMTS-13) and the diagnosis of thrombotic thrombocytopenic purpura. *Pathophysiol. Haemost. Thromb.* *33*:417–21, 2003/2004.
3. MOAKE, J. L.: Thrombotic thrombocytopenic purpura and the hemolytic uremic syndrome. *Arch. Pathol. Lab. Med.* *126*:1430–3, 2002.
4. SCULLY, R. E., ed.: Case records of the Massachusetts General Hospital. *N. Engl. J. Med. 325*:265, 1991.
5. KNUPP, C. L.: Thrombotic thrombocytopenic purpura in older patients. *J. Am. Geriatr. Soc. 36*:331, 1988.
6. DUNEA, G., MURHRCKE, R. C., NAKAMOTO, S., AND SCHWARTZ, F. D.: Thrombotic thrombocytopenic purpura and acute renal failure. *Am. J. Med. 41*:1000, 1966.
7. NEWMAN, D. J. AND PRICE, C. P.: Renal Function and nitrogen metabolites. In: *Teitz Textbook of Clinical Chemistry*, C. A. BURTIS AND E. R. ASHWOOD, eds., Saunders, Philadelphia, 1999, pp. 1204–70.

Case 6

Oliguria with Metabolic Acidosis after Renal Transplantation

C. Darrell Jennings

A 37-year-old white male with end-stage renal disease and on chronic hemodialysis presented 10 days after receiving a 1 B locus, 2 DR locus mismatch for a three of six HLA antigen mismatched kidney transplant (see section on *HLA matching* below). The kidney functioned within the first 48 hours with good urine output and a rapid decline of serum creatinine to 1.5 mg/dL (133 μmol/L) and urea nitrogen to 23 mg/dL (8.2 mmol urea/L). The patient had been placed on routine antirejection prophylactic therapy consisting of a calcineurin inhibitor and mycophenolate mofetil.

The patient presented 10 days posttransplant with complaints of pain and tenderness over the site of the graft with fever and reduced urine output. The following laboratory values were obtained:

Analyte	Value, Conventional Units	Reference Interval, Conventional Units	Value, SI Units	Reference Interval, SI Units
Urea nitrogen	72 mg/dL	7–18	25.7 mmol urea/L	2.5–6.4
Creatinine	7.0 mg/dL	0.8–1.4	619 μmol/L	71–124
Urea nitrogen/ creatinine ratio	10. 3:1	12–20:1	41:6:1	48.5–80.8:1
Sodium	142 mmol/L	136–145	Same	
Potassium	5.9 mmol/L	3.8–5.1	Same	
Chloride	99 mmol/L	98–108	Same	
CO₂, total	13 mmol/L	23–29	Same	
Phosphorus	9.5 mg/dL	2.7–4.5	3.07 mmol/L	0.87–1.45
Urate	14.0 mg/dL	4.5–8.0	833 μmol/L	268–476

Tietz's Applied Laboratory Medicine, Second Edition. Edited by Mitchell G. Scott, Ann M. Gronowski, and Charles S. Eby

Analyte	Value, Conventional Units	Reference Interval, Conventional Units	Value, SI Units	Reference Interval, SI Units
Calcium, total	8.0 mg/dL	8.4–10.2	2.00 mmol/L	2.10–2.55
Cyclosporine, trough	50 ng/mL	Therap.: 100–200	42 nmol/L	83–166
Creatinine clearance	18 mL/min	90–130	$0.17\ \text{mLs}^{-1}\ \text{m}^{-2}$	0.87–1.25
pH (aB)	7.28	7.35–7.45	Same	
$p\text{CO}_2$ (aB)	29 mm Hg	35–48	3.9 kPa	4.7–6.4
$p\text{O}_2$ (aB)	98 mm Hg	83–108	13.1 kPa	11.1–14.4
Urinalysis				
pH	5.0	4.0–8.0	Same	
Glucose	1+	Negative		
Leukocytes	3–5 hpf	None		

Because of the low cyclosporine trough level, it was felt that calcineurin inhibitor toxicity was not likely the cause of the acute renal dysfunction. The urea nitrogen/creatinine ratio of 10 : 1 did not suggest pre-renal causes. Consequently, a renal biopsy was obtained and showed diffuse lymphocytic infiltration of the interstitium. There was interstitial edema and some loss of tubules. Renal vessels were patent, and there was no acute intimal injury. The patient's cyclosporine dose was increased, and he was given high-dosage steroids and the immunosuppressant rabbit antithymocyte globulin, a polyclonal antibody preparation against T-cell lymphocytes. This treatment resulted in an improvement in his overall state. The steroids were then rapidly tapered, and the antithymocyte globulin course was completed. Several days later the patient presented for a routine follow-up and complained of feeling weak, tired, and somewhat nauseated, but his urine output was normal. Laboratory results obtained at this visit were as follows:

Analyte	Value, Conventional Units	Reference Interval, Conventional Units	Value, SI Units	Reference Interval, SI Units
Urea nitrogen	19 mg/dL	7–18	6.8 mmol urea/L	2.5–6.4
Creatinine	1.6 mg/dL	0.8–1.4	141 µmol/L	71–124
Urea nitrogen/ creatinine ratio	82 mL/min	90–130	0.79 mL/s per m²	0.87–1.25
Sodium	139 mmol/L	136–145	Same	
Potassium	4.0 mmol/L	3.8–5.1	Same	
Chloride	112 mmol/L	98–108	Same	
CO_2, total	15 mmol/L	23–29	Same	
pH (aB)	7.31	7.35–7.45	Same	
$p\text{CO}_2$ (aB)	31 mm Hg	35–48	4.1 kPa	4.7–6.4
Urinalysis				
pH	5.0	4.6–8.0		
Glucose	2+	Negative		
Leukocytes	1–2 hpf	None		

Because of the persistent acidosis, the patient was given bicarbonate orally. After 48 hours, repeat laboratory studies revealed the following:

Analyte	Value, Conventional Units	Reference Interval, Conventional Units	Value, SI Units	Reference Interval, SI Units
Sodium	141 mmol/L	136–145	Same	
Potassium	3.1 mmol/L	3.8–5.1	Same	
Chloride	112 mmol/L	98–108	Same	
Bicarbonate (aB)	17 mmol/L	18–23	Same	
pH (aB)	7.33	7.35–7.45	Same	
pCO_2 (aB)	33 mm Hg	35–48	4.4 kPa	4.7–6.4
Urinalysis				
pH	7.0	4.6–8.0		
Glucose	2+	Negative		
Leukocytes	1–2 hpf	None		
β_2-Microglobulin	Increased			

The persistent acidosis was felt to be a manifestation of tubulointerstitial disease secondary to acute renal allograft rejection. Despite further therapy, allograft rejection continued, and creatinine clearance further declined. After 10 months, the patient returned for chronic hemodialysis.

HLA Matching[1]

In 2003, more than 25,000 organs were transplanted in the United States, over 18,000 from deceased and almost 7000 from living donors. Unfortunately over 7000 patients died while awaiting transplant. All immunocompetent individuals, except identical twins, reject tissues from other human beings. The vigor of the rejection is related to the immune competence of the recipient (host) and the immunogenicity of the graft (donor tissue). The less similar the donor and recipient, the greater the immunogenicity of the graft. The dominant system in immune recognition is the HLA (human leukocyte antigen) system, which consists of several closely linked loci on the short arm of chromosome six. Three loci—the A, B, and DR—are evaluated in clinical solid organ transplantation. The degree of mismatch is expressed as the number of mismatched antigens out of a possible six; the patient in this case was mismatched for three out of six. Because of improvements in immunosuppression and changes in renal allocation guidelines, increasing numbers of patients are being transplanted with four, five, or six antigen mismatches; indeed, in 2003, 62% of recipients had four or more HLA mismatches. While the degree of matching plays a less important role in first-year survival, it remains a predictor of 5-year graft survival with a 10% difference between zero (74%) and six (64%) antigen mismatches. Unfortunately, even allografts with six of six matches can be rejected, albeit usually less vigorously. Thus, all recipients except identical twins are treated with immunosuppressive agents.

Calcineurin Inhibitor Effects and Toxicity[1,2]

Since the first edition of this book, major changes have occurred in immunosuppressive maintenance therapy. Calcineurin inhibitors and antimetabolites remain the mainstays, but there has been a progressive migration from the calcineurin inhibitor, cyclosporine, to another calcineurin inhibitor, tacrolimus, and from azathioprine (antiproliferative by incorporating thioguanine nucleotides into DNA) to mycophenolate mofetil (an inhibitor of inosine monophosphate dehydrogenase). In 2003, 67% of kidney patients received tacrolimus and 81% received mycophenolate mofetil as maintenance therapy. These newer therapies have translated into improved first-year graft survival rates and decreased incidence of acute rejection from >50% in 1996 to 15% in 2002. Use of calcineurin inhibitors to suppress renal allograft rejection also exposes the patient to these drugs' toxicities. Acute toxicity results from increased renal vascular resistance with resulting decreased blood flow and glomerular filtration rate (GFR) and is associated with little morphological change. Thus, development of oliguric dysfunction in renal transplant recipients may be the result of allograft rejection due to insufficient drug levels or the result of drug toxicity. The problem is compounded by the fact that in calcineurin inhibitor-treated patients, the classic signs of rejection (graft tenderness and fever) may be suppressed. The clinical and anatomic pathology laboratories can be useful in resolving this question by performing therapeutic drug monitoring assays and renal biopsy.

Calcineurin inhibitors block induction of interleukin-2 (IL-2) mRNA in T cells and thus inhibit the cascade leading to T-cell activation and proliferation. Since they may cause renal toxicity and dysfunction, monitoring trough levels in blood is very important. The choice of sample and methodology for measurement of drug levels is somewhat variable. Whole blood is the preferred specimen, since these drugs diffuse variably into red cells in a temperature- and hematocrit-dependent fashion. Measurement may be done by either immunoassay, HPLC, or more recently high-performance liquid chromatography tandem mass spectroscopy (LC-MS/MS). HPLC and LC-MS/MS can distinguish active parent drug from metabolites. Immunoassays vary in their ability to distinguish parent drug from metabolites. LC-MS/MS methods are rapidly becoming the gold standard for determining parent concentrations of calcineurine inhibitors and other immunosuppressants such as sirolimus and everolimus. The therapeutic range of immunosuppressants often depends on the particular assay utilized and its specificity for the parent molecule and/or active metabolites. A typical therapeutic range for cyclosporine use in renal transplantation patients is 100–200 ng/mL (83–166 nmol/L). Thus, the patient in this case was actually below the therapeutic range and was unlikely to have had drug toxicity. (see also Case 72).

Allograft Rejection[2]

The biopsy in the case presented above suggested that the renal allograft was being rejected. A rejection that occurs several days posttransplant with a predominantly cellular type of immune response is termed *acute rejection*. Hyperacute rejection occurs within minutes to hours and involves predominantly the humoral arm of the immune response. This occurs in patients with preformed antibody to antigens expressed in the graft, particularly those on endothelial cells. Hyperacute rejections have been nearly eliminated by the laboratory performance of a crossmatch of the recipient's sera against lymphocytes from the donor.

The clinical laboratory findings resulting from acute renal allograft rejection are the same as those from acute renal failure and thus do not distinguish among rejection, acute tubular necrosis, and drug toxicity. Consequently, renal biopsy and a favorable response to antirejection therapy may be the best indicators of rejection. Renal biopsy is associated with significant morbidity. As an alternative, fine-needle aspiration cytology has been tried, but with limited success. Attempts to monitor immunological events by measurement of activation antigens and lymphocyte subsets by flow cytometry have generally been disappointing.

The patient in this case had classic findings of renal allograft rejection with azotemia, oliguria, fever, and graft tenderness. Glomerular filtration was markedly reduced, and the histological picture was compatible with acute rejection. Secondary changes of hyperkalemia and metabolic acidosis were also present.

Uremic Acidosis[3,4]

Metabolic acidosis of renal failure develops when the kidney is unable to excrete the endogenously generated acid load of approximately 1 mEq/kg body weight per day. The metabolic acidosis that develops in the presence of diffuse renal disease associated with significant reduction of GFR is sometimes referred to as *uremic acidosis*. It is important to distinguish this entity from the more specific deficit of renal urine acidification in renal tubular acidosis (RTA) that is associated with well-preserved GFR. Because of the accumulation of organic acids, the acidosis of renal failure is usually a normochloremic acidosis with increased anion gap. RTA is typically a hyperchloremic non-anion-gap acidosis. However, some studies have suggested that as many as 30% of patients with renal failure may have some component of hyperchloremic acidosis. In addition, potassium retention and hyperkalemia are common in renal failure, whereas some forms of proximal and distal RTA are characterized by potassium loss and hypokalemia.

The vast majority of patients with GFR <20 mL/min will have some degree of acidosis manifested by a reduction in plasma bicarbonate. In general, the more severe the reduction of GFR, the lower the plasma bicarbonate concentration will be. The basic defect is a failure of tubular function resulting in less net acid excretion than daily endogenous acid production. If glomerular function is relatively less compromised than tubular function, the filtration and excretion of organic anions occur, and a non-anion-gap acidosis is the result. If glomerular and tubular function are proportionately reduced, as might be expected in the diffuse injury of advanced renal failure, the organic anions are retained in proportion to the deficit in hydrogen ion excretion, resulting in an increased anion gap acidosis. In many cases the acidosis will be a mixed-anion-gap and non-anion-gap acidosis. Additional electrolyte findings in uremia include hyperkalemia, hyperphosphatemia, and hypocalcemia. Generally, in chronic renal failure there is reasonable preservation of residual distal tubular hydrogen ion excretion so that acidification of the urine occurs appropriately. The major deficit in chronic renal failure is a reduction in ammonium formation and excretion, which is considerably greater than the reduction in titratable acid excretion. The reduction in ammonium excretion appears to be a direct result of the loss of functioning nephron mass.

Renal Tubular Acidosis (RTA)[5,6]

After resolution of this patient's episode of graft rejection, much of his renal function tests returned to near-normal values. In addition, other electrolytes returned to normal except for chloride, which remained moderately elevated. This picture was not consistent with persisting metabolic acidosis from renal failure. Furthermore, this is a hyperchloremic metabolic acidosis, which is not the typical form of acidosis seen in renal failure. Certainly, a nonrenal cause of hyperchloremic acidosis could be considered.

Many of the conditions that give rise to hyperchloremic metabolic acidosis can be viewed as secondary to either loss of bicarbonate in urine or stool or the addition of hydrochloric acid or hydrochloric acid–generating compounds. A discussion of the differential of extrarenal causes is not included, but some are noted in Reference 6. Renal causes include proximal and distal RTA, aldosterone deficiency, hyperkalemia, defective ammoniagenesis, and renal insufficiency. This patient did not have the electrolyte pattern of either aldosterone deficiency (hyperkalemia) and did not at this point have renal insufficiency. Patients with distal RTA have an inability to acidify urine in the distal tubule. There is some controversy as to whether this deficit is secondary to backward leak of secreted H^+ or inability to secrete H^+. The patient in this case had a urine pH of 5.0, demonstrating the ability to acidify the urine. A significant clue to the underlying problem was obtained when the patient was placed on bicarbonate therapy. In response to bicarbonate therapy, the plasma bicarbonate increased only minimally, and the urine became alkaline despite the preserved ability of the distal tubules to acidify. This must have been due to proximal tubular wasting of bicarbonate and thus represented the proximal form of RTA.

Healthy individuals excrete very little bicarbonate in their urine. Patients with proximal RTA have a reduced proximal renal threshold for bicarbonate reabsorption, typically between 15 and 20 mmol/L. When plasma bicarbonate is below the renal threshold, urine pH may be appropriately acidic because of preserved distal tubular mechanisms. However, once plasma bicarbonate levels increase, bicarbonate wasting occurs and eventually overwhelms the acid-excreting capacity of the distal nephron, and alkaline urine is produced (pH > 6.0). Most of these patients have significant bicarbonate wasting with fractional excretion[*] > 15%; occasional patients may have more moderate wasting with fractional excretion[*] between 3% and 15%.[7] Many patients have, as did this patient, additional evidence of proximal renal tubular dysfunction such as glucosuria, amino aciduria, and β_2-microglobulinuria. These findings all reflect disordered proximal tubular transport. In addition, because of reduced proximal sodium and bicarbonate resorption, there is increased distal delivery of sodium, which exchanges with potassium and leads to urinary potassium wasting and hypokalemia. Further bicarbonate administration may aggravate the hypokalemia.

Proximal RTA as a pure defect in bicarbonate transport is usually seen only in children. Much more often the defect is a component of a generalized defect in proximal tubular transport with wasting of glucose, phosphate, urate, amino acids, and others (i.e., Fanconi syndrome). Thus, hypophosphatemia and hypouricemia are frequent

---

[*]*Fractional excretion* of a compound is the renal clearance of that compound expressed as a percentage of creatinine clearance or of some other measure of GFR. Clearance is calculated as concentration of analyte in urine divided by its concentration in serum and multiplied by the urine flow rate in mL/min. For example

$$\text{Creatinine clearance, mL/min} = \frac{\text{creatinine (U), mg/dL}}{\text{creatinine (S), mg/dL}} \times \text{flow rate (U), mL/min}$$

For example, fractional clearance of bicarbonate is determined from assay of bicarbonate and creatinine on the same urine and serum specimens. The value is calculated as the bicarbonate clearance divided by the creatinine clearance in an equation simplified by the cancellation of units and flow rate:

$$\text{Fractional excretion (bicarbonate), \%} = \frac{\text{creatinine (S), mg/dL} \times \text{bicarbonate (U), mmol/L}}{\text{creatinine (U), mg/dL} \times \text{bicarbonate (S), mmol/L}} \times 100$$

Since bicarbonate is normally almost completely reabsorbed, fractional excretion is <3%. Patients with proximal RTA, however, have significant bicarbonate wasting; thus, fractional excretion is typically >15%.

laboratory findings. The hypokalemia may result in muscle weakness or cramps, paresthesias, polyuria, and thirst. One of the most common symptoms of RTA in children is failure to thrive, presumably secondary to the chronic acidosis. The causes of proximal RTA are numerous.[6]

In this particular case, proximal RTA was part of a generalized defect in proximal tubular transport brought about by tubulointerstitial injury secondary to renal allograft rejection. The proximal renal tubule is normally very rich in class II major histocompatibility antigens, possibly because of their role in oligopeptide transport, and is thus a vulnerable target for immune attack in patients receiving incompatible renal allografts.

References

1. 2004 Annual Report of the U.S. Organ Procurement and Transplantation Network and the Scientific Registry of Transplant Recipients: Transplant Data. Department of Health and Human Services, Health Resources and Services Administration, Healthcare Systems Bureau, Division of Transplantation, Rockville, MD; United Network for Organ Sharing, Richmond, VA; University Renal Research and Education Association, Ann Arbor, MI, 1994–2003.

2. MAGEE, C. C. AND MILFORD, E.: Clinical aspects of renal transplantation. In *Brenner & Rector's The Kidney*, 7th ed., Saunders, Philadelphia, 2004, pp. 2805–48.

3. URIBARRI, J.: Acidosis in chronic renal insufficiency: Acid-base in renal failure. *Semin. Dialysis 13*:232–4, 2000.

4. KOVACIC, V., ROGULJIC, L., AND KOVACIC, V.: Metabolic acidosis of chronically hemodialyzed patients. *Am. J. Nephrol. 23*:158–64, 2003.

5. WAGNER, C. A. AND GEIBEL, J. P.: Acid-base transport in the collecting duct. *J. Nephrol. 15*:S112–27, 2002.

6. NEWMAN, D. J. AND PRICE, C. P.: Renal function and nitrogen metabolites. In *Teitz Textbook of Clinical Chemistry*, C. A. BURTIS AND E. R. ASHWOOD, eds., Saunders, Philadelphia, 1999, pp. 1204–70.

Case 7

A Woman with Uremia, Pulmonary Infiltration, and Hemoptysis

C. Darrell Jennings

A 47-year-old white female developed severe nausea and vomiting 4 weeks prior to her current hospital admission. There had been no pain, but she had experienced a 7-lb (3.2-kg) weight loss. Her serum urea nitrogen was 40 mg/dL (14.3 mmol urea/L) and her creatinine 3.2 mg/dL (283 μmol/L). Urinalysis revealed numerous erythrocytes and granular casts, but an intravenous pyelogram (IVP) showed no structural abnormalities or obstruction. Five days later the creatinine rose to 6.8 mg/dL (60 μmol/L), the serum urea nitrogen rose to 72 mg/dL (25.7 mmol urea/L), and the creatinine clearance was 13 mL/min (reference range, 72–114). Past history was unrevealing, and there were no abnormal physical findings.

The patient was referred to the university hospital because of the significant deterioration of renal function. On admission the patient had the following laboratory findings:

Analyte	Value, Conventional Units	Reference Interval, Conventional Units	Value, SI Units	Reference Interval, SI Units
Hemoglobin	11.0 g/dL	12–16	6.83 mmol/L	7.45–9.93
Creatinine	6.3 mg/dL	0.7–1.2	557 μmol/L	62–106
Urea nitrogen	70 mg/dL	7–18	25.0 mmol/L	2.5–6.4
Sodium	135 mmol/L	136–145	Same	
Potassium	4.6 mmol/L	3.8–5.1	Same	
Chloride	97 mmol/L	98–108	Same	
CO$_2$, total	21 mmol/L	23–29	Same	
Urinalysis				

Tietz's Applied Laboratory Medicine, Second Edition. Edited by Mitchell G. Scott, Ann M. Gronowski, and Charles S. Eby

Analyte	Value, Conventional Units	Reference Interval, Conventional Units	Value, SI Units	Reference Interval, SI Units
Specific gravity	1.010	1.003–1.040		
pH	6.0	4.6–8.0		
Protein; Granular cast and numerous erythrocytes present in sediment	1+	Negative		
24-hour protein	518 mg/day	0–100 mg/day		

Other tests showed platelet count, WBC, C3 complement, antistreptolysin O (ASO), and antinuclear antibodies (ANA) to be within normal limits. A chest x-ray examination revealed a right middle lobe infiltrate.

The patient was treated with intravenous fluids for acid–base, electrolyte, and fluid management. Subsequently the serum creatinine decreased to 4.4 mg/dL (389 μmol/L). She was discharged with a diagnosis of acute renal failure induced by the IVP and super-imposed on renal insufficiency of undetermined cause. Plans were made to determine the etiology of the renal insufficiency on an outpatient basis.

Five days after discharge, the patient presented with increasingly severe nausea and vomiting. Physical examination was unchanged except for an increased temperature of 100.2°F (37.9°C). The serum creatinine was now 7.8 mg/dL (690 μmol/L) and the serum urea nitrogen was 88 mg/dL (31.4 mmol urea/L). Prothrombin and partial thromboplastin times were normal, and erythrocyte casts were seen on urinalysis.

Shortly after her second admission, a renal biopsy provided findings of crescentic glomerulonephritis. Immunofluorescence studies were indeterminate, and the patient was placed on immunosuppressive therapy. Over a 2-week period, the creatinine fell to 1.9 mg/dL (168 μmol/L). An attempt to decrease the immunosuppression therapy resulted in a rise of the serum creatinine to 2.4 mg/dL (212 μmol/L). At this time the patient developed hemoptysis and showed bilateral pulmonary infiltrates on the chest film. Arterial blood gas studies gave the following results:

Analyte	Value, Conventional Units	Reference Interval, Conventional Units	Value, SI Units	Reference Interval, SI Units
pH	7.50	7.35–7.45	Same	
pO_2	60 mm Hg	83–108	8.0 kPa	11.1–14.4
pCO_2	38 mm Hg	32–45	5.1 kPa	4.3–6.0

Pulmonary function continued to deteriorate with pO_2 falling to 45 mm Hg (6.0 kPa) despite increase in the fraction of inspired oxygen (FI O_2) up to 100%.

Creatinine values continued to rise, urine output decreased progressively, and the creatinine clearance fell to 7 mL/min (reference range, 72–114). By the 29th hospital day recurrent hemoptysis had developed, and aggressive plasmapheresis (plasma exchange) was initiated because open biopsy revealed lung findings that included focal necrosis of alveolar walls with intraalveolar hemorrhage. Immunofluorescence studies of lung tissue showed linear fluorescence along the alveolar basement membranes.

The patient's respiratory status slowly improved over the next 2 weeks. However, her renal function improved only minimally as evidenced by a creatinine clearance of

15 mL/min. She was discharged home and, on an outpatient basis, underwent plasmapheresis weekly for one month. Two months later at a clinic visit, she had complaints of nausea and vomiting, diffuse itching, weakness and fatigue, and sharp left-sided pleuritic pain. On physical examination, she was hypertensive with 1+ to 2+ pedal edema. A pleural friction rub was heard on auscultation. Her skin had a sallow color.

Laboratory tests at that time revealed the following:

Analyte	Value, Conventional Units	Reference Interval, Conventional Units	Value, SI Units	Reference Interval, SI Units
Sodium	139 mmol/L	136–145	Same	
Potassium	5.5 mmol/L	3.8–5.1	Same	
Chloride	102 mmol/L	98–108	Same	
CO_2, total	19 mmol/L	23–29	Same	
Urea nitrogen	95 mg/dL	7–18	33.9 mmol urea/L	2.5–6.4
Creatinine	9.1 mg/dL	0.7–1.2	804 μmol/L	62–106
Glucose	105 mg/dL	75–105	5.8 mmol/L	4.2–5.8
Calcium	6.2 mg/dL	8.4–10.2	1.55 mmol/L	2.10–2.54
Phosphorus	5.6 mg/dL	2.7–4.5	1.81 mmol/L	0.87–1.45
Urate	8.8 mg/dL	2.5–6.2	523 μmol/L	149–369
Hemoglobin	9.7 g/dL	12–16	6.02 mmol/L	7.45–9.93
Hematocrit	28%	37–47	0.28	0.37–0.47

Erythrocyte indices were as follows: MCV, 91 fL (reference range, 81–99); MCH, 29 pg (reference range, 27–31); MCHC, 35 g Hg/dL (22 mmol Hb/L; reference range, 33–37; 20–23). The corrected reticulocyte count was <1%. The patient was clearly uremic and was considered a candidate for chronic hemodialysis and ultimately renal transplantation.

Nephritic Syndrome

This patient's case presents the problem of rapidly deteriorating renal function, terminating in uremia with coexistent pulmonary hemorrhage and hemoptysis. The presence of erythrocytes in the urine indicated hemorrhage into the urinary tract. Whereas hemorrhage may occur at any point from the glomerulus to the urethra, the presence of erythrocyte casts localizes the process within the kidney, most likely high in the nephron. Additional evidence of reduced glomerular filtration rate (GFR), namely, rising serum urea nitrogen and creatinine, oliguria, and acidosis (decreased total CO_2 and increased anion gap) supports the inference that the glomeruli are the site of injury. The combination of hematuria with manifestations of reduced GFR constitutes the nephritic syndrome, which is the result of diffuse injury to the glomeruli.

Most glomerulopathies are the result of immunological injury of either the immune complex type or antibody-dependent type. The injury may be either a primary manifestation of a disease or part of a systemic process such as Goodpasture's disease.

A hallmark of glomerulonephritis is severe injury to the glomerular filtration apparatus such that erythrocytes are lost into Bowman's space and then appear in the urine. Less severe forms of glomerular injury may allow loss of protein but not of cellular elements. If protein loss is massive, the nephrotic syndrome may result.

Other features of glomerulonephritis are a reduction of blood flow through the glomeruli and a reduction in GFR because of compromise of the capillaries by the inflammatory process. If the injury involves only a few glomeruli, the result is generally asymptomatic hematuria and proteinuria. Alternatively, if the injury is diffuse, the nephritic syndrome results. The nephritic syndrome consists of hematuria plus evidence of reduced GFR. Reduced GFR is accompanied by hypertension, edema, azotemia, oliguria, and electrolyte and acid–base disturbances, most commonly metabolic acidosis and hyperkalemia.

When injury to the glomeruli is particularly severe, activated clotting factors enter Bowman's space with resulting deposition of fibrin. The fibrin appears to stimulate a proliferative response from the parietal epithelial cells and infiltrating macrophages. The capsular proliferation may compress the glomerulus or obstruct the opening into the proximal renal tubule. In either case, severe compromise of nephron function is the result.

Some patients present with the clinical and laboratory findings of acute nephritis and suffer a progressive loss of renal function over a matter of weeks. The clinical term *rapidly progressive glomerulonephritis* (RPGN) is then used. Frequently these patients have severe oliguria or even anuria. Electrolyte disturbances, particularly hyperkalemia, may become an urgent problem, and metabolic acidosis may develop as seen in this patient.

In early glomerulonephritis, tubular function may remain relatively unchanged, and the urine and serum biochemical pattern can resemble prerenal causes of azotemia with concentrated, low-sodium urine and an increased serum urea nitrogen/creatinine ratio due to tubular reabsorption of Na^+ and urea. As injury progresses, the urine becomes more isosthenuric (specific gravity of urine similar to that of unmodified glomerular filtrate, 1.010 ± 0.002), and the serum urea nitrogen/creatinine ratio becomes more typical of intrinsic renal disease.

Rapidly progressive glomerulonephritis (RPGN) is a clinical syndrome with many causes. These may be divided into three groups: postinfectious RPGN, RPGN associated with systemic disease, and idiopathic RPGN. The most common form occurring after infection is poststreptococcal. Common systemic diseases associated with RPGN include systemic lupus erythematosus, Wegener's granulomatosis, vasculitis, and Goodpasture's syndrome.[1] The pulmonary findings of linear fluorescence along alveolar basement membranes confirm that this patient had Goodpasture's syndrome. Goodpasture's syndrome is associated with antibodies to a component of the α_3 chain of type IV collagen preferentially expressed in basement membranes of pulmonary alveoli and renal glomeruli.[2,3] This antibody explains the clinical picture of RPGN with associated pulmonary hemorrhage. In both organs there is an acute necrotizing inflammatory lesion resulting in loss of basement membrane integrity with subsequent hemorrhage.

Approximately 50–70% of patients with Goodpasture's syndrome present with pulmonary symptoms. A smaller percentage of patients, as in this case, have initial renal findings. Therapy includes plasmapheresis and immunosuppressive drugs.[4] Despite good responses to plasma exchange, some patients, as in this case, may still eventually require dialysis or transplantation. Transplantation may be delayed until anti-GBM titers have been negative for 6–12 months to reduce the risk of recurrent disease posttransplantation. The diagnosis of Goodpasture's is based on the finding of a linear fluorescent pattern in pulmonary or glomerular basement membrane. The demonstration of antiglomerular basement membrane (anti-GBM) antibodies, present in over 90% of patients in peripheral blood,[5] is generally the initial laboratory test.

The uremic syndrome is the result of extensive loss of nephron function including both glomerular and tubular components. The typical uremic syndrome is generally seen when GFR is less than 20–25% of normal. The cause is inadequate functional renal mass. It may be regarded as loss of the kidney's normal excretory, regulatory, and endocrine functions.

Failure of excretory function results in retention of nitrogenous wastes, most commonly measured as serum urea nitrogen and creatinine concentrations. There is also failure to excrete the daily endogenous acid load with a resulting metabolic acidosis. This acidosis usually results in an elevated anion gap acidosis secondary to diminished NH_3 production; it is reflected in a decreased serum bicarbonate and pH. The patient may exhibit constitutional symptoms and compensatory hyperventilation. Retention of additional, presently uncharacterized wastes probably contributes to gastrointestinal ulceration; abnormal skin coloration and itching; neuromuscular abnormalities ranging from peripheral neuropathy to seizures, stupor, or coma; and episodes of pleuritis and pericarditis. There is also an acquired deficit of platelet function that may give rise to a prolonged bleeding time and may contribute to gastrointestinal hemorrhage.

Regulatory failure is manifested by failure to regulate electrolytes and water, blood pressure, and acid–base status. Inability to concentrate or dilute the urine adequately leads to inability to handle either a salt load or free water load. An increased salt load results in volume expansion with aggravation of hypertension, edema, and possibly congestive heart failure. An increased free water load causes hyponatremia and may contribute to edema and volume overload. Failure to regulate electrolytes may lead to life-threatening hyperkalemia. Inability to concentrate may give rise to hypovolemia with salt and water deprivation. Poor regulation of the renin–angiotensin system, with resulting salt and water retention and hypervolemia, contributes to hypertension, which is common in the uremic syndrome. Hypertension contributes to further renal injury.

Last, failure of important endocrine function also occurs in chronic renal failure with uremia and may help to separate it clinically from acute renal failure. Inadequate secretion of erythropoietin causes a normochromic, normocytic anemia with low reticulocyte count. The uremia may be aggravated by gastrointestinal hemorrhage. Failure of proper synthesis of 1,25-dihydroxyvitamin D and hyperphosphatemia give rise to hypocalcemia with consequent stimulation of parathyroid glands, which ultimately culminates in the complex metabolic bone disease called *renal osteodystrophy* (see Cases 10 and 29). The anatomical features of renal osteodystrophy resemble a combination of osteomalacia and osteitis fibrosa cystica.

In summary, this patient presented with acute nephritis with a rapidly progressive course and associated pulmonary hemorrhage. A renal biopsy showed a crescentic glomerulonephritis but indeterminate immunofluorescent staining. A subsequent lung biopsy revealed linear immunofluorescent staining for immunoglobulins characteristic of Goodpasture's syndrome. Although the patient responded initially to plasma exchange, she ultimately developed end-stage renal disease with uremic syndrome and required hemodialysis; she now awaits renal transplantation.

Additional Reading

JARA, L. J., VERA-LASTRA, O., AND CALLEJA, M. C.: Pulmonary-renal vasculitic disorders: differential diagnosis and management. *Curr. Rheumatol. Rep.* 5:107–15, 2003.

HUDSON, B. G., TRYGGVASON, K., SUNDARAMOORTHY, M., AND NEILSON, E. G.: Alport's syndrome, Goodpasture's syndrome, and Type IV collagen. *N. Eng. J. Med.* 348:2543–56, 2003.

BORZA, D.-B., NEILSON, E. G., AND HUDSON, B. G.: Pathogenesis of Goodpasture syndrome: A molecular perspective. *Semin. Nephology.* 23:522–31, 2003.

WINTERS, J. L., PINEDA, A. A., MCLEOD, B. C., and GRIMA, K. M.: Therapeutic apheresis in renal and metabolic diseases. *J. Clin. Apheresis* 15:53–73, 2000.

SHAH, M. K. and HUGGHINS, S. Y.: Characteristics and outcomes of patients with Goodpasture's syndrome. *South Med. J.* 95:1411–18, 2002.

Case 8

Young Man with Edema and Decreased Urine Output

H. William Schnaper

A 19-year-old man presented to the hospital complaining of swelling of his ankles, abdomen, and eyelids for the past 4 days. He had been in good health until several months ago when he noted a "bloated" sensation after eating. He also thought that he had gained weight recently, noting that his jeans seemed tighter. Four days before presentation, he experienced headaches and mild abdominal pain. At bedtime, there were depressions in his legs from the elastic in his socks. In the morning his legs were less swollen, but his eyes appeared "puffy." These symptoms abated somewhat by evening, but lower extremity swelling recurred. He noticed that his urine appeared a bit darker than usual, and he thought that he might be urinating less frequently. Except for some mild upper respiratory congestion, which he had attributed (along with the initial eye "puffiness") to allergies, he reported no other symptoms. He denied blurred vision, rashes, joint pains, fevers, or grossly bloody urine. The past medical history and the rest of the review of systems were noncontributory.

Physical examination revealed a muscular, well-nourished, 185-lb (84-kg) black male in no acute distress. Temperature was 99°F (37.2°C), heart rate was 78 bpm, respiratory rate was 28/min, and blood pressure was 110/68 mm Hg. There was mild edema of the eyelids. The head, eyes, ears, nose, and throat were all normal. The thyroid was not enlarged. There was a 4-cm span of shifting dullness appreciated on percussion of the posterior thorax. No rales or rhonchi were noted on auscultation of the lungs. Cardiac examination was unremarkable. The abdomen was soft without organomegaly; there was a sense of "fullness" to the abdomen, although no fluid wave could be observed. The genitalia showed mild, nontender scrotal swelling. There was 2–3+ pitting edema two-thirds of the way from the ankle to the knee. The ankles were markedly edematous, with depressions in the edema made by the tops of the patient's shoes. The nailbeds were pale, but edema of the hands was minimal. A chest film was obtained and showed bilateral pleural effusions. There was no evidence of infiltration, consolidation, or pulmonary overcirculation.

Tietz's Applied Laboratory Medicine, Second Edition. Edited by Mitchell G. Scott, Ann M. Gronowski, and Charles S. Eby
Copyright © 2007 John Wiley & Sons, Inc.

The following laboratory studies were obtained:

Analyte	Value, Conventional Units	Reference Interval, Conventional Units	Value, SI Units	Reference Interval, SI Units
Sodium	135 mmol/L	136–145	Same	
Potassium	4.5 mmol/L	3.5–5.0	Same	
Chloride	97 mmol/L	96–106	Same	
CO_2, total	24 mmol/L	24–30	Same	
Urea nitrogen	25 mg/dL	11–23	8.9 mmol urea/L	3.9–8.2
Creatinine	1.0 mg/dL	0.6–1.2	88 μmol/L	53–106
Glucose	87 mg/dL	70–105	4.8 mmol/L	3.9–5.8
Calcium	7.9 mg/dL	8.4–10.2	1.98 mmol/L	2.10–2.54
Protein, total	4.6 g/dL	6.0–8.0	46 g/L	60–80
Albumin	1.2 g/dL	3.5–5.5	12 g/L	35–55
Urate	4.2 mg/dL	1.5–7.0	250 μmol/L	89–416
Cholesterol, total	322 mg/dL	<200	8.34 mmol/L	<5.18
Triglyceride	270 mg/dL	40–150	3.05 mmol/L	0.45–1.69
Urinalysis				
pH	6.0	4.6–8.0	Same	
Specific gravity	1.050	1.001–1.036	Same	
Protein	3+ (confirmed by sulfosalicylic acid precipitation)	Negative		
Glucose	Negative	Negative		
Ketones	Negative	Negative		
Microscopic				
Erythrocytes	0–2/hpf	Rare		
Hyaline casts	1–2/hpf	Rare		
Granular casts	None	None		
Erythrocyte casts	None	None		
Amorphous crystals	None	Rare		
Urine protein: creatinine ratio	5.6			

These data indicated that the patient had urinary protein loss, with decreased serum albumin concentration, peripheral edema, and elevated serum cholesterol concentration. This tetrad of findings defines the nephrotic syndrome. Additional tests were performed to help elucidate the etiology of the nephrosis:

Analyte	Value, Conventional Units	Reference Interval, Conventional Units	Value, SI Units	Reference Interval, SI Units
C3 complement	98 mg/dL	87–150	980 mg/L	870–1500
C4 complement	15 mg/dL	13.8–27.0	150 mg/L	138–270
Antinuclear antibody titer	<1:20	<1:20	2.30 g/L	
Anti-DNA titer	Negative	Negative		
IgM	230 mg/dL	45–145	2.30	0.45–1.45
IgG	320 mg/dL	550–1900	3.20 g/L	5.50–19.00
IgA	127 mg/dL	60–333	1.27 g/L	0.60–3.33
Urine protein	5.3 g/day	100 mg/day		

The absence of values indicating inflammation strongly suggested that the patient did not have an underlying nephritic lesion. Percutaneous renal biopsy was performed, showing moderate glomerular enlargement and mild mesangial expansion with increased extracellular matrix. The tubules and interstitium were unremarkable in appearance. Immunofluorescence microscopy showed trace mesangial staining for IgM but was negative for IgG, IgA, C3, or fibrin. Electron microscopy showed patchy effacement of the glomerular epithelial podocytes but no electron-dense deposits. A diagnosis of early focal segmental glomerulosclerosis (FSGS) was made.

The patient was started on oral prednisone, 80 mg/day. A sodium-restricted diet with mild fluid restriction and treatment with furosemide, 60 mg daily, were instituted. After 3 days, the patient's edema had decreased significantly, although the urine albumin remained 4+. Five weeks after initiating treatment, a urine dipstick reading was 2+ and his urine protein:creatinine ratio was 2.1. His weight was 5 lb (2.3 kg) less than when he was first seen. Prednisone was continued.

Clinical Findings

This patient had a fairly typical presentation of the nephrotic syndrome, a condition that is characterized by significant urinary loss of albumin, hypoproteinemia, peripheral edema, and hypercholesterolemia. The most striking finding in nephrotic patients is the peripheral edema that develops first in areas with insufficient tissue turgor to resist infiltration by extravasated fluid (e.g., eyelids or scrotum). Dependent areas, such as the lower extremities, may also show prominent pitting edema. Edema may have an insidious onset; frequently its manifestations are attributed to nonspecific "fluid retention" (lower extremities) or allergies (eyelid edema) when first noted. Nonspecific complaints that may indicate edema include weight gain, headache, abdominal pain, or malaise. The degree of edema and its extent above the ankle roughly correspond to disease severity, the amount of sodium and water intake, and whether the patient has maintained the extremities in an elevated or a dependent position (illustrated by shifting of the edema between the face and the legs as reported by the patient). Pleural effusion, indicated by shifting dullness on thoracic examination in the present case, and abdominal ascites are frequent findings. Additional physical findings that have been observed include softening of the ear cartilage and horizontal lines (Muehrcke's lines) in the nailbeds.

Nephrotic patients should be evaluated for a skin rash, which would raise the possibility of collagen vascular diseases such as systemic lupus erythematosus, and also for fever, which would suggest that the patient may have either renal inflammation or intercurrent infection. Nephrotic patients are susceptible to bacterial infections, mostly pneumococcal, including otitis, pneumonia, or primary peritonitis (the latter is more common in children). The absence of fever, especially after initiation of corticosteroid treatment, does not rule out infection.

Pathophysiology of Nephrotic Syndrome

It is important to differentiate between the terms *nephrosis* and *nephritis*. Nephrosis is a clinical disorder defined by the following: (1) proteinuria, (2) hypoalbuminemia, (3) peripheral edema, and (4) hyperlipidemia. In contrast, nephritis is a pathologically defined process involving inflammation in the kidney. It is possible (although not the case for the patient described here) that a patient could be nephrotic because of glomerulonephritis that causes significant urinary protein loss. Thus, *nephritis* and *nephrosis* are different, but not mutually exclusive, diagnoses.

The symptoms of nephrosis represent an "appropriate" physiological response to abnormal circumstances within the body. For example, fluid retention and edema result from an alteration in the normal balance of hydrostatic and oncotic forces in the vascular space. Even under normal circumstances, the capillary wall is not watertight. Fluid is extruded from the proximal part of the capillary but is drawn back in by a combination of oncotic pressure and a reduction in the internal hydrostatic pressure along the length of the capillary. By weight, albumin constitutes approximately half of the serum protein mass. However, because it is one of the smaller proteins (MW 68 kD) in the serum, it makes up well over half of the number of macromolecules present in the vascular space and is therefore the major oncotic agent contributing to retaining fluid within the vessel. It is thought that urinary loss of albumin alters the balance of pressure ("Starling forces") maintaining capillary integrity (Fig. 8.1). Extravasated fluid is not reabsorbed, leading to peripheral edema. Because vascular volume is reduced, renal perfusion is decreased. This causes the kidney to produce renin, which induces thirst, activates angiotensin to constrict blood vessels and maintain blood pressure, and finally leads to aldosterone activity that stimulates distal tubular reabsorption of sodium. These physiological responses have the effect of leading to further edema. Thus, fluid retention in nephrosis represents an appropriate physiological response of the kidney rather than a true loss of renal function.[1]

The etiology of FSGS is uncertain. There clearly is a genetic component in idiopathic FSGS, with several single-gene mutations affecting the kidney in Mendelian fashion. The involved genes are often expressed uniquely or primarily in the podocyte, a specialized

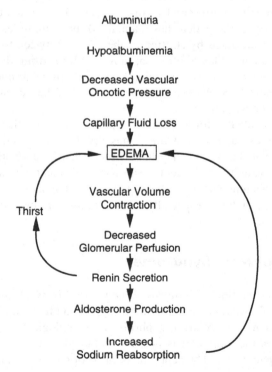

Figure 8.1   Proposed pathogenesis of the nephritic syndrome.

epithelial cell in the renal glomerulus that supports the glomerular capillary and itself builds the final barrier to macromolecular passage through the glomerulus. The proteins expressed by these genes include the transcription factor WT-1; proteins that contribute to the stability of the structures in the glomerular filtration barrier such as podocin (encoded by *NPHS2*), CD2-associated protein (encoded by *CD2AP*) and α-actinin-4 (encoded by *ACTN4*); genes that regulate renal development, such as Pax-2 (encoded by *PAX2*); and mitochondrial proteins.

FSGS may also occur in response to adaptive changes by the kidney that cause hypertrophy, resulting in an increase in per nephron workload. Such adaptations occur after a reduction in renal mass, or in the setting of sickle cell anemia or obesity. This "postadaptive" form of FSGS[1] often is associated with glomerular enlargement (glomerulomegaly).

Differential Diagnosis

Hypoalbuminemia may on rare occasions result from congenital analbuminemia, an inherited defect. However, this disorder seldom causes edema. Patients with acquired hypoalbuminemia have either decreased synthesis, as would be seen in malnutrition or severe hepatic failure, or increased losses. Massive losses most often occur through the gut or the kidney. Thus, in order to confirm a diagnosis of nephrotic syndrome in a patient who has edema, it is essential to establish the presence of proteinuria. If the patient is voiding infrequently because of renal effects of decreased intravascular volume, confirmation of proteinuria may be difficult. It is not unusual for nephrotic patients to go more than 24 hours without voiding, even when normal or near-normal serum urea nitrogen and creatinine concentrations suggest a normal glomerular filtration rate.

The diseases causing nephrosis can be divided into those that are systemic and those that affect mainly the kidney. Systemic diseases include urologic disorders, cancer (the kidneys may be affected by circulating immune complexes), congestive heart failure, and systemic inflammatory diseases such as systemic lupus erythematosus and Henoch–Schönlein purpura. Immunity-mediated diseases of the kidney that cause nephrotic syndrome include membranoproliferative glomerulonephritis (MPGN), membranous nephropathy, or chronic immune complex glomerulonephritis. Another group of idiopathic renal diseases causing nephrosis is not accompanied by inflammatory changes and may thus be considered as examples of "primary" nephrotic syndrome. These include minimal change disease, mild mesangial proliferation, and FSGS.

Selection and Interpretation of Laboratory Results

Laboratory tests in nephrotic patients have four purposes: to establish the clinical syndrome, to evaluate renal function, to define the underlying etiological process as well as possible, and to monitor the effects of therapy. In the present case, the protein loss proved to be urinary, as indicated by the positive urine "dipstick" test that was confirmed by the turbidemetric sulfosalicylic acid test. The amount of proteinuria in glomerular disease (including both nephrosis and nephritis) represents the filtered load from the glomerulus minus the protein reabsorbed by the renal tubule. It is usually fairly constant throughout the day and is thus called "fixed" proteinuria. In contrast, the absolute amount of protein excreted in other conditions may vary throughout the day. Since protein determination by dipstick reflects concentration and is affected by urine volume (e.g., results will be lower with effective diuretic therapy), proteinuria is more accurately evaluated by measurements of protein on a timed (12- or 24-hour) urine collection. A quick test that provides a rough estimate of absolute proteinuria per unit time is the urine protein:creatinine ratio. Healthy adults excrete about 1 g/m^2 per day of creatinine (exact amount depends on muscle mass), so the protein:creatinine ratio approximates 24-hour urine protein excretion in grams. To rule out postural proteinuria, the patient should remain supine during the collection period or the spot urine for protein:creatinine should be obtained from the first void after rising in the morning.

The other findings required for a diagnosis of nephrotic syndrome are low serum albumin and hyperlipidemia. Although findings vary from patient to patient, edema usually becomes apparent when the serum albumin concentration drops to around 2 g/dL (20 g/L). Depending on the glomerular filtration rate and the degree of protein loss, the serum albumin may even drop below 1 g/dL (10 g/L). When such low concentrations are reached, the amount of albuminuria may decrease because of the lower filtered load. The causes for the elevated plasma cholesterol and triglycerides include increased hepatic synthesis of lipoproteins, abnormal lipid transport, and abnormalities in function of lipolytic enzymes.[2] Lipiduria may lead to the presence of oval fat bodies in the urine.

Decreased renal function in nephrotic patients at initial presentation, as indicated by high serum creatinine and serum urea nitrogen, usually suggests the presence of nephritis or other renal disease. Renal failure is indicated by increased serum urea nitrogen and serum creatinine concentrations and may be accompanied by hyperkalemia, hypertension, and fluid overload culminating in congestive heart failure. Urine output is not a reliable sign of renal failure, since decreased urine volume usually results from the physiological response to hypoalbuminemia. Because of their apparently volume-contracted state, patients with nephrotic syndrome may increase tubular reabsorption of urea and exhibit mild to moderate increases in serum urea nitrogen concentrations without concomitant increases in creatinine (which is not reabsorbed). Rarely, intrarenal edema and low renal blood flow rates may cause a marked decrease in glomerular filtration.[3] This decrease is difficult to differentiate from acute renal failure and is a diagnosis that should be reached only by exclusion of other possibilities such as bilateral renal vein thrombosis or the presence of nephritis.

Once the diagnosis of nephrotic syndrome is established and the patient is stable, it is important to determine whether there is any evidence for inflammatory renal disease. Although a few erythrocytes may be seen in the urine in primary forms of nephrotic syndrome, and can be a sign of renal vein thrombosis, gross hematuria or cylindruria (presence of granular or erythrocyte casts) strongly suggests the presence of nephritis. The urine specific gravity should be high, reflecting both the patient's volume-contracted state and high urine protein concentration. Relatively low specific gravity (1.010–1.020) should raise concern about urine concentrating ability and the possibility of renal tubular disease. The type of protein found in the urine is also of potential interest. In primary nephrotic syndrome, proteinuria is relatively "selective", with loss mostly of albumin. In patients with nephritic lesions, the larger molecules in the globulin fraction of serum proteins are lost as well. Thus, low serum globulins (IgG in particular), is also suggestive of a nephritic lesion.

Antinuclear antibody and anti-DNA antibody titers are obtained to screen for collagen vascular disease, usually lupus. Low serum C4 concentrations reflect activation of the classical complement pathway, and C3 is decreased when either the classical or alternative pathway is activated. Such activation is most common in lupus or membranoproliferative glomerulonephritis. Complement is also consumed in acute glomerulonephritis, which only infrequently causes nephrotic syndrome. In children age 1.5–10, minimal change nephropathy is so likely to be the cause of nephrosis that patients with no laboratory or clinical evidence supporting an alternative diagnosis are usually given a therapeutic trial of corticosteroid therapy.[4] In older children and adults, a renal biopsy is performed to determine the diagnosis and to indicate appropriate therapeutic measures. In the present case, the mesangial expansion and glomerulomegaly along with extracellular matrix accumulation in the absence of evidence for renal inflammation or scarring, strongly support the diagnosis of FSGS. This lesion is the primary cause of acquired chronic kidney disease in children[5] and has been increasing in incidence in both children and adults.[6,7] In 2004 a new diagnostic classification was proposed for various histological subtypes of FSGS.[8]

Treatment

FSGS presents a challenging treatment problem. A significant percentage of patients progress to renal failure over a period of one to many years. The main determinant of whether patients are likely to experience chronic deterioration of renal function is response to therapy by a complete (full cessation of proteinuria) or partial (at least 50% decrease in proteinuria) response.[1] Initial treatment is usually oral prednisone at a daily dose of 2 mg/kg or 60 mg/m^2 (maximum 80–100 mg). Corticosteroids have significant side effects, including truncal obesity, acne, hirsutism, bone demineralization, and increased gastric acid secretion leading to hyperphagia and peptic ulceration. Pediatric patients who do not respond are given a trial of either oral cyclosporine; or high-dose, intravenous methylprednisolone boluses (500 mg/m^2) with an oral alkylating agent such as cyclophosphamide or chlorambucil for up to 12 weeks. Both of these treatments are more immunosuppressive than oral prednisone and have more significant toxic effects. Adults may require months to enter remission after starting oral prednisone,[9] so this treatment is continued for a much more extended duration than in children, where an often more aggressive disease course indicates a more aggressive approach to find an effective treatment. Many internists prefer alternative treatments such as prednisone for adults as well.

An important part of the management of FSGS is genetic testing, which is now commercially available for mutations of *NPHS2* and *WT1*. *NPHS2* mutations are felt by some, although not all, authorities to be treatment-resistant.[10] Thus, identification of relevant mutations may suggest alternative approaches to management that might avoid unnecessary toxicity. *WT1* mutations can also be associated with sexual reversal phenotypes or genotype abnormalities that require further evaluation.[11]

Over time, proteinuria and serum creatinine levels must be followed to ascertain disease control and to monitor progression to renal failure. An ominous sign of progression is tubulointerstitial involvement, which may be suggested by consistently low urine-specific gravities and is confirmed by biopsy. It is generally believed that intraglomerular hypertension may contribute to disease progression. Particularly in patients such as the present one with glomerulomegaly on biopsy, an angiotensin converting enzyme inhibitor or angiotensin receptor blocker is given as adjunctive therapy.

Symptomatic treatment for nephrotic patients includes restriction of sodium and water intake. Bed rest or other means of elevating the lower extremities may help mobilize pedal edema. There are two indications for pharmacological diuresis. In patients with massive ascites or acute respiratory distress from pleural effusions, intravenous infusion of albumin and furosemide to force diuresis of edema fluid is of some benefit. In patients with steroid-unresponsive disease, oral diuretics may help decrease fluid retention. However, since the kidneys are responding to a perceived volume-depleted state, diuretics are often less effective than they would be in a patient without nephrosis. As is always the case with diuretic therapy, attention should be given to ensuring that the patient is not overly diuresed nor become hypokalemic.

Helpful Notes

All the findings and problems associated with nephrosis can best be understood when viewed as a consequence of protein loss. Thus, it is important to consider the pathophysiological mechanism of nephrotic syndrome in evaluating the patient. For example, the symptomatic treatments suggested above reflect the need to deplete fluid from the tissue space rather than from the vascular space. Trace minerals that are protein bound (e.g., zinc) may be depleted because of albuminuria. Loss of other proteins may cause alterations in laboratory values, such as the decreased serum calcium concentration that reflects loss of albumin as a binding protein and the decreased serum total thyroxine that reflects loss of thyroxine-binding globulin. These changes are seldom of physiological consequence since ionized calcium concentrations and free thyroxine should be normal. However, vitamin D binding protein is lost in the urine, so 25-OH vitamin D_3 and 1,25-$(OH)_2$ vitamin D_3 levels may be low[12] and contribute to decreased bone density.[13] Further, infants with congenital nephrotic syndrome may have significant hypothyroidism. Urinary loss of naturally occurring, circulating anticoagulants may contribute to a relatively high incidence of thrombotic events in nephrotic patients.

Changes may also occur in concentrations of drugs, such as digoxin, that are bound mostly to circulating proteins; these measurements must be interpreted with care in nephrotic patients.

References

1. SCHNAPER, H. W., ROBSON, A. M. AND KOPP, J. B.: Nephrotic syndrome: Minimal change nephropathy, focal segmental glomerulosclerosis and collapsing glomerulopathy. In *Diseases of the Kidney and Urinary Tract*, 8th ed., R. W. SCHRIER, ed., Lippincott, Williams & Wilkins, Philadelphia, 2007, pp. 1585–1672.

2. KAYSEN, G. A.: Hyperlipidemia in the nephrotic syndrome. *Am. J. Kidney Dis.* 12:548–51, 1988.

3. LOWENSTEIN, J., SCHACHT, R. G., AND BALDWIN, D. S.: Renal failure in minimal change nephrotic syndrome. *Am. J. Med.* 70:227–33, 1981.

4. International Study of Kidney Disease in Children: The primary nephrotic syndrome in children. Identification of patients with minimal change nephrotic syndrome from initial response to prednisone. *J. Pediatr.* 98:561–4, 1981.

5. U. S. Renal Data System: *2004 Annual Data Report: Atlas of End-Stage Renal Disease in the United States.* National Institutes of Health, National Institute of Diabetes and Digestive and Kidney Diseases, Department of Health and Human Services, Bethesda, MD, 2004.

6. BONILLA-FELIX, M., PARRA, C., DAJANI, T., FERRIS, M. ET AL.: Changing patterns in the histopathology of idiopathic nephrotic syndrome in children. *Kidney Int.* 55:1885–90, 1999.

7. HAAS, M., SPARGO, B. H., AND COVENTRY, S.: Increasing incidence of focal-segmental glomerulosclerosis among adult nephropathies: A 20-year renal biopsy study. *Am. J. Kidney Dis.* 26:740–50, 1995.

8. D'AGATI, V. D., FOGO, A. B., BRUIJN, J. A., AND JENNETTE, J. C.: Pathologic classification of focal segmental glomerulosclerosis: A working proposal. *Am. J. Kidney Dis.* 43:368–82, 2004.

9. RYDEL, J. J., KORBET, S. M., BOROK, R. Z., AND SCHWARTZ, M. M.: Focal segmental glomerulosclerosis in adults: Presentation, course and response to treatment. *Am. J. Kidney Dis.* 25:534–42, 1995.

10. RUF, R. G., LICHTENBERGER, A., KARLE, S. M., HAAS, J. P. ET AL.: Patients with mutations in NPHS2 (podocin) do not respond to standard steroid treatment of nephrotic syndrome. *J. Am. Soc. Nephrol.* 15:722–32, 2004.

11. SAYLAM, K. AND SIMON, P.: WT1 gene mutation responsible for male sex reversal and renal failure: The Frasier syndrome. *Eur. J. Obstet. Gynecol. Reprod. Biol. 110*:111–13, 2003.

12. GRYMONPREZ, A., PROESMANS, W., VAN DYCK, M., JANS, I. ET AL.: Vitamin D metabolites in childhood nephrotic syndrome. *Pediatr. Nephrol. 9*:278–81, 1995.

13. LEONARD, M. B., FELDMAN, H. I., SHULTS, J., ZEMEL, B. S. ET AL.: Long-term, high-dose glucocorticoids and bone mineral content in childhood glucocorticoid-sensitive nephrotic syndrome. *N. Engl. J. Med. 351*:868–75, 2004.

Case 9

A New Doctor for a Man with Diabetes and Hypertension

Michael E. Hull

A recently retired 65-year-old African-American man with a 10-year history of type 2 diabetes mellitus (DM) moved to a new city to be near his grandchildren. He presented to his new primary care physician's office for routine evaluation. Over the preceding 12 months he had been making efforts to increase his physical activity with a daily 30-minute brisk walk. He had received extensive instruction regarding an optimal diet for diabetes, but he admitted to frequent indiscretions. He produced a diary of his self-monitored whole-blood glucose values that was incomplete, and indicated sporadically inadequate control, with most fasting values in the 100–125 mg/dL range, but some above 160 mg/dL. His prior medical records indicated a history of microalbuminuria of 100 mg/day on several occasions.

In addition to diabetes, other medical issues included chronic hypertension and gastroesophageal reflux disease. His daily medications were insulin, hydrochlorothiazide, enalapril, aspirin, and omeprazole. He was a nonsmoker. His mother had a history of chronic hypertension and died at age 71 of complications of end-stage renal disease and congestive heart failure.

The patient's vital signs showed a temperature of 36.8°C, blood pressure of 148/86 mm Hg, heart rate of 72/min, and respiratory rate of 12/min. He weighed 97 kg and was 185 cm tall, with a body mass index of 28.3 kg/m^2.

The patient had a generally healthy appearance. Of note on physical examination were fundoscopic findings of macular edema and focal dot–blot hemorrhages. Laboratory values obtained at the office visit were as follows:

Analyte	Value, Conventional Units	Reference Interval, Conventional Units	Value, SI Units	Reference Interval, SI Units
HA1c	9.7%	4.6–6.2	Same	Same
Sodium	141 mmol/L	136–145	Same	Same
Potassium	4.5 mmol/L	4.0–4.9	Same	Same
Chloride	108 mmol/L	98–108	Same	Same

Tietz's Applied Laboratory Medicine, Second Edition. Edited by Mitchell G. Scott, Ann M. Gronowski, and Charles S. Eby
Copyright © 2007 John Wiley & Sons, Inc.

Analyte	Value, Conventional Units	Reference Interval, Conventional Units	Value, SI Units	Reference Interval, SI Units
Carbon dioxide	24 mmol/L	23–31	Same	Same
Urea nitrogen	25 mg/dL	8–25	8.9 mmol/L	2.9–8.9
Creatinine	1.4 mg/dL	0.8–1.4	124 μmol/L	71–124
Glucose	187 mg/dL	70–110	10.3 mmol/L	3.9–6.1
Calcium	8.4 mg/dL	8.6–10.3	2.10 mmol/L	2.15–2.58
Alanine transaminase	33 IU/L	13–40	0.55 μkat/L	0.22–0.67
Aspartate transaminase	28 IU/L	19–48	0.47 μkat/L	0.32–0.80
Alkaline phophatase	75 IU/L	38–126	1.78 μkat/L	0.9–1.98
Bilirubin	1.0 mg/dL	0.2–1.1	15 μmol/L	3–19
Albumin	4.7 g/dL	3.6–5.0	47 g/L	36–50
Hb	14 g/dL	14–18	140 g/L	140–180
Hct	41%	40–50	0.41	0.40–0.50
Platelets	$352 \times 10^2/\mu l$	150–450	$352 \times 10^9/L$	150–450
Urinalysis				
Specific gravity	1.020			
pH	6			
Protein	2+	Negative		
Nitrite	Negative	Negative		
Leukocyte esterase	Negative	Negative		
Glucose	Negative	Negative		
Ketones	Negative	Negative		
Urine microscopy				
RBC	5/hpf	Negative		
WBC	0/hpf	Few		
No bacteria or yeast;				
No casts				

The physician diagnosed mild, nonproliferative diabetic retinopathy and mild chronic renal disease secondary to diabetes mellitus and hypertension. She was interested in quantifying the current renal dysfunction and stratifying the patient's risk for future end-stage renal disease. Incorporating knowledge of the patient's plasma creatinine, age, and African-American race, she estimated a glomerular filtration rate (GFR) of 65 mL/min per 1.73 m^2 using the Modification of Diet in Renal Disease study (MDRD) equation [see Eq. (9.3)] that she had recently read about. She used the "GFR calculator" on the National Kidney Foundation Website to perform the calculation. She also ordered a 24-hour urine protein determination and started the patient on a low-salt, low-protein diet. The urine protein determination was 1.0 g/24 hours; normal was 0–150 mg/24 hours.

Definition of Chronic Kidney Disease

Chronic kidney disease (CKD; also *chronic renal failure* or *chronic renal insufficiency*) is broadly defined as a decrease in renal function that precedes end-stage renal disease (ESRD). ESRD is a diagnosis that implies dependence on renal replacement therapy in the form of either dialysis or transplantation. The pathophysiology of the disorder is related to the irreversible loss of nephron units caused by a wide array of insults, with diabetes and hypertension as the most common etiologies in Western, industrialized countries. Others include immune-complex-mediated disease, infectious nephropathies, and heritable renal disease. The detailed mechanisms by which nephrons are irreversibly damaged are beyond the scope of this discussion.

Each kidney contains approximately one million nephrons whose function is to filter and excrete wastes and to regulate water, acid–base, and electrolyte homeostasis. Daily, the adult kidneys must perform this task on an average of 170–200 L of blood that arrives via the renal arteries. As nephrons are lost, the capacity to regulate electrolytes and acid–base balance is progressively impaired. Clinically observable renal dysfunction occurs when the number of healthy nephrons decreases by ~50–60%. Some compensation for these defects occurs in the early stages of disease through hyperfiltration effected by hypertrophy of the remaining nephrons and through increases in glomerular capillary pressure and flow, both mediated by vasoactive molecules, cytokines, and growth factors. Eventually, however, these mechanisms fail and the descent to ESRD begins. ESRD is also referred to by the clinical term *uremia*, the culmination of progressive electrolyte and nitrogenous waste imbalances. This leads to a variety of cardiac, musculoskeletal, dermatologic, psychiatric, and neurologic sequelae, collectively referred to as the *uremic syndrome*. In the case outlined above, the physician has identified a patient who is likely in the early stages of renal failure, based on the findings of proteinuria and a decreased estimated GFR. An emerging area of very high interest in nephrology is early identification of patients such as this one, who are showing only minimal laboratory and clinical evidence of renal dysfunction. Ultimately, it would be desirable to halt or delay the progression of early renal failure with more aggressive treatment of the underlying etiology with dietary and pharmacological interventions.

Chemistry and Hematologic Abnormalities in Chronic Kidney Disease

In contrast to acute renal failure (see Case 5), in which physical signs and symptoms related to fluid overload can be obvious, CKD develops insidiously and laboratory methods are essential for identifying the process so that interventions to arrest the decline in function can be made before frank uremia develops. The earliest change observable in the laboratory is usually urinary protein excretion. Increased serum creatinine and urea appear somewhat later, but can likely be detected in preclinical CKD in some cases. Because serum creatinine values are dependent on factors such as sex, age, and race, equations such as the MDRD equation have been proposed to estimate GFR when changes in creatinine values may not seem significant. Electrolyte abnormalities, acidosis, and hematological abnormalities such as anemia are almost never the initial findings of CKD in patients who are receiving adequate routine care by physicians.

Proteinuria

Normally, little albumin (66 kDa) and almost no proteins larger than albumin should pass the selectively permeable glomerular barrier. Smaller proteins may gain passage into the tubules, but the total protein excretion is less than 150 mg/day in health. Active reabsorption and catabolism of filtered low-molecular-weight proteins in the proximal tubules normally keeps frank proteinuria from developing. An example of a low-molecular-weight protein that is fully filtered but reabsorbed and catabolized is the cysteine protease cystatin C. Incidentally, measurement of serum cystatin C has been proposed as an alternative to creatinine as a means to estimate GFR, but interpretation of these values also requires incorporation of some demographic and nonlaboratory clinical variables. The presence of heavy proteinuria (>1000 mg/day) indicates a disruption of the glomerular barrier, but levels of greater than 300 mg/day are considered to indicate early pathology. In CKD, damage to the remaining nephrons results in impairment of both glomerular and tubular function. An increase in urinary excretion of proteins of all sizes follows. In particular, an increase in albumin excretion to 30–300 mg/day, termed *microalbuminuria*, is predictive of eventual overt nephropathy in diabetics if documented on two separate occasions, as in this case. This may occur years before excretion of albumin exceeds 1 g/day, so it has become routine to uncover this laboratory finding in diabetics in order to predict future renal function at a time when effective dietary and medical interventions will be beneficial.

Azotemia

Elevations in blood urea nitrogen (BUN) and creatinine concentrations occur as the number of functional nephrons decreases. With fewer nephrons, the capacity for filtration of these renally cleared substances declines. In addition, some reabsorption of BUN occurs in the renal tubules, which can result in a faster increase in BUN to variable degrees, depending on the underlying process responsible for the renal insufficiency. With major caveats that will be discussed below, azotemia can be followed as a measure of GFR as there is an inverse relation between GFR and plasma creatinine and urea concentrations.

Electrolyte Abnormalities

Greater than 70% of filtered sodium is reabsorbed in the proximal tubule by the action of an energy dependent Na^+-K^+ transporter. It is an osmotically and charge-neutral process, such that as sodium is absorbed, anions (mainly chloride) and water passively follow. In the ascending loop of Henle, active transport via the $Na^+-K^+-2Cl^-$ cotransporter results in reabsorption of about 25% of the filtered load of sodium. Further reabsorption in the distal tubule and collecting ducts maintains an overall balance of sodium excretion with ingestion. Distal reabsorption of sodium is increased by the action of the renin–angiotensin–aldosterone axis, while water retention at the collecting ducts is effected by increases in antidiuretic hormone (ADH).

Total body sodium and water content are generally increased in patients with moderate to severe chronic renal disease due to an overwhelming salt and water load imposed on the kidneys. In early CKD the effective loss of nephrons is initially offset by hyperfiltration and nephron hypertrophy. Eventually, water and sodium begin to be cleared at a lower rate. When this happens, remaining healthy nephrons face a threshold for the amount of sodium that they can handle. Sodium and water are retained approximately equally, so normonatremia is the rule. In the case presented above, the mild edema shown in the patient's lower extremities may be a result of his early CKD, but severe electrolyte abnormalities are seldom seen prior to moderate to severe renal disease.

Potassium excretion, likewise, is impaired in the setting of CKD and as the disease progresses, failure to manage this can result in dangerous cardiac arrhythmias due to acute hyperkalemia. Hyporeninemic hypoaldosteronism (especially characteristic of diabetic nephropathy), angiotensin-converting enzyme (ACE) inhibitor administration, or both, can further complicate this picture.[1]

Calcium and phosphate derangements develop in CKD by multiple and complex mechanisms. Phosphate retention begins early in CKD due to a decrease in filtered and excreted phosphate. This brings about the development of hyperparathyroidism by feedback mechanisms that are peripheral to this discussion (see Case 31). High levels of urinary phosphate also suppress renal hydroxylation of 25-hydroxyvitamin D, decreasing plasma levels of calcitriol, a principal enhancer of calcium absorption from the gastrointestinal tract. Thus, the classic hypocalcemia of CKD develops. In response to low calcium, hyperparathyroidism develops and can lead to dramatic bony changes due to the action of parathyroid hormone on osteoclasts directed toward increasing plasma calcium, (see Cases 10 and 29). This renal osteodystrophy will occur in unchecked hyperparathyroidism of renal disease, but is rarely seen in settings where aggressive electrolyte correction is pursued.

Acidosis

This becomes an important sequela of CKD in its later stages. Tubular damage can result in a reduced ability to secrete ammonium, which is a key mechanism that prevents hydrogen ions from being reabsorbed. The result is a metabolic acidosis manifested by a decrease in plasma carbon dioxide and an elevated anion gap. Again, in patients with CKD due to diabetes, hyporeninemic hyperaldosteronism is common, and in such cases, the acidosis is accompanied by hyperkalemia and hyperchloremia.

Anemia

As a result of decreased in output of erythropoietin, a renally produced hormone responsible for erythropoiesis, a normocytic, normochromic anemia develops in later stages of CKD.

Diagnosis of CKD

Diagnosis of CKD is often preceded by the recognition of other disease entities that place the patient at risk. In the case of hypertension and diabetes, the development of renal failure is one of many risks that mandate regular follow-up with primary care physicians. As noted above, microalbuminuria may be observed for years, alerting physicians to the possibility of future renal failure. When patients exhibit frank albuminuria (≥ 1 g/day), this provides conclusive evidence of some degree of early renal damage. It is felt that this level of proteinuria is reached 10–15 years after the onset of diabetes at a point when the serum creatinine concentrations may still not reflect markedly impaired filtration, as observed in the current patient.[2]

Estimation of GFR

Determining GFR is done by measuring a substance in both blood and urine that has the following properties: produced at a constant rate in the body, completely filtered at the glomerulus (i.e., is of low molecular weight), excreted only by the kidneys, and not reabsorbed or secreted by the renal tubules. Alternatively, an exogenous substance that exhibits these properties can be measured in the blood and urine after administration of a known amount. The classic exogenous "gold standard" for determining GFR was inulin, but this has been replaced by measuring the clearance of more readily available substances such as the contrast agent iohexol or ^{125}I-*iothalamate*. Since none of the gold standard methods are practical or economical for routine purposes, the surrogate for GFR in clinical practice has been the clearance of creatinine. Clearance of an analyte, x, is defined as follows:

$$C_x = \frac{U_x * U_{vol}}{P_x * t} \qquad (9.1)$$

where C is clearance, U_x is the concentration of x in urine, U_{vol} is the volume of urine, P_x is the concentration of x in plasma, and t is the time of urine collection. When x is an ideal analyte, such as inulin or ^{125}I-iothalamate, C_x = GFR.

While creatinine clearance has been considered an adequate estimate of GFR, it is flawed because it is not an ideal analyte according to the criteria listed above. Specifically, proximal tubular secretion of creatinine through an organic cation pathway occurs. This secretion of creatinine will result in falsely elevated values for creatinine clearance, especially in the setting of markedly decreased GFR. In addition, plasma or serum creatinine can vary considerably as a result of clinical and demographic variables. Higher muscle mass and male sex are associated with higher plasma creatinine levels. Dietary intake of protein can also lead to variability in plasma creatinine levels among patients with equivalent renal function. Even the inverse relationship between GFR and plasma creatinine is not straightforward. GFR must fall to approximately 60% of its normal value before a rise in creatinine above most adult reference intervals may be detected.[3] These variations complicate the interpretation of GFR estimates made from plasma and urine creatinine measurements using Equation (9.1). A further drawback to analyzing urine to determine the clearance of any substance is that urine must be collected over a defined period, usually 24 hours. This is cumbersome and is fraught with errors of over- or undercollection that raise questions about the usefulness of the results.

In order to overcome these potential pitfalls, mathematical estimations, including the Cockcroft–Gault (CG) equation, were developed to estimate GFR from only the serum or plasma creatinine concentrations:

Cockcroft–Gault equation

$$C_{creat} = \frac{(140 - age) * (weight,\ kg)}{72 * P_{creat,\ mg/dL}} \qquad (9.2)$$

If female, multiply C by 0.85 (units mL/min). This equation was validated against 24-hour creatinine clearance values, not against a gold standard method, so it is not truly a GFR estimate, but rather an estimated 24-hour creatinine clearance.[4] However, it is often treated in clinical practice as a GFR estimate and compared with other estimates of GFR such as the MDRD equation, which were validated against gold standard GFR measurements (e.g., ^{125}I-iothalamate clearance). A benefit of the CG equation is that it limits the required laboratory data to plasma creatinine, while making adjustments for demographics and body mass. Continual reassessment of the performance of this and other formulae used to estimate GFR resulted in the development of the MDRD equation in 1999.

MDRD Equation for GFR

The Modification of Diet in Renal Disease Study (MDRD) was a randomized, multicenter clinical trial that followed the effects of three different amounts of dietary protein and phosphorus intake and two different doses of blood pressure control on the rate of loss of kidney function in persons with various chronic kidney diseases. All patients in this study had GFR determined by ^{125}I-iothalamate clearance to monitor their renal function.[5] Within this study, new equations for GFR were developed from a large randomized training set ($n = 1628$) using the patients' laboratory and demographic data and their measured GFRs. Important excluded groups in this study to note were type 1 diabetics, type 2 diabetics taking insulin, and patients with normal renal function. Several equations using demographic and laboratory values such as creatinine, urea nitrogen, and albumin were developed and validated against actual GFR in a different set of patients in the study.[6] The most widely used MDRD equation to emerge from this effort, referred to as the "abbreviated MDRD," and the equation that this patient's physician used to estimate his GFR, is as follows:

MDRD, abbreviated

$$GTR = 186 * (P_{Cr})^{-1.154} * (age)^{-0.203} \tag{9.3}$$

If black, multiply GFR by 1.210; if female, multiply GFR by 0.742 (units mL min^{-1} 1.73 m^{-2}).

The MDRD equation differs from the Cockcroft–Gault equation in several ways. The MDRD equation does not require a weight variable because it normalizes the GFR for a standard body surface area of 1.73 m^2 and factors in racial differences between Caucasian and African-Americans. The utility of this equation and its good correlation with actual GFRs below 60 mL/min has been validated in numerous studies. In 2002, the National Kidney Foundation (NKF) and the National Kidney Disease Education Program (NKDEP) recommended that all creatinine values reported by clinical laboratories be accompanied by an estimated GFR calculated using the MDRD equation.[7] According to these guidelines, such population screening would allow earlier detection of chronic kidney disease.

Screening Utility of MDRD Equation

It is hoped that the power of the MDRD equation or any other estimate of GFR will be in earlier identification of renal disease. Because of the morbidity associated with the development of CKD and the relative irreversibility of the process once it has progressed to ESRD, there is an impetus to identify asymptomatic patients that may not be identified by routine serum creatinine values. For this reason, the MDRD equation has been put forward as a means to identify asymptomatic patients with risk factors for the development of renal disease at the beginning of the downward trend of their GFR. Studies have indicated that such early intervention may be effective in delaying the progression of CKD.[5]

A staging system based on the demonstration of renal damage and stratified by GFR has been developed (Table 9.1). Identification of stage 1 or stage 2 chronic renal disease in

Table 9.1 GFR Staging

Stage	Clinical disease manifestations	GFR (mL min^{-1} 1.73 m^{-2})
1	Kidney damage without decreased GFR Possible microalbuminuria	≥ 90
2	Kidney damage with mildly decreased GFR Microalbuminuria to frank proteinuria	60–89
3	Moderately decreased GFR Frank proteinuria, electrolyte abnormalities, anemia	30–59
4	Severely decreased GFR Progression of stage 3 manifestations	15–29
5	ESRD Uremic syndrome, dialysis requirement	<15

patients with minimal symptoms is the driving force behind the search for more accurate formulas for estimating GFR. As stated earlier, the serum creatinine will not change significantly in stages 1 and 2. A reasonable assumption has been made that treating underlying disease processes more aggressively in these patients may slow the progression to higher stages and to ESRD.[7]

The utility of the MDRD equation for such an application has been debated for several reasons:

1. None of the equations developed from the MDRD have been validated in normal individuals because such patients were excluded from the study by design. Comparison of the MDRD equation performance in normals and patients with mild chronic kidney disease has shown considerable underestimation of GFR in normals,[8] which would translate into false-positive diagnoses of early renal dysfunction if applied to a wide, asymptomatic population.

2. The equations perform optimally in patients with true GFRs of less than 60. Therefore, the utility of the equation in the target population for screening (i.e., stages 1 and 2 chronic renal disease) may be limited. Indeed, current NKF recommendations now suggest any estimated GFR value >60 mL min^{-1} 1.73 m^{-2} be reported as ">60" and not as an exact GFR value.[10]

3. The exclusion of a large segment of the diabetic population in the MDRD raises issues about the generalization of the equations to that group, which comprises a high percentage of the population with CKD. Finally, from the laboratory perspective there is considerable variability in creatinine methods that may affect the estimated GFR value.[11,12]

As noted above, the MDRD equation is most reliable in its estimation of GFR when actual GFR is less than 60 mL min^{-1} 1.73 m^{-2}. However, in mid- to late-stage chronic renal disease, clinical and laboratory findings are rarely subtle, and decisions about when to begin renal replacement therapy are usually not based on the GFR, but rather on the presence of intractable volume overload, hyperkalemia, or uremic complications such as encephalopathy. Therefore, the full value of estimating GFR may be debatable in patients in mid- to late-stage renal failure.

Creatinine Assays

Any discussion of the suitability of GFR estimates must take into account the variability in creatinine assays. Variability between creatinine methods has several causes. The Jaffe assay based on the alkaline picrate reaction is the most commonly used method for determining creatinine. Creatinine reacts with the picrate ion in an alkaline medium to give an orange-red complex. But since the Jaffe reaction is not specific for creatinine, other Jaffe complexes ("noncreatine chromagens") can be produced by the reaction of picrate with other compounds in plasma, such as glucose, ketone bodies, and serum proteins. Current Jaffe creatinine assays are based on kinetic measurement of the formed chromagens that are able to more specifically measure creatinine, but their values are still elevated slightly by noncreatinine chromagens, mainly serum proteins. A "compensated" Jaffe assay based on kinetic measurements is one that is calibrated to read $\sim$0.2 mg/dL lower to account for the nonspecific contribution of serum proteins. The assay used in the MDRD study was an "uncompensated" Beckman Rate Jaffe/CX3 Synchron assay based on the kinetic alkaline picrate reaction. Other, more specific assays for creatinine include enzymatic and HPLC methods that will produce values $\sim$0.2–0.3 mg/dL lower than Jaffe methods. These are not as commonly used as the Jaffe methods, even though they are more specific. It should be clear that assays not calibrated to match the assay used to develop the MDRD study or any non-Jaffe creatinine assay will give higher results for estimated GFR by the MDRD equation. For example, using plasma creatinine values obtained from a compensated Jaffe assay in the MDRD equation will result in an overestimation of GFR. In this situation, up to 50% overestimation of the GFR has been observed in individuals with serum creatinine values less than 1.75 mg/dL (155 μmol/L).[11] Recently, the impact of these calibration variations was investigated using the range of calibration differences observed between clinical laboratories in the 1994 College of American Pathologists (CAP) survey. It was shown that calibration differences result in much more error in GFR estimation at GFRs greater than 60 mL min^{-1} 1.73 m^{-2} than at GFRs below that threshold.[12] This is consistent with the recommendation to report estimated GFRs over 60 mL min^{-1} 1.73 m^{-2} as simply ">60 mL min^{-1} 1.73 m^{-2}," but it also makes it difficult to accomplish the goal of identifying those in early stages of CKD. Efforts at standardization of creatinine assays are under way.[10] Without improvements in the assays, it is unlikely that any reformulation of the equations estimating either creatinine clearance or GFR will be able to yield reliable results for detecting the early stages of CKD when plasma creatinine is $\leq$1.5 mg/dL.

Currently, evaluation of urine for protein and sediment may be the first-line approach in screening patients deemed to be at risk for chronic renal disease.[3] Frank proteinuria both precedes severe declines in GFR and occurs at a disease stage in which GFR estimations are not particularly accurate for the reasons noted above. Hopefully the addition of newer GFR estimates will eventually help to bring into sharper focus the risk level of patients in early renal failure. This desirable advance, however, awaits better standardization of creatinine assays as much as it awaits an equation validated for a wider range of disease entities (including diabetes) and normal individuals.[8,9] Such efforts are currently ongoing.

Treatment of CKD

The treatment of CKD in its early stages is a combination of tighter control of the underlying etiology, usually hypertension and/or diabetes, and dietary restrictions of sodium, potassium, and protein due to the imbalances in the renal handling of these substances. Pharmacologically, ACE inhibitors have been important for both their antihypertensive effects and their activity on the afferent arterioles, which decreases intraglomerular pressure. In cases of extacellular fluid excess, loop diuretics are appropriate in the predialysis stages. Theses drugs also effect a kaliuresis. In some cases, potassium-sparing diuretic such as spironolactone is also an option. Calcium must frequently be administered in these patients, but care must be taken to avoid a high-calcium-phosphate product, which can result in metastatic calcification.

The later stages of CKD are treated similarly to the early stages, but diuresis becomes more important as fluid volume expands. Eventually, the need for renal replacement therapy becomes evident as volume overload, electrolyte imbalance, and uremic symptoms become impossible to treat by other medical means.

Conclusion

The case presented here will be played out more often in primary care medicine in the future as efforts intensify to diagnose and treat chronic renal disease at an earlier stage and as renal failure incidence increases with the population's age. The goal for patients such as this one would be to detect a significant decrease in GFR during his microalbuminuric stage. However, improvements in the standardization of creatinine assays are one of the major hurdles to ushering in a new era of developing better estimates and improving early renal failure treatment.

References

1. SKORECKI, K., GREEN, J., AND BRENNER, B. M.: Chronic renal failure. In *Harrison's Principles of Internal Medicine*, 16th ed., D. L. KASPER, A. S. FAUCI, D. L. LONGO, E. BRAUNWALD, S. L. HAUSER, AND J. L. JAMESON, eds., McGraw-Hill, New York, 2005, pp. 1653–63.

2. MOLITCH, M. E.: Management of early diabetic nephropathy. *Am. J. Med. 102*:392–8, 1997.

3. DE JONG, P. E. AND GANSEVOORT, R. T.: Screening techniques for detecting chronic kidney disease. *Curr. Opin. Nephrol. Hypertens. 14*:567–72, 2005.

4. COCKCROFT, D. W. AND GAULT, M. H.: Prediction of creatinine clearance from serum creatinine. *Nephron 16*:31–41, 1976.

5. KLAHR, S., LEVEY, A. S., BECK, G. J. ET AL.: The effects of dietary protein restriction and blood-pressure control on the progression of chronic renal disease. *N. Engl. J. Med. 330*:877–84, 1994.

6. LEVEY, A. S., BOSCH, J. P., LEWIS, J. B. ET AL.: A more accurate method to estimate glomerular filtration rate from serum creatinine: A new prediction equation. *Ann. Intern. Med. 130*:461–70, 1999.

7. National Kidney Foundation K/DOQI Workgroup: Clinical practice guidelines for chronic kidney disease: Evaluation, classification and stratification. *Am. J. Kidney Dis. 39*:S1–153, 2002.

8. RULE, A. D., LARSON, T. S., BERGSTRALH, E. J. ET AL.: Using serum creatinine to estimate glomerular filtration rate: Accuracy in good health and in chronic kidney disease. *Ann. Intern. Med. 141*: 929–37, 2004.

9. STEVENS, L. A. AND LEVEY, A. S.: Clinical implications of estimating equations for glomerular filtration rate. *Ann. Intern. Med. 141*:959–61, 2004.

10. MYERS, G. L., MILLER, W. G., CORESH, J. ET AL.: Recommendations for improving serum creatinine measurement: A report from the laboratory working group of the national kidney disease education program. *Clin. Chem. 52*:5–18, 2006.

11. CHAN, M. H., NG, K. F., SZETO, C. C. ET AL.: Effect of a compensated Jaffe creatinine method on the estimation of glomerular filtration rate. *Ann. Clin. Biochem. 41*:482–4, 2004.

12. MURTHY, K., STEVENS, L. A., STARK, P. C., AND LEVEY, A. S.: Variation in the serum creatinine assay calibration: a practical application to glomerular filtration rate estimation. *Kidney Int. 68*:1884–7, 2005.

Case 10

A Pain in the Back

Kevin J. Martin and Esther A. González

A 64-year-old woman had been on hemodialysis 3 times a week for the past 5 years. At the time of her annual physical examination, she noted that she had had a gradual increase in aches and pains over the past 2 years, which appeared to be increasing in severity. The pain was mostly in her lower back, but also in her legs, and was associated with a decreased ability to stand up from a sitting position. She was utilizing nonsteroidal analgesic agents to control the discomfort. The cause of her renal disease was IgA nephropathy, which had had a reasonably rapid course, with her renal function deteriorating over the 5 years prior to starting dialysis. She had no other significant complaints and appeared to be compliant with her medications. Her appetite was good, and the parameters of adequacy of dialysis were also satisfactory. As part of her routine hemodialysis monitoring, she had monthly chemistry profiles, and quarterly measurement of parathyroid hormone (PTH). Serum calcium concentrations ranged between 9.2 and 9.6 mg/dL (2.3 and 2.4 mM) over the preceding year, and serum phosphorus had ranged from 5.4 to 6.1 mg/dL (1.74 to 1.97 mM). Measurements of intact PTH ranged from 329 to 447 pg/mL (329 to 447 ng/L) over the preceding year. It was noted that when she started on hemodialysis, intact PTH was 214 pg/mL. BUN concentration ranged from 74 to 89 mg/dL (26.9 to 32.5 mM), and serum creatinine concentrations were 8.6–9.2 mg/dL. The remainder of the serum chemistry testing was within normal reference intervals, with the exception of alkaline phosphatase, which was elevated at 212 IU/mL.

Physical examination revealed that the patient was in no distress. The chest was clear on auscultation, cardiac examination revealed an absence of volume overload, and there was a loud 4/6 systolic ejection murmur at the base of the heart, radiating to the carotids. The liver was not enlarged, and the spleen was not palpable. Abdominal examination was unremarkable. Examination of the extremities revealed an absence of peripheral edema, and there was no tenderness to palpation. She had mild kyphosis (outward curvature of the spine) and had demonstrable difficulty in rising from a sitting position, and had some leg pain when asked to walk.

Definition of Disease

Renal osteodystrophy is the term used to describe the abnormalities of the skeleton that can occur in association with chronic kidney disease. A wide spectrum of skeletal

Tietz's Applied Laboratory Medicine, Second Edition. Edited by Mitchell G. Scott, Ann M. Gronowski, and Charles S. Eby
Copyright © 2007 John Wiley & Sons, Inc.

abnormalities may be seen in this setting, which range from high-turnover bone disease due to secondary hyperparathyroidism, known as *osteitis fibrosa* in its severe form, to the opposite end of the spectrum of bone turnover, where it can be excessively low and give rise to a skeletal abnormality known as *adynamic bone disease*. Some patients may also have mineralization defects in the skeleton, which may be manifested as osteo-malacia. In many patients, there is evidence of both high bone turnover together with min-eralization defects of bone, and this is termed *mixed renal osteodystrophy*. Abnormalities of the skeleton are extremely common in patients with advanced kidney diseases, even in the absence of symptoms, and symptomatic bone disease in this patient population is relatively unusual nowadays. It is important to recognize that other forms of skeletal disease may also coexist in these patients, and therefore, this patient, who is a postmeno-pausal female, who had been treated with corticosteroids in the past, is also likely to have a component of osteoporosis from either of these causes. Accordingly, these complex bony abnormalities may cause significant problems in this setting of chronic kidney disease.

Differential Diagnosis

There are several considerations in this patient that could account for her symptoms. The initial consideration is that she had hyperparathyroid bone disease, as a result of sec-ondary hyperparathyroidism. In this regard, measurements of intact PTH had ranged within 300–400 pg/mL, which is clearly above the normal interval for these PTH assays, in which the upper limit of normal would be approximately 65 pg/mL. While at first glance this may indicate severe hyperparathyroidism, it is important to note that in the setting of advanced chronic kidney disease, there is known to be skeletal resistance to the actions of PTH, and higher than normal concentrations of PTH appear to be required to maintain bone turnover. In recent times, clinical practice guidelines have been intro-duced for the control of the abnormalities of mineral metabolism in patients with chronic kidney disease, and it is recommended that intact PTH should ideally be main-tained between 150 and 300 pg/mL in order to maintain normal bone turnover. Thus, in the patient under consideration, PTH concentrations are only marginally increased above the desired therapeutic range. Although measurement of intact PTH is useful to assess the effects of hyperparathyroidism on bone, there is a considerable range of concen-trations that may be seen and this patient's PTH concentration is in a "gray zone" where prediction of the effects of PTH on bone may be difficult. Other biochemical determi-nations may be helpful in conjunction with the PTH assay. In this particular patient, the elevated alkaline phosphatase suggests evidence of increased osteoblast activity, which could potentially be due to the effects of excess PTH on bone. However, most patients with hyperparathyroid bone disease sufficient to cause symptoms have higher concen-trations of intact PTH, the elevated alkaline phosphatase raises that concern in this patient. An additional consideration is that this patient had osteoporosis accounting for her back pain from microfactures. She was postmenopausal and had been treated with cor-ticosteroids in the past, both of which can be significant contributors to decreased bone density and osteoporosis. Osteoporosis, however, rarely results in pain in the lower limbs associated with proximal muscle weakness, as was seen in this patient.

In recent times there have been refinements in the assay for PTH as a result of the observation that so-called "intact" PTH assays are now known to also measure aminoterm-inally truncated PTH fragments, such as PTH 7-84. This has led to assays that are specific for the full-length 84-amino-acid PTH molecule. Examples of commercially available assays of this type are the Bio-Intact PTH assay (Nichols Diagnostics Institute) and the Whole PTH assay (Scantibodies Clinical Laboratories). It is hoped that these assays will have improved clinical performance and allow for better reproducibility between assays from various manufacturers.

An additional consideration is that this patient had an osteomalacic lesion of bone, due to defective bone mineralization. Most symptomatic osteomalacia in the setting of chronic kidney disease has been the result of accumulation of aluminum in bone in the era where aluminum-based phosphate binders were utilized to try to prevent hyperphosphatemia. This patient had never received aluminum-containing compounds, and accordingly, this is an unlikely possibility.

However, the patient had a long history of proteinuria, which is associated with significant loss of vitamin D–binding protein in the urine, and was likely vitamin D–deficient. Therefore, the possibility exists that she had vitamin D deficiency–induced impaired mineralization in bone.

Accordingly, on clinical grounds, it is not possible to make a specific diagnosis of bone disease in this patient, and accordingly, a decision was made to perform bone biopsy following double tetracycline labeling to allow for the measurement of dynamic parameters of bone mineralization. She therefore received two short courses of tetracycline for 2 days, each at 14-day intervals, and had a transiliac bone biopsy performed 5 days after the second course. The bone core was analyzed for histomorphometry and revealed the presence of severe osteitis fibrosa cystica with evidence of markedly increased bone resorption, some delayed mineralization, and markedly decreased trabecular bone. The diagnosis, therefore, was osteitis fibrosis cystica.

Treatment

With a firm histological diagnosis, it was possible to proceed with efforts to try to control and decrease the concentrations of parathyroid hormone in this patient. Serum calcium was in the lower part of the normal reference interval, within the clinical practice guidelines, and serum phosphorus was slightly above the clinical practice guideline recommended concentrations; therefore the initial approach to treatment was to further control hyperphosphatemia by the prescription of non-calcium-containing phosphate binders with meals, which was successful in lowering serum phosphorus values to approximately 5 mg/dL. At this time, a vitamin D analog, paricalcitol, was added to her regimen. This was administered intravenously 3 times a week during hemodialysis, and the dose titrated according to its effect on PTH concentrations. The injectible vitamin D analog, paricalcitol, has a direct effect to decrease the transcription of the PTH gene and will lower PTH secretion. During this therapy, it was necessary to monitor the concentrations of serum calcium and phosphorus on a frequent basis in order to avoid hypercalcemia or hyperphosphatemia. The vitamin D analog was chosen on the basis of experimental data, suggesting that this analog had a lesser ability to increase calcium and phosphorus absorption from the intestine than the native active vitamin D sterol, calcitriol. The decision was made to try to decrease PTH concentrations in this patient to approximately 150 pg/mL, which is toward the lower end of the target range for clinical practice guidelines. This therapy was associated with a marked improvement in her symptoms over the subsequent 3–6 months of therapy, and she no longer required the use of nonsteroidal drugs for pain control.

The principles of treatment of hyperparathyroid bone disease are to control serum phosphorus, while keeping serum calcium values within the normal range, and to limit the calcium intake in this patient group, such that calcium balance is not excessively positive or persistently negative. Vitamin D sterols such as paricalcitol are often used to take advantage of its direct effect to suppress PTH on bone, and this has less calcemic and phosphatemic potential than does the native hormone, calcitriol. Additional agents are also available that may be suitable in other patients, such as the calcimimetic agent cinacalcet hydrochloride, which is an allosteric activator of the calcium-sensing receptor in the parathyroid gland, and directly decreases PTH secretion by this mechanism. Monitoring the parameters of mineral metabolism, including calcium, phosphorus, and PTH, is necessary in all patients on dialysis in order to prevent and treat both the skeletal and extraskeletal consequences and disorders of mineral metabolism in this patient group.

Additional Reading

EKNOYAN, G., LEVIN, A., AND LEVIN, N. W.: Bone metabolism and disease in chronic kidney disease. *Am. J. Kidney Dis. 42*:1–201, 2003.

GONZALEZ, E. A., SACHDEVA, A., OLIVER, D. A., AND MARTIN, K. J.: Vitamin D insufficiency and deficiency in chronic kidney disease. A single center observational study. *Am. J. Nephrol. 24*:503–10, 2004.

MARTIN, K. J., GONZALEZ, E. A., AND SLATOPOLSKY, E.: Renal osteodystrophy. In *The Kidney*, 7th ed., B. M. BRENNER, ed., Saunders, Philadelphia, 2004, pp. 2255–304.

MARTIN, K. J., AKHTAR, I., AND GONZALEZ, E. A.: Parathyroid hormone: New assays, new receptors. *Semin. Nephrol. 24*:3–9, 2004.

MARTIN, K. J. AND GONZALEZ, E. A.: Vitamin D analogs: Actions and role in the treatment of secondary hyperparathyroidism. *Semin. Nephrol. 24*:456–9, 2004.

SLATOPOLSKY, E., GONZALEZ, E., AND MARTIN, K.: Pathogenesis and treatment of renal osteodystrophy. *Blood Purif. 21*:318–26, 2003.

Case 11

Refractory Hyponatremia with Lung Cancer

Manish J. Gandhi

A 59-year-old white female was admitted for evaluation of refractory chronic hyponatremia, an ongoing problem for the past 6 months. The patient reported an 11-lb weight gain and increased fluid intake over the past 10 days prior to admission. Family members also reported that the patient had become increasingly confused during this time. The patient was previously admitted to the hospital for hyponatremia approximately one month ago and had been discharged 10 days prior to this admission. Serum sodium on previous admission was 122 mol/L and following treatment had risen to 136 mmol/L on discharge.

Past history is significant for schizophrenia diagnosed 15 years ago and for oat cell carcinoma of the left lung diagnosed 3 years ago with the patient subsequently undergoing left pnuemonectomy followed by chemotherapy. One month prior to this admission, CT scan of the chest and abdomen revealed recurrent oat cell carcinoma of the left hemithorax that is currently being treated by radiotherapy. CT scan of the head at the time revealed no evidence of brain metastasis. Physical examination revealed a confused, agitated, and moderately obese white female. Vital signs: temperature 36.7°C, respiratory rate 24, blood pressure 150/90 mm Hg, pulse 104 bpm. Slight ankle edema was noted, but the remainder of the physical examination was unremarkable. Relevant laboratory investigations at admission revealed the following:

Analyte	Value, Conventional Units	Reference Interval, Conventional Units	Value, SI Units	Reference Interval, SI Units
Sodium	121 mmol/L	135–148	Same	
Potassium	4.4 mmol/L	3.0–5.5	Same	
Chloride	81 mmol/L	95–107	Same	
Urea nitrogen	9 mg/dL	7–18	3.2 mmol urea/L	2.5–6.4
Creatinine	0.7 mg/dL	0.6–1.2	61.8 umol/L	53–106
Glucose, fasting	97 mg/dL	70–110	5.3 mmol/L	3.8–6.1
Uric acid	3.2 mg/dL	3–8.2	0.19 mmol/L	0.18–0.48
Osmolality calculated	230 mOsm/kg	275–295	230 mmol/kg	275–295

Tietz's Applied Laboratory Medicine, Second Edition. Edited by Mitchell G. Scott, Ann M. Gronowski, and Charles S. Eby

Analyte	Value, Conventional Units	Reference Interval, Conventional Units	Value, SI Units	Reference Interval, SI Units
TSH	1.5 μIU/ml		1.5 mIU/L	
Urine osmolality	303 mOsm/kg	NA	303 mmol/kg	NA
Urine sodium	31 mmol/L	NA	Same	NA

Thyroid function tests and serum cortisol values were all within normal limits.

The patient was treated with a high-sodium diet and fluid restriction of 1000 mL/24 hours, and 4 days after treatment the laboratory values were as follows:

Analyte	Value, Conventional Units	Reference Interval, Conventional Units	Value, SI Units	Reference Interval, SI Units
Sodium	127 mmol/L	135–148	Same	
Potassium	4.5 mmol/L	3.0–5.5	Same	
Chloride	86 mmol/L	95–107	Same	
Calculated osmolality	272 mOsm/kg	275–295	230 mmol/kg	275–295

The patient was discharged after another 2 days, when her mental status had improved and the serum sodium had risen to 135 mmol/L. She was sent home and told to restrict fluid intake to 1000 mL/24 hours.

Differential Diagnosis of Hyponatremia

Hyponatremia, one of the more common fluid and electrolyte disturbances, can be the result of multiple causes and is highly prevalent in critically ill patients.[2,3] It is defined as a serum sodium concentration of less than 135 mmol/L. Conceptually, hyponatremia can be classified into dilutional and depletional causes. Dilutional hyponatremia is the result of increased extracellular fluid (ECF) in the presence of normal or an increased total body sodium (Na^+) that is less than the increase in ECF volume. Depletional hyponatremia is found when Na^+ is lost in the presence of normal ECF volume or when there is a greater decrease in total body Na^+ than a decrease in ECF volume.

Clinically, hyponatremia is often classified into three basic types depending on the ECF status of the patient (Table 11.1). Thus, a careful physical exam to assess the patient's volume status is critical. The exam should note signs of either excess volume (recent weight gain, edema, swelling) or decreased ECF (dry skin and mucous membranes, lack of skin targor, and flat jugular veins). Appropriate laboratory tests to help differentiate the hyponatremia include serum and urine electrolytes, serum and urine osmolality, and thyroid and adrenal hormones.

Hyponatremic plasma can be either hyperosmotic, isotonic, or hypoosmotic, making the measurement of plasma osmolality an important initial step in the assessment of hyponatremia. Of these, the most common is hypoosmotic hyponatremia since Na^+ is the primary determinant of plasma osmolality. When hyponatremia occurs in the presence of increased plasma osmolality, this can only be due to an increased amount of other

Table 11.1 Clinical Classification of Hyponatremia

Volume status	Hypovolemic	Normovolemic	Hypervolemic
Mechanism	Loss of both water and Na^+ Na loss > water loss	Total body water increased, normal to mild decrease in Na^+; prevention of free water excretion	Excess of both total body water and Na^+
			Water retention > renal Na^+ loss
Causes	Gastrointestinal fluid loss	SIADH	Heart failure
	Burns	Hypothyroidism	Nephrotic syndrome
	Salt-losing nephritis	Psychogenic polydipsia, beer-drinker's potomania	
	Addison's disease	Diuretics	Renal failure

solutes in the ECF that causes an extracellular shift of water or an intracellular shift of Na^+ to maintain osmotic balance between the extra- and intracellular. The most common cause of this type of hyponatremia is severe hyperglycemia. In fact, "true" plasma Na^+ in the setting of hyperglycemia can be calculated by adding 1.6 mmol/L of Na^+ for every 100 mg/dL increase of glucose above 100 mg/dL.

If the measured Na^+ concentration in plasma is decreased, but measured plasma osmolality, glucose, and urea are normal, the only explanation is pseudohyponatremia caused by the *electrolyte exclusion effect*. This can occur in patients with severe hyperlipidemia or hyperproteinemia (e.g., paraprotein, multiple myeloma) when Na^+ is measured by either flame emission spectrophotometry or by an indirect ion-selective electrode (see discussion below).

Most often when hyponatremia is present the plasma osmolality will also be low. As stated above, this type of hyponatremia can be due to either excess loss of Na^+ (*depletional hyponatremia*) or increased extracellular volume (*dilutional hyponatremia*). Differentiating causes of this type of hyponatremia initially requires a clinical assessment of volume status. This is best accomplished by a history and physical examination.

Depletional hyponatremia (excess loss of Na^+) is almost always accompanied by a loss of water but to a lesser extent than the loss of Na^+. Hypovolemia is apparent in the physical examination (orthostatic hypotension, tachycardia, decreased skin turgor, flat jugular veins). Loss of fluid is the cause of the hyponatremia, and this can occur through either renal or extrarenal losses. If urine Na^+ is low (generally <10 mmol/L), the loss will be extrarenal most typically from the gastrointestinal tract or the skin. If, on the other hand, urine Na^+ is elevated in this setting (generally >20 mmol/L), renal loss of Na^+ is occuring. Renal loss of Na^+ can occur with osmotic diuresis, thiazide diuretics, adrenal insufficiency (the absence of aldosterone and cortisone prevents distal tubule reabsorption of Na^+), or "potassium-sparing" diuretics, such as spironolactone, which block aldosterone-mediated distal reabsorption of Na^+. Renal loss of Na^+ in excess of H_2O will also occur in metabolic alkalosis as a result of prolonged vomiting, because the increased renal HCO_3^- excretion that occurs with alkalosis is accompanied by Na^+ ions.

Dilutional hyponatremia is a result of excess H_2O retention and can sometimes be detected during the physical examination. When total body water (TBW) is increased, but the central intravascular volume is decreased, as in congestive heart failure, hepatic cirrhosis, or the nephrotic syndrome, and a vicious cycle is established. The decreased blood volume is sensed by peripheral baroreceptors and results in increased aldosterone and antidiarectic hormone (ADH) even though TBW is excessive. The kidneys properly reabsorb Na^+ and H_2O in response to the increased aldosterone and ADH to restore the blood volume, but this simply results in further increases in TBW and further dilution of Na^+. In this setting urine Na^+ will be low.

In hypoosmotic hyponatremia with normal volume status, the most common etiologies are the syndrome of inappropriate ADH (SIADH), primary polydypsia, hypothyroidism, or adrenal insufficiency. SIADH is usually a result of ectopic or otherwise "inappropriate" ADH production arising from a variety of conditions and results in excessive H_2O retention. SIADH often is diagnosed by a urine osmolality that is greater than plasma osmolality in the setting of hyponatremia, but only when renal, adrenal, and thyroid functions are normal.

In this patient the clinical findings indicate a relatively normovolemic hyponatremia in the presence of a hypoosmolar plasma and an inappropriately high excretion of Na^+ in the urine. Her history of recurrent oat cell carcinoma and chronic refractory hyponatremia, together with normal thyroid and adrenal function, would place SIADH high on the differential diagnosis for this patient.

Definition of the Disease

SIADH is a relatively common cause of refractory hyponatremia that is due to an autonomous and sustained production of ADH the absence of known stimuli for its release. Clinically SIADH is characterized by[1]

1. Hyponatremia and hypoosmolar plasma
2. Clinical euvolemia and absence of severe edema
3. Urine osmolality greater then plasma osmolality
4. Inappropriate excretion of sodium (Na^+) in the urine usually greater then 20 mmol/L
5. Absence of other causes of hyponatremia such as adrenal insufficiency, renal insufficiency, nephrotic syndrome, congestive heart failure, and liver cirrhosis

Pathogenesis

ADH, also known as *arginine vasopressin*, is normally released from the pituitary in response to osmotic receptors in the hypothalamus. If plasma osmolality increases above 280 mOsm/L, the cells of the osmoreceptors shrink and stimulate release of ADH, which acts on the collecting ducts of the nephron to render them permeable to water. When the collecting ducts are water-permeable, water is reabsorbed passively because of the concentration gradient within the medulla of the kidney. If excess ADH is secreted when the osmolality is less than 280 mOsm/L, excess water is reabsorbed and hyponatremia will develop. The absence of ADH will lead to water loss, polyuria, and hypernatremia. This condition, which is essentially the opposite of SIADH, is referred to as diabetes insipidus.

Table 11.2 Causes of SIADH

Neoplasms
  Carcinoma of lung, pancreas, bladder, colon, kidney, prostate
  Leukemia
  Thymoma
  Lymphomas
  Sarcomas
  Brain tumor
Neurological disorders
  Head trauma
  Stroke
  Subarachnoid hemorrhage
  Meningitis
  Encephalitis
  Hydrocephalus
  Guillain–Barré syndrome
  Acute intermittent porphyria
Lung disease
  Pneumonia, tuberculosis
  Bronchiectasis
  Positive-pressure ventilation
Drugs
  Increased ADH production
    Antidepressants: tricyclics, MAO inhibitors, SSRI
    Antineoplastic: cyclophosphamide
    Carbamazepine
    Ecstasy
    Nicotine
  Potentiate ADH action
    Chlopromamide
    NSAIDs
    Cyclophosphamide
Miscellaneous
  Postoperative state
  AIDS
  Stress, pain

Source: Adapted from *Current Medical Diagnosis and Treatment*, 2003.

The dilutional hyponatremia of SIADH in most cases results from either increased circulating ADH produced ectopically by malignancies or from a "reset osmostat" for ADH secretion, such that ADH is released at a lower than normal threshold of plasma osmolality. An example of the former is the current patient, while the latter can be observed in quadriplegia (in which effective volume depletion may result from venous pooling in the legs), psychosis, tuberculosis, and chronic malnutrition. Increased antidiuretic activity promotes increased reabsorption of water in the collecting ducts of the nephron, resulting in a decreased urine volume with increased urine sodium excretion and increased urine osmolality. The resulting reabsorption of excess water leads to a dilutional hyponatremia and a low plasma osmolality. Furthermore, the intravascular volume expansion due to the excess reabsorbed water results in decreased renal sodium reabsorption and additional urine sodium excretion. Many conditions have been associated with SIADH, which may be classified into four major groups, neoplasia, neurological disorders, lung disease (nonmalignant), and a wide variety of drugs that are beyond the scope of discussion here (Table 11.2).

Clinical Features

Clinical features usually depend on the rate at which hyponatremia develops. In general, slowly progressive hyponatremia is associated with fewer and less severe clinical symptoms than is an equivalent degree of hyponatremia that is acute in onset.[4] Mild, chronic hyponatremia may be asymptomatic. When the serum sodium concentration falls below 125 mmol/L, mild CNS symptoms such as confusion, lethargy, fatigue, anorexia, nausea, and muscle cramps may develop. More severe CNS symptoms can occur with a further fall in serum sodium and include hypothermia, delirium, coma, seizures, Cheyne–Stokes respiration, and pathologic reflexes. Sudden death can occur when there has been rapid development of hyponatremia to values below 115 mmol/L.

Laboratory Investigation of SIADH

Ruling Out Pseudohyponatremia

A first step in documenting hyponatremia is to confirm that it is truly a pathologic hyponatremia by ruling out conditions causing pseudohyponatremia by the electrolyte exclusion effect. If osmolality is normal in the setting of hyponatremia this must be considered.

Pseudohyponatremia occurs when the nonaqueous volume of plasma is markedly increased, usually as a result of severe hyperlipidemia or a high concentration of paraprotein, either of which excludes electrolytes from a portion of the total plasma volume and leads to low concentrations of sodium in the total plasma.[2,3] The indirect ion-specific electrode and flame photometry both include dilution of samples before the analysis and thus measures the concentration in the total plasma volume. The activity of sodium in the aqueous fraction of plasma is measured by direct ion-specific electrodes and is not affected by high triglyceride or protein concentrations as no sample dilution is performed.

Instruments designed to perform multiple tests with a high sample throughput often measure sodium by indirect ion-specific electrodes. These methods first dilute the sample, thus determining the sodium concentration in the total plasma volume rather than its activity in water as done by a direct ion-specific electrode. The most recent report of the College of American Pathologists[1] indicates that the majority of clinical laboratories perform Na^+ measurements with indirect ion-specific electrodes after diluting the samples, making the analysis subject to pseudohyponatremia.

Serum Osmolality

Since hyponatremic plasma can be either hyperosmotic, isotonic, or hypoosmotic, the measurement of plasma osmolality is an important initial step in the assessment of hyponatremia. As described above, in hypoosmotic hyponatremia with normal volume status, the most common etiologies are SIADH, primary polydypsia, hypothyroidism, or adrenal insufficiency. In this patient the mild edema suggests slight excess of TBW.

In a typical SIADH patient there will be a hyposomolar plasma (<270 mOsm/kg), inappropriate urine response to hypoosmolality (urine osmolality $>$ plasma osmolality), and an inappropriately elevated urine sodium concentration (>20 mmol/L in a random urine sample). In other patients with dilutional hyponatremia secondary to excess fluid intake, there will be true plasma hyposomolality, but unlike SIADH, these patients will make an appropriately dilute urine (urine osmolality $<$ plasma osmolality) and urine sodium concentration will usually be <20 mmol/L. In contrast, in patients with depletional hyponatremia due to extra renal sodium losses such as profuse sweating will have hypotonic plasma, a low urine sodium concentration (<20 mmol/L), and a urine osmololality that is greater than that of plasma, while patients who have depletional hyponatremia due to impaired renal conservation as in mineralocorticoid

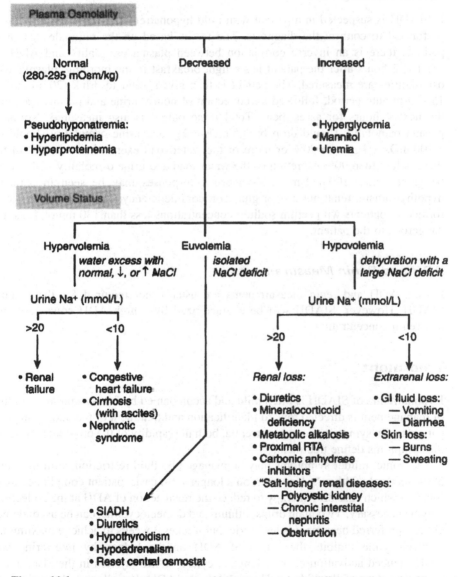

Figure 11.1   Algorithm for interpretation of laboratory tests in the differential diagnosis of hyponatremia.

deficiencies will have increased urine sodium concentrations. The algorithm in Figure 11.1 is often helpful for interpreting laboratory tests in the differential diagnosis of hyponatremia.

Other Tests

SIADH is essentially a diagnosis of exclusion, and thus a complete diagnosis necessitates laboratory tests to exclude cardiac, hepatic, renal, adrenal, or thyroid failure; and clinical history to determine the effects of pituitary surgery, diuretic therapy, or medications that can stimulate ADH release.

Water-Loading Test

If SIADH is suspected in a patient with mild hyponatremia, a water-loading test can be performed to confirm the diagnosis. The test is based on the rationale that in normal patients there is an inverse correlation between plasma osmolality and ADH release. Briefly, 2 hours after the patient has a light breakfast in the morning, plasma and urine osmolalities are measured. The patient is then given water to drink (20 mL/kg) over a 15–30-minute period, followed by collection of hourly urine and plasma specimens for the next 4 hours for assessment. Total urine output is also measured. Normally, the plasma osmolality should drop by ≥5 mOsm/kg, and urine osmolality should drop to ≤100 mOsm/kg, with 90% or more of the water load excreted in 4 hours. In SIADH, there is less then 90% excretion of the water load and urine osmolality will consistently be greater then 100 mOsm/kg. Subnormal responses may be seen in patients with hypothyroidism, renal disease, or glucocorticoid deficiency. This test should not be performed in patients with serum sodium concentrations less than 130 mmol/L as it can be dangerous to the patient.

ADH and Renin Measurements

Plasma ADH and renin measurements are usually not required for the diagnosis of SIADH. However, SIADH will be characterized by a high ADH concentration and a low renin concentration.

Treatment

Hyponatremia of SIADH is often mild and accompanied by few symptoms, and the focus of management is directed toward identification and treatment of the underlying cause. In patients with symptomatic hyponatremia, both the rapidity of the onset and the severity of the symptoms define treatment.

Chronic, milder symptoms may be managed by fluid restriction, with fluid intake of 500–1000 mL/24 hours. However, on a longer-term basis, patient compliance may be an issue, in which case drug therapy to reduce the renal action of ADH at the collecting ducts may be necessary. Two main drugs, lithium and demeclocycline, can be used; demeclocycline is preferred because it is less toxic, but it takes 3 weeks to achieve maximum effect. Demeclocyline inhibits the action of ADH on the kidney by interfering with the ADH-induced activation of the adenylate cylase–cAMP system in the distal tubule and collecting duct of the kidney. This inhibits the ADH-dependent reabsorption of water and can result in excess loss of water but not sodium. Thus demeclocycline acts by producing a condition that is conceptually the opposite of SIADH. Doses range from 600 to 1200 mg/day. Similarly, Li^+ also blocks the end-organ effect of ADH and, in fact, one of the side effects of Li^+ therapy is nephrogenic diabetes insipidus.

Saline infusion (3% hypertonic or even isotonic) is usually reserved for symptomatic acute hyponatreamia of less than 3 days' duration or in the rare significantly symptomatic patient with chronic hyponatremia. In either case the extreme caution needs to be exercised as rapid correction of hyponatraemia can lead to serious, permanent, neurological manifestations, central pontine myelinolysis (osmotic demyelination syndrome), and death.[5] The therapeutic objective is to increase serum sodium by no more than 12 mmol/L in the first 24 hours of treatment at the rate of 0.5–1 mmol/L per hour to a target level of approximately 125 mmol/L.[4] Thereafter, further treatment should be maintained using more traditional modes of therapy, such as fluid restriction.

References

1. BARTTER, F. C. AND SCHWARTZ, W. B.: The syndrome of inappropriate secretion of antidiuretic hormone. *Am. J. Med.* 42:790–806, 1967.

2. ADROGUE, H. J., AND MADIAS, N. E.: Hyponatremia. *N. Engl. J. Med.* 342:1581–9, 2000.

3. SMITH, D. M., McKENNA, K., AND THOMPSON, C. J.: Hyponatraemia. *Clin. Endocrinol.* (Oxford) 52:667–78, 2000.

4. FRASER, C. L. AND ARIEFF, A. I.: Epidemiology, pathophysiology, and management of hyponatremic encephalopathy. *Am. J. Med.* 102:67–77, 1997.

5. STERNS, R. H., RIGGS, J. E., AND SCHOCHET, S. S. JR., Osmotic demyelination syndrome following correction of hyponatremia. *N. Engl. J. Med.* 314:1535–42, 1986.

Part Four

Liver Diseases

Cases of Wilson's disease, cirrhosis/hematochromatosis, hepatitis C,
and nonalcoholic fatty liver disease are presented in Cases 12, 13, 15, and 16
(all edited by MGS), respectively; Gilbert's disease is the topic of Case 14
(edited by AMG).

Tietz's Applied Laboratory Medicine, Second Edition. Edited by Mitchell G. Scott, Ann M. Gronowski, and
Charles S. Eby
Copyright © 2007 John Wiley & Sons, Inc.

Case 12

Adolescent Female with Tremor, Depression, and Hepatitis

Steven I. Shedlofsky

A 16-year-old white female presented to her pediatrician with tremor and depression. Approximately 8 months previously, her mother noted a mild lack of muscle coordination, which slowly progressed. As a result, the patient failed to be reelected as a school cheerleader just one month prior to presentation. A depressed affect with fatigue and malaise had developed and was thought to be secondary to this failure. However, when a tremor was noted along with mild dysarthria, the patient's mother decided to seek medical attention for her. Prior to this time, the patient had been healthy except for an appendectomy at age 9. There was no history of head trauma or neonatal jaundice, nor was there a history of neurological disease in her family. The patient has three younger siblings who are all healthy.

On initial examination, the patient had a flat affect. She weighed 108 lb (49 kg) and had normal vital signs. There was a fine tremor of both hands and arms, which worsened with voluntary actions, but no focal neurological deficits. Mild scleral icterus was noted, and the patient had several spider angiomata on her chest and several ecchymoses on each of her shins. Her liver was palpable 2 cm below the right costal margin with a dull edge, and there was tenderness to fist percussion. Her spleen was barely palpable under the left costal margin.

The following initial laboratory results were obtained:

Analyte	Value, Conventional Units	Reference Interval, Conventional Units	Value, SI Units	Reference Interval, SI Units
Hemoglobin	10.2 g/dL	12–16	6.33 mmol/L	7.45–9.93
Hematocrit	32%	37–47	0.32	0.37–0.47
Leukocyte count	$12.0 \times 10^3/\mu L$	4.8–10.8	$12.0 \times 10^9/L$	4.8–10.8
MCV	98 fL	80–94	Same	
Platelet count	$78 \times 10^3/\mu L$	150–450	$78 \times 10^9/L$	150–450
Prothrombin time: INR[a]	1.94	0.8–1.2		

Tietz's Applied Laboratory Medicine, Second Edition. Edited by Mitchell G. Scott, Ann M. Gronowski, and Charles S. Eby
Copyright © 2007 John Wiley & Sons, Inc.

Analyte	Value, Conventional Units	Reference Interval, Conventional Units	Value, SI Units	Reference Interval, SI Units
Sodium	137 mmol/L	136–145	Same	
Potassium	4.7 mmol/L	3.8–5.1	Same	
Chloride	99 mmol/L	98–107	Same	
CO_2, total	23 mmol/L	23–31	Same	
Urea nitrogen	10 mg/dL	8–21	3.6 mmol/L	2.9–7.5
Creatinine	0.8 mg/dL	0.7–1.3	71 μmol/L	62–115
Glucose	118 mg/dL	80–115	6.5 mmol/L	4.4–6.4
Calcium	118 mg/dL	4.2–5.1	2.35 mmol/L	2.10–2.55
Phosphorus	4.7 mEq/L	2.7–4.5	0.68 mmol/L	0.87–1.45
Protein, total	2.1 mg/dL	6.2–7.6	68 g/L	62–76
Albumin	6.8 g/dL	3.2–4.6	29 g/L	32–46
Cholesterol	2.9 g/dL	120–210	3.94 mmol/L	3.11–5.44
Urate	2.1 mg/dL	2.5–6.2	125 μmol/L	149–362
Bilirubin, total	7.7 mg/dL	0.2–1.0	131 μmol/L	3–17
AST	211 U/L	19–48	3.52 μkat/L	0.32–0.80
ALT	195 U/L	13–40	3.24 μkat/L	0.22–0.67
ALP	34 U/L	30–100	0.56 μkat/L	0.5–1.7
Urinalysis	Negative for protein, blood, and cells; glucose, 2+; bilirubin, 2+; amorphous phosphate and urate crystals present	Negative for all		

[a]International Normalized Ratio.

Because of the patient's anemia and elevated bilirubin, further studies were ordered to rule out hemolytic disease. The patient's conjugated bilirubin was 4.0 mg/dL (68 μmol/L), and a corrected reticulocyte count was 4.2% (reference range 0.5–1.5), confirming the presence of hemolysis. A Coombs test was negative. Despite her glycosuria, a haemoglobin A_1c was normal at 5.4%, and 2-hour postprandial serum glucose was only 114 mg/dL (6.3 mmol/L). Ultrasonographic examination of her abdomen showed a normal gallbladder without stones and no dilated intra- or extrahepatic ducts. Her liver was inhomogeneous and slightly enlarged with a prominent portal vein, suggesting cirrhosis with active inflammation. The spleen was slightly enlarged at 13.5 cm. A small amount of ascitic fluid was noted. Further evaluation of the abnormal liver studies included the following:

Analyte	Value, Conventional Units	Reference Interval, Conventional Units	Value, SI Units	Reference Interval, SI units
HBsAg	Negative	Negative	Same	
IgM anti-HB core Ab	Negative	Negative	Same	
IgM anti-HA Ab	Negative	Negative	Same	
Antihepatitis C Ab	Negative	Negative	Same	
$\alpha_1$1-Antitrypsin	182 mg/dL	78–200	1.82 g/L	0.78–2.00
Ceruloplasmin	16 mg/dL	20–45	160 mg/L	200–450
Antinuclear Ab	Negative	Negative	Same	
Anti-smooth-muscle Ab	Negative	Negative	Same	
Antiliver/kidney microsomal Ab	Negative	Negative	Same	

The slightly low ceruloplasmin level in the setting of elevated transaminases and neurologic symptoms raised the suspicion of hepatolenticular degeneration (Wilson's disease). A serum copper was obtained but at 171 µg/dL (26.9 µmol/L) was within the normal range of 60–190 (9.4–29.9). A more careful eye examination showed a golden brown band of pigment encircling the posterior cornea near the limbus of both eyes. An ophthalmologist performed a slit-lamp examination confirming the presence of Kayser–Fleischer rings. An MRI of the brain with T2 weighting demonstrated possible hyperintensity of the basal ganglia, a finding often seen in Wilson's disease. A baseline 24-hour urine collection was assayed for copper to further support the presumptive diagnosis of Wilson's disease, and a complete urine collection was documented by volume (840 mL/day) and urine creatinine (0.9 g/day). Baseline urinary copper excretion was elevated at 154 µg/day (2.43 µmol/day); (reference range, <40–100; <0.60–1.5). Because this elevation could also occur in other forms of liver injury, such as autoimmune hepatitis, an adjunctive urinary copper excretion test was performed several days later by giving 500 mg of the copper chelating drug D-penicillamine at 0 hour and 12 hour of the 24-hour collection. Finding an excretion of 2250 µg copper/day (35.2 µmol/day; reference range, <1600; <25) made Wilson's disease much more likely.[1]

To unequivocally establish the diagnosis, a liver biopsy was performed. Because of the patient's poor coagulation status, this was done by the transjugular approach with a prior infusion of fresh frozen plasma that normalized the patient's prothrombin time. Platelet infusions were not felt to be necessary. Macronodular cirrhosis was found with several regenerative nodules demonstrating ballooning degeneration of hepatocytes and pyknotic nuclei. An orcein stain for copper was positive, but showed variable staining between cirrhotic nodules. (A hepatic copper level was sent and came back 10 days later elevated at 264 µg/g dry weight liver; the normal was <50 µg/g and >250 was "diagnositic" of Wilson's disease.)

On the basis of the clinical and laboratory findings, therapy with D-penicillamine and a low-copper diet was initiated. Although abdominal distention due to ascites developed, the patient responded to a low-sodium diet and spironolactone. Her bilirubin decreased to 2.4 mg/dL (41 µmol/L) after 2 months, and her AST and ALT levels decreased to normal. Her hematocrit increased to 36% (0.36), and the reticulocytosis disappeared. Several 24-hour urine specimens obtained during the first 6 months of her D-penicillamine therapy showed marked cupruresis of 3000–5000 µg/day (47.2–78.7 µmol/day).

The patient's neurologic and psychiatric findings improved dramatically on therapy, although she was left with a fine tremor. After 10 months she developed a rash, arthralgias, and proteinuria. These symptoms were believed to indicate a lupuslike syndrome secondary to her D-penicillamine therapy. She was then started on oral zinc acetate therapy, but had too much abdominal discomfort. This prompted a switch to trientine therapy, which she has followed for the last 2 years without problems. An esophagogastroduodenoscopy showed no varices, but portal hypertensive gastropathy was noted. Because of her cirrhosis with its continued evidence of portal hypertension, the patient has been evaluated by the liver transplantation service. However, she has remained with a stable, relatively low MELD (model of end-stage liver disease) score of 12 based on a prothrombin time INR of 1.3, total bilirubin of 1.8 mg/dL, and creatinine of 0.9 mg/dL (see calculation at www.mayoclinic.org/gi-rst/mayomodel6.html).

The patient's parents were advised to have no more children and the parents and the patient's three younger siblings have all been screened with medical history, examination, routine laboratories, serum ceruloplasmin, slit-lamp examination, and 24-hour urinary copper excretion. No abnormalities have been found. But arrangements are being made to perform genotyping/haplotype studies at a specialized molecular laboratory.

Definition of Disease[1-3]

Pathophysiology of Wilson's Disease

Wilson's disease, also called *hepatolenticular degeneration*, is a rare autosomal recessive disorder of copper metabolism due to mutations in the ATP7B gene, which encodes a copper-transporting P-type ATPase expressed in hepatocytes. Over 200 mutations have been described, and most patients seen in the United States are compound heterozygotes. The incidence of Wilson's disease is estimated to be only 0.5–3 per 100,000. But the disease is invariably fatal unless the patient is identified and copper accumulation prevented. The defect in the ATP7B protein blocks the hepatocyte from excreting excess copper into bile for elimination in feces, the normal route for excess copper excretion. The defect also decreases the incorporation of copper into liver-synthesized protein, ceruloplasmin. Apoceruloplasmin has a short half-life compared with copper-containing ceruloplasmin, and that is why ceruloplasmin is usually low in Wilson's disease patients. The copper that accumulates within hepatocytes is toxic and eventually causes necrosis with release of the copper into the serum as "nonceruloplasmin"-bound copper. This excess copper is redistributed to the central nervous system, cornea, kidneys, and red blood cells, causing a wide spectrum of clinical manifestations.

Normal mechanisms of copper absorption, utilization, and excretion are complex. There is usually a large excess of dietary copper, most of which is absorbed in the intestine and rapidly transported to the liver by the portal venous system. However, if the intestinal enterocyte is exposed to large doses of another divalent cation metal such as zinc, the protein, metallothionein, is induced in the enterocyte that preferentially binds and sequesters copper, preventing copper absorption. Once in the liver cell, copper can be either temporarily sequestered by various cytosolic proteins or stored in lysosomes. But most excess copper is excreted into bile by the ATP7B protein. The copper secreted into bile can't be reabsorbed within the intestine. Copper that is incorporated into ceruloplasmin within the liver cell is released into the serum and normally represents ∼90% of serum copper. Ceruloplasmin transports copper to other cells for use in many important cellular enzymes such as cytochrome *c* oxidase, cytosolic superoxide dismutase, and monoamine oxidase. The ceruloplasmin in serum also has an important ferrioxidase function that converts highly reactive ferrous iron to the safer ferric form.

Manifestations of Wilson's Disease

Wilson's disease patients present after age 6 (usually between the ages of 12 and 30) with either neurologic/psychiatric problems, or at slightly earlier ages with manifestations of liver disease. Fifteen percent have acute intravascular hemolytic anemia, renal disease (Fanconi-like syndrome), or bone disease (osteomalacia). Approximately 25% of cases present with two or more manifestations, as did this patient.

The hepatic involvement of Wilson's disease can take several forms, including the insidious onset of cirrhosis, chronic active hepatitis, or fulminant liver failure. In the first and most common presentation, patients develop complications of *cirrhosis* such as ascites, bleeding esophageal varices, and liver failure (e.g., coagulopathy, spider angiomata, hyperbilirubinemia, encephalopathy). The liver is usually small and not palpable; often there is little hepatocellular necrosis, and serum aminotransferases may even be normal. When patients present with a *chronic active hepatitis* like picture, the liver is usually enlarged, and aminotransferase elevations are 2-4X ULN with AST usually > ALT. Histological examination of the liver seldom can distinguish between wilsonian cirrhosis or chronic active hepatitis and other causes (e.g., viral, autoimmune diseases, or drug toxicity). Copper studies are essential for the differential diagnosis of these patients. *Fulminant liver failure* due to Wilson's disease is also difficult to differentiate from other causes since serum ceruloplasmin can be low and urinary copper excretion high in other forms of fulminant liver disease. However, in Wilson's disease, liver failure appears to be associated with relatively low serum alkaline phosphatase activities and very high bilirubin values, so that an alkaline phosphatase/bilirubin ratio of <2.0 (alkaline phosphatase in U/L/bilirubin, total in mg/dL) has been proposed as evidence for wilsonian fulminant liver failure.

The neurological and psychiatric presentations of Wilson's disease are insidious and often misdiagnosed. Poor coordination, resting and intention tremor, excessive salivation, and dysarthria are commonly seen. The more severe dystonic manifestations are now rarely seen because of earlier diagnosis and institution of therapy. Psychiatric manifestations can be quite varied but are always progressive. Unfortunately, once well established, psychiatric manifestations do not respond as well to copper removal.

The hemolytic anemia of Wilson's disease is often episodic, probably owing to intermittent release of free copper from the liver that affects red blood cell membranes. An intravascular hemolytic anemia often accompanies fulminant hepatic failure and should strongly suggest Wilson's disease as the cause of the liver failure. Renal involvement can be significant with a Fanconi-like syndrome characterized by aminoaciduria, glycosuria, phosphaturia, hypercalciuria, and high uric acid excretion with low serum urate levels (as occurred in the case presented). It is probably this chronic renal involvement that leads to the osteomalacia sometimes seen.

Comments[1-3]

The most commonly used laboratory study to screen for Wilson's disease is the serum ceruloplasmin assay. A value of <20 mg/dL (<0.2 g/L) suggests the diagnosis. However, a more recent prospective study showed that a low ceruloplasmin has only 6% positive predictive value. Therefore, a normal ceruloplasmin does not rule out the disorder, and a subnormal value doesn't confirm the diagnosis. If suspicion is high, two other important diagnostic steps are indicated:

1. An examination for Kayser–Fleischer rings is performed. These copper deposits in Deçemet's membrane near the limbus of the cornea will be seen in most, but not all patients with neurological symptoms if carefully sought with a slit-lamp examination. Kayser–Fleischer rings are absent 38–50% of the time when there is only hepatic involvement.

2. One must obtain a 24-hour urine for copper, which primarily reflects levels of non-ceruloplasmin-bound copper. If urine copper is >100 μg/day (>1.6 μmol/day), Wilson's disease is highly likely, especially in symptomatic patients. But a value >40 μg/day (>0.6 μmol/day) is still suggestive of the diagnosis. Especially for children, measuring the urinary excretion after D-penicillamine challenge (500 mg per os at the beginning and after 12 hours of the 24-hour collection) provides further evidence for Wilson's disease if the value is >1600 μg/day (>25 μmol/day).

Confirmation of the diagnosis of Wilson's disease usually requires a liver biopsy with quantitation of the liver copper. All patients with Wilson's disease will have a markedly elevated hepatic copper, >250 μg/g dry weight. Values <40 μg/g dry weight are felt to exclude the diagnosis. Cautions include using disposable biopsy needles and placing the sample in copper-free plasticware. Variable copper distribution in patients with cirrhosis can give inaccurate results if too small a biopsy core (<1 cm) is analyzed. Heterozygotes for the Wilson's disease gene often have low serum ceruloplasmin but usually have intermediate hepatic copper concentration. However, other cholestatic liver disorders such as primary biliary cirrhosis, sclerosing cholangitis, biliary obstruction or atresia, and Indian childhood cirrhosis can also display high liver copper concentrations. These entities are usually associated with normal or high serum ceruloplasmin and have other distinguishing features.

Treatment[1-3]

Because Wilson's disease is invariably fatal if untreated and because effective treatment resolves most problems and allows prolonged survival, every patient with Wilson's disease must begin uninterrupted lifelong therapy. A low copper diet is most important during the first year of therapy, with avoidance of such foods as shellfish, nuts, mushrooms, legumes, and organ meats such as liver. The mainstay of therapy is chelation of copper and the drug D-penicillamine is usually started first. Dosing of 250–500 mg/day is escalated in 250-mg increments every 4–7 days to a total of 1–1.5 g/day in divided doses given 1 hour before or 2 hours after meals. The drug chelates hepatic copper and allows rapid urinary excretion. Although most patients tolerate D-penicillamine, it often has hypersensitivity-type side effects, some of which are too serious to allow its continued use. In such cases another effective chelating agent, trientine, can be used. A third orally active chelating agent, tetrathiomolybdate, is being studied and may be available soon.

Oral zinc therapy has also been demonstrated as effective in lowering copper stores. Zinc works by inducing enterocyte metallothionein, which sequesters dietary copper, preventing absorption and promoting elimination as the enterocyte sloughs into the intestinal lumen. Although zinc was originally promoted only as maintenance therapy after successful chelation, it has also been effective for initial therapy in asymptomatic patients and is better tolerated than D-penicillamine. Zinc acetate 50 mg 3 times daily, and taken away from meals is the most popular form and may have slightly less gastric irritation that the gluconate or sulfate salts. Some patients, including the young girl presented, have too much dyspepsia and cannot tolerate zinc. Sometimes giving the doses with meals improves tolerance, but higher doses may be required to control copper. Adding oral zinc to chelation therapy is also being studied.

Monitoring Wilson's disease patients on therapy includes routine checking of liver function and injury tests, CBC, and checking for recurrence of neurologic and psychiatric symptoms. Although determining the total serum copper and calculation of the "nonceruloplasmin-bound copper" is not particularly helpful in making the diagnosis of Wilson's disease, it may be helpful in monitoring therapy. Total copper in μg/dL (reference range 60–190) minus 3 times the ceruloplasmin (in mg/dL) estimates the nonceruloplasmin copper and is <15 μg/dL in normals and in successfully treated Wilson's patients. Annual 24-hour urines for copper should be performed. Patients on chelation therapy should be excreting 200–500 μg/day (3–8 μmol/day) and if on zinc therapy, urinary copper excretion should be <75 μg/day (1.2 μmol/day).

Liver transplantation has been performed in a number of Wilson's disease patients, usually for fulminant liver failure. Transplantation is also indicated in patients who do not respond to chelation therapy or who cannot be managed with oral chelation therapy because of either noncompliance or drug sensitivities. The fact that liver transplantation completely resolves copper accumulation is further evidence that the defect of Wilson's disease is primarily one of hepatic excretion.

References

1. ROBERTS, E. A. AND SCHILSKY, M. L.: A practice guideline on Wilson's disease. *Hepatology* 37:1475–92, 2003.
2. GITLIN, J. D.: Wilson's disease. *Gastroenterology* 125:1868–77, 2003.
3. DHAWAN, A., TAYLOR, R. M., CHEESMAN, P., DE SILVA, P., KATSIYIANNAKIS, L., AND MIELI-VERGANI, G.: Wilson's disease in children: 37-year experience and revised King's score for liver transplantation. 11:441–8, 2005.

Case 13

Adult Male with New-Onset Ascites

Steven I. Shedlofsky

A 56-year-old white male presented with abdominal and ankle swelling of several months' duration. There was no history of chronic medical problems, except for impotence over the past 3–4 years for which he occasionally took sildenafil. The patient was on no other medications. He was a successful accountant, married with three children. He was a $\frac{1}{2}$-pack/day smoker and drank two or three beers each day. His father had been killed during World War II, and he had an uncle who died of liver cirrhosis 10–15 years previously. He had two brothers and two sisters who were all in good health.

On physical examination the patient was well developed, looked tanned even though it was winter, weighed 196 lb (89 kg), and had normal vital signs. The patient had several prominent stigmata of chronic liver disease, including spider angiomata on his chest, palmar erythema, Dupuytren's contractures, testicular atrophy, and female escutcheon; however, he was anicteric. He had normal chest and normal cardiac findings, and his abdomen was protuberant, but not tense. There was no palpable or ballotable liver edge, but his spleen was felt just under the left costal border. On digital rectal examination he had prominent hemorrhoids and a normal prostate. A stool sample was brown and negative for occult blood. He had 2+ pitting ankle edema.

Initial laboratory results were as follows:

Analyte	Value, Conventional Units	Reference Interval, Conventional Units	Value, SI Units	Reference Interval, SI Units
Hemoglobin	14.5 g/dL	14–18	9.0 mmol/L	8.69–11.17
Hematocrit	43%	40–54	0.43	0.40–0.54
Leukocyte count	$4.9 \times 10^3/\mu L$	4.8–10.8	$4.9 \times 10^9/L$	4.8–10.8
MCV	92 fL	80–94	Same	
Platelet count	$93 \times 10^3/\mu L$	150–450	$93 \times 10^9/L$	150–450
Ethanol	0.0 mg/dL	0	0.0 mmol/L	0
Prothrombin	16.5 s	11–15	Same	
time, INR	1.34	0.8–1.2		

Tietz's Applied Laboratory Medicine, Second Edition. Edited by Mitchell G. Scott, Ann M. Gronowski, and Charles S. Eby

Analyte	Value, Conventional Units	Reference Interval, Conventional Units	Value, SI Units	Reference Interval, SI Units
Sodium	134 mmol/L	136–14	Same	
Potassium	3.6 mmol/L	3.8–5.1	Same	
Chloride	99 mmol/L	98–107	Same	
CO_2, total	27 mmol/L	23–31	Same	
Urea nitrogen	8 mg/dL	8–21	2.8 mmol urea/L	2.8–7.5
Creatinine	0.8 mg/dL	0.7–1.37	1 μmol/L	62–115
Glucose	148 mg/dL	80–115	8.2 mmol/L	4.4–6.4
Protein, total	6.4 g/dL	6.2–7.6	64 g/L	62–76
Albumin	2.9 g/dL	3.2–4.6	29 g/L	32–46
Cholesterol	182 mg/dL	140–220	4.70 mmol/L	3.62–5.69
Bilirubin, total	1.3 mg/dL	0.2–1.0	22 μmol/L	3–17
AST	62 U/L	19–48	1.03 μkat/L	0.32–0.80
ALT	71 U/L	13–40	1.18 μkat/L	0.22–0.67
ALP	82 U/L	56–119	1.4 μkat/L	0.9–2.0
GGT	27 U/L	10–50	0.45 μkat/L	0.17–0.83
Urinalysis	Within normal limits			
Urine sodium, random	5 mmol/L			Same

An ultrasonographic scan of the abdomen showed marked ascites with an inhomogeneous, coarsened liver not containing any intrahepatic masses, an intact gallbladder without gallstones, and an enlarged spleen of 17.5 cm. Seven liters of peritoneal fluid was drained and the patient received albumin (42 g) after the procedure. Analysis of the fluid demonstrated a total leukocyte count of $75 \times 10^3/\mu L$ ($75 \times 10^9/L$), 20% of which were granulocytes; total protein, 0.9 g/dL (9 g/L); albumin, <0.8 g/dL (<8 g/L); glucose, 120 mg/dL (6.7 mmol/L); amylase, 81 U/L (1.35 μkat/L); and LDH, 80 U/L (1.33 μkat/L). The Gram stain was negative, as was cytological examination for malignant cells. The serum ascites albumin gradient (SAAG) was >2.1 g/dL (2.9 minus <0.8) and deemed to be due to portal hypertension.

The patient was started on spironolactone (200 mg/day) and furosemide (20 mg bid) and placed on a diet of 2 g sodium/day. There was a rapid diuresis of 20 lb (9 kg) over the next 2 weeks with resolution of his ankle edema as well as less abdominal fullness. Further laboratory studies to evaluate causes for chronic liver disease were reported as follows:

Analyte	Value, Conventional Units	Reference Interval, Conventional Units	Value, SI Units	Reference Interval, SI Units
HbsAg	Negative	Negative	Same	
Anti–hepatitis C Ab	Negative	Negative	Same	
Antinuclear Ab	Negative	Negative	Same	
Anti-smooth-muscle Ab	Negative	Negative	Same	
Antiliver/kidney microsomal Ab	Negative	Negative	Same	
α_1-Antitrypsin	132 mg/dL	78–200	1.3 g/L	0.8–2.0
Phenotype	M_1M_1			
Ceruloplasmin	30 mg/dL	18–45	300 mg/L	180–450
Iron, total	316 μg/dL	65–170	57 μmol/L	12–30
TIBC	312 μg/dL	250–425	56 μmol/L	45–76

Analyte	Value, Conventional Units	Reference Interval, Conventional Units	Value, SI Units	Reference Interval, SI Units
Transferrin saturation	98%	20–50	0.98	0.20–0.50
Ferritin	4675 ng/mL	17–270	4675 μg/L	17–270

Because of his abnormal serum iron and transferrin saturation values, a diagnosis of hereditary hemochromatosis (HH) causing cirrhosis and portal hypertension was suspected. Confirmation of HH was made by molecular analysis for the G845A (C282Y) mutation of the HFE gene[1] using PCR amplification of peripheral WBC DNA followed by enzymatic digestion with Rsa1. The patient was homozygous for this common mutation.

A liver biopsy was planned to confirm the diagnosis of cirrhosis and assess the degree of hepatic iron overload, but could not be performed until the patient's ascites was resolved. After several weeks of diuresis and a repeat ultrasonographic examination that showed no residual ascites, his liver biopsy revealed cirrhosis with marked iron deposition (4+) in hepatocytes and Kupffer cells. A quantitative iron determination on the biopsy sample showed 360 μmol/g dry weight (reference range, 5–22), and his "iron index" (liver iron divided by age) was $360/56 = 6.4$ (see Discussion section). His serum α-fetoprotein concentration was 1.2 ng/mL (1.2 μg/L; reference range, <15). HFE molecular analysis of his siblings revealed that one sister was homozygous for C282Y mutation and a sister and brother were each heterozygous. Neither of the heterozygous siblings had the H63D mutation. None of the patient's siblings had evidence of excess iron, although the homozygote sister had a transferrin saturation of 80% (0.80).

The patient stopped all alcohol intake. An esophagogastroduodenoscopy (EGD) was normal with no esophageal or gastric varices noted. Weekly to biweekly phlebotomies of 500 mL were begun. After 17 months, and removal of 45 units of blood, the patient's serum ferritin was 24 ng/mL (24 μg/L), his transferrin saturation was 27%, and his hematocrit had fallen to 37% (0.37). His AST and ALT returned to normal. Although his initial glucose had been high on presentation, he never developed overt diabetes, and a hemoglobin A_1c was 5.7%. After several years of taking spironolactone (50 mg/day), the patient discontinued the drug. His ascites recurred, and a repeat paracentesis again showed a low leukocyte count with a wide SAAG. He responded to reinstitution of therapy but required larger doses. He continued to have therapeutic phlebotomies 3–5 times a year and has remained relatively stable with serum ferritins in the 30–50 ng/mL range, eight years after his diagnosis was made. Unfortunately he has been unable to work for the past 2 years owing to weakness and difficulty concentrating. Results of biannual determinations of α-fetoprotein have remained low and annual ultrasounds remain unchanged. However, a repeat EGD showed the development of varices and the patient was placed on a nonselective β-blocker (nadolol 40 mg/day).

Evaluation and Management of New-Onset Ascites

Although cirrhosis of the liver with resulting portal hypertension is the most common cause of ascites, there are many other possible etiological factors, such as right-sided heart failure, constrictive pericarditis, malignancies, chronic peritoneal infection (especially tuberculosis), pancreatic duct leak, and hypothyroidism. Therefore, every patient with ascites should have an examination of the ascitic fluid obtained by paracentesis that assesses cell and differential count, cytology, glucose, LDH, amylase, total protein, and albumin.[2] Determining the difference between serum and ascitic fluid albumin concentrations (the "serum-ascites albumin gradient") has been found particularly useful for differential diagnosis; a "wide gradient" (>1.1 g/dL) suggests that the ascites is due to chronic liver disease or cardiac failure, whereas a "narrow gradient" (<1.2 g/dL) suggests peritoneal carcinoma, peritoneal inflammation, or a hollow organ leak.

The goal of therapy in patients with portal hypertensive ascites is to eliminate the peritoneal fluid accumulation, which not only is uncomfortable for the patient and can cause respiratory compromise but also puts the patient at increased risk of a peritoneal infection. Indeed, the most important reason for performing a paracentesis on all patients who present with ascites is to determine whether they have spontaneous bacterial peritonitis (SBP).[2] Poor coagulation status is *not* a contraindication to performing the paracentesis. SBP has a very poor prognosis unless aggressively treated with antibiotics. A diagnosis of SBP is made immediately if the peritoneal fluid *granulocyte* count (not total leukocyte count) is $>250 \times 10^3/\mu L$ ($>250 \times 10^9/L$). Culture of peritoneal fluid can be 91% sensitive for diagnosis of SBP; but the culture medium must be inoculated at the bedside and results are often not available for several days. Gram stain of peritoneal fluid is not very sensitive for detecting and identifying organisms. Prophylactic use of antibiotics in selected patients with recurrent SBP is recommended, but routine use in all patients with ascites only leads to SBP with resistant organisms.

Fortunately for the patient under discussion, his ascites was due to portal hypertension and was noninfected with a low granulocyte count. It resolved relatively easily with diuretics and a sodium-restricted diet.

Pathophysiology, Diagnosis, and Management of Hereditary Hemochromatosis

Hereditary hemochromatosis (HH) is a relatively common homozygous recessive disorder with variable penetrance due to a cysteine to tyrosine substitution at amino acid 282 (C282Y) of the HFE protein.[1] The HH genotype can be detected in approximately 1:250–1:400 Caucasians, but less than 1% of HFE homozygotes and compound heterozygotes appear to have a clinically significant iron overload phenotype.[3-7] The incidence of the C282Y mutation in non-Caucasian populations is very low. But many other genetic causes of iron overload occur at much lower rates in both Caucasians and non-Caucasians as a result of mutations in other iron-metabolism proteins. However, the wide availability of molecular testing has made the identification of C282Y and H63D HFE mutations an important part of the evaluation of iron-overloaded Caucasian patients and has replaced HLA testing. The H63D mutation is relevant only if there is heterozygosity for C282Y, since "compound heterozygotes" are at risk for iron overload. Heterozygotes for C282Y and heterozygotes and homozygotes for the H63D mutation alone are not at risk.

In normal individuals, all dietary iron is absorbed from the duodenum and proximal jejunum where enterocytes regulate the amount of iron transported across the basolateral membrane into the body on the basis of the body's iron requirements.[5] Unneeded iron is sequestered within the enterocyte as cellular ferritin and is lost into the GI tract as the enterocyte migrates to the villus tip and is sloughed. However, in HH the ability to regulate this process is lost and there is abnormally high duodenal absorption of dietary iron over the subject's lifetime. There may also be dysregulation of iron sequestration within macrophages throughout the body. These defects lead to iron deposition and damage to a number of organs, including the liver, pancreas, heart, pituitary, and synovium.

Much new and exciting information has been learned about absorption, transport, and cellular iron regulation since the mid-1990s, with the molecular identification not only of the HFE protein but also of most of the iron uptake and transport proteins. Excellent detailed reviews are available.[5,6] Hepcidin is a 25-amino-acid liver-derived peptide that negatively regulates intestinal iron absorption and also regulates macrophage iron metabolism. Patients with HH have inappropriately low serum hepcidin. But how the mutant HFE protein causes this situation is still unclear. Decreased hepatic hepcidin production might also explain the mild iron overload often seen in patients with various liver diseases such as alcoholic and hepatitis C–induced liver disease.

The appropriate way to screen for HH is to determine serum iron and total iron-binding capacity (TIBC), with calculation of the percent transferrin saturation.[7] Because of the diurnal variation in serum iron concentrations, *fasting* morning specimens are recommended. HH is suspected if the transferrin saturation is >60% in men and >50% in women. Ferritin, an important iron-binding and intracellular iron storage protein, should also be measured in the serum of patients with suspected HH. Serum ferritin is *not* an iron transport protein, and the presence of ferritin in the serum probably represents protein that "leaks" out of macrophages that are processing iron. Serum ferritin does not become elevated early in HH and only increases with heavy iron loading when iron spills over from hepatocytes into the reticuloendothelial system. In non-HH patients, serum ferritin is increased with acute hepatocyte damage (acute hepatitis) or if there is a systemic inflammatory reaction or certain hematologic malignancies. Therefore, an elevated serum ferritin value should be interpreted with caution. But in most HH patients serum ferritin is a good reflection of total body iron stores and is used to monitor iron reduction therapy.

Iron loading in HH can affect several organs, with the manifestations of end-organ damage usually appearing in the 40s–60s age range in men and slightly later in women. Women are somewhat protected since they lose iron over many years with menses. In the liver, iron overload can lead first to occult, then clinically evident cirrhosis, and eventually to development of malignant hepatoma. In the pancreas, iron loading of the islets of Langerhans causes glucose intolerance or frank diabetes. Cardiomyopathies and arrhythmias can develop with iron deposition in cardiac myocytes. Testicular atrophy and impotence occur in men as a result of decreased gonadotropin production by the iron-loaded pituitary. Women can develop secondary amenorrhea. Chondrocalcinosis develops in joint synovia and leads to a pseudogout picture. Hyperpigmentation of skin may be observed, but is actually due to increased melanin rather than iron deposition. Because each of these manifestations more often are caused by factors other than HH, a physician must cultivate a high index of suspicion for the disease and utilize screening tests.

On finding a high percent transferrin saturation and homozygosity for the C282Y mutation, the degree of hepatic injury is assessed with a liver biopsy with special stains for iron deposits (Prussian blue or Perls' stain) and by quantitative determination of iron content of liver tissue. If the patient is relatively young, <age 30, liver biopsy is probably not necessary as long as all other liver tests are normal. An "iron index" can be calculated from the iron content of liver (in μmol/g of dry liver) divided by the age of the subject, and an index >1.9 is usually found in HH homozygotes. But the importance of calculating the iron index is much less now that HFE genetic testing is available. Once the diagnosis of HH is made on the basis of laboratory (including HFE analysis), biopsy, and clinical results, one should not forget to screen siblings with iron studies and HFE molecular testing. It is less important to screen children who are obligate heterozygotes as they generally have no significant risk of iron overload (unless the patient's spouse is an HFE heterozygote or homozygote).

Fortunately for iron-overloaded HH patients, phlebotomy therapy is a highly effective method for lowering body iron stores. Every 500 mL of blood removed contains ∼250 mg of iron. Phlebotomies are usually instituted every 1–2 weeks while keeping the patient on a high-protein and folate-supplemented diet. Immediately prior to the phlebotomy, patients should have a light snack and take in fluids. The removed blood can be used by blood banks (although some centers post "warnings" that the blood was obtained for therapeutic reasons). The goal of phlebotomy therapy is to lower the serum ferritin to < 100 ng/mL (< 100 µg/L) and a transferrin saturation around 30% and then find a phlebotomy frequency (usually every 2–4 months) that keeps the ferritin and transferrin saturation within normal range without causing iron deficiency or anemia. Treated precirrhotic HH patients have been shown to have a normal life expectancy. But once cirrhosis or diabetes develops, HH patients have markedly shortened lifespans. Occasionally HH patients require liver transplantation, but often do poorly afterwards because of cardiac problems and infections.

The importance of identifying HH in patients who present with cirrhosis, diabetes, cardiomyopathy, chondrocalcinosis, or impotence cannot be overstressed because iron removal therapy is safe and generally effective if instituted early. Usually cirrhosis, diabetes, and impotence are not reversible. If homozygotes are recognized early, prior to development of symptoms of end-organ damage, preventive (prophylactic) treatment is easily initiated by prescribing regular blood donation to reduce the rate of iron loading. Serum iron determination as part of a *fasting* morning chemistry screening panel was shown to help in early identification of iron-overloaded homozygotes and was cost-effective.[8] In this study identifying serum irons of ≥ 180 µg/dL led to further testing in 1% of patients that included transferrin saturation and ferritin. Eight of 127 identified patients were recommended for a liver biopsy, with four unsuspected cases of clinically significant HH discovered. However, only a few large institutions such as the Kaiser-Permanente Health Care System have adopted screening for iron overload.[5] Screening with HFE mutational analysis is too expensive and will not identify patients who are iron-overloaded because of the low penetrance of this mutation.

References

1. FEDER, J. N., GNIRKE, A., THOMAS, W. ET AL.: A novel MHC class I-like gene is mutated in patients with hereditary hemochromatosis. *Nat. Genet. 13*:399–408, 1996.
2. RUNYON, B. A.: Management of adult patients with ascites due to cirrhosis. *Hepatology 39*:841–56, 2004.
3. PIETRANGELO, A.: Hereditary hemochromatosis—a new look at an old disease. *N. Engl. J. Med. 350*:2383–97, 2004.
4. BEUTLER, E., FELITTI, V. J., KOZIOL, J. A., HO, N. J., AND GELBART, T.: Penetrance of 845G->A (C282Y) HFE hereditary hemochromatosis mutation in the USA. *Lancet 359*:211–18, 2002.
5. HEENY, M. M. AND ANDREWS, N. C.: Iron homeostasis and inherited iron overload disorders: An overview.

Am. Hematol. Oncol. Clin. North Am. 18:1379–403, 2004.
6. SHARMA, N., BUTTERWORTH, J., COOPER, B. T., TSELEPIS, C., AND IQBAL, T. H.: The emerging role of the liver in iron metabolism. *Am. J. Gastroenterol. 100*:201–6, 2005.
7. FLEMING, R. E., BRITTON, R. S., WAHEED, A., SLY, W. S., AND BACON, B. R.: Pathogenesis of hereditary hemochromatosis. *Clin. Liver Dis. 8*:755–73, 2004.
8. BALAN, V., BALDUS, W., FAIRBANKS, V., MICHELS, V., BURRITT, M., AND KLEE, G.: Screening for hemochromatosis: A cost-effectiveness study based on 12,258 patients. *Gastroenterology 107*:453–9, 1994.

Case 14

An Unexpected Finding . . . .

Nathan C. Walk

A 30-year-old Caucasian medical student with no past medical history underwent a routine checkup by his primary care provider. History was as follows:

Review of systems — No complaints—"just want to make sure everything is okay"
Past medical history — Broken leg at age 17
Family history — Hypertension in mother, lung cancer in deceased grandfather (smoker)
Social history — Denies smoking, alcohol, or drug use
Medications — None
Allergies — No known drug allergies

On physical examination, his vitals signs were stable with a blood pressure of 118/70 and a heart rate of 74. He appeared anxious, but well nourished and healthy. Auscultation of the chest demonstrated a regular cardiac rate and rhythm. The lungs were clear bilaterally. The abdomen was soft, nontender, and nondistended; no hepatomegaly or splenomegaly was appreciated. Peripheral extremities were unremarkable.

A complete blood count (CBC) and complete metabolic panel (CMP) were ordered *at the student's request*. The student admitted to being a bit "overly cautious." The CBC was normal and the CMP results were as follows:

Analyte	Value, Conventional Units	Reference Interval, Conventional Units	Value, SI Units	Reference Interval, SI Units
Sodium	144 mmol/L	132–146	Same	
Potassium	4.3 mmol/L	3.5–5.1	Same	
Chloride	105 mmol/L	98–107	Same	
CO_2, total	25 mmol/L	22–28	Same	
BUN	11 mg/dL	6–20	3.9 mmol/L	2.1–7.1
Glucose	84 mg/dL	74–100	4.7 mmol/L	4.1–5.6
Protein, total	7.5 g/dL	6.4–8.3	75 g/L	64–83
Albumin	5.3 g/dL	3.5–5.2	53 g/L	35–52
AST	17 U/L	<35	0.29 μkat/L	<0.60
ALT	22 U/L	<45	0.37 μkat/L	<0.77
Bilirubin, total	4.7 mg/dL	0–2.0	80.4 μmol/L	0–34
Bilirubin, conjugated	0.4 mg/dL	0.0–0.2	6.8 μmol/L	0.0–3.4

Tietz's Applied Laboratory Medicine, Second Edition. Edited by Mitchell G. Scott, Ann M. Gronowski, and Charles S. Eby
Copyright © 2007 John Wiley & Sons, Inc.

The elevated unconjugated hyperbilirubinemia was noted, and several follow-up tests were ordered. Although the patient had no upper quadrant pain, a RUQ (right upper quadrant) ultrasound was performed to evaluate for cholelithiasis and/or liver pathology. It was unremarkable.

The patient's blood was sent for DNA testing for Gilbert's syndrome and came back positive for the homozygous polymorphism, A(TA)$_7$TAA, in the promoter of the UGT1A1 gene. The UGT1A1 gene encodes the similarly named protein, the hepatic enzyme necessary for conjugation of bilirubin.

Definition of Disease

Gilbert's syndrome was first described in 1901 by Augustine Gilbert and Pierre Lereboullet. Patients with Gilbert's syndrome have mild, chronic unconjugated hyperbilirubinemia in the absence of liver disease or hemolysis; the bilirubin typically ranges within 3–6 mg/dL (51.3–102.6 μmol/L). Gilbert's syndrome is the most common inherited cause of unconjugated hyperbilirubinemia (Gilbert's syndrome and other causes are listed in Table 14.1); 3–10% of the population are estimated to have Gilbert's syndrome.[1,2]

Gilbert's syndrome is harmless in adults. It is important to recognize, however, because detection of hyperbilirubinemia may raise the possibility of subclinical liver disease and instigate an extensive and unnecessary laboratory workup. Patients will occasionally complain of abdominal discomfort and general fatigue, but neither these nor any other symptoms have been definitively linked to Gilbert's syndrome. Typically, jaundice in these patients fluctuates, with exacerbations following prolonged fasting, surgery, infection, excessive exercise, or ethanol consumption. The patient is often unaware of the jaundice until it is detected by physical examination or routine laboratory testing. Liver function tests are normal, and the liver appears normal on microscopic examination.

Table 14.1   Hereditary Hyperbilirubinemias

Disorder	Inheritance[a]	Defect in metabolism of bilirubin	Clinical course
Unconjugated hyperbilirubinemia			
Crigler–Naijar syndrome, type I	Ar	Absent UGT1 activity	Fatal in neonatal period
Crigler–Naijar syndrome, type II	AD, variable penetrance	Decreased UGT1 activity	Mild, occasional kernicterus
Gilbert's syndrome	Ar	Decreased UGT1 activity	Innocuous
Conjugated hyperbilirubinemia			
Dubin–Johnson syndrome	Ar	Impaired biliary excretion of bilirubin	Innocuous
Rotor syndrome	Ar	Impaired biliary excretion of bilirubin	Innocuous

[a]Ar, autosomal recessive; AD, autosomal dominant.

Differential Diagnosis

The disorders of bilirubin metabolism can be divided into five major categories: (1) increased production, (2) decreased hepatic uptake, (3) impaired hepatic conjugation, (4) decreased secretion into the biliary tract, and (5) decreased excretion into the small intestine. The first three of these are associated with unconjuated hyperbilirubinemia and the latter two, with a conjugated hyperbilirubinemia.

In general, the diagnosis of Gilbert's syndrome is made by exclusion of other entities associated with elevated unconjugated bilirubin. Although the list of diseases that can cause an elevation in unconjugated hyperbilirubinemia is rather extensive, the differential diagnosis in most cases comes down to hemolysis, liver disease, and Gilbert's syndrome. This is in part because most other causes of hyperbilirubinemia typically cause a concomitant and more pronounced rise in the conjugated form.

Diagnosis of Gilbert's syndrome typically is one of exclusion, made in the presence of (1) unconjugated hyperbilirubinemia noted on several occasions; (2) normal CBC, reticulocyte count, and blood smear; (3) normal liver function test results; and (4) absence of other disease processes. A diagnosis of exclusion is always less satisfactory than a positive confirmation; particularly in situations where the clinical scenario is more nebulous, a physician may seek harder to exclude liver problems. Additional testing is frequently performed. Perhaps the most promising of additional testing modalities, in caucasian patients whom Gilbert's is suspected, is the PCR-based test for the polymorphism in the promoter of the UGT1A1 gene (discussed below). Other tests which may be useful in the evaluation include

- *Fasting*—when placed on a 300 kcal diet per day for 2 days, patients with Gilbert's will increase their serum bilirubin by approximately 1.5 mg/dL (25 μmol/L); the major increase is in the unconjugated fraction. Healthy controls and patients with hemolysis do not show a significant increase.
- *RUQ ultrasound*—exclusion of lithiasis, evaluation of gross liver pathology.
- *Liver biopsy*—definitive exclusion of active liver disease.
- *HPLC measurement of conjugated/unconjugated bilirubin*—provides a more specific measurement than enzymatic methods.

Pathogenesis

In order to understand the pathogenesis of Gilbert's syndrome, it is necessary for a brief overview of bilirubin metabolism. As mentioned previously, disorders of bilirubin metabolism can be divided into five major categories. Of note, the secretion of bilirubin into the biliary tract is rate-limiting, and most susceptible to impairment with liver damage[3]—hence, most cases of liver disease will see a rise in *both* conjugated and unconjugated bilirubin.

Production

Bilirubin is the end product of heme metabolism. The daily production of heme in healthy individuals ranges from 0.2 to 0.3 g, the majority the result of breakdown of senescent red blood cells by the mononuclear phagocyte system. The remainder of heme is derived from turnover of hepatic heme or hemoproteins and from premature destruction of newly formed red blood cells in the bone marrow. Within the phagocytic system, heme is degraded to biliverdin by heme oxygenase, then to bilirubin by biliverdin reductase. Unconjugated bilirubin is nonpolar, and must be complexed with albumin in the blood to make it water soluble for delivery to the liver.

Uptake

Uptake into hepatocytes is via diffusion or facilitated transport. This involves binding of bilirubin to anion-binding proteins. This step is usually not an important point of impairment in bilirubin metabolism, although some drugs, such as rifampin, are known to interfere at this step.

Conjugation

Bilirubin, still in its unconjugated form at this point, is then glucuronidated, or conjugated, to make it water-soluble. This is necessary for the release and solubilizing of bilirubin in bile, as no albumin is present in bile for binding. The enzyme responsible for glucuronidation of bilirubin in human liver is UDP–glucuronosyltransferase (bilirubin/uridine diphosphoglucuronate–glucuronosyltransferase), or UGT. This enzyme is located in the endoplasmic reticulum. Of the two isoforms reported, only UGT1A1 contributes significantly to bilirubin glucuronidation.[4,5]

Secretion

Conjugated bilirubin is then secreted by an energy-dependent process into bile. This process is still incompletely understood, but is the rate-limiting step in hepatic metabolism of bilirubin. Impairment in secretion is present in Rotor's and Dubin–Johnson syndromes, which present with a conjugated hyperbilirubinemia.

Excretion

Excretion of conjugated bilirubin into the small intestine occurs via the biliary tract with delivery of bile to the ampulla of Vater. Any disruption of this delivery pathway by compression, blockage, or obliteration of the biliary ducts will result in bile backup, consequent reabsorption of bilirubin, and a conjugated hyperbilirubinemia.

Unconjugated hyperbilirubinemia in Gilbert's syndrome is the result of decreased hepatic glucuronidating activity. The molecular basis for Gilbert's syndrome lies in one of two types of mutations associated with the UGT1A1 gene. The first, which occurs in nearly all cases in Caucasians, is a dinucleotide polymorphism in the TATA box promoter of the UGT1A1 gene, where A(TA)$_7$TAA replaces A(TA)$_6$TAA.[6-8] The insertion of the extra TA in the promoter decreases transcription of the gene; patients who are homozygous for the A(TA)$_7$TAA allele have UGT1A1 production that is approximately 30% of normal.[9] In the Caucasian population, the frequency of the A(TA)$_7$TAA allele is approximately 35%; almost all Caucasian patients with Gilbert's syndrome are associated with homozygosity for this polymorphism and *no* associated coding mutation (discussed below).[6,7] On the other hand, the frequency of this polymorphism in the Japanese population is only 11%, and only one-third of Japanese patients with Gilbert's syndrome are associated with homozygosity at this site without an associated coding mutation.

The second type of mutation, rare in Caucasians but common in Asians, is caused by missense mutations in the coding region of the UGT1A1 gene.[10] Several missense mutations have been described, including G71R and P229Q.[11] The possibility of coding mutations, for which a patient may be heterozygous, homozygous, or compound heterozygous, and one or both copies of the A(TA)$_7$TAA promoter allele, allows for a range of phenotypes in this population. In addition, an additional missense mutation, Y486D, with or without the accompanying G71R mutation, has been associated with Crigler–Naijjar syndrome type II.[12] It is clear that in the Asian population the range of mutations affecting the UGT1A1 gene are more diverse, the phenotypes more complex, and as of yet, the situation not fully understood.

Treatment

The course for Gilbert's syndrome is benign, and hence no treatment is necessary. Definitive diagnosis via genetic testing can prevent an extensive and unnecessary clinical workup and provide patients with some peace of mind.

References

1. OWENS, D. AND EVANS, J.: Population studies on Gilbert's syndrome. *J. Med. Genet. 12*:152–6, 1975.
2. BAILEY, A., ROBINSON, D., AND DAWSON, A. M.: Does Gilbert's disease exist? *Lancet 1*:931–3, 1977.
3. KAPLAN, L. M., AND ISSELBACHER, K. J.: Jaundice. In *Harrison's Principles of Internal Medicine*, 14th ed., A. S. FAUCI, E. BRAUNWALD, AND K. J. ISSELBACHER, ET AL., eds., McGraw-Hill, New York, 1998, pp. 249–54.
4. RITTER, J. K., CRAWFORD, J. M., AND OWENS, I. S.: Cloning of two human liver bilirubin UDP-glucuronosyltransferase cDNAs with expression in COS-1 cells. *J. Biol. Chem. 266*:1043–7, 1991.
5. BOSMA, P. J., SEPPEN, J., GOLDHOORN, B. ET AL.: Bilirubin UDP-glucuronosyltransferase 1 is the only relevant bilirubin glucuronidating isoform in man. *J. Biol. Chem. 269*:17960–4, 1994.
6. BOSMA, P. J., CHOWDHURY, J. R., AND BAKKER, C. ET AL.: The genetic basis of the reduced expression of bilirubin UDP-glucuronosyltransferase 1 in Gilbert's syndrome. *N. Engl. J. Med. 333*:1171–5, 1995.
7. MONAGHAN, G., RYAN, M., SEDDON, R., HUME, R., AND BURCHELL, B.: Genetic variation in bilirubin UPD-glucuronosyltransferase gene promoter and Gilbert's syndrome. *Lancet 347*:578–81, 1996.
8. JANSEN, P. L., BOSMA, P. J., BAKKER, C., LEMS, S. P., Slooff, M. J., AND HAAGSMA, E. B.: Persistent unconjugated hyperbilirubinemia after liver transplantation due to an abnormal bilirubin UDP-glucuronosyltransferase gene promoter sequence in the donor. *J. Hepatol. 27*:1–5, 1997.
9. BLACK, M., AND BILLING, B. H.: Hepatic bilirubin UDP-glucuronyl transferase activity in liver disease AND Gilbert's syndrome. *N. Engl. J. Med. 280*:1266–71, 1969.
10. KOIWAI, O., NISHIZAWA, M., HASADA, K. ET AL.: Gilbert's syndrome is caused by a heterozygous missense mutation in the gene for bilirubin UDP-glucuronosyltransferase. *Hum. Mol. Genet., 4*:1183–6, 1995.
11. KAMISAKO, T.: What is Gilbert's syndrome? Lesson from genetic polymorphisms of UGT1A1 in Gilbert's syndrome from Asia. *J. Gastroent. Hepatol. 19*:955–57, 2004.
12. TAKEUCHI, K., KOBAYASHI, Y., TAMAKI, S. ET AL.: Genetic polymorphism of bilirubin UDP-glucuronosyltransferase in Japanese patients with Crigler Najjar syndrome or Gilbert's syndrome as well as in healthy Japanese subjects. *J. Gastroenterol. Hepatol. 19*:1023–8, 2004.

Case 15

I Did It Just Once—A 37-Year-Old Man with Hepatitis C

Alvaro Koch and Luis R. Peña

This 37-year-old white male, a native of Appalachia, worked as a banker and was married with two children. He had no significant past medical history. The bank closed the local branch and laid him off while transferring others. He could not find a job despite multiple efforts and interviews. He started frequenting bars and became acquainted with a group of people who used drugs. After much insistence from his peers, he decided to try a dose of intravenous cocaine. A partner injected him with a needle that had been previously used by others in the group. Three weeks later, and because of concerns about infections, he visited his primary care physician (PCP), who ordered acute hepatitis and HIV viral serologies and liver tests. The hepatitis C antibody (anti-HCV) and anti-HIV were negative, and liver enzymes were mildly elevated to less than 2 times the upper limit of normal (ULN). His PCP discussed these findings and the clinical history with a specialist in a close tertiary center. Because of the high index of suspicion, the specialist recommended obtaining a qualitative reverse transcriptase polymerase chain reaction (RT-PCR) for hepatitis C (HCV) RNA, which was positive. Five weeks later the patient started experiencing significant malaise, myalgias, and flulike symptoms. His appetite was poor. He visited his PCP again. He did not report fever, acholic stools, choluria, jaundice, or icterus. He did complain of some nausea but not vomiting. Physical examination demonstrated the patient to be a well-developed, well-nourished man appearing his stated age. He stated that he had not used drugs again, claiming he did it just the one time. Blood pressure was 126/67 mm Hg, pulse 75 bpm, respirations 16/min, and temperature 98.6°F (37°C). The patient was hydrated with no jaundice or icterus. The abdomen was soft and nondistended but mildly tender to palpation in the right upper quadrant; the liver was enlarged to 8 cm below the costal margin. The spleen was not palpable. There was pain to punch percussion in the lower ribcage. The rest of the physical examination was unremarkable. A hemogram, prothrombin time,

Tietz's Applied Laboratory Medicine, Second Edition. Edited by Mitchell G. Scott, Ann M. Gronowski, and Charles S. Eby

and comprehensive metabolic panel were obtained. Because of abnormalities, additional tests were immediately requested. Relevant results are listed below:

Analyte	Value, Conventional Units	Reference Interval, Conventional Units	Value, SI Units	Reference Interval, SI Units
Leukocyte count	$7.5 \times 10^3/\mu L$	4.0–10.5	$75 \times 10^9/L$	4–10.5
Hemoglobin	14.5 g/dL	13.5–17.2	9.06 mmol/L	7.45–9.93
Platelet count	$198 \times 10^3/\mu L$	150–450	$198 \times 10^9/L$	150–450
Prothrombin time (INR)	1.1	0.8–1.2		
Bilirubin, total	2.1 mg/dL	0.4–1.5	35.9 μmol/L	6.8–25.6
ALP	125 U/L	40–110	2.1 μkat/L	0.7–1.9
AST	1156 U/L	18–43	19.6 μkat/L	0.3–0.7
ALT	1689 U/L	17–60	28.7 μkat/L	0.3–1.0
GGT	68 U/L	12–43	1.2 μkat/L	0.2–0.7
Anti-HCV[a]	Positive	Negative		
HCV RNA$_{Qual}$PCR[b]	Positive	Negative		
HBsAg[c]	Negative	Negative		
Anti-HBc[d]	Negative	Negative		
Anti-HCV[e]	Negative	Negative		
RPR	Negative	Negative		

[a]Antibodies against hepatitis C virus.
[b]Qualitative RT-PCR for HCV RNA.
[c]Hepatitis B surface antigen.
[d]IgG and IgM antibodies against hepatitis B core antigen.
[e]Antibodies against HIV-1 and HIV-2.

On reviewing the chart, the result of the previous RT-PCR for HCV was found to be positive and the anti-HCV negative. With these findings the diagnosis of anicteric, acute hepatitis C was made. The case was reported to the local healthcare department. An appointment was made at a tertiary center to see a hepatologist for further management.

By the time the patient was seen by the hepatologist, almost 9 weeks had passed since his exposure, which in this case was easily identifiable due to the lack of other risk factors. The patient was feeling somewhat better but still complained of malaise. This physical exam revealed hepatomegaly, but not as painful and of a lesser degree. The patient was counseled about the risk of transmission and precautions to avoid it. The possibility of treatment was brought to discussion by the patient. The specialist advised him to wait until 12 weeks had passed since the time of the exposure before attempting treatment. The patient was advised to return in 3 weeks to obtain a new HCV RNA$_{Qual}$ PCR. The patient did not follow the recommendation. Five years later the patient showed up at the hepatologist's clinic. An update on his social and medical history revealed that the patient was divorced shortly after the time of infection and had started drinking heavily, about 2–3 fifths of vodka a week. He denied using drugs except for just the one time. He had also lost about 10 lb since his last visit. Updated tests showed the following:

Analyte	Value, Conventional Units	Reference Interval, Conventional Units	Value, SI Units	Reference Interval, SI Units
Leukocyte count	$5.3 \times 10^3/\mu L$	4.0–10.5	$5.3 \times 10^9/L$	4.4–10.5
Hemoglobin	13.5 g/dL	13.5–17.2	8.33 mmol/L	7.45–9.93

Analyte	Value, Conventional Units	Reference Interval, Conventional Units	Value, SI Units	Reference Interval, SI Units
MCV	109 fL	80–95	Same	
Platelet count	173 × 10³/μL	150–450	173 × 10⁹/L	150–450
Prothrombin time (INR)	1.1	0.8–1.2		
Bilirubin, total	1.5 mg/dL	0.4–1.5	25.6 μmol/L	6.8–25.6
ALP	145 U/L	40–110	2.5 μkat/L	0.7–1.9
AST	187 U/L	18–43	3.2 μkat/L	0.3–0.7
ALT	172 U/L	17–60	2.9 μkat/L	0.3–1.0
GGT	126 U/L	12–43	2.1 μkat/L	0.2–0.7
Anti-HCV	Positive	Negative		
HCV RNA$_{Qual}$PCR	Positive	Negative		
HBsAg	Negative	Negative		
Anti-HBc	Negative	Negative		
Anti-HCV	Negative	Negative		
RPR	Negative	Negative		

These results were discussed with the patient. He was interested in pursuing treatment. The patient was advised to stop drinking and return to the clinic after he had completed 6 months of complete sobriety. A prescription was written for vitamin B$_{12}$ 1000 μg subcutaneously once a month for 4 months, folic acid 1 mg daily for 30 days, and thiamine 100 mg daily for 30 days. He also received his first dose of hepatitis A and B vaccine and was instructed to complete the series.

The patient followed the physician's recommendations and presented to the clinic 6 months later for follow-up and to discuss treatment possibilities. Repeated blood tests showed the following:

Analyte	Value, Conventional Units	Reference Interval, Conventional Units	Value, SI Units	Reference Interval, SI Units
Leukocyte count	6.8 × 10³/μL	4.0–10.5	6.8 × 10⁹/L	4.0–10.5
Hemoglobin	13.9 g/dL	13.5–17.2	8.68 mmol/L	7.45–9.93
MCV	93 fL	80–95	Same	
Platelet count	184 × 10³/μL	150–450	184 × 10⁹/L	150–450
Prothrombin time (INR)	1.1	0.8–1.2	Same	
Bilirubin, total	1.3 mg/dL	0.4–1.5	22.2 μmol/L	6.8–25.6
ALP	105 U/L	40–110	1.8 μkat/L	0.7–1.9
AST	109 U/L	18–43	1.9 μkat/L	0.3–0.7
ALT	127 U/L	17–60	2.2 μkat/L	0.3–1.0
GGT	55 U/L	12–43	0.9 μkat/L	0.2–0.7
Hepatitis C genotype	1a			

An abdominal ultrasound showed increased echogenicity with an otherwise normal exam. A liver biopsy was performed and showed mild fatty changes, rare Mallory hyaline, grade 2–3 portal inflammation, grade 2 lobular inflammation, and stage 2 fibrosis.

The patient was started on treatment with a form of pegylated interferon (PEG) plus ribavirin (RIB). Baseline blood tests on day one before he received his first dose of PEG and RIB showed the following:

Analyte	Value, Conventional Units	Reference Interval, Conventional Units	Value, SI Units	Reference Interval, SI Units
Leukocyte count	$7.9 \times 10^3/\mu L$	4.0–10.5	$7.9 \times 10^9/L$	4.0–10.5
Absolute neutrophil count	$4.76 \times 10^3/\mu L$	1.7–8.4	$4.76 \times 10^9/L$	1.7–8.4
Hemoglobin	13.9 g/dL	13.5–17.2	8.68 mmol/L	7.45–9.93
MCV	84 fL	80–95		
Platelet count	$271 \times 10^3/\mu L$	150–450	$271 \times 10^9/L$	
TSH	2.34 μIU/mL	0.6–4.5	2.34 mIU/L	0.6–4.5
HCV RNA$_{Quant}$ PCR (viral load)[a]	837,000[b] IU/mL			

[a]HCV RNA$_{Quant}$ PCR: Quantitative RT-PCR for HCV RNA or viral load.
[b]4,017,600 copies/mL.

He tolerated treatment fairly well; major side effects were malaise and myalgias around the day of the injection that decreased in severity as the treatment progressed, weight loss of about 8 lb, and moderate insomnia. He also developed neutropenia and anemia as low as $0.865 \times 10^3/\mu L$ and 10.1 g/dL, respectively, which were well tolerated and did not require dose reduction. At the end of week 12 of treatment his viral load had dropped to 1850 IU/mL, and by the end of week 24 his HCV RNA$_{Qual}$ PCR was negative and remained negative throughout the remaining 24-week of treatment completing a total of 48 weeks. A repeated HCV RNA$_{Qual}$ PCR 24-week after finishing his treatment was also negative.

Types of Hepatitis

The liver responds to any injury in three different ways: (1) inflammation, generically called *hepatitis*, which can be of different nature (leukocytic, lymphocytic, plasmo[a]cytic, etc.); (2) cholestasis, which represents an impairment of the bile flow at any point from the sinusoidal membrane to the extrahepatic bile ducts; and (3) a combination of both. Cholestasis can be caused by drugs, toxins, virus, and blockage of the biliary tree at any level and from multiple causes (stones, strictures, tumors, etc.). A cholestatic injury is characterized by elevation of alkaline phosphatase and bilirubin, which is normally secreted into bile. Cholestatic injury may occur in a pure form with no evident parenchymal damage or may be accompanied by hepatocellular damage.[1] A hepatitic injury is characterized by an elevation of transaminases and represents hepatocellular damage and necrosis. It can be related to multiple causes such as bacteria, drugs, toxins, virus, autoimmunity, metabolic disorders, or circulatory failure. Hepatitis presents clinically with findings that are nonspecific and insufficient to identify the cause; laboratory studies are essential for doing so.

Hepatitis can present in three different forms—fulminant, acute or chronic—and may range in severity from a completely asymptomatic condition to a fatal fulminant hepatic failure. Viruses are the most common cause of hepatitis and among them hepatitis A, B, and C are the most common. For viral hepatitis, the routes of transmission and the epidemiology, as well as the morbidity and mortality, vary among these three agents.

Hepatitis A virus (HAV) is one of the most common causes of acute viral hepatitis and it is closely related to sanitary conditions and therefore endemic in developing countries.

The route of transmission is fecal–oral through contaminated water and food. Most cases of hepatitis A are asymptomatic or exhibit only minor and nonspecific constitutional or gastrointestinal symptoms that abate within a few days. The asymptomatic form occurs in most children and in up to 10% of adults, and it usually goes undiagnosed. Hepatitis A can also presents as fulminant hepatic failure. Acute hepatitis A is diagnosed by the presence of IgM antibodies (IgM anti-HAV), which can be detected early before the patient becomes symptomatic, and represents a marker of acute infection. The IgM anti-HAV decrease very rapidly and are replaced by IgG antibodies (IgG anti-HAV), which persist for life and confer lifelong immunity. Clinically there are two tests available: (1) IgM anti-HAV, whose presence makes the diagnosis of acute hapatitis A; and (2) total (IgG + IgM) anti-HAV, whose presence represents acute or past exposure to hepatitis A and will also be positive in vaccinated individuals. Hepatitis A does not evolve to a chronic form and there is no carrier state for HAV. Currently there is a vaccine available for HAV with a vaccination efficacy rate of 94–100%.

Hepatitis B (HBV)[2] is one of the most common infectious diseases in the world, affecting 5% of the world's population. Approximately 70–80% of infected individuals reside in Asia and the western Pacific, where it represents a major public health problem. Vertical transmission from mother to neonate accounts for the majority of new infections in the world today, and it is the main form of transmission in highly

Interpretation of the Hepatitis B Panel.[9]

Tests	Results	Interpretation
HBsAg	Negative	Susceptible
Anti-HBc	Negative	
Anti-HBs	Negative	
HBsAg	Negative	Immune due to natural infection
Anti-HBc	Positive	
Anti-HBs	Positive	
HBsAg	Negative	Immune due to hepatitis B vaccination
Anti-HBc	Negative	
Anti-HBs	Positive	
HBsAg	Positive	Acutely infected
Anti-HBc	Positive	
IgM anti-HBc	Positive	
HBsAg	Positive	Chronically infected
Anti-HBc	Positive	
IgM anti-HBc	Negative	
Anti-HBs	Negative	
HBsAg	Negative	Four interpretations possible[a]
Anti-HBc	Positive	
Anti-HBs	Positive	

[a]Interpretations: (1) may be recovering from acute HBV infection, (2) may be distantly immune and test not sensitive enough to detect very low level of anti-HBs in serum, (3) may be susceptible with a false-positive anti-HBc, or (4) may be undetectable level of HBsAg present in the serum and the person is actually a carrier.

endemic areas. In less endemic areas (North America), hepatitis B is horizontally transmitted mainly through sexual contact, occupational exposure to contaminated blood or blood products, and sharing intravenous drug paraphernalia. Other less common sources of infection include household contact with an HBV carrier, hemodialysis, tattooing, body piercing, exposure to infected healthcare workers, and transplanted organs. HBV can also be found in saliva, semen, breast milk, and most other body fluids, with the exception of stool. About 95% of acutely infected immunocompetent adults will recover completely, with only 1–5% of cases becoming chronically infected. By contrast, ~95% of infected neonates become chronic carriers. Hepatitis B infection is one of the leading causes of cirrhosis and hepatocellular carcinoma (HCC). Definitive diagnosis of hepatitis B requires the understanding of HBV serologies and the information each test provides as described in the Table.

Hepatitis B surface antigen (HBsAg) is commonly used for diagnosing acute HBV infection or detecting carriers. It is the first viral marker to appear during an acute infection. Its persistence beyond 6 months typically characterizes the state of chronic carrier. The presence of HBsAg indicates that a person is infectious.

Hepatitis B surface antibody (HBsAb or anti-HBs) is a protective, neutralizing antibody and a marker of recovery or immunization. Its presence, in the absence of other positive HBV serologies, is seen in successfully immunized individuals.

Hepatitis B core total antibody (anti-HBc) is a combination of IgG and IgM antibodies. It develops in all HBV infections and indicates HBV infection at some undefined time in the past. It generally persists for life, is not a marker for acute infection, and does not develop in persons whose immunity to HBV is from vaccine.

Hepatitis B core IgM antibody (IgM anti-HBc) appears in persons with acute disease and tends to disappear several weeks after initial exposure. It is a marker of acute infection with HBV although it can also be seen during flares or exacerbation episodes of chronic HBV.

Hepatitis B "e" antigen (HBeAg) is a marker of replication and infectivity. Its absence does not ensure that there is no replication or infectivity as in the precore mutant strain of HBV, which does not produce HBeAg, but it still successfully replicates.

Hepatitis B "e" antibody (HBeAb or anti-HBe) appears when infected individuals lose the HBeAg, a process called *seroconversion*. This is often associated with the disappearance of hepatitis B DNA (HBV DNA) in serum and remission of liver disease.

Hepatitis B DNA is a marker of replication and infectivity. It can be detected and quantified by using a nucleic acid test (NAT). This marker is used to determine the need for treatment and to assess the response to therapy.

Treatment of HBV has experienced remarkable progress since the mid-1990s. Current therapies approved by the Food and Drug Administration (FDA) include interferon-α, pegylated interferons (α-2a or α-2b), lamivudine, adefovir, and entecavir. Other drugs under study are clevudine and telbivudine. The main obstacle to treatment of hepatitis B with nucleot(s)ide analogues has been the development of drug resistance, the most common of which is the YMMD mutant that can develop during treatment with lamivudine.

Hepatitis B can be successfully prevented by active immunization with vaccination efficacy rates of 90% in adults and 95% in infants, children, and adolescents. Widespread use of hepatitis B vaccine is responsible for the recent decreased mortality from HCC in Asia.

Hepatitis C (HCV) is the most common blood borne disease in the United States and the leading cause of cirrhosis, HCC, and liver transplantation in the Western world. HCV infection is an important risk factor for development of HCC. Before 1992, transfusion of blood products was the main source of infection. Currently, most new cases come from

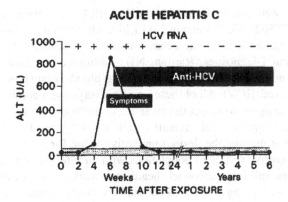

Figure 15.1 Serological course of a typical case of acute, self-limited hepatitis C.[3]

sharing drug paraphernalia as in this case. The clinical spectrum of hepatitis C is diverse in terms of presentation and natural history. Hepatitis C carriers are usually asymptomatic and are diagnosed by the incidental finding of elevated transaminases that prompts further testing or positive serological tests found when donating blood. Another common but unfortunate form of presentation is decompensated end-stage liver disease characterized by ascites, portal hypertension-related gastrointestinal bleeding, and/or hepatic encephalopathy. In most patients (80%) acute hepatitis C (Fig. 15.1) is anicteric and presents with no or few symptoms and therefore is rarely recognized. When clinically apparent, the illness usually lasts for 2–12 weeks and resembles other forms of acute viral hepatitis with an onset of malaise, nausea, and right abdominal pain, followed by choluria and mild jaundice.[3] The average incubation period of posttransfusion hepatitis C is 7–8 weeks (range 2–26 weeks).[4] The first marker of infection is HCV RNA, which can be detected in serum as early as one week after exposure. Specific antibodies appear within 20–150 days after exposure, with a mean of 50 days. Elevation of aminotransferases generally occur after week 4, shortly before symptoms appear, and reach peak levels 10 times the ULN in the great majority of cases. Full recovery from acute hepatitis C occurs in only 15% of patients. The propensity to chronic infection is the most distinguishing characteristic of hepatitis C, occurring in at least 85% of patients. The chronic state (Fig. 15.2) is characterized by persistence of detectable levels of HCV RNA in serum and aminotransferase levels that can fluctuate widely from normal to several times the ULN.

The diagnosis of hepatitis C is simple but requires the understanding of the information that each test provides and its correct interpretation. FDA-licensed or approved anti-HCV screening test kits being used in the United States comprise three

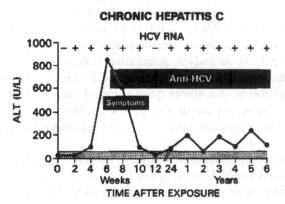

Figure 15.2 Serological course of a typical case of chronic hepatitis C.[3]

immunoassays; two enzyme immunoassays (EIA) (Abbott HCV EIA 2.0, Abbott Laboratories, Abbott Park, IL, and ORTHO® HCV Version 3.0 ELISA, Ortho-Clinical Diagnostics, Raritan, NJ), and one enhanced chemiluminescence immunoassay (CIA) (VITROS® Anti-HCV assay, Ortho-Clinical Diagnostics, Raritan, NJ). Additional kits have been approved by the FDA but are not intended for use in screening blood, plasma, or tissue donors (e.g., Abbott AxSYM® Anti-HCV). All of these immunoassays use a combination of recombinant HCV-encoded antigens to detect the presence of antibodies in serum to a mixture of these HCV-specific antigens. Their overall specificity is ≥99%. Despite the high specificity, the test does not provide the desired predictive value for a positive test in low-risk population. False-positive results in populations with an infection prevalence <10% (volunteer blood donors, military personnel, healthcare workers, etc.) averages approximately 35%. A person with a negative result should be considered uninfected. If positive, this test tells that the patient has been exposed to the virus at an unknown time in the past and can indicate past or current infection. An anti-HCV positive test *does not* make the diagnosis of active infection. A positive immunoassay should be followed by a confirmatory test that confirms the actual presence of the virus. The best alternative is to use a NAT such as RT-PCR, branched chain DNA (bDNA) detection, or transcription-mediated amplification (TMA) to detect the presence of HCV RNA in the blood. A positive NAT for HCV RNA confirms the diagnosis of active infection with HCV.[5]

Non-nucleic acid confirmatory test rely on the use of immunoblot assays that employ five different recombinant HCV-specific antigens immobilized on nitrocellulose strips (recombinant immunoblot assay [RIBA]). Recombinant human superoxide dismutase is included as a control band. Binding of anti-HCV antibodies can then be demonstrated by enzyme-labeled anti-IgG, the pattern of binding indicating the specific anti-HCV reactivity. Reactivity with one band is considered an "indeterminate" reaction and reactivity with two or more bands a confirmed positive. Indeterminate anti-HCV RIBA test results have been observed in recently infected persons who are in the process of seroconversion, and occasionally in persons chronically infected with HCV. Indeterminate results also might indicate a false-positive screening test result, which is the most common interpretation among those at low risk. Another sample should be collected for repeat anti-HCV testing (>1 month later) or for HCV RNA testing. Confirmatory tests that detect antibodies, such as RIBA, are not clinically useful and its use is currently recommended only when EIA tests are "weakly positive" and to differentiate between individuals who have recovered from an infection (anti-HCV positive, NAT for HCV RNA repeatedly negative, and HCV RIBA positive) and those who have a false-positive anti-HCV test (anti-HCV positive, NAT for HCV RNA repeatedly negative, and HCV RIBA negative).

NATs are used in clinical practice to diagnose acute infection, confirm chronic active infection, and to monitor a patient's response to therapy. NATs can be qualitative (HCV RNA$_{Qual}$ RT-PCR) or quantitative (HCV RNA$_{Quant}$ RT-PCR) and are based on RT-PCR technology. The main difference between these is the lower level of detection; the qualitative test is the more sensitive. More recently a quantitative, homogeneous TaqMan® RT-PCR test for HCV RNA has been developed. This new, real-time PCR is based on the TaqMan® 5'-nuclease assay format that allows quantitation of the viral load within a very broad dynamic range, allowing the use of a single test for both purposes. NATs are also used to determine HCV genotypes, an important element influencing the treatment duration and response.

The role of the liver biopsy in the management of patients with chronic hepatitis C has been one of the most controversial topics. Liver enzymes have shown little value in predicting fibrosis. Noninvasive tests based on panels of serum markers for assessment of fibrosis are available but not widely accepted. Our personal approach on this subject is to offer a liver biopsy to all patients with hepatitis C, in particular those with genotypes 1 or 4. We use the information provided by the liver biopsy, in terms of severity of inflammation and more importantly the degree of fibrosis, to counsel patients with hepatitis C genotype 1 regarding the need of treatment. The higher the degree of fibrosis the stronger we feel about recommending treatment. For those patients with genotype 1 with none or minimal fibrosis that do not want to be treated, we recommend repeating a liver biopsy every 4 years to evaluate progression of fibrosis and reassess the need for treatment.

In patients with HCV infection, alcohol consumption is known to cause accelerated progression of liver fibrosis, higher frequency of cirrhosis, and increased incidence of HCC. These patients also have decreased survival as compared with patients with either alcohol abuse or HCV liver injury alone. Alcohol abuse causes decreased response to interferon treatment in HCV patients. It is therefore necessary for patients with HCV infection to abstain from alcohol consumption.[6]

Treatment

There is broad agreement that treatment of acute hepatitis C is highly effective. Several controlled and uncontrolled studies have clearly demonstrated that interferon treatment of acutely infected patients is effective in preventing progression to chronicity.[7,8] Where there is not agreement is the optimum timing for therapy and the most effective treatment dose and duration. The limited evidence available supports the idea of delaying therapy for 12–14 weeks from onset of symptoms or time of exposure. This approach would avoid treating an excessive number of patients who will otherwise clear the virus spontaneously. Data regarding the other two conflicting points is heterogeneous but most clinicians seem to be using pegylated interferon at standard doses for 24 weeks. The response rates with this approach can reach sustained viral response (SVR) greater than 80%. The addition of ribavirin to this regimen in the setting of *acute* hepatitis C is not yet justified.

According to the 2002 National Institutes of Health consensus on hepatitis C management, all patients with chronic hepatitis C are potential candidates for antiviral therapy. Treatment is recommended for patients with an increased risk of developing cirrhosis. These patients are characterized by detectable HCV RNA levels, a liver biopsy with portal or bridging fibrosis, and at least moderate inflammation and necrosis. The current standard of care for treatment of chronic hepatitis C is a combination of a form of pegylated interferon (α-2a [Pegasys®, Hoffmann-La Roche Inc, Nutley, NJ] or α-2b [PEG-Intron®, Schering Corp., Kenilworth, NJ) plus ribavirin. Peginterferon α-2a has a fixed dose, and peginterferon α-2b is dosed based on the patient's weight. Both are administered subcutaneously once a week. Ribavirin is taken orally twice a day, and the dose depends on the patient's weight and genotype. HCV genotypes 1 and 4 are treated for 48 weeks and genotypes 2 and 3 for 24 weeks. For genotype 1 and 4, response to treatment is first assessed at the end of week 12 of treatment where a drop of the HCV RNA $>2 \log_{10}$ of the initial value is considered as early virological response (EVR). Patients who achieve EVR continue on therapy and are retested again at the end of week 24, where a positive HCV RNA$_{Qual}$ PCR will prompt discontinuation of treatment and those who test negative will complete 48 weeks of treatment. Patients who test negative by a HCV RNA$_{Qual}$ PCR test at the end of week 48 are considered to have end-of-treatment response (ETR). Additional follow-up off therapy, irrespective of the genotype, is continued for 24 more weeks. Those who continued to be HCV RNA negative after 24 weeks off therapy have achieved a SVR and are considered cured. EVR is not assessed in patients with genotypes 2 and 3, and they are all treated for 24 weeks. Response to treatment depends mainly on the genotype and viral load. Additional factors such as race, weight, and presence of cirrhosis also play an important role. Difficult-to-treat patients are those with genotype 1 and high viral load ($>2 \times 10^6$ copies/mL). Patients with genotype 1 as a group achieve 52% SVR (47–65%); SVR for genotypes 2 and 3 can be as high as 84%.

References

1. RAMKUMAR, D. AND LABRECQUE, D. R.: *Drug-induced liver disease and environmental toxins*, In: ZAKIM, D., BOYER, T. D., editors. Hepatology – A Textbook of Liver Disease. Philadelphia, Saunders; 2003. p. 755–832.
2. NAIR, S. AND PERRILLO, B.: *Hepatitis B and D*, In: ZAKIM, D., BOYER, T. D., editors. Hepatology – A Textbook of Liver Disease. Philadelphia, NJ: Saunders; 2003. p. 959–1016.
3. HOOFNAGLE, J. H.: Hepatitis C: The clinical spectrum of disease. *Hepatology 26*:15S–20S, 1997.
4. MARCELLIN, P.: Hepatitis C: The clinical spectrum of the disease. *J. Hepatol. 31*:S9–16, 1999.
5. ALTER, M. J., KUHNERT, W. L., AND FINELLI, L.: Guidelines for laboratory testing and result reporting of antibody to hepatitis C virus. *MMWR Recomm. Rep. 52*:1–15, 2003.
6. SAFDAR, K. AND SCHIFF, E. R.: Alcohol and hepatitis C. *Semin. Liver Dis. 24*:305–15, 2004.
7. MYERS, R. P., REGIMBEAU, C., THEVENOT, T. ET AL.: Interferon for acute hepatitis C. *Cochrane Database Syst. Rev. CD000369*, 2001.
8. ZEKRY, A., PATEL, K., AND MCHUTCHISON, J. G.: Treatment of acute hepatitis C infection: More pieces of the puzzle? *J. Hepatol. 42*:293–6, 2005.
9. Centers for Disease Control and Prevention. Atlanta: National Center for Infectious Diseases. *Hepatitis B Frequently Asked Questions—Serology.* Available from http://www.cdc.gov/ncidod/diseases/hepatitis/b/faqb.htm#serology (updated 12/1/2005; cited 1/17/2006).

Case 16

Obese Woman with Persistently Abnormal Liver Enzymes

Iliana Bouneva, M.D.

A 58-year-old Caucasian woman with type 2 diabetes was sent for evaluation to the hepatology clinic with persistent elevation of liver enzymes and complaints of fatigue, dull right upper quadrant abdominal pain, nausea without vomiting, and mild leg swelling for the past 3–4 months. From routine laboratory data 3–4 years ago the patient was found to have mildly elevated liver enzymes, which was attributed to a lipid-lowering agent (niacin), which was stopped at that time. Since then she has not been on lipid-lowering medication. Laboratory work was not repeated until recently, when she was found again to have elevated aminotransferase levels.

The patient denied jaundice, pruritus, and change in appetite, but reported a 6–7-lb weight gain. Additionally, she denied a history of hepatitis and any other liver or gallbladder disease in the past. The patient never smoked, used alcohol, or illicit drugs. There was no history of blood transfusions, tattoos placed, or multiple sexual partners. She had not been recently exposed to anyone with known viral hepatitis. Her family history was positive for hypertension, heart disease, and diabetes mellitus, but negative for liver and biliary tract disease. Her current medications included metformin, glipizide, losartan, metoclopramide, and aspirin. She used no over-the-counter medications, including herbal or dietary supplements.

On physical examination the patient's vital signs were normal and her height was 5 ft 6 in., with weight 228 lb for a calculated body mass index (BMI) of 37. She was an obese white female. Her skin was warm and dry without rash, jaundice, or palmar erythema; but there were a few spider angiomata present on the neck and anterior chest wall. There was no lymphadenopathy, thyroid enlargement, or jugular venous distention. The lungs and heart were normal on auscultation. The abdomen was obese, soft, and nontender. The liver was palpable about 2–3 cm below the right costal margin and was smooth and nontender to palpation. There was no shifting dullness, and bowel sounds were normal. Lower extremities showed mild, 1 (+) pitting pedal edema. The patient

Tietz's Applied Laboratory Medicine, Second Edition. Edited by Mitchell G. Scott, Ann M. Gronowski, and Charles S. Eby

was alert and fully oriented without focal neurologic deficit and no asterixis. Initial laboratory studies from blood and urine were as follows:

Analyte	Value, Conventional Units	Reference Interval, Conventional Units	Value, SI Units	Reference Interval, SI Units
Hemoglobin	13.4 g/dL	12–16	8.32 mmol/L	7.45–9.93
Hematocrit	39%	37–47	0.39	0.37–0.47
Leukocyte count	$4.7 \times 10^3/\mu L$	4.8–10.8	$4.7 \times 10^9/L$	4.8–10.8
MCV	85 fL	80–94	Same	
Platelet count	$110 \times 10^3/\mu L$	150–450	$110 \times 10^9/L$	150–450
Prothrombin time (INR)	1.31	0.8–1.2	Same	
Sodium	138 mmol/L	136–145	Same	
Potassium	3.9 mmol/L	3.8–5.1	Same	
Chloride	103 mmol/L	98–107	Same	
CO_2, total	29 mmol/L	23–31	Same	
Urea nitrogen	10 mg/dL	8–21	9.6 mmol/L	2.9–7.5
Creatinine	0.7 mg/dL	0.7–1.3	71 μmol/L	62–115
Glucose	221 mg/dL	80–115	12.2 mmol/L	4.4–6.4
Calcium	8.8 mg/dL	8.4–10.2	2.20 mmol/L	2.10–2.55
Phosphorus	3.4 mg/dL	2.7–4.5	1.10 mmol/L	0.87–1.45
Protein, total	6.8 g/dL	6.2–7.6	68 g/L	62–76
Albumin	3.2 g/dL	3.5–5.0	32 g/L	35–50
AST	67 U/L	16–48	1.13 μkat/L	0.27–0.80
ALT	89 U/L	13–40	1.51 μkat/L	0.22–0.67
ALP	166 U/L	30–100	2.77 μkat/L	0.50–1.67
GGT	70 U/L	10–50	1.19 μkat/L	0.17–0.83
Urinalysis				
pH	6.8	4.6–8.0		
Specific gravity	1.028	1.001–1.036		
Protein	Negative			
Glucose	Negative			
Leukocytes	Negative			
Ketones	Negative			

Additional tests to assess the possible etiology of the patient's liver injury were also obtained:

Analyte	Value, Conventional Units	Reference Interval, Conventional Units	Value, SI Units	Reference Interval, SI Units
HBsAg	Negative	Negative	Same	
Anti–hepatitis C Ab	Negative	Negative	Same	
Antinuclear Ab	Negative	Negative	Same	
Anti-smooth-muscle Ab	Negative	Negative	Same	
Antiliver/kidney microsomal Ab	Negative	Negative	Same	
α_1-Antitrypsin phenotype	137 mg/dL M_1M_1	78–200	1.3 g/L	0.8–2.0
Ceruloplasmin	32 mg/dL	18–45	320 mg/L	180–450
Ferritin	253 ng/mL	17–270	253 μg/L	17–270

Analyte	Value, Conventional Units	Reference Interval, Conventional Units	Value, SI Units	Reference Interval, SI Units
α-Fetoprotein	4.2 mg/dL	<8.5	4.2 μg/L	<8.5
Total cholesterol	212 mg/dL	<200	5.49 mmol/L	<5.18
LDL cholesterol	144 mg/dL	<130	3.73 mmol/L	<3.37
Triglycerides	316 mg/dL	<250	3.57 mmol/L	<2.83

An abdominal ultrasound revealed increased echogenicity of the liver with somewhat prominent caudate lobe suggestive of cirrhosis but no focal liver lesions. The spleen was slightly enlarged, at 14 cm in size. There was also a small amount of free fluid seen in the perihepatic region. Color flow Doppler ultrasound imaging showed patent hepatic vasculature with normal directional flow. A subsequent upper endoscopy was performed that showed only mild portal hypertensive gastropathy but no esophageal or gastric varices.

Because of the presence of several clinical, laboratory, imaging, and endoscopic findings that were suggestive, but not definitive, for cirrhosis, a percutaneous liver biopsy was performed. The biopsy revealed significant fatty change (60%) within the liver parenchyma. Portal areas showed mild chronic lymphocytic infiltration without interface changes. Hepatic lobules showed significant hepatocyte degeneration (balloon degeneration and Mallory hyaline) and moderate inflammatory infiltrate consisting of lymphocytes and neutrophils. There was extensive fibrosis present on trichrome stain, including bridging fibrosis and incomplete regenerative nodules formation consistent with early cirrhosis.

A weight loss program, including diet, exercise, and behavioral modification, was started. Better control of her diabetes was advised, and the patient's dose of metformin was increased. Treatment of hyperlipidemia with atorvastatin was recommended as well. The patient was also started on treatment with vitamin E. Since she did not have signs of decompensated cirrhosis (no ascites, hepatic encephalopathy, or esophageal varices), a liver transplant evaluation was not offered at this time.

Nonalcoholic Fatty Liver Disease (NAFLD)

Definition

Nonalcoholic fatty liver disease (NAFLD) is a spectrum of histological changes in the liver in patients who drink <20–30 g of alcohol per day, ranging from simple fatty infiltration (steatosis) to a pattern of injury characterized by inflammation, hepatocyte degeneration, and fibrosis, known as *nonalcoholic steatohepatitis* (NASH), and to frank cirrhosis. The histological changes in NAFLD are indistinguishable from those observed in alcoholic liver disease. Although the quantity of alcohol considered harmful is >30 g/day in men and >20 g/day in women, there is no consensus on the amount necessary to cause liver damage. Additionally, patients' self-reporting of alcohol consumption is frequently inaccurate.

Epidemiology

NAFLD has been increasingly recognized as an important public health problem. Since it is closely linked to obesity, its significance is expected to increase even further with the current obesity epidemic. NAFLD is seen most commonly in middle age—in the fourth decade of life in men, and in the sixth decade in women—but can occur at any age, including in children. The prevalence of NAFLD shows equal distribution in men and women and is seen in all ethnic groups. An increased prevalence in African-Americans and Hispanics has been reported, possibly because obesity and diabetes mellitus are more frequent in these two populations.

The strongest risk factor for NAFLD is *obesity*. NAFLD may occur in 75% of obese people, and 20% of them may have NASH. The severity and the type of obesity (in particular, a central type with increased waist-to-hip circumference) are associated with the degree of steatosis and with increased frequency and severity of NASH. *Diabetes mellitus type 2* (DM) is seen in 10–55% of patients with NAFLD. This association probably is not simply a result of the more common occurrence of DM in obese individuals because it has been shown that the degree of steatosis is positively associated with DM independent of the degree of obesity. *Hyperlipidemia*, and particularly hypertrigyceredemia, is also an important risk factor seen in 20–81% of patients with NAFLD.

These risk factors are components of the so-called metabolic syndrome, which is associated with increased risk of atherosclerosis. The syndrome is characterized by abdominal obesity (waist circumference >40 in. in men and >35 in. in women), atherogenic dyslipidemia (elevated triglycerides >150 mg/dL, low HDL <40 mg/dL in men and <50 mg/dL in women), hypertension (blood pressure >130/85 mm Hg), insulin resistance with or without glucose intolerance or overt diabetes (fasting glucose >100 mg/dL), a prothrombotic and a proimflammatory state. NAFLD is recognized as the liver's manifestation of the metabolic syndrome.

Natural History

In general, simple steatosis is considered a reversible condition. However, NASH may progress to cirrhosis in up to 10–15% of patients. In fact, NASH is currently considered the major cause of cryptogenic cirrhosis. As NASH progresses to cirrhosis, steatosis and hepatocyte degeneration often decrease as fibrous bridges develop and the original pericentral nature of fibrosis becomes less apparent. In the absence of characteristic features, a diagnosis of "cryptogenic" cirrhosis is made. NASH-associated cirrhosis may decompensate, progress to hepatocellular carcinoma, and may recur after liver transplantation.

It is not clear why some patients progress to more advanced forms of NAFLD and others remain stable for years. The most important risk factors for progression are also obesity and diabetes mellitus. But other risk factors have been identified as well, including age >45 years, ALT >40 IU/L, an AST/ALT ratio >0.8, increased triglyceride, increased iron, extent of steatosis and degree of inflammation on liver biopsy. Based on these data, a patient who is, for example, younger than 40 years, does not have obesity or DM, and has an AST/ALT ratio <0.8, has minimal risk of having significant fibrosis. On the other hand, two-thirds of patients older than 45 years of age, with obesity, DM, and an AST/ALT ratio >0.8, will likely have significant fibrosis.

Pathology

NAFLD is a histologic diagnosis. The earliest and the most important histologic feature is *steatosis*, which is usually of a macrovesicular type. Steatosis is considered grade 1 if 25–33% of hepatocytes are involved, grade 2 if 33–64% are involved, and grade 3 if more than 66% are involved. The term *NASH* implies that in addition to steatosis, there is also inflammation, hepatocyte degeneration, and fibrosis. Inflammation is more pronounced in the lobules than in the portal tracts. It is composed of mixed acute (neutrophils) and chronic (lymphocytes) inflammatory cells. The most important features of hepatocyte degeneration are cytologic ballooning and Mallory bodies. Mitochondrial abnormalities are frequently observed on electron microscopy and include megamitochondria, multilamellar mitochondria, and intramitochondrial crystalline inclusions.

The fibrosis of NASH begins as pericellular fibrosis, in which the extracellular collagen matrix is deposited along hepatocytes in the space of Disse and is more prominent in the centrilobular and perivenular areas. Individual hepatocytes may by outlined by a rim of fibrosis, giving the so called "chicken wire" appearance of the fibrous tissue on trichrome stain. Fibrosis eventually may progress to formation of central–central and central–portal bridging and, ultimately, to *cirrhosis*. Often steatosis disappears with the development of cirrhosis.

Recently the Pathology Committee of the NASH Research Network designed a scoring system addressing the full spectrum of lesions in NAFLD and proposed a NAFLD activity score (NAS). The scoring system includes 14 histologic features: 4 were evaluated semi-quantitatively (steatosis 0–3, lobular inflammation 0–2, hepatocellular ballooning 0–2, and fibrosis 0–4), and 9 others (microvesicular steatosis, microgranulomas, lipogranulomas, portal inflammation, acidophil bodies, pigmented macrophages, megamitochondria, Mallory's hyaline, glycogenated nuclei) were recorded as present or absent. NAS ≥ 5 correlates with diagnosis of NASH.

Pathogenesis

Insulin resistance (IR) is a hallmark of the metabolic syndrome and plays a central role in the pathogenesis of NAFLD as well. The main abnormality in carbohydrate metabolism is decreased glucose uptake by the muscle, resulting in increased blood glucose concentration. In addition, IR leads to increased fatty acid uptake by the liver, which inhibits the Krebs cycle and stimulates gluconeogenesis. This leads to increased hepatic glucose output. The hyperglycemic state is sensed by the pancreatic β cells, which increase insulin production to restore euglycemia. Over time the increased insulin supply declines and overt diabetes develops.

With IR the principal abnormality in lipid metabolism is resistance to the insulin-mediated suppression of lipolysis, which leads to increased output of free fatty acids from adipose tissue. The fatty acids are delivered to the liver, where they undergo reesterification to triglycerides, resulting in their accumulation in the hepatocytes (steatosis) and increased β-oxidation in mitochondria leads to generation of reactive oxygen species (ROS). Other hepatic oxidative pathways also may be involved (e.g., peroxisomes, cytochromes P450).

Oxidative stress is believed to serve as a "second hit" that is of a paramount importance for progression of steatosis to NASH. ROS attracts inflammatory cells that release various cytokines and chemokines (e.g., tumor necrosis factor α, TNFα), which further increases hepatic inflammation. In addition, ROS and TNFα directly stimulate hepatic stellate cells to produce extracellular matrix, leading to development of fibrosis. ROS are also responsible for the development of the characteristic mitochondrial abnormalities observed in NASH since they cause lipid peroxidation of mitochondrial membranes and oxidative damage to mitochondrial DNA. There is also evidence that depletion of antioxidants (e.g., paraoxonase −1, vitamin E) contributes to the oxidative damage.

Clinical Presentation

Patients with NAFLD usually have other findings of the metabolic syndrome—obesity, diabetes, and hyperlipidemia. The majority of patients with steatosis and NASH are asymptomatic at presentation. About a third of them may have nonspecific complaints of fatigue, malaise, and vague right upper quadrant (RUQ) abdominal pain. The most common finding on physical exam is hepatomegaly, seen in about 75% of patients. Patients with the most advanced stages of NAFLD have the typical clinical findings of cirrhosis (palmar erythema, spider angiomata, hepatosplenomegaly, jaundice, ascites, hepatic encephalopathy, variceal bleeding, etc.).

Usually, the first clues to the diagnosis of NAFLD are incidentally found abnormal liver enzymes, most commonly mild to moderate elevations (two- to five-fold) of aminotrasnferases—alanine aminotransferase (ALT) and aspartate aminotransferase (AST). The AST/ALT ratio is typically <1; a ratio >1 may suggest advanced fibrosis or cirrhosis. Alkaline phosphatase may also be mildly increased (usually no more than two- to three-fold). Bilirubin and albumin are almost always normal, unless cirrhosis has developed. Liver enzymes can be completely normal in any form of NAFLD, and the degree of the laboratory abnormality does not correlate with the severity of histologic injury.

It is important to screen for other common causes of chronic liver disease that is associated with hepatic steatosis such as alcoholic liver disease, viral hepatitis (particularly hepatitis C, genotype 3), autoimmune hepatitis, genetic diseases (Wilson's disease, galactosemia), and drug-induced liver injury (e.g., corticosteroids, estrogens, amiodarone).

Abdominal imaging such as ultrasound (US), computed tomography (CT), and magnetic resonance imaging (MRI) are also helpful diagnostic tools. Ultrasound is used most commonly since it is noninvasive, inexpensive, and not associated with radiation exposure. It typically shows hepatomegaly (in 85% of patients), increased echogenicity of the liver ("bright liver"), presence of liver–kidney contrast, vascular blurring, and deep attenuation of the ultrasound beam.

The gold standard for diagnosis of NAFLD is liver biopsy. There is no consensus at present on the necessity to perform a liver biopsy in all the patients with suspected NAFLD. Liver biopsy will distinguish the different histological types of NAFLD, estimate prognosis, and exclude other causes of liver disease. But it is an invasive test, associated with risks and increased cost. It is generally recommended that ALT and US be used for screening patients with risk factors for NAFLD. If they are abnormal, a liver biopsy should be considered, especially in patients with hepatomegaly.

Treatment

Traditionally, treatment of NAFLD has been directed at correction of the components of metabolic syndrome (obesity, DM, hyperlipidemia). Only recently, therapies aimed at the underlying pathophysiological mechanisms of the disease (insulin resistance, oxidative stress) have been used. The goal of treatment is not simply normalization of the liver enzymes, but improvement of steatosis, inflammation, and fibrosis. There is no FDA-approved medical treatment of NAFLD at present. Proponents of bariatric surgery for obesity (e.g., gastric bypass) are hopeful that long-term weight loss induced by surgery will markedly benefit NAFLD patients. But this has not yet been confirmed.

Treatment of Medical Conditions Associated with Metabolic Syndrome and NAFLD

Obesity. Because of the strong association between NAFLD and obesity, weight reduction seems to be the most logical first therapeutic approach. It should include a combination of diet, exercise, behavioral modifications, and pharmacological treatment. Medications are indicated in morbid obesity with BMI >40 or in severe obesity with BMI >35 in the presence of obesity-associated comorbid conditions. Gradual weight loss of at least 10% of body weight has been shown to improve insulin resistance, serum aminotransferases, and liver histology. However, rapid weight loss may be associated with a worsening of the inflammation and fibrosis. Treatment of obesity with orlistat (a reversible inhibitor of gastric and pancreatic lipases) has been shown to improve, steatosis, necroinflammatory activity, fibrosis and lower serum aminotranferases. Other weight loss medications (phentermine, sibutramine) have not been studied in patients with NAFLD.

Diabetes mellitus. Insulin sensitizers, such as thiazolidindiones and biguanides, have been studied as potential therapies for NASH. Thiazolidindiones (troglitazone, pioglitazone, rosiglitazone) have been shown to improve, hepatic steatosis, necroinflammatory activity, mitochondrial morphology, fibrosis and decrease aminotransferases in patients with NASH. The main drawback of these medications is their potential hepatotoxicity (troglitazone was withdrawn from the market for this reason). Only pioglitazone has not been reported to have major hepatotoxicity. Treatment with the biguanide metformin has also been shown to lead to improvement of insulin sensitivity and serum aminotransferases, but without beneficial effect on liver histopathology.

Hyperlipidemia. Studies with 3-hydroxy-3-methylglutaryl coenzyme-A (HMG-CoA) reductase inhibitors, in particular atorvastatin, have shown improvement in hepatic steatosis, inflammatory activity, and fibrosis. A recent trial with another lipid-lowering agent with antioxidant properties, probucol, showed improvement of aminotransferases and serum lipids, but liver histology was not studied.

Treatment of NASH with Antioxidants   Since chronic oxidative stress plays a central role in the development of NASH, different antioxidants have been tried. Vitamin E has been shown to decrease serum aminotransferases and to improve hepatic inflammation and fibrosis. Betaine, a component of the methionine metabolic cycle, has been shown to improve aminotransferases and to decrease steatosis, necroinflammation, and fibrosis. The biliary cytoprotective medication ursodeoxycholic acid (UDCA) has also been studied. The precise mechanism of action of UDCA is unknown, but it is believed to reduce oxidative stress at the level of mitochondrial membrane leading to decreased cellular apoptosis and necrosis. The most recent studies have shown however that UDCA is not useful for treatment of NAFLD, at least as a monotherapy.

In summary, NAFLD is a common and increasingly important cause of liver disease. Efforts to promote healthier diets, encourage exercise and active lifestyles, and better manage the metabolic syndrome are the most important components of therapy. The precise role of pharmacologic treatment of NAFLD still remains to be established. It is possible that there may be different causes of NAFLD, each requiring a distinctive treatment. Further larger prospective, randomized, double-blind, placebo-controlled, and well-conducted studies supported by liver biopsies are needed before any routine therapy is recommended.

Additional Reading

FALCK–YTTER, Y., YOUNOSSI, Z. M., MARCHESINI, G., AND McCULLOUGH, A. J.: Clinical features and natural history of nonalcoholic steatosis syndromes. *Semin. Liver Dis. 21*:17–26, 2001.

McCULLOGH, A. J.: Update on nonalcoholic fatty liver disease. *J. Clin. Gastroenterol. 34*:155–62, 2002.

NEUSCHWANDER-TETRI, B. A., AND CALDWELL, S. H.: Nonalcoholic steatohepatitis: Summary of an AASLD single topic conference. *Hepatology 37*:1202–9, 2003.

ALBA, L. M. AND LINDOR, K.: Review article: Nonalcoholic fatty liver disease. *Aliment Pharmacol. Ther. 17*:977–86, 2003.

SANYAL, A. J. (guest editor), AND GITLIN, N. (consulting editor): Nonalcoholic fatty liver disease. *Clinics Liver Dis. 8*:481–734, 2004.

KLEINER, D. E., BRUNT, E. M., VAN NATTA, M., ET AL.: Design and validation of a histological scoring system for nonalcoholic fatty liver disease. *Hepatology 41*:1313–21, 2005.

Part Five

Thyroid Diseases

Cases 17, 18, and 19 (all edited by AMG) report and discuss cases of Graves disease, Hashimoto's thyroiditis, and papillary thyroid carcinoma, respectively.

Tietz's Applied Laboratory Medicine, Second Edition. Edited by Mitchell G. Scott, Ann M. Gronowski, and Charles S. Eby
Copyright © 2007 John Wiley & Sons, Inc.

Case 17

The Irritable Wife

William E. Winter

A 33-year-old Caucasian woman presented to her primary healthcare provider with complaints of anxiety and a "racing heartbeat." She was in good health until these symptoms began approximately one year ago. Over the same period of time, her menstrual periods had become irregular, she had lost 15 lb (7 kg) unintentionally, and she was having social problems with her spouse and coworkers because of "irritability." She slept poorly, complained of occasional loose stools, and was easily overheated. She insisted at night that the air conditioner be set to 65°C. She also complained that her lower neck was "bulging," as were her eyes.

Prior to one year ago, her past medical history was unremarkable. She had had no serious illnesses, hospitalizations for illnesses, or surgeries. She gave birth to a healthy boy 8 years previously following a normal pregnancy, labor, and delivery. She took no chronic medications and reported no allergies, and her immunizations were up to date.

Her family history was striking for hypothyroidism in her 64-year-old mother and pernicious anemia in her 29-year-old sister. She was said to have a distant relative with Graves disease. There was no family history of premature cardiovascular disease, hypertension, cancer, or diabetes.

Her review of symptoms was negative for complaints of visual disturbances, headaches, nausea, vomiting, diarrhea, or constipation.

Physical examination revealed a thin, somewhat distraught, 33-year-old Caucasian woman who was in no cardiac or respiratory distress. Her height was 168 cm, and her weight was 45 kg. Her body mass index was 16 kg/m^2. Her vital signs were as follows: temperature = 36.8°C, pulse = 110 beats per minute and regular, respirations = 16 breaths per minute, blood pressure = 125/62 mm Hg. Repeat blood pressure measurement in the opposite arm was measured at 124/58 mm Hg. HEENT examination revealed bilateral proptosis and elevation of the upper eyelid exposing an increased amount of white sclera. The disks and fundi were normal. The neck was supple without masses or lymphadenopathy. The thyroid gland was diffusely enlarged and smooth. The thyroid was nontender, was not attached to any underlying neck structures, and moved freely with swallowing. A thyroid bruit was not appreciated by auscultation. The lungs were clear to auscultation and percussion. Other than tachycardia and bounding (3+ to 4+), symmetric pulses in the upper and lower extremities, the cardiovascular examination was normal. No murmurs or gallop were noted. The abdomen was soft without masses or hepatosplenomegaly. Normal bowel

Tietz's Applied Laboratory Medicine, Second Edition. Edited by Mitchell G. Scott, Ann M. Gronowski, and Charles S. Eby
Copyright © 2007 John Wiley & Sons, Inc.

sounds were present. She had Tanner IV breasts and pubic hair. Her pelvic examination was normal. Mild nonpitting pretibial edema was noted bilaterally. Her skin was smooth and slightly wet with perspiration. Her hair was fine. Cranial nerves II–XII were grossly intact. A mild tremor was appreciated. Reflexes were 3+ to 4+ and symmetric in the upper and lower extremities. There were no focal neurologic deficits.

Based on the history of "nervousness," personality change, oligomenorrhea, heat intolerance, loose stools, and weight loss and the physical examination findings of tachycardia, a bounding (hyperdynamic) pulse, warm skin, exophthalmos, pretibial myxedema, and smooth skin and hair, the diagnosis of hyperthyroidism appeared certain. Thyroid-stimulating hormone (TSH; thyrotropin) and free thyroxine (thyroxine = tetraiodothyronine; free T4 = FT4) measurements were obtained:

Analyte	Value, Conventional Units	Reference Interval, Conventional Units	Value, SI Units	Reference Interval, SI Units
TSH	0.01 μIU/mL	0.35–4.2	0.01 mIU/L	0.35–4.2
Free T4	3.2 ng/dL	0.8–2.7	41.3 pmol/L	2.3–9.0

In the patient, the suppressed TSH and elevated FT4 concentrations were consistent with the diagnosis of primary (autonomous) hyperthyroidism. If the FT4 were normal, the physician had planned to order a total 3,5,3′-triiodothyronine (T3) measurement. However, this was not necessary because the FT4 was elevated.

Therapy was initiated with 4× daily doses of oral propylthiouracil (PTU). Within 6 weeks, there was a decline in the heart rate to 90 bpm and a weight gain of 4 lb. The patient's "irritability" had declined, and her interpersonal relations had improved. It was too soon to note whether her menstrual cycle had returned to normal.

Definition of the Disease

Hyperthyroidism and *thyrotoxicosis* are synonymous terms. Excess thyroid hormone elevates the basal metabolic rate (e.g., causing weight loss) and causes the classic findings exhibited in this patient involving the nervous system (e.g., personality changes, tremor, hyperreflexia), cardiovascular system (tachycardia with a hyperdynamic heart, bounding pulses and wide pulse pressure), and gastrointestinal tract (e.g., loose stools or diarrhea). In extreme cases, high output heart failure can result. Many other systems can be affected such as the tissues of the retroorbital space, the skin, the hair, and the reproductive system. The patient's oligomenorrhea is likely a consequence of her disordered metabolism, the stress of illness and weight loss.

Goiter with hyperthyroidism, exophthalmos, and pretibial myxedema are the pathognomonic triad of Graves disease. Graves disease is a classic organ-specific autoimmune disease where there is a humoral autoimmune response to the TSH receptor. In Graves disease goiter [i.e., hyperplasia of the thyroid with palpable (and often visible) gland enlargement] and hyperthyroidism (i.e., hyperfunction of the thyroid) result from IgG autoantibodies that bind to and stimulate the TSH receptor. Such agonist autoantibodies [i.e., thyroid-stimulating immunoglobulins (TSIs)] can be identified in 80–100% of subjects with Graves disease. In contrast, TSIs are detected in 0–10% of control populations and up to 20% of subjects with Hashimoto thyroiditis.

Exophthalmos results from edema of the retroorbital muscles and adipose tissue hyperplasia. While the etiopathogenesis of exophthalmos is controversial, TSIs are believed to be involved. Some investigators have demonstrated TSH receptors on retro-orbital tissues. Pretibial myxedema is a marker of autoimmune thyroid disease (AITD) in general because pretibial myxedema can be observed in both Graves disease and Hashimoto thyroiditis. TSIs have also been implicated in the genesis of pretibial myxedema.

Susceptibility to autoimmune thyroid disease, both Graves disease and Hashimoto thyroiditis, appears to be inherited in an autosomal dominant pattern with increased pene-trance in women. The genetic locus providing this susceptibility has eluded definitive identification. Onset of AITD can occur during childhood or adulthood. Both Graves disease and Hashimoto thyroiditis are strongly familial and can occur in the same family. Among female siblings, mothers and offspring within a single family, some individuals can exhibit Graves disease whereas other individuals can display Hashimoto thyroiditis. Because HLA-DR3 is associated with Graves disease and HLA-DR4 or DR5 are associated with Hashimoto thyroiditis, an interactive model of the development of AITD can be created. Hypothetically the "AITD" gene plus DR3 in a single individual favors a T-helper-2-cell-type CD4 T cell response (Th2) to the TSH receptor producing agonistic TSH receptor autoantibodies (i.e., Graves disease). In contrast, the "AITD" gene plus DR4 or DR5 favors a T-helper-1-cell-type CD4 T cell response (Th1) with cell-mediated immunity against the thyroid follicular cells that causes their destruction (i.e., Hashimoto thyroiditis).

As organ-specific autoimmune diseases, both Graves disease and Hashimoto thyroiditis are commonly associated with pernicious anemia and even type 1 (autoimmune) diabetes mellitus. Less commonly Graves disease or Hashimoto thyroiditis can be associated with autoimmune Addison disease or adrenal autoantibodies. The association of AITD (or type 1 diabetes mellitus) and Addison disease/adrenal autoantibodies is termed *autoimmune poly-glandular syndrome type 2*. The older literature referred to the association of adrenal and thyroid autoimmunity as *Schmidt syndrome*. The coexistence of AITD, Addison disease/adrenal autoantibodies, and type 1 diabetes mellitus was termed *Carpenter syndrome*.

In the present case, there was a family history of Graves disease, Hashimoto thyroid-itis, and pernicious anemia. Because of the recognized associations among autoimmune endocrinopathies, it is prudent that all patients with AITD be tested for autoantibodies to the gastric parietal cells. Testing for gastric parietal cell autoantibodies can be per-formed by indirect immunofluorescence using snap-frozen human stomach as substrate. If gastric parietal cell autoantibodies are detected, yearly measurements of vitamin B_{12} (or better yet, methyl malonic acid) and ferritin should be carried out to detect early-onset pernicious anemia and iron deficiency. Recall that achlorhydria is a consequence of chronic lymphocytic gastritis (the cause of pernicious anemia) and this will deter normal iron absorption.

Differential Diagnosis

Similar to many endocrine conditions, the individual differential diagnoses of weight loss, tachycardia, loose stools and behavioral changes are very broad. Considerations in cases of weight loss include cancer, malnutrition, malabsorption, infectious, autoimmune and inflammatory disorders, or any significant focal or systemic disease. Tachycardia can result from exercise, pain, anxiety, hypovolemia, anemia, cardiac arrhythmias, or heart failure as well as endocrine conditions such as hyperthyroidism or pheochromocytoma. Whereas pheochromocytoma is a rare condition (annual incidence $\sim$1 per 10^6), hyperthyroidism is common, affecting up to 1 in 100 women. Loose stools or diarrhea suggest malabsorption or intestinal inflammatory or infectious disease. Rare endocrine causes of secretory diarrheas encompass somatostatinoma, VIPoma, and glucagonoma. Behavioral changes can reflect intrinsic neurologic or psychiatric disease or almost any serious focal or systemic disorder.

The specific differential diagnosis of hyperthyroidism entails primary and central disorders. Central hyperthyroidism can be "secondary" from TSH excess or "tertiary" from thyrotropin-releasing hormone (TRH) excess. Both conditions are extremely rare even though TSH-secreting pituitary adenomas are clearly described in the medical literature. Even rarer are individuals with true clinical hyperthyroidism who suffer from isolated pituitary resistance to thyroid hormone but exhibit peripheral responsiveness to thyroid hormone.

The causes of primary hyperthyroidism include Graves disease, the destructive phase of Hashimoto thyroiditis, postpartum thyroiditis, toxic thyroid nodules (either single or multiple), viral thyroiditis (subacute thyroiditis; also known as *de Quervain thyroiditis*), pregnancy-induced hyperthyroidism (i.e., from an hCG-sensitive TSH receptor mutation), hCG-secreting tumors (e.g., choriocarcinoma), struma ovarii (i.e., ectopic thyroid tissue in an ovarian teratoma), and exogenous administration of excess thyroid hormone (e.g., factitious hyperthyroidism). Functional thyroid nodules (i.e., "hot" nodules) are almost never malignant. Iodine-induced primary hyperthyroidism appears to result when an otherwise hyperthyroid patient is euthyroid, at least in part, because of iodine deficiency. Iodine replenishment then allows the clinical expression of hyperthyroidism as more thyroid hormone can now be synthesized. Iodine-induced hyperthyroidism can be referred to as the "Jod Basedow syndrome."

The differentiation of Graves disease from the destructive phase of Hashimoto thyroiditis is an interesting challenge. Not all patients with Hashimoto thyroiditis will display a destructive phase. When this does occur, hyperthyroidism results from increased release of thyroid hormone from tissue damage and follicular necrosis. Whereas patients with Graves disease are persistently hyperthyroid if untreated, the destructive phase of Hashimoto thyroiditis occurs in somebody who has previously been hypothyroid. Thus a transition from hypothyroid to transiently hyperthyroid suggests Hashimoto thyroiditis and not Graves disease. A destructive phase of Hashimoto thyroiditis in the postpartum period is possible and not altogether uncommon. Using other diagnostic modalities, TSIs are more common in Graves disease than Hashimoto thyroiditis. Radioactive iodine uptake in Graves disease is elevated whereas in Hashimoto thyroiditis radioactive iodine uptake is reduced and/or patchy in distribution.

Diagnosis

TSH and free T4 are the two first-line tests used to diagnose hyperthyroidism. TSH assays in almost all laboratories currently represent third-generation assays with lower limits of detection for TSH near 0.01 μU/mL. FT4 assays have greatly improved since the early 1990s. Rarely is a dialysis equilibrium measurement of FT4 required. If serum TSH is suppressed and FT4 is normal, T3 toxicosis can be diagnosed by finding an elevated T3. While some laboratories offer unbound (free) T3 measurements (FT3), a total T3 measurement is usually satisfactory because T3 testing is not a first-line screening test for thyroid dysfunction. Furthermore, because of its higher concentration, in analytical terms total T3 is more easily measured than FT3. T3 (or FT3) should usually only be measured to rule in or rule out T3 toxicosis. Even in the setting of hypothyroidism, a low T3 in addition to a low FT4 provides no additional diagnostic or therapeutic information. Isolated depressions in T3 with normal TSH and FT4 concentrations are not uncommon in sick inpatients displaying sick euthyroid syndrome (e.g., nonthyroidal illness). To avoid confusion with sick euthyroid, inpatient thyroid function testing should only be performed when myxedema coma or heart failure, or thyroid storm are clinical considerations that would require immediate medical therapy if recognized. Furthermore while FT4 and T3 are both elevated in thyroid storm, the diagnosis of "storm" is not based on laboratory values but is based on the clinical status of the patient (e.g., "Is a hyperthyroid patient in acute high-output heart failure from hyperthyroidism?").

T3 toxicosis is a legitimate form of hyperthyroidism that deserves treatment similar to classic cases of hyperthyroidism with a suppressed TSH and elevated FT4. T3 toxicosis may occur in the setting of iodine deficiency or may be a very early stage in the development of hyperthyroidism. When the TSH receptor is stimulated by either TSH or an autoantibody, T3 synthesis and release increases to a greater extent than the increased synthesis and release of T4. Therefore with any form of thyroid stimulation through the TSH receptor, T3 rises more rapidly than T4.

If the T3 and FT4 are both normal in the face of a persistent suppression in TSH not otherwise explained (e.g., dopamine or high-dose glucocorticoid use, pituitary or hypothalamic insufficiency), subclinical hyperthyroidism is diagnosed. Increased prevalence of atrial arrhythmias and osteoporosis have been observed in individuals with subclinical hyperthyroidism.

A progression from euthyroidism to hyperthyroidism is outlined below:

	TSH	FT4	T3
Euthyroid	Normal	Normal	Normal
Subclinical hyperthyroidism	Decreased	Normal	Normal
T3 Thyrotoxicosis	Decreased	Normal	Increased
Hyperthyroidism	Decreased	Increased	Increased

Because the most common cause of hyperthyroidism is Graves disease, thyroperoxidase autoantibodies (TPOA) were sought in this patient and were found to be positive at a high concentration. This confirmed an autoimmune etiology for the patient's hyperthyroidism and the presence of Graves disease. Thyroglobulin autoantibodies (TGA) are less commonly positive than TPOA in Graves disease but would have been ordered next if TPOA were negative. Positivity for TPOA and/or TGA do not distinguish Graves disease from Hashimoto thyroiditis.

If the clinical diagnosis of Graves disease were in question and TPOA and TGA were negative, thyroid stimulating immunoglobulins (TSI) would have been ordered. TSI testing was not ordered in this case because the clinical, laboratory, and TPOA findings were collectively diagnostic for Graves disease and the absence or presence of TSIs would not alter the diagnosis or treatment.

The thyrotropin-binding inhibitory immunoglobulin (TBII) assay is an appropriate diagnostic test in cases of suspected atrophic thyroiditis where antagonist TSH receptor autoantibodies produce thyroid gland atrophy and hypothyroidism. However, in cases of Graves disease the TBII assay is theoretically inferior to the TSI assay. While the TBII assay does recognize autoantibodies that can bind to the TSH receptor, the TBII assay does not distinguish agonist from antagonist TSH receptor autoantibodies.

Treatment

The first line of therapy in treating Graves disease is the administration of antithyroid medications that block thyroid hormone synthesis and release. Such drugs include PTU (as used in this patient) and methimazole. Because PTU blocks the peripheral conversion of T4 to T3, it has a theoretical advantage over methimazole. However methimazole need only to be taken 3 times daily, instead of four, which would allow higher compliance. If the symptoms of hyperthyroidism are severe, a catecholamine β blocker can be administered such as propranolol.

After 1–2 years of controlling hyperthyroidism on oral antithyroid medications, the physician can withdraw antithyroid medications to determine whether the patient has entered into a remission. Indeed, anywhere from ~20% to ~60% of subjects will remain euthyroid. Of the patients who relapse back into hyperthyroidism, a second trial of oral antithyroid medications can be prescribed. Alternatively, the patient can be offered radioactive iodine therapy to ablate the thyroid gland. Such therapy is safe and effective. The long-term sequela is the development of hypothyroidism. However, hypothyroidism is easier to treat pharmacologically than Graves disease because thyroid hormone replacement need be given only once daily. If the thyroid gland is damaged by radioiodine but not completely ablated, there is concern that differentiated thyroid cancer might develop in the future.

As an alternative to radioiodine, a definitive therapy for hyperthyroidism is surgical thyroidectomy. The issues here concern cost, the completeness of the thyroidectomy, possible damage to the recurrent laryngeal nerves that control the vocal cords, and inadvertent parathyroidectomy. Most authorities recommend radioiodine over surgery as definitive therapy for hyperthyroidism. However, surgery will produce a euthyroid state more rapidly that radioiodine. Furthermore, radioiodine is not an option if definitive therapy of hyperthyroidism is required during pregnancy. Radioiodine administered to a pregnant woman can cross the placenta and ablate the fetal thyroid gland producing congenital hypothyroidism. Surgery is an important option if coexistent thyroid cancer were a consideration. Finally, there are some studies to support the hypothesis that radioiodine may worsen Grave ophthalmopathy.

If surgery is undertaken, the surgeon and anesthesiologist should be highly experienced to avoid surgical complications as noted above. Preoperatively high doses of iodine may be administered to decrease vascularity of the thyroid gland that would reduce surgical bleeding. High-dose iodine can also induce a euthyroid state which should be achieved preoperatively.

Additional Reading

ANDO, T., LATIF, R., AND DAVIES, T. F.: Thyrotropin receptor antibodies: New insights into their actions and clinical relevance. *Best Pract. Res. Clin. Endocrinol. Metab.* *19*:33–52, 2005.

SCHATZ, D. A. AND WINTER, W. E.: Autoimmune polyglandular syndromes. In *Pediatric Endocrinology*, 2nd ed., M. SPERLING, ed., Sanders, Philadelphia, 2002, pp. 671–88.

WINTER, W. E.: Autoimmune endocrinopathies. In *Pediatric Endocrinology*, 4th ed., F. LIFSHITZ, ed., Marcel Dekker, New York, 2003, pp. 683–720.

BARTALENA, L., WIERSINGA, W. M., AND PINCHERA, A.: Graves' ophthalmopathy: State of the art and perspectives. *J. Endocrinol. Invest.* 27:295–301, 2004.

BURMAN, K. D.: Hyperthyroidism. In *Principles and Practice of Endocrinology and Metabolism*, 3rd ed., K. L. BECKER ET AL., eds., Lippincott, Williams & Wilkins, Philadelphia, 2001, pp. 409–28.

COOPER, D. S.: Hyperthyroidism. *Lancet 362*:459–68, 2003.

WINTER, W. E. AND SIGNORINO, M. R.: Autoimmune endocrinopathies. In *Immunologic Disorders in Infants and Children*, 5th ed., E. R. STIEHM, ed., Saunders, Philadelphia, 2004, pp. 1179–221.

LARSEN, P. R., DAVIES, T. F., HAY, I. D.: The thyroid gland. In *Williams Textbook of Endocrinology*, 9th ed., J. D. WILSON ET AL., eds., Saunders, Philadelphia, 1998, pp. 389–515.

LAZARUS, J. H.: Thyroid disorders associated with pregnancy: Etiology, diagnosis, and management. *Treat. Endocrinol. 4*:31–41, 2005.

WHITLEY, R. J.: Thyroid function. In *Tietz Textbook of Clinical Chemistry*, 3rd ed., C. A. BURTIS AND E. R. ASHWOOD, eds., Saunders, Philadelphia, 1999, pp. 1496–527.

Case 18

The Fatigued Attorney

Kenneth B. Ain

A 28-year-old attorney reported for her yearly physical examination complaining of tiredness, difficulty concentrating on her work, and a noticeable decline in her memory over the past several months. She attributed many of these symptoms to the severe stress generated by her legal caseload. Further questioning by her physician revealed that the frequency of her bowel movements had decreased from once daily, 6 months ago, to once every 2 or 3 days. She was having difficulty keeping her weight down, and despite warm weather, she felt chilled without a light sweater. Her only medication was an oral contraceptive. Family history was significant for hypothyroidism in her mother and older sister.

Physical examination revealed a well-proportioned woman, 65 in. (1.65 m) in height, 125 lb (56.7 kg) in weight, and with sparse eyebrows (particularly at the lateral margins). Her facial features appeared slightly puffy in comparison to the photograph on her driver's license taken 3 years before. The pulse rate was 58 bpm and the blood pressure 138/88 mm Hg. Examination of her neck disclosed a small goiter of 25 g (normal, 15–20 g) with a palpable pyramidal lobe and a firm, bosselated texture. Her deep tendon reflexes were normally contractive but showed a delayed relaxation phase.

The initial clinical impression was that of moderate hypothyroidism of several months' duration. The texture of her thyroid gland and the occurrence of hypothyroidism in her family suggested an autoimmune etiological factor. The following serum values were reported:

Analyte	Value, Conventional Units	Reference Interval, Conventional Units	Value, SI Units	Reference Interval, SI Units
Free T4	0.7 ng/dL	0.9–1.6	9.3 pmol/L	12–21
Total T4	11.4 µg/dL	5–11.5	147 nmol/L	64–148
TSH	22.0 µU/mL	0.6–4.5	22.0 mU/L	0.6–4.5
Antithyroperoxidase antibodies	6280.0 IU/mL	0–70	6280.0 IU/mL	0–70
Cholesterol	230 mg/dL	140–225	5.95 mmol/L	3.62–5.82

Tietz's Applied Laboratory Medicine, Second Edition. Edited by Mitchell G. Scott, Ann M. Gronowski, and Charles S. Eby
Copyright © 2007 John Wiley & Sons, Inc.

The laboratory results, low free thyroxine (free T4) and increased TSH (thyrotropin), confirmed the clinical impression of hypothyroidism. The elevated TSH with a concordantly low free T4 indicates primary hypothyroidism. The etiology of this thyroid dysfunction appears likely to be autoimmune thyroiditis (Hashimoto's thyroiditis) as evidenced by the elevated concentration of antithyroperoxidase (TPO) antibodies. The patient was started on 112 μg L-thyroxine (levothyroxine) daily and 2 months later reported resolution of all of her symptoms. Laboratory studies at that time showed the following:

Analyte	Value, Conventional Units	Reference Interval, Conventional Units	Value, SI Units	Reference Interval, SI Units
Free T4	1.5	0.9–1.6 ng/dL	20.0	12–21 pmol/L
TSH	2.0	0.6–4.5 μU/mL	2.0	0.6–4.5 mU/L

Definition of the Disease

The cause of hypothyroidism may be primary (thyroid dysfunction), secondary (pituitary dysfunction), or tertiary (hypothalamic dysfunction). Primary hypothyroidism is 1000-fold more common than secondary or tertiary causes.[1] Hypothyroidism is associated with cold intolerance, weight gain, constipation, dry skin, bradycardia, hoarseness, and slow mental processing.[1] In adults, the characteristic signs and symptoms of hypothyroidism may have an insidious onset. Chronic cutaneous changes include dry, puffy skin with a yellowish complexion as well as a thickening of the subcutaneous tissues due to accumulation of mucopolysaccharides. The hair becomes dry and brittle and is often sparse. The voice may deepen in pitch, and hypoventilation has been observed. Hypothyroid patients can show decreased pulse rate, decreased cardiac stroke volume, and decreased myocardial contractility that causes decreased cardiac output. Since peripheral metabolism is slowed, arteriovenous oxygen may not show a significant difference. Pleural and pericardial effusions may develop as a result of increased capillary permeability to serum proteins. This leakage of protein, as well as decreased renal glomerular filtration rate and free water clearance, may contribute to generalized edema and hyponatremia. Gastrointestinal hypomotility with associated constipation is frequently seen, and the effects of hypothyroidism on hepatic metabolism may be reflected in the decreased degradation rate of certain drugs as well as by the degree of hypercholesterolemia. Neuromuscular effects are evidenced by increased muscular volume and stiffness with slow contractility and relaxation. Mental symptoms include decreased ability to concentrate, impaired memory, and hypersomnolence; behavioral manifestations range from depression to frank psychosis. Severe long-term hypothyroidism, particularly with additional insults such as systemic infections, may progress to coma with significant associated mortality.

Etiology

Worldwide, iodine deficiency is still the most common cause of hypothyroidism; an estimated 400 million people are at risk. In regions with sufficient iodine, particularly North

America and Europe, autoimmune thyroid disease (primarily Hashimoto's thyroiditis) is the usual cause of hypothyroidism.

The incidence of congenital hypothyroidism (cretinism), in iodine-sufficient countries, is approximately one in 4000 births and may be associated with the most severe neuropsychological abnormalities.[1] This high incidence has resulted in the institution of neonatal screening programs in many developed countries. Clinical features include feeding problems, hypotonia, umbilical hernia, constipation, enlarged tongue, dry skin, characteristic facies, and open posterior fontanelle. On radiological examination, poor skeletal maturation can be seen as retardation in the appearance of ossification centers. Failure to institute early treatment with thyroid hormone leads to significant brain damage. Even with early therapy, there may still be a residual effect to lower the intelligence quotient.

Hashimoto's thyroiditis (lymphocytic thyroiditis) is the most frequent cause of primary hypothyroidism in developed countries, occurring with a prevalence of approximately 15% in women aged 18–24 and in 25% of women between the ages of 55 and 64. It is about a third as common in men. Hashimoto's thyroiditis is characterized by lymphocytic infiltration of the thyroid gland and the production of antibodies that recognize thyroid-specific antigens. It is currently believed that the disease occurs as a consequence of abnormalities in suppressor T-lymphocyte function that cause a localized cell-mediated immune response, although the pathogenesis is still not completely understood.[2] The study of Hashimoto's thyroiditis has served as a general model for inquiry into the mechanisms of autoimmune disease.

Most patients with Hashimoto's thyroiditis present with some thyroid enlargement (goiter) that has a bosselated texture on palpation. There is usually some degree of hypothyroidism, although transient hyperthyroidism may result from inflammatory release of preformed thyroid hormones. The immune processes underlying Hashimoto's disease are similar to the processes causing hyperthyroidism from thyroid-stimulating antibodies in Graves disease. Both conditions show a significant concordance with other autoimmune disease as well as frequent familial concordance. Findings that are associated with this condition include the presence of circulating autoantibodies directed against thyroid peroxidase (TPO or microsomal antigen) and thyroglobulin. Histopathological diagnosis is not usually necessary, although fine-needle aspiration biopsy may provide diagnostic cellular material if needed.

Diagnosis

TSH is the most sensitive way to assess thyroid function.[3] Elevated serum TSH concentrations usually indicate primary hypothyroidism irrespective of its cause or severity. Very rare pituitary tumors secreting TSH are distinguished by inappropriate TSH elevations in the face of elevation of the free T4 and clinical thyrotoxicosis. Alternatively, rare syndromes of resistance to thyroid hormone may be seen with inappropriate TSH elevations, and also with elevations of free T4, but without thyrotoxic symptoms. Persistent mild elevations of TSH, even when free T4 is normal, warrant therapy with thyroid hormone. The reference interval for TSH is undergoing reevaluation considering that, in the past, individuals with subclinical hypothyroidism were inappropriately included in the normal reference population. This is likely to result in changes in the reference interval with lowering of the upper limits of normal. If associated with elevated concentrations of TPO antibodies, patients are at increased risk of progression to overt hypothyroidism. When elevated TSH concentrations are measured in a clinically hypothyroid patient, or a patient undergoing routine screening, TSH should be repeated with a serum free T4 measurement.

As demonstrated in this case, total T4 measurement alone can be inadequate and misleading as a measure of metabolically active thyroxine. Free T4, the portion of T4 that circulates free in the serum, represents only 0.03% of the total T4. The majority of circulating T4 is protein-bound to thyroxine-binding globulin, thyroxine-binding prealbumin, lipoproteins, and albumin. Increased concentrations of thyroxine-binding globulin, caused by estrogen during pregnancy or in oral contraceptive pills, as in this case, can cause the total T4 concentration to be elevated, even though the concentration of free T4 is low. Considering the widespread availability of free T4 assays, it is no longer appropriate to use the total T4 level for clinical assessments.

TSH can be misleading when the cause of hypothyroidism is secondary or tertiary, due to disease of the pituitary gland or hypothalamus. In these cases TSH can be low, normal, or modestly elevated. When the index of suspicion for hypothyroidism is high, free T4 testing should be performed concomitantly with TSH. Likewise, TSH can be transiently elevated in euthyroid patients with seizure disorders and falsely elevated as a result of heterophile antibody interference. Again, measurement of free T4 can be useful.

Although not essential, the diagnosis of autoimmune hypothyroidism can be confirmed by detection of thyroid autoantibodies such as antithyroperoxidase (TPO) antibodies. These antibodies have also been reported to increase prior to the onset of clinical disease and thus can be used to identify patients at risk of developing hypothyroidism.

Treatment

Patients presenting with hypothyroidism should be treated with L-thyroxine (levothyroxine) at dosages sufficient to restore the TSH concentration to the lower half of the reference interval. In patients with normal thyroid function, the size of a goitrous thyroid may be reduced by such replacement therapy. Laboratory monitoring should begin 6–8 weeks after therapy begins and each year thereafter, once the target TSH concentration is achieved. Use of thyroid antibody measurement for monitoring treatment of autoimmune disease is not recommended.

References

1. ROBERTS, C. G. AND LADENSON, P. W.: Hypothyroidism. *Lancet 363*:793–803, 2004.
2. WEETMAN, A. P. AND McGREGOR, A. M.: Autoimmune thyroid disease: Further developments in our understanding. *Endocrine Rev. 15*:788–830, 1994.
3. L. A. DEMERS AND C. A. SPENCER, eds., *Laboratory Support for the Diagnosis and Monitoring of Thyroid Disease*, The National Academy of Clinical Biochemistry Laboratory Medicine Practice Guidelines, 2003.

Case 19

The Reluctant Chef

Kenneth B. Ain

A general internist in the community referred a 42-year-old woman to an endocrinologist for evaluation of a newly discovered 1.0-cm right-sided thyroid nodule. The patient failed to appear for her appointment and for two rescheduled visits. Ten months later, she appeared at the clinic, apprehensive because she had noticed the appearance of another neck mass lateral to the thyroid nodule. The patient was employed as a pastry chef at a local hotel and otherwise felt well. She was healthy except for recently diagnosed mild diastolic hypertension, under current treatment with a small, daily dose of lisinopril.

Physical evaluation revealed a thin, nervous woman with a blood pressure of 136/86 mm Hg and a pulse rate of 96 bpm. Examination of her neck disclosed a firm nodule, 3.6×2.4 cm, in the medial aspect of the right thyroid lobe. Two lymph nodes, 2.0 cm each, were palpable in the right anterior cervical triangle. Other features of the examination disclosed no further abnormalities. Fine-needle aspiration biopsies of the thyroid nodule and both lymph nodes were performed at this initial visit, and blood was drawn for the following studies:

Analyte	Value, Conventional Units	Reference Interval, Conventional Units	Value, SI Units	Reference Interval, SI Units
Free T4	1.2 ng/dL	0.9–1.6	16 pmol/L	12–21
TSH	1.4 μU/mL	0.6–4.5	1.4 mU/L	0.6–4.5
Antithyroglobulin antibodies	<2.2 IU/mL	0–2.2	<2.2 IU/mL	0–2.2
Antithyroperoxidase antibodies	<70 IU/mL	0–70	<70 IU/mL	0–70

These laboratory results confirmed the clinical impression of euthyroidism and gave no serological evidence for autoimmune thyroid disease. Evaluation of the thyroid biopsy smears revealed clusters of pleomorphic cells with eccentrically located nuclei and presence of intranuclear cytoplasmic inclusions. Immunoperoxidase staining identified calcitonin granules in the cytoplasm. The cytological diagnosis was medullary carcinoma of the thyroid. Biopsies of the cervical lymph nodes revealed the presence of cells identical to

Tietz's Applied Laboratory Medicine, Second Edition. Edited by Mitchell G. Scott, Ann M. Gronowski, and Charles S. Eby
Copyright © 2007 John Wiley & Sons, Inc.

those seen on the thyroid biopsy. With these results in mind, the physician ordered the following laboratory tests:

Analyte	Value, Conventional Units	Reference Interval, Conventional Units	Value, SI Units	Reference Interval, SI Units
Calcitonin, basal (P)[a]	98 pg/mL	<20	98 ng/L	<20
Carcinoembryonic antigen (S)	12.0 ng/mL	<3.0	12.0 μg/L	<3.0
Calcium, total (S)	9.2 mg/dL	8.4–10.2	2.30 mmol/L	2.10–2.55
Calcium, ionized (P)	4.62 mg/dL	4.48–4.92	1.16 mmol/L	1.12–1.23
Norepinephrine (24 hour, U)	12.5 μg/day	15–100	74 nmol/day	89–591
Vanillylmandelic acid (24 hour, U)	2.4 mg/day	<6.8	12 μmol/day	<34
Metanephrine (24 hour, U)	96 g/day	45–290	524 nmol/day	245–1583

[a]Formerly, pentagastrin stimulation provided a more sensitive measure of calcitonin, but this agent is no longer available.

The patient underwent total surgical thyroidectomy and modified radical right cervical node resection. All detectable tumor was removed, and her recovery was uneventful. Pathological analysis of the operative specimen confirmed the diagnosis of medullary thyroid carcinoma with an intrathyroidal primary tumor, 4.0 × 2.5 cm in size, and 7 of 37 resected lymph nodes containing metastatic tumor. Follow-up evaluation with biannual physical examination, chest and abdomen CT scans, serum calcitonin and CEA measurements, and nuclear scanning using radiolabeled octreotide was planned.

Definition of the Disease

Medullary thyroid carcinoma (MTC) is a malignancy of the parafollicular cells of the thyroid gland and represents 5–8% of thyroid cancers.[1] Parafollicular cells are derived from the embryonic neural crest and do not concentrate iodine or secrete thyroid hormones. MTC cells may produce calcitonin, prostaglandins, serotonin, histaminase, carcinoembryonic antigen (CEA), and occasionally corticotropin (ACTH). Eighty percent of cases of MTC are sporadic; the remaining cases are familial, presenting either as multiple endocrine neoplasia (MEN) syndromes 2A or 2B or as isolated medullary thyroid carcinoma. The familial forms are inherited as an autosomal dominant trait, which is consequent to a mutation of the RET protooncogene of chromosome 10. Inherited MTC is frequently bilateral; it may be diagnosed in the precursor stage (C-cell or calcitonin-secreting parafollicular cell hyperplasia) in affected relatives of an index case by genetic testing of peripheral blood cells for the RET mutation identified in the index patient.[2] Sporadic (nonhereditary) MTC more often presents as a unilateral thyroid mass not associated with the features that characterize MEN syndromes. The MTC of MEN2a is associated with hyperparathyroidism, often presenting as four-gland hyperplasia, and with pheochromocytoma, the adrenal medullary tumor that secretes catecholamines. The MTC of MEN2b is usually a more aggressive malignancy and is associated with pheochromocytoma, marfanoid body habitus, mucosal neuromas, and intestinal ganglioneuromas.

Differential Diagnosis

In this patient, MTC became evident as a unilateral thyroid mass with local lymph node involvement. The key diagnostic tests at the time of presentation were tests for pheochromocytoma and hyperparathyroidism so that the probability of a MEN syndrome could be assessed. This approach is important for two reasons: (1) surgical removal of a thyroid mass in a patient with untreated pheochromocytoma is risky and potentially fatal and (2) if the patient has a familial form of MEN, evaluation of asymptomatic relatives is central to their early diagnosis and cure. Normocalcemia in this patient tended to rule out concurrent hyperparathyroidism, and normal urinary catecholamine values suggested absence of pheochromocytoma. Some physicians recommend computed axial tomography of the adrenal glands for additional evidence of absence of pheochromocytoma. The familial connection for this patient was impossible to pursue by evaluating the family history, since she was an adopted child and knew of no blood relatives to be screened; however, commercial gene sequencing of DNA obtained from peripheral blood can usually reveal the RET mutation of familial disease. It is an appropriate standard of care to evaluate each index case of MTC for these mutations so that affected families can be genetically screened. Family members with the mutation are provided a prophylactic thyroidectomy.

The basal calcitonin concentration served in this case as a tumor marker for MTC and would serve after primary resection of the tumor as an index for recurrence or progression of neoplasia. Detection of MTC is made more sensitive by use of stimulation tests utilizing intravenous calcium gluconate or pentagastrin (no longer available). Because a definitive diagnosis for this case was already recorded, based on an elevated basal calcitonin level and biopsy findings, a stimulation test was unnecessary. Persistently elevated calcitonin concentrations, occurring in the patient after apparently successful surgical treatment, would raise concern for local recurrence or metastatic dispersal of tumor. Elevation of the CEA concentration, as seen in this patient, is not surprising in view of the diagnosis but would not of itself be sufficient to support a diagnosis of MTC.

Treatment

Once an associated pheochromocytoma has been either excluded or recognized and surgically treated, treatment of MTC requires total thyroidectomy and appropriate lymphadenectomy.[3] Since efficacy of chemotherapeutic agents has not been well established for this disease, as complete as possible surgical removal of the entire thyroid and tumor is critical. Assertive and meticulous lymph node dissection may provide greater disease-free survival in selected patients with only local disease. [131]I treatment for distant, unresectable, metastatic MTC is totally ineffective since these tumor cells cannot concentrate iodine. Radiation therapy may be used to treat locally recurrent, unresectable tumor, but this therapy usually proves merely palliative and often fails to improve survival. The patient with apparently successful surgical ablation must be followed indefinitely with calcitonin and CEA blood tests as well as other examinations. If there are elevations of these tumor markers, the patient should be restaged to determine the site(s) of recurrent or metastatic disease. Appropriate methods include: CT scanning, ultrasound, MRI scanning, PET scans, and radiolabeled octriotide scans. The onset of manifestations of MEN syndromes may not be synchronous; consequently, familial

MTC patients without hyperparathyroidism or pheochromocytoma at their initial presentation must be regularly screened for development of these conditions, particularly if they have been seen in other affected family members.

When diagnosed, sporadic MTC is usually more advanced than is familial MTC detected by genetic screening. A thyroidectomy, performed in the earliest stages of C-cell hyperplasia, may be curative. Survival in MTC after treatment is approximately 80% at 5 years, although persons with more advanced tumors do worse and those with less advanced tumors at the time of diagnosis do better. Morbidity and mortality from this cancer may occur decades after initial presentation, making lifelong follow-up a necessity.

References

1. L. A. DEMERS AND C. A. SPENCER, eds., *Laboratory Support for the Diagnosis and Monitoring of Thyroid Disease*, The National Academy of Clinical Biochemistry Laboratory Medicine Practice Guidelines, 2003.
2. MASSOLL, N. AND MAZZAFERRI, E. L.: Diagnosis and management of medullary thyroid carcinoma. *Clin. Lab. Med. 24*:49–83, 2004.
3. ORLANDI, F., CARACI, P., MUSSA, A., SAGGIORATO, E., PANCANI, G., AND ANGELI, A.: Treatment of medullary thyroid carcinoma: an update. *Endocrine Related Cancer 8*:135–47, 2001.

Part Six

Adrenocortical Diseases

Cases of congenital adrenal hyperplasia, Cushing syndrome, Addison disease with chronic adrenal insufficiency, Conn's syndrome (primary hyperaldosteronism), multiple endocrine neoplasia, and pheochromocytoma are presented and discussed in Cases 20, 21, 22, 23, 24, and 25, respectively (all edited by AMG).

Tietz's Applied Laboratory Medicine, Second Edition. Edited by Mitchell G. Scott, Ann M. Gronowski, and Charles S. Eby
Copyright © 2007 John Wiley & Sons, Inc.

Case 20

Child with Rapid Growth and Precocious Sexual Maturation

Phyllis W. Speiser

A 6-year-old boy was admitted to the medical center with a 4-year history of rapid somatic growth and a 6-month history of pubic hair growth. The patient was the full-term product of a normal vaginal delivery following an uncomplicated first gestation in a 34-year-old healthy female. Birth weight was 8 lb 9 oz (3.9 kg) and length 21.5 in. (54.6 cm). There were no neonatal problems. The mother ceased breastfeeding the infant at 10 days of life and changed to formula because he did not seem to gain weight. Thereafter, weight gain was normal. Between 9 and 18 months of age, the patient's linear growth was just above the 95th percentile, but by $2\frac{1}{2}$ years of age, his height was average for a $4\frac{1}{2}$-year-old child. His tall stature was disregarded by his family and pediatrician, who considered this normal since his parents were tall [father 74 in. (1.90 m) and mother 66 in. (1.68 m)]. When the patient was 3 years old, his mother observed that his penis was larger than that of age-matched peers, and by the age of 4 some acne had developed. Pubic hair developed at $5\frac{1}{2}$ years of age, at which time he was referred to a pediatric endocrinologist for evaluation.

Physical examination revealed a tall, well proportioned, muscular boy with mild facial acne. His height at 54.6 in. (1.39 m) was average for a boy of 10 years 3 months; his weight of 68 lb (31 kg) was average for 9 years 10 months. Blood pressure was normal (100/64 mm Hg). Dentition was advanced for age. The thyroid was not palpable. Examination of the chest and abdomen was unremarkable. The penis measured 7 cm semierect; fine, dark pubic hair was observed at the base of the phallus (Tanner stage II). Testes were each 3 mL in volume, without palpable masses. There were no pigmented cutaneous lesions. Neurological examination was normal.

Tietz's Applied Laboratory Medicine, Second Edition. Edited by Mitchell G. Scott, Ann M. Gronowski, and Charles S. Eby
Copyright © 2007 John Wiley & Sons, Inc.

Laboratory results were as follows:

Analyte	Value, Conventional Units	Reference Interval, Conventional Units	Value, SI Units	Reference Interval, SI Units
Sodium	138 mmol/L	135–145	Same	Same
Potassium	4.0 mmol/L	3.5–4.7	Same	Same
Chloride	103 mmol/L	99–108	Same	Same
Bicarbonate	25 mmol/L	24–32	Same	Same
Luteinizing hormone (LH), basal	1.7 mU/mL	<1 (prepuberty)	1.7 U/L	<1
Follicle-stimulating hormone (FSH), basal	<1 mU/mL	<1 (prepuberty)	<1 U/L	<1
Testosterone	172 ng/dL	2–12	5.9 nmol/L	0.07–0.46 nmol/L
17-Hydroxyprogesterone, basal	11,690 ng/dL	<100	354 nmol/L	<3 nmol/L
17-Hydroxyprogesterone, 60 minutes after ACTH stimulation	22,000 ng/dL	<200	666.6 nmol/L	<7.5 nmol/L
Cortisol, basal	7 g/dL	5–20	193 nmol/L	138–552
Cortisol, after ACTH stimulation	10 g/dL	2–3 × basal	276 nmol/L	2–3 × basal

Computed tomography of the head was normal. Bone age based on x-ray examination of the wrist was read as compatible with a maturation of 12 years 9 months. Ultrasonographic examination of the testes showed no masses. The history of chronic accelerated growth velocity accompanied by signs of sexual maturation, the presence of relatively small testes for the degree of masculinization, and markedly elevated concentrations of serum 17-hydroxyprogesterone, the principal substrate for 21-hydroxylase, led to the diagnosis of congenital adrenal hyperplasia due to 21-hydroxylase deficiency.

The patient was started on treatment with hydrocortisone. Reevaluation following 3 months of medical therapy indicated that linear growth was still accelerated, the testes had enlarged slightly, and the testosterone concentration had further increased. Repeat measurement of serum gonadotropins during sleep showed an LH of 19.9 mU/mL (19.9 U/L) and an FSH of 3.5 mU/mL (3.5 U/L), indicating pituitary stimulation of the testes. A gonadotropin-releasing hormone analog was added to the medical regimen to suppress central puberty.

Definition of the Disease

Congenital adrenal hyperplasia (CAH) is a group of diseases that result from reduced or absent activity of one of the five enzymes of cortisol synthesis in the adrenal cortex (Fig. 20.1). Each enzyme deficiency produces characteristic alterations in the concentrations of the particular steroid hormones that are substrates for, or products of, metabolism by the defective enzyme.[1,2] Approximately 90% of cases of CAH are attributable to deficiency of 21-hydroxylase, a microsomal cytochrome P450 enzyme required in the pathways leading to cortisol and aldosterone but not required in the production of sex steroids. In the presence of a defect in 21-hydroxylase, the synthesis of cortisol is blocked. This leads to disruption of the normal feedback mechanisms and overproduction of ACTH. The result is adrenal hyperplasia, the oversecretion of

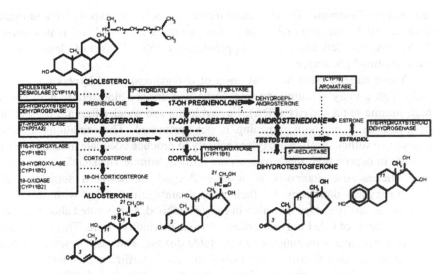

CLASS: MINERALOCORTICOIDS   GLUCOCORTICOIDS   **SEX STEROIDS**

ZONE: GLOMERULOSA   FASCICULATA   RETICULARIS

Figure 20.1   Pathways of steroidogenesis within the adrenal gland. Enzyme nomenclature is given inside boxes; common names of steroid intermediates are listed. Steroid structures are shown for cholesterol (upper left), aldosterone, cortisol, testosterone, and estradiol (bottom of figure). Adrenal precursors hormones such as androstenedione are converted to sex steroids in the periphery by various additional enzyme pathways. There are alternative metabolic pathways within the adrenal gland as well.

precursors of potent androgens such as androstenedione, and pre- and postnatal virilization. Deficiency of 21-hydroxylase may also interfere with the synthesis of aldosterone, which leads to salt-wasting.

The disease has an autosomal recessive mode of inheritance. The gene (termed *CYP21A2*) encoding the active 21-hydroxylase enzyme and a highly homologous pseudo-gene are located on the short arm of the sixth chromosome in the midst of the HLA complex (chromosome 6p21.3). A combination of two severe mutations in each of the *CYP21A2* alleles produces the classic form of the disease (e.g., deletion–deletion), whereas two milder mutations (exon 7 valine-281 to leucine–exon 7 valine-281 to leucine) or a combination of a severe and a mild deficiency allele produces mild or nonclassic CAH. Numerous other mutations, aside from these two mentioned, have been detected in patients with 21-hydroxylase deficiency. Heterozygotes have reduced enzymatic activity that is detectable only by the mildly elevated 17-hydroxyprogesterone concentration after ACTH stimulation.

Clinical Features

The most prominent feature of CAH is progressive virilism with advanced somatic development. In the classic or severe form of the disease, this process begins in utero, manifesting in affected females as varying degrees of genital ambiguity that range from mild clitoral enlargement, through fusion of the labioscrotal folds and urogenital sinus (common opening onto the perineum of both urethra and vagina), to a penile urethra. Internal genitalia, including upper vagina, cervix, uterus, fallopian tubes, and ovaries, are structurally normal. Because male fetuses are normally exposed to androgen in utero, both internal and external genital formations are normal in males affected with 21-hydroxylase deficiency CAH. Approximately 75% of cases of classic cases have the "salt-wasting" phenotype.

These patients have neonatal onset of hyponatremia and hyperkalemia, inappropriately high urinary sodium, and low serum and urinary aldosterone with concomitantly high plasma renin activity (PRA). Hypovolemia and shock often are present at the time of diagnosis if newborn screening is not performed. The remaining 25% of classic cases have sufficient 21-hydroxylase activity to produce adequate aldosterone in response to sodium deprivation; these patients are termed "simple virilizers".

Whereas the diagnosis is usually flagged in newborn females with classic 21-hydroxylase deficiency by their genital ambiguity, males with this form of the disease can easily escape detection in early childhood, and as noted above, those with salt-wasting forms of CAH may experience serious morbidity or die. This is among the rationales for neonatal screening for this treatable disease. The case presented here is entirely typical of the clinical history of a male with simple virilizing 21-OHD.

The nonclassic form of CAH presents with less severe virilization of postnatal onset and fewer growth problems. Nonclassic CAH may also be distinguished from the classic form of the disease by lesser elevation of serum 17-hydroxyprogesterone and different mutations.

Diagnosis

The diagnosis of CAH is now most often made through newborn screening programs, which have been implemented in the vast majority of states in the United States. Most programs use a radioimmunoassay for filter paper 17-hydroxyprogesterone, however, because of the low positive predictive value for this assay, second-tier testing with either tandem mass spectrometry or genotyping is now being considered.

Confirming the hormonal diagnosis of 21-hydroxylase deficiency is straightforward; baseline and ACTH-stimulated serum concentrations of 17-hydroxyprogesterone are abnormally high, generally greater than 10,000 ng/dL. In order to improve specificity, it is important to measure a panel of several adrenocortical hormones. This effectively rules out other forms of virilizing adrenal hyperplasia (see Table 20.1). Normative data for both the basal and ACTH-stimulated values of these hormones are age- and sex-specific.

Administration of glucocorticoids to the patient with advanced bone age due to chronic hypersecretion of adrenal androgens will rapidly suppress ACTH and thereby suppress adrenal secretion of these hormones. Such fluctuations in adrenal sex steroid hormones may release the hypothalamic–pituitary axis from tonic suppression. Therefore, if testicular enlargement or breast development indicative of ovarian estrogen secretion is observed in young children, gonadotropins should be measured to ascertain whether central puberty is in progress.

The salt-wasting form of 21-OHD is accompanied by the metabolic derangements described in the preceding text. Normal individuals or patients affected with the simple virilizing form of 21-OHD, when stressed with severe sodium deprivation (dietary intake of 10 mmol/day), excrete more than 22 mmol/m^2 of aldosterone daily. Salt-wasting patients, however, excrete negligible aldosterone despite markedly elevated concentrations of plasma renin activity and angiotensin II, which are the primary stimuli of de novo aldosterone synthesis. A patient with 21-0HD who demonstrates signs of virilism

Table 20.1 Characteristics of Different Forms of Congenital Adrenal Hyperplasia

Disease	21-Hydroxylase deficiency	11β-Hydroxylase deficiency	Aldosterone synthase deficiency	17α-Hydroxylase deficiency	3β-Hydroxysteroid dehydrogenase deficiency	Lipoid hyperplasia
Defective gene	CYP21A2	CYP11B1	CYP11B2	CYP17	HSD3B2	STAR
Enzyme	P450c21	P450c11	P450aldo	P450c17	3β-HSD	
Chromosomal location	6p21.3	8q24.3	8q24.3	10q24.3	1p13.1	8p11.2
Ambiguous genitalia	+in females	+in females	No	+in males No puberty in females	+in males Mild in females	+in males No puberty in females
Addisonian crisis	+	Rare	Salt-wasting only	No	+	++
Incidence (general population)	1 : 10–15,000	1 : 100,000	Rare	Rare	Rare	Rare
Hormones						
Glucocorticoids	Low	Low	Normal	Corticosterone normal	Low	Low
Mineralocorticoids	Low	High	Low	High	Low in males High in females	Low
Androgens	High	High	Normal	Low	Low in males High in females	Low
Estrogens	Relatively high in females	Relatively high in females	Normal	Low	Low	Low
Physiology						
Blood pressure	Low	High	Low	High	Low	Low
Na balance	Low	High	Low	High	Low	Low
K balance	High	Low	High	Low	High	High
Acidosis	+	± Alkalosis	+	± Alkalosis	+	+
Elevated metabolites	17-OHP	DOC 11-deoxycortisol	Corticosterone, ± 18-hydroxycorticosterone	DOC corticosterone,	DHEA, $17\text{-}\delta^5$Preg	None

Key: 17-OHP, 17-hydroxyprogesterone; DOC, deoxycorticosterone; DHEA, dehydroepiandrosterone; $17\text{-}\delta^5$ Preg, $17\text{-}\delta^5$ pregnenolone.

Source: Adapted from White, P. C. and Speiser, P. W., *Endocrine Rev. 21*:245, 2000.

but has no history of electrolyte abnormalities or dehydration, such as in this case, is likely to have normal aldosterone synthesis.

Genotyping may serve as an adjunct to hormonal diagnosis, particularly in the genetic counseling of family members and to perform prenatal diagnosis.

Treatment

The aim of medical treatment is to replace cortisol and thus reduce ACTH secretion. This suppresses adrenal androgens and restores normal somatic growth and sexual maturation. The drug of choice in young children is hydrocortisone given in slightly larger than physiological doses. Hydrocortisone is preferred over more potent and long-acting steroids such as prednisone or dexamethasone, because the hydrocortisone is less likely to result in growth suppression. Patients with evidence of precocious central puberty may also require pituitary suppression with a gonadotropin-releasing hormone analog. In salt-wasting patients with deficiency of aldosterone, mineralocorticoid replacement must be added. The drug of choice is oral 9a-fludrocortisone, often given with oral sodium chloride supplements. If life-threatening shock ("adrenal crisis") should occur, both hydrocortisone and isotonic sodium chloride are administered intravenously, along with cardiotonic medications until normotension is restored.

Surgical treatment is often recommended to correct the genital ambiguity in females with classic disease. This procedure is usually done within the first few months of life. It consists of clitoroplasty to reduce the size of the erectile tissue, and vaginoplasty if there is a combined urethra and vagina (urogenital sinus). In this operation, the surgeon separates the distal urethra and vagina. Besides ameliorating the stenotic vagina, this also helps avoid urinary tract infections.

Helpful Diagnostic Notes

Ambiguous genitalia in the newborn may be caused by a number of different conditions, including the incomplete form of androgen resistance syndrome (testicular feminization), gonadal dysgenesis, and inability to convert testosterone to its active metabolite, dihydrotestosterone, due to deficiency of the nonadrenal enzyme 5α-reductase. Initial evaluation of all such patients should include karyotype analysis, radiographic imaging of the pelvis to identify internal genital anatomy, and basal and appropriately stimulated concentrations of hormones in the mineralocorticoid, glucocorticoid, and sexsteroid pathways. The diagnosis of 21-hydroxylase deficiency is strongly suspected in a female when the karyotype is 46,XX, a uterus is detected, and there are no male (wolffian) internal genital structures. In newborn males, the first manifestation of the disease is salt-wasting adrenal crisis. Clues to the diagnosis in older males are usually rapid linear growth and signs of androgen excess with disproportionately small testes. The latter sign differentiates gonadal from extragonadal pseudopuberty, as in congenital adrenal hyperplasia.

References

1. P. W. SPEISER, AND P. C. WHITE: Congenital adrenal hyperplasia. *N. Engl. J. Med. 349*:776–88, 2003.
2. Congenital adrenal hyperplasia. In *Endocrinology and Metabolism Clinics of North America*, P. W. SPEISER, ed., 2001, Vol. 30 (the entire volume is devoted to CAH), p. 1.

Case 21

Weight Gain, Infertility, and Hypertension

William E. Winter

A 30-year-old African-American woman with a complex medical history presented to her private physician with complaints of emotional lability and depression over the previous 12–18 months. During this period, she gained 25–30 lb (11–14 kg), despite her best attempts to maintain her weight through regular exercise. She also complained of infertility as she had not conceived after a year of unprotected intercourse with her spouse of 10 years. She did have a 5-year-old daughter from her current marriage. That pregnancy was complicated by preeclampsia. At presentation, she reported that her menstrual periods were irregular and in the last 6 months she had had only had two menstrual periods; the last was 6 weeks ago.

Her past medical history was significant for a spontaneous rib fracture 12 months ago. She had reached for a book located on the floor and developed acute chest pain. Chest x-ray in the emergency department revealed the fracture. The fracture was treated conservatively with rest and external support. The radiology report noted some demineralization of the spine and ribs in addition to the fracture. Follow up bone mineral density (BMD) measurements via dexa scan revealed the following findings consistent with a decline in bone mineral density (SD—standard deviation):

Location	BMD
Lumbar spine	− 1.93 SD below the mean
Left hip	− 1.18 SD below the mean

Concerning her past medical history, other than tonsillectomy and adenoidectomy at age 6 for recurrent pharyngitis, the patient had no past hospitalizations for medical illnesses. Her childhood illnesses included chicken pox. Other than preeclampsia as noted in her first and only pregnancy, prior to 18 months ago, she reported no serious illnesses. Her immunizations were up-to-date. She took no chronic medications and used no medicinal creams. She denied glucocorticoid use.

Regarding her family history, the patient's 62-year-old mother had migraine headaches. Her 72-year-old father was alive and well. There was no family history of

Tietz's Applied Laboratory Medicine, Second Edition. Edited by Mitchell G. Scott, Ann M. Gronowski, and Charles S. Eby
Copyright © 2007 John Wiley & Sons, Inc.

depression or other forms of psychiatric illness. There was no family history of endocrine disorders including thyroid disease and diabetes mellitus.

Review of systems was positive for polyuria and polydipsia, tiredness, weakness, and easy bruisability. She voided 2–3 times per night. She suffered headaches 1–2 times per week that were relieved with aspirin or acetaminophen. She did not complain of cough, shortness of breath, or wheezing. She did not complain of nausea, vomiting, diarrhea, or constipation. She did report that she always felt hungry.

Physical examination revealed an obese 30-year-old African-American woman who was in no acute distress. Her height was 157 cm, and her weight was 81 kg. Her body mass index was 33 kg/m². Her vital signs were as follows: temperature = 36.5°C, pulse = 95 beats per minute, respirations = 18 breaths per minute, blood pressure = 155/95 mm Hg. Repeat blood pressure measurement in the opposite arm revealed 160/92 mm Hg. Her facial appearance was plethoric with prominent checks (i.e., "moon facies"). Mild facial hirsutism involving the temporomandibular areas was identified. Her HEENT examination revealed normal discs and fundi. There was no papilledema or arterial narrowing. There was no thyromegaly or cervical lymphadenopathy. There was a prominent collection of adipose tissue over her upper back below her neck consistent with a "buffalo hump." She had distinct, visible, and palpable supraclavicular fat pads. Her pulmonary and cardiac exams were normal. Her breasts were Tanner stage 4, and no masses or discharge were appreciated. She displayed central adiposity. The abdomen was obese and nontender with normal bowel sounds. By palpation, modest hepatomegaly was appreciated. The spleen was not palpable. The arms and legs were relatively thin and had minimal muscle mass. All peripheral pulses were 2+ and symmetric in the upper and lower extremities. Her pelvic examination was normal. Her skin was oily and slightly wet with perspiration. Neurologic examination revealed decreased strength in the arms and legs. Cranial nerves II–XII were grossly intact. There were no focal neurologic deficits. Her visual fields were intact by confrontation.

Because of her "moon facies," plethora, buffalo hump, supraclavicular fat pads, centripetal obesity, stria, hypertension, and history of depression, infertility, and polyuria/polydipsia/nocturia, the differential diagnosis of her problems focused on Cushing syndrome.

Baseline CBC and serum and urine chemistries were ordered after an overnight fast. To evaluate the potential cause of infertility, serum prolactin, testosterone, estradiol, luteinizing hormone (LH), and follicle-stimulating hormone (FSH) were measured. A 24-hour urinary free cortisol (UFC) concentration was determined to detect hypercortisolism. Like many 24-hour collections, proper sample preservation was necessary.

Analyte	Value, Conventional Units	Reference Interval, Conventional Units	Value, SI Units	Reference Interval, SI Units
Sodium	142 mEq/L	135–145	142 mmol/L	135–145
Potassium	3.4 mEq/L	3.5–5.0	3.4 mmol/L	3.5–5.0
Chloride	95 mEq/L	95–105	95 mmol/L	95–105
CO$_2$, total	34 mEq/L	24–32	34 mmol/L	24–32
Creatinine	0.8 mg/dL	0.5–1.2	71 umol/L	44–106
BUN	18 mg/dL	10–20 mg/dL	6.4 mmol urea/L	3.6–7.1
Glucose	128 mg/dL	65–99 mg/dL	7.1 mmol/L	3.6–5.5
Prolactin	18 ng/mL	3–20 ng/mL	18 ug/L	3–20
Testosterone	56 ng/dL	<62 ng/dL	1.94 nmol/L	<2.15

Analyte	Value, Conventional Units	Reference Interval, Conventional Units	Value, SI Units	Reference Interval, SI Units
Estradiol	82 pg/mL	≤145 pg/mL (follicular phase)	285 pmol/L	≤503
FSH	2.5 mIU/mL	1.1–9.6 mIU/mL (follicular phase)	2.5 IU/L	1.1–9.6 IU/L (follicular phase)
LH	0.6 mIU/mL	0.8–25.8 mIU/mL (follicular phase)	0.6 IU/L	0.8–25.8 IU/L (follicular phase)
Urinary free cortisol	216 μg/24 hours	20–90	596 nmol/day	55–248

Her CBC revealed a mild normocytic, normochromic anemia, mild lymphopenia, and no detected eosinophils. Hypokalemia was identified. Her urinalysis was unremarkable except for a urine pH of 5.5 in the freshly voided sample. Based on the elevated total CO_2, low normal chloride, and acidified urine, a metabolic alkalosis was apparent. The gonadotropin levels ruled against primary gonadal failure. Neither testosterone or prolactin were elevated.

To supplement the elevated urinary free cortisol measurement, which was consistent with cortisol excess, an overnight dexamethasone suppression test was next performed, with the following results:

Analyte	Value, Conventional Units	Reference Interval, Conventional Units	Value, SI Units	Reference Interval, SI Units
Cortisol	15 μg/dL	<5	414 nmol/L	<138

The patient was queried to ensure that she took the prescribed dexamethasone, which she reported that she did.

Together with the patient's history and physical examination (1) the elevated urinary free cortisol and (2) the elevated postdexamethasone 8:00 am cortisol were consistent with Cushing syndrome (e.g., hypercortisolism). Recognizing that a variety of conditions can mimic Cushing syndrome ("pseudo-Cushing syndrome"), a "formal" dexamethasone suppression test was performed.

The results of the formal dexamethasone suppression test are given below:

	Baseline Day 1	Baseline Day 2	Low Dose Day 3	Low Dose Day 4	High Dose Day 5	High Dose Day 6
Urinary free cortisol	250 μg	210 μg	175 μg	235 μg	155 μg	145 μg
Creatinine	1.1 g	1.0 g	1.1 g	1.0 g	1.1 g	0.9 g

The degree of UFC suppression on high-dose dexamethasone was borderline. However, basal fasting ACTH concentrations drawn on two consecutive days approximately one week prior to the above formal dexamethasone suppression test revealed measurable ACTH concentrations despite hypercortisolism (note the corresponding elevated am and pm cortisol concentrations with loss of diurnal variation). Measurable ACTH concentrations would exclude an autonomous source of cortisol production by the adrenal cortex.

Analyte	Value, Conventional Units	Reference Interval, Conventional Units	Value, SI Units	Reference Interval, SI Units
Day 1				
0800h				
ACTH	113 pg/mL	<70	25 pmol/L	<15.4
Cortisol	34 μg/dL	7–25	938 nmol/L	193–690
2200h				
Cortisol	31 μg/dL	2–9	856 nmol/L	193–690
Day 2				
0800h				
ACTH	59 pg/mL	<70	13 pmol/L	<15.4
Cortisol	28 μg/dL	7–25	773 nmol/L	193–690

Magnetic resonance imaging (MRI) of the pituitary was next carried out in search of a pituitary adenoma with and without gadolinium contrast enhancement. The MRI report is summarized as follows: "Overall, the pituitary gland did not appear definitively enlarged. There was a suggestion of asymmetry and prominence of the left side of the gland when compared to the right. The gadolinium-enhanced scan demonstrated a fairly homogeneous contrast enhancement except for a questionable small (~5 mm) focus of slightly increased signal in the most anterior left portion of the pituitary. However, there was no definite evidence for pituitary microadenoma."

If imaging had revealed an adenoma, the diagnosis of Cushing disease would have been established. In the absence of definitive MRI evidence of a pituitary adenoma, inferior petrosal venous sinus sampling (IPSS) was carried out in radiology. Results are listed in Table 21.1.

At baseline (−15 minutes and 0 minute), the IPSS-R sample is more than 10 fold greater than the peripheral and the IPSS-L concentrations. The magnitude of these differences was amplified by CRH injection. IPSS to peripheral blood ACTH ratios of ≥3 are consistent with a pituitary source of the ACTH. The average ratio of IPSS ACTH to peripheral ACTH in Cushing disease is 15 with the lower limit of normal near 1.5–1.7. These data are consistent with an ACTH-secreting pituitary adenoma even in the presence of ambivalent MRI findings.

Review of the clinical and laboratory data supported the diagnosis of Cushing disease: lymphopenia, eosinopenia, and hypokalemia, and a metabolic alkalosis with hypertension, fasting hyperglycemia and reduced bone mineral density.

Neurosurgery was consulted. Prior to surgery her hypertension was managed with benazepril HCl and hydrochlorothiazide. Benazepril HCl is an angiotensin-converting enzyme inhibitor, whereas hydrochlorothiazide is a diuretic.

Transplenoidal removal of a ~4-mm pituitary mass was accomplished. The tumor was localized to the right side of the pituitary gland. Immunohistochemistry was positive for ACTH staining in the microadenoma.

The patient's postoperative course was unremarkable. From 6 weeks to 12 weeks postoperatively she was weaned off replacement doses of oral glucocorticoids. Over the next year, regular menses returned, she was weaned off her antihypertensives, she lost weight and her psychological disposition improved.

Table 21.1 Corticotropin-Releasing Hormone (CRH) Stimulation Test

Time	ACTH (pg/mL) peripheral	ACTH (pg/mL) IPSS-R[a]	ACTH (pg/mL) IPSS-L[b]	ACTH ratio: IPSS-R/ peripheral	ACTH ratio: IPSS-L/ peripheral	ACTH ratio: IPSS-R/IPSS-L	Cortisol (μg/dL) pheripheral
−15	15	170	13	11.3	0.87	13.1	10
0	20	285	18	14.2	0.90	15.8	8.8
+3	21	836	48	39.8	2.3	17.4	8.3
+5	40	729	78	18.2	1.95	9.3	7.5
+10	45	585	56	13.0	1.24	10.4	12.6
+15	70	747	81	10.7	1.16	9.2	18.8
+30	94	797	105	8.5	1.12	7.6	26.3
+60	132	784	221	5.9	1.67	3.5	30.8

[a]IPSS-R = right inferior petrosal venous sinus sample.
[b]IPSS-L = left inferior petrosal venous sinus sample.
Note: ACTH pg/mL × 0.22 = ACTH pmol/L.

Definition of the Disease

Cushing syndrome results from cortisol excess. While excess cortisol secretion is usually a chronic condition in Cushing syndrome, some cases display episodic secretion of hypercortisolism, for example, only after meals. Such cases can be extremely perplexing and require the most vigorous investigation for the identification and confirmation of hypercortisolism.

Excess cortisol affects many systems in the body. Concerning the central nervous system (CNS), appetite is increased with consequent weight gain. Emotional lability can result in such an extreme form that Cushing syndrome patients may present with psychosis.

Cortisol in excess redistributes body fat to centripetal locations in the face, upper back, supraclavicular fossa, and abdomen. As a catabolic agent, muscle breakdown supplies carbon skeletons that the liver uses to synthesize glucose via gluconeogenesis. The combination of cortisol-induced insulin resistance at peripheral tissues such as muscle and adipose tissue, and increased hepatic glucose output produce abnormal glucose tolerance or frank diabetes. Muscle breakdown in the arms and legs leads to a myopathy manifested as reduced muscle size and weakness. Bone catabolism can be expressed as back pain, osteopenia, and pathologic fractures. Catabolism with thinning and structural weakness of the skin induces purple stria. Bruisability is a manifestation of vascular fragility from protein catabolism. Weakness of the abdominal muscles and increased intrabdominal fat produce a protuberant abdomen.

Eosinopenia is a consequence of the immunomodulating effects of glucocorticoids. In pharmacologic doses, glucocorticoids can produce lymphocyte lysis. This is one component of certain chemotherapy regiments used in the treatment of leukemia (e.g., childhood acute lymphoblastic leukemia).

High cortisol concentrations will interact with the mineralocorticoid receptor, inducing a state of hypermineralocorticoidism. This is manifested in increased urinary potassium loss and hypokalemia in the plasma; increased hydrogen ion excretion in the urine, inducing a metabolic alkalosis; and sodium retention, leading to hypertension. Cortisol's interaction with the androgen receptor appears to be responsible for hirsutism in women with Cushing syndrome. Insulin resistance and hyperandrogenism interfere with normal menstrual cycling manifested as oligomenorrhea, amenorrhea, and even infertility.

Most cases of Cushing syndrome result from excess intake of exogenous glucocorticoids. High-dose glucocorticoids may be part of an intended pharmacologic regimen for treatment of asthma, severe inflammatory, autoimmune, or neoplastic conditions. Alternatively, excess glucocorticoids may be self-administered by the patient and not the intention of the treating physician. The physician seeing a patient with possible Cushing syndrome must first exclude exposure to exogenous glucocorticoids before launching into an expensive and potentially invasive workup.

Endogenous Cushing syndrome can result from (1) a pituitary adenoma producing excess ACTH (e.g., Cushing disease), (2) ectopic ACTH or CRH secretion, or (3) autonomous excess cortisol production by the adrenal (e.g., an adrenal tumor).

Cushing disease accounts for about 70% of endogenous Cushing syndrome cases. In a patient with documented hypercortisolism who has suppression of cortisol secretion with high-dose dexamethasone, an elevated ACTH, and a pituitary lesion on MRI, the diagnosis of Cushing disease is straightforward. This case illustrates what must be done when the clinical features do not clearly distinguish Cushing disease from ectopic ACTH/CRH. A microadenoma is a pituitary tumor <10 mm in diameter whereas a macroadenoma is 10 mm in diameter or greater.

Cases of ectopic ACTH (or ectopic CRH, which is less common than ectopic ACTH) may not present with classic findings of Cushing syndrome because the underlying malignancy responsible for the ectopic ACTH secretion dominates the clinical presentation with weight loss, weakness, inanition, and other symptoms. Ectopic ACTH may also present very abruptly, whereas patients with Cushing disease or cortisol-secreting adrenal tumors have histories of disease prolonged over months or years. ACTH concentrations in ectopic ACTH can range from 200 to 1000 pg/mL. The classic condition producing ectopic ACTH is an oat cell carcinoma of the lung. Other tumors producing the ectopic ACTH syndrome include carcinoid, thymoma, islet cell tumors, medullary thyroid carcinoma, and pheochromocytoma. CRH measurements are available for clinical use if ectopic CRH is a clinical consideration. Very rarely, patients will have both ectopic ACTH and CRH production.

Autonomous cortisol hypersecretion from the adrenal cortex can result from (1) adrenocortical adenoma, (2) adrenocortical carcinoma, (3) bilateral micronodular hyperplasia, or (4) bilateral macronodular hyperplasia. The identification of these disorders depends on differentiation of unilateral versus bilateral disease [e.g., using computed tomography (CT) or MRI and bilateral adrenal vein sampling for cortisol], identification of metastases (which, if present, indicate a carcinoma), and ultimately gross and microscopic examination of the surgically removed gland(s). With bilateral adrenal hypercortisolism, plasma cortisol is elevated in both adrenal veins. In unilateral adrenal disease, one adrenal vein exhibits high cortisol concentrations whereas the other adrenal vein cortisol is suppressed or at least no more than the systemic cortisol concentrations.

Cortisol-producing adrenocortical adenomas are typically unilateral, circumscribed, brown-yellow in color, and homogeneous in consistency. They weigh less than 30 g. Histologically, the cells appear normal surrounded by a fibrous capsule. This form of Cushing syndrome displays a longer duration of disease prior to discovery because of its subtle nature.

Grossly, cortisol-producing adrenocortical carcinomas are irregular and histologically display hemorrhage, necrosis, nuclear pleomorphism, and mitotic figures. Invasion of the capsule and blood vessels is pathognomonic for carcinoma. The clinical history is of shorter duration (e.g., 4–6 months) compared with cortisol-producing adrenocortical adenomas. Tumor weight is often greater than 100 g and the tumors may be palpable during abdominal physical examination. Hepatomegaly can develop when metastases are present.

Cortisol-producing adrenocortical carcinomas can be occasionally associated with Li–Fraumeni syndrome, which includes sarcomas, brain tumors, leukemia, lymphomas, and/or early-onset breast cancer. Clinical onset is before age 45. P53 mutations are observed in Li–Fraumeni syndrome.

Bilateral micronodular hyperplasia is also known as *primary nodular hyperplasia* or *adrenocortical dysplasia*. Grossly, 2–3-cm nodules are visible in both adrenal glands. The nodules may be pigmented. Bilateral macronodular hyperplasia is also known as *massive macronodular hyperplasia* or *macronodular adrenal dysplasia*. In this condition, the nodules can vary between 0.2 and 4 cm and may weigh over 100 g. Some of these tumors display activating G_S mutations. In some cases displaying postmeal hypercortisolism, the adrenal tumors have been found to express receptors for gastric inhibitory polypeptide, which is secreted by the intestine in response to meals. This can lead to episodic Cushing syndrome and diagnostic difficulties.

Differential Diagnosis

Each of the symptoms and signs of Cushing syndrome has an extensive differential diagnosis. The most common issues concern distinguishing exogenous obesity from Cushing syndrome. In cases of exogenous obesity the arms and legs are not thin and do not demonstrate a loss of muscle mass. In exogenous obesity, stria appear more pink in color and not purple. If the physician cannot clearly exclude Cushing syndrome in an obese patient, laboratory evaluation would be required. Other pathologic causes of weight gain and/or increased adipose tissue include hypothyroidism, growth hormone deficiency, pseudohypoparathyroidism, pseudopseudohypoparathyroidism, Prader–Willi syndrome, and Laurence–Moon–Biedle syndrome.

Hypokalemic hypertension with metabolic alkalosis encompasses ~2% of all cases of hypertension. The differential diagnosis includes aldosteronoma (also termed *aldosterone-producing* adenoma), bilateral adrenal hyperplasia with aldosterone hypersecretion (also known as *idiopathic primary hyperaldosteronism*), adrenal adenomas secreting desoxycorticosterone, glucocorticoid-remedial hypertension (or *dexamethasone-suppressible hypertension*), apparent mineralocorticoid excess, Liddle syndrome (a gain-of-function mutation in the β or γ subunits of the epithelial sodium channel of the distal convoluted tubule and collecting duct), renin-secreting juxtaglomerular apparatus tumors, and secondary hyperaldosteronism from renovascular disease or intrinsic renal disease.

Diabetes mellitus can be autoimmune (type 1), insulin-resistant (type 2), gestation-induced [gestational diabetes mellitus (GDM)] or secondary to an underlying etiology (e.g., "other specific types of diabetes"). The causes of "other specific types of diabetes" include (1) intrinsic β-cell defects (e.g., mitochondrial diabetes, maturity-onset diabetes of youth), (2) inborn errors in the insulin receptor (e.g., leprachaunism), (3) chronic pancreatic diseases (e.g., chronic pancreatitis, cystic fibrosis), (4) diabetes associated with infection, (5) drug-induced diabetes (e.g., glucocorticoid-induced),

(6) genetic conditions associated with diabetes, (7) other autoimmune forms of diabetes (e.g., insulin receptor autoantibodies), and (8) diabetes secondary to endocrine disorders (e.g., Cushing syndrome, acromegaly, pheochromocytoma).

Pathologic fractures as observed in Cushing syndrome can result from cancers, osteomalacia, osteoporosis, or other forms of osteopenic bone disease.

Diagnosis

Screening Tests for Cushing Syndrome

24-hour urinary free cortisol. Initially, baseline serum and urine electrolytes should be measured as well as 24-hour UFC. Hyperglycemia and hypokalemic metabolic acidosis support the diagnosis of Cushing syndrome. UFC concentrations two- to threefold greater than the upper limit of normal (>120 μg/day) suggest true hypercortisolism. Concentrations <100 μg/day exclude the diagnosis of Cushing syndrome.

Overnight dexamethasone supression test. Either a 24-hour urinary free cortisol or an overnight dexamethasone suppression test can be used as a screening test for Cushing syndrome. The overnight dexamethasone suppression test is carried out by administering 1 mg of dexamethasone orally at 2200 and measuring a fasting serum cortisol concentration at 0800-h the next morning. Dexamethasone is employed in an attempt to induce suppression of the hypothalamic–pituitary–adrenal cortical axis because dexamethasone, a synthetic glucocorticoid, is not detected in currently used cortisol immunoassays. A normal response to dexamethasone suppression of the hypothalamic–pituitary–adrenal cortical axis is considered to be an 0800 cortisol of <5 μg/dL (<138 nmol/L). Cortisol concentrations >10 μg/dL (>276 nmol/L) are interpreted as a failure to respond to dexamethasone suppression consistent with cortisol excess. Cortisol concentrations of $5-10$ μg/dL demonstrate only borderline suppression. In such cases, further laboratory investigation to rule in or rule out Cushing syndrome is indicated. One reason for "failed suppression" is failure to take the 2200 dexamethasone dose; another reason is abnormally rapid dexamethasone metabolism. If this is a clinical consideration when the am (morning) cortisol is not suppressed, the test can be repeated and a serum dexamethasone concentration measured in the morning in addition to the cortisol concentration. An inappropriately low am dexamethasone concentration indicates an increased rate of dexamethasone metabolism or a failure to take the dexamethasone.

Midnight cortisol. Measuring a midnight (mn) cortisol is another appropriate screening test for Cushing syndrome in addition to the 24-hour UFC collection or 0800 cortisol following pm dexamethasone administration. A mn cortisol concentration of <5 μg/dL (<138 nmol/L) essentially rules out Cushing syndrome. This is well documented in the research literature. However, the challenge and expense is that an indwelling heparinized intravenous catheter must be placed prior to the subject falling asleep and the sample must be obtained while the subject is still asleep. The expense of hospitalization to carry out this test would appear to be excessive and unjustified since there are other laboratory alternatives for screening for Cushing syndrome. Furthermore, there is generally no outpatient setting where intravenous cannulation, monitoring, and blood drawing can be carried out on sleeping patients.

There is convincing data that salivary cortisol measurements are useful in the diagnosis of Cushing syndrome. However, few laboratories are prepared to measure salivary cortisol. Such assays must have very low limits of detection.

Diagnostic Testing

Positive screening tests may suggest the presence of Cushing syndrome, but further testing is needed. Various conditions such as alcoholism, obesity, and depression are well recognized causes of pseudo-Cushing syndrome where there is basal hypercortisolism in the absence of true Cushing syndrome (e.g., in pseudo-Cushing syndrome cortisol suppression typically occurs in response to "low dose" dexamethasone; see discussion below).

The "formal" dexamethasone suppression test is carried out in three stages: baseline (2 days), "low dose" dexamethasone suppression (2 days), and "high dose" dexamethasone suppression (2 days). First, two baseline 24-hour urine specimens are collected for UFC excretion or 17-hydroxycorticosteroid (17-OHCS) excretion. 17-OHCS are the urinary breakdown products of 11-desoxycortisol and cortisol. Urinary creatinine excretion is also determined to validate that a 24-hour urine collection was obtained. On days 3 and 4, 0.5 mg of dexamethasone is administered orally every 6 hours. In patients with true Cushing syndrome, neither UFC nor 17-OHCS decline by 50% or more compared with the average baseline excretions. While 50% suppression is used as a cutpoint by many experts, a greater degree of suppression (e.g., a decline in UFC or 17-OHCS of $\geq 65-90\%$) is even more convincing that the hypothalamic–pituitary adrenal axis is suppressible. Either UFC or 17-OHCS should be ordered, but not both.

The low-dose portion of the test can be performed as an outpatient if the patient is reliable. On the other hand, if the collections are performed when the patient is an inpatient, the nursing staff must be extensively counseled as to the necessity of a complete collection. For example, a bottle for urine collection must accompany the patient on any extended trips throughout the hospital.

If low dose dexamethasone fails to suppress the cortisol, the test is continued onto days 5 and 6 by administering high-dose dexamethasone at 2 mg every 6 hours. The total 6-day test is termed the "formal dexamethasone supression test" or the "low-dose–high-dose dexamethasone suppression test." Again, suppression is sought on days 5 and 6. If suppression occurs on high-dose dexamethasone, Cushing disease (e.g., an ACTH-secreting pituitary adenoma) can be diagnosed. In the majority of patients with Cushing disease, the hypothalamic setpoint for cortisol-negative feedback is elevated and suppression can be achieved only with high dexamethasone doses. Some clinicians will undertake a "super-high-dose dexamethasone suppression test" (e.g., 8 mg every 6 hours) if the results of the "regular" high-dose dexamethasone suppression are equivocal or there is a high index of suspicion for Cushing disease. Only $\sim 60\%$ of patients with Cushing disease will suppress on high-dose dexamethasone. Therefore this test is helpful if suppression on high-dose dexamethasone occurs; however, failure to achieve suppression on high-dose dexamethasone does not rule out Cushing disease. Failure to suppress on high-dose dexamethasone is clearly typical of Cushing syndrome resulting from ectopic adrenocorticotrophic hormone (ACTH; corticotrophin) production, ectopic corticotrophin-releasing hormone (CRH) production, and cortisol-secreting adrenal tumors.

One proposal to improve the differentiation of Cushing disease and adrenal adenoma is to measure peripheral ACTH 30, 45, and 60 minutes after administering intravenous ovine corticotrophin-releasing hormone (CRH) on completing the low-dose dexamethasone suppression test (e.g., days 3 and 4). In the routine CRH test using 1 μg/kg of CRH injected over 1 minute, Cushing disease patients display ACTH concentrations of >10 pg/mL (>2.2 pmol/L), whereas other forms of Cushing syndrome display ACTH concentrations of <10 pg/mL. However like so many tests that assess adrenal function, this CRH test is not infallible.

ACTH

Serum ACTH concentrations can help determine the etiology of Cushing syndrome. While loss of diurnal variation is typical of Cushing syndrome, the presence of diurnal variation does not rule out Cushing syndrome. On occasion both am and pm cortisol concentrations are elevated, yet the pm is no more than 50% of the am concentration. The measurements of am and pm serum cortisol and ACTH, by themselves, are not recommended as screening tests for Cushing syndrome. However once the diagnosis of Cushing syndrome is established an elevated ACTH concentration excludes cortisol-secreting adrenal tumors and narrows the differential diagnosis of Cushing syndrome to ectopic ACTH/CRH versus Cushing disease. Serum ACTH concentrations >300 pg/mL (>66 pmol/L) are usually suggestive of an ACTH-secreting tumor.

MRI

MRI should not be obtained until the biochemical diagnosis of Cushing syndrome is established because 5–15% of the otherwise healthy general population can exhibit MRI findings suggestive of a pituitary adenoma. Such MRI findings can be referred to as "incidentomas" (e.g., incidental findings).

Inferior Petrosal Venous Sinus Sampling (IPSS)

In this procedure the venous system is entered from a femoral vein and three catheters are placed; one peripheral catheter is located in the inferior vena cava for measurement of systemic ACTH concentrations, and individual catheters are placed in each of the inferior petrosal sinuses. This is not a benign procedure and should be undertaken only by highly trained and experienced neuroradiologists. Bleeding or blood vessel perforation in the CNS can produce grave consequences.

Venous blood from the pituitary drains into the inferior petrosal venous sinuses that next drain into the internal jugular veins. This test is performed by obtaining baseline samples in the inferior vena cava (IVC) and inferior petrosal venous sinuses at −15 minutes and at time 0. Subsequently, 100 μg of reconstituted ovine corticotropin-releasing hormone (CRH) is injected intravenously for pituitary stimulation. Blood samples are then drawn simultaneously from each inferior petrosal venous sinus catheter and from the IVC at +3 minutes, +5 minutes, +10 minutes, +15 minutes, +30 minutes, and +60 minutes following CRH injection.

Localization of right versus left adenomas is correct in only ~60% of cases. This is likely accounted for by the fact that blood flow into the left and right sinuses is not 100% localized to either side. For example, one IPSS may drain more blood than the other IPSS, and the sinuses are not perfectly symmetric.

Treatment

Proper therapy depends on the specific cause of Cushing syndrome. Cushing disease is treated surgically via removal of the pituitary adenoma. The surgical repeat rate for transphenoidal pituitary surgery is approximately 1%. Ectopic ACTH or CRH is treated by managing the primary neoplasia. Likewise, adrenal disorders producing hypercortisolism are managed surgically with the diagnosis confirmed by gross and microscopic examination of the excised adrenal glands. In cases of adrenal carcinoma or ectopic ACTH/ CRH that cannot be treated surgically, there are drugs that poison the adrenocortical tissue inhibiting cortisol secretion (e.g., aminoglutethimide, ketoconazole, mitotane). In cases of adrenal tumors with ectopic hormone receptor expression, receptor blocking therapies are under development.

Additional Reading

ASA, S. L., HORVATH, E., AND KOVACS, K.: Pituitary neoplasms: An overview of the clinical presentation, diagnosis, treatment, and pathology. In *Endocrine Tumors*, E. L. MAZZAFERRI AND N. A. SAMAAN, eds., Blackwell Scientific Publications, Oxford, UK, 1993, pp. 77–112.

BEAUREGARD, C., DICKSTEIN, G., AND LACROIX, A.: Classic and recent etiologies of Cushing's syndrome: Diagnosis and therapy. *Treat. Endocrinol. 1*:79–94, 2002.

DEMERS, L. M. AND WHITLEY, R. J.: Function of the adrenal cortex. In *Tietz Textbook of Clinical Chemistry*, 3rd ed., C. A. BURTIS, AND E. R. ASHWOOD, eds., Saunders, Philadelphia, 1999, pp. 1530–69.

FINDLING, J. W. AND RAFF, H.: Screening and diagnosis of Cushing's syndrome. *Endocrinol. Metab. Clin. North. Am. 34*:385–402, 2005.

GARCIA, C., BILLER, B. M. AND KLIBANSKI, A.: The role of the clinical laboratory in the diagnosis of Cushing's syndrome. *Am. J. Clin. Pathol. 120*:S38–45, 2003.

Laboratory approaches to diseases of the adrenal cortex and adrenal medulla. In *Handbook of Diagnostic Endocrinology*, W. E. WINTER, I. JIALAL, AND D. W. CHAN, eds., AACC, Inc., 1999, pp. 49–88.

LINDSAY, J. R. AND NIEMAN, L. K.: Differential diagnosis and imaging in Cushing's syndrome. *Endocrinol. Metab. Clin. North Am. 34*:403–21, 2005.

OLDFIELD, E. H., DOPPMAN, J. L., NIEMAN, L. K. ET AL.: Petrosal venous sampling with and without corticotropin-releasing hormone for the differential diagnosis of Cushing's syndrome. *N. Engl. J. Med. 325*:897–905, 1991.

ORTH, D. N., KOVACS, W. J., AND DEBOLD, C. R.: The adrenal cortex. In *Williams Textbook of Endocrinology*, 8th ed., J. D. WILSON AND D. W. FOSTER, eds., Saunders, Philadelphia, 1992, pp. 489–620.

SCHTEINGART, D. E.: Cushing syndrome. In *Principles and Practice of Endocrinology and Metabolism*, 3rd ed., K. L. BECKER, J. P. BILEZIKIAN, W. J. BREMNER ET AL., eds., Lippincott Williams & Wilkins, Philadelphia, 2001, pp. 723–38.

TABARIN, A., GRESELLE, J. F., SAN-BALLI, F., LEPRAT ET AL.: Usefulness of the corticotropin-releasing hormone test during bilateral inferior petrosal sinus sampling for the diagnosis of Cushing's syndrome. *J. Clin. Endocrin. Metabol. 73*:53–9, 1991.

WILLIAMS, G. H., AND DLUHY, R. G.: Diseases of the adrenal cortex. In *Harrison's Principles of Internal Medicine*, 12th ed., J. D. WILSON, E. BRAUNWALD, K. J. ISSELBACHER, R. G. PETERSDORF, A. S. FAUCI, AND R. K. ROOT, eds., McGraw-Hill, New York, 1991, pp. 1713–34.

YANOVSKI, J. A., CUTLER, G. B., DOPPMAN, J. L. ET AL.: The limited ability of inferior petrosal sinus sampling with corticotropin-releasing hormone to distinguish Cushing's disease from pseudo-Cushing states or normal physiology. *J. Clin. Endocrin. Metabol. 77*:503–9, 1992.

Case 22

The Tired Teenager

William E. Winter

A 15-year-old Caucasian male presented with chief complaints of weakness, fatigue, weight loss, and nausea that had developed slowly over the last 6 months. Nonspecific "tiredness" had been a problem for at least 9 months. His appetite was poor, but he did have a craving for table salt. A 15-lb (6.8-kg) unintended weight loss was reported over the last 9 months.

His past medical history was unremarkable. He had had no serious illnesses, no hospitalizations, and no surgeries. His immunizations were up-to-date. He took no chronic medications and had no allergies.

Review of his family history revealed that his 42-year-old mother developed Hashimoto thyroiditis at age 16. The maternal aunt had Graves disease that was diagnosed at age 22.

His review of systems was negative for polyuria, polydipsia, and nocturia. He suffered from "heat intolerance" and became easily dehydrated, although this could be treated by aggressive oral replenishment with Gatorade. He was never hospitalized for dehydration. He did not complain of headaches, cough, shortness of breath, or wheezing. While he did experience episodic nausea, there were no complaints of vomiting, diarrhea, or constipation.

Physical examination revealed a gaunt 15-year-old male in no acute distress. His height was 180 cm, and his weight was 50 kg. His body mass index (BMI) was 15 kg/m^2. His vital signs were as follows: temperature = 37.1°C, pulse = 110 beats per minute at rest, respirations = 22 breaths per minute, blood pressure = 90/50 mm Hg. Repeat blood pressure measurement in the opposite arm revealed 88/43 mm Hg. HEENT examination was benign. Disks and fundi were normal. The neck was supple without masses, thyromegaly, or lymphadenopathy. The lungs were clear to auscultation and percussion. The abdomen was soft without masses or hepatosplenomegaly. Bowel sounds were present but reduced. He had Tanner IV genitalia and pubic hair. The pulses were weak (only 1+) and rapid in the upper and lower extremities. Capillary refill was delayed, suggesting reduced cardiac output. The patient's sallow skin displayed a mottled hyperpigmented in sun-exposed and non-sun-exposed areas. The skin creases were more deeply hyperpigmented as was a scar on his leg from a minor bicycle accident that occurred some years ago. The nailbeds and oral mucosal also exhibited hyperpigmentation. The lips were pale as were the nailbeds. Cranial nerves II–XII were grossly intact.

Tietz's Applied Laboratory Medicine, Second Edition. Edited by Mitchell G. Scott, Ann M. Gronowski, and Charles S. Eby
Copyright © 2007 John Wiley & Sons, Inc.

There were no focal neurologic deficits. Reflexes were 1+ and symmetrical in the upper and lower extremities.

The complaint of tiredness aroused an initially diverse differential diagnosis that included endocrine disorders, hematologic disorders, cardiovascular, infectious diseases, hepatic and renal disorders, as well as psychiatric disorders. The astute primary care physician noted several findings in the patient's history and physical examination that focused her workup on the possibility of Addison disease (i.e., primary adrenal insufficiency): salt craving, weight loss, borderline hypotension with tachycardia, and hyperpigmentation. Hypotension in adults is considered to be a systolic blood pressure of less than 90 mmHg or a blood pressure 40 mmHg less than their baseline blood pressure.

CBC, fasting basic metabolic panel (BMP), urinalysis (including the spot urine sodium concentration), and am (morning) cortisol were ordered. His CBC revealed a mild normocytic, normochromic anemia with a modestly increased eosinophil count but was otherwise unremarkable. His BMP is given below:

Analyte	Value, Conventional Units	Reference Interval, Conventional Units	Value, SI Units	Reference Interval, SI Units
Sodium	128 mEq/L	135–145	128 mmol/L	135–145
Potassium	5.8 mEq/L	3.5–5.0	5.8 mmol/L	3.5–5.0
Chloride	105 mEq/L	95–105	105 mmol/L	95–105
CO_2, total	19 mEq/L	24–32	19 mol/L	24–32
Creatinine	1.3 mg/dL	0.5–1.2	114.9 μmol/L	44–106
Blood urea nitrogen	26 mg/dL	10–20	9.3 mmol/L	3.6–7.1
Glucose	60 mg/dL	65–99	3.3 mmol/L	3.6–5.5

These studies were consistent with a (relatively) hyperchloremic, normal anion gap acidosis that most likely resulted from reduced mineralocorticoid activity based on the patient's hyponatremia and hyperkalemia. The urinalysis showed a urine specific gravity of 1.025 with a urine sodium of 40 mEq/L. This latter finding is pathologic as in the face of hyponatremia in the plasma, the urine sodium should generally be reduced to less than 10 mEq/L. Inappropriate urinary sodium loss was consistent with mineralocorticoid deficiency.

Hyperpigmentation together with mineralocorticoid deficiency were consistent with primary adrenal insufficiency. With deficient cortisol concentrations in the bloodstream, there is a lack of normal suppression of hypothalamic corticotrophin-releasing hormone (CRH) release leading to a subsequent elevation in adrenocorticotrophic hormone (ACTH; corticotropin) release. The first 13 amino acids of ACTH share sequence identity with α-melanocyte-stimulating hormone (MSH). Thus a chronic elevation in ACTH can induce hyperpigmentation.

The patient's modest hypoglycemia was consistent with glucocorticoid insufficiency. Cortisol stimulates the production of gluconeogenic enzymes. The cortisol concentration was 5 μg/dL (138 nmol/L; am reference interval: 7–25 μg/dL; 193–690 nmol/L). This was consistent with glucocorticoid deficiency. Combined glucocorticoid and mineralocorticoid deficiencies can contribute to hypovolemia and hypotension, resulting in a compensatory tachycardia. A prerenal azotemia was recognized in the elevations in the both the plasma creatinine and BUN concentrations with a BUN:creatinine ratio of 20:1 (0.08:1 mmol of urea/μmol of creatinine).

A confirmatory cosyntropin (Cortrosyn) stimulation test was performed:

Analyte	Value, Conventional Units	Reference Interval, Conventional Units	Value, SI Units	Reference Interval, SI Units
Cortisol				
Baseline	6 μg/dL	7–25	166 nmol/L	193–690
+30 min	9 μg/dL	≥ 20 ($\delta \geq 7$)	248 nmol/L	≥ 552 ($\delta \geq 193$)
+60 min	11 μg/dL	≥ 20 ($\delta \geq 7$)	304 nmol/L	≥ 552 ($\delta \geq 193$)
Baseline				
Plasma renin activity (supine)	9.3 ngmL^{-1}h^{-1}	0.2–1.6	9.3 μg L^{-1} h^{-1}	0.2–1.6

δ = change over baseline

The deficient peak cortisol and the deficient change in cortisol over baseline, of only 5 μg/dL, confirmed hypocortisolism (e.g., glucocorticoid insufficiency). The elevated renin result supported the diagnosis of mineralocorticoid insufficiency, and primary adrenal insufficiency was diagnosed.

A tuberculin skin test was placed to exclude tuberculus adrenalitis. The skin test was nonreactive 48 hours later. Testing for adrenal cell cytoplasmic autoantibodies (ACA) was positive, consistent with an autoimmune etiology for the patient's Addison disease.

In light of the family history of autoimmune thyroid disease, the finding of primary autoimmune adrenal failure as the etiology of the patient's Addison disease is not unexpected. Because multiple autoimmune endocrine diseases can occur in the same individual, the reference laboratory was asked to test the patient's serum sample for islet autoantibodies [e.g., islet cell cytoplasmic autoantibodies (ICA), glutamic acid decarboxylase autoantibodies (GADA), and insulin-associated 2-autoantibodies (IA-2A)], thyroperoxidase autoantibodies (TPOA), and steroidal cell autoantibodies (SCA). Whereas ICA, GADA, IA-2A, and SCA were negative, TPOA was strongly positive. Thyroid function studies revealed the following results:

Analyte	Value, Conventional Units	Reference Interval, Conventional Units	Value, SI Units	Reference Interval, SI Units
TSH	2.3 μIU/mL	0.35–4.2	2.3 mIU/L	0.35–4.2
Free T4	1.1 ng/dL	0.8–2.7	14.2 pmol/L	10.3–34.8

These data are consistent with the biochemical euthyroid state. The physician planned to repeat the TSH measurement on a yearly basis in an effort to detect thyroid gland insufficiency.

Based on the diagnosis of Addison disease, the physician prescribed replacement doses of oral glucocorticoids and an oral mineralocorticoid: 9-α-fluorohydrocortisone. During times of stress the patient was told to triple his glucocorticoid dose. He was also instructed concerning the parenteral injection glucocorticoids in the event of severe illness when he should also seek immediate medical care.

Over a period of a few weeks, his strength and vigor improved. Over 3 months, he gained 20 lb (9 kg). His nausea resolved. Repeat BMP displayed resolution of the patient's hyponatremia, hyperkalemia, hypoglycemia.

Definition of the Disease

Primary adrenal insufficiency (i.e., Addison disease) results from adrenal gland failure. This will be reviewed shortly. Deficiencies of CRH (tertiary) or ACTH (secondary) can result in central adrenal insufficiency. However, the pathology is limited to glucocorticoid insufficiency because aldosterone secretion is not controlled by the hypothalamus and anterior pituitary but is, instead, controlled by the renin–angiotensin system. Primary adrenal insufficiency is therefore a much more serious disorder than central adrenal insufficiency. Patients with ACTH deficiency may exhibit hyponatremia from a decreased ability to excrete a free water load, but do not experience hyperkalemia because mineralocorticoid secretion is essentially intact.

Patients with isolated glucocorticoid deficiency from ACTH (or CRH) deficiency harbor many of the same complaints as patients with primary adrenal insufficiency: tiredness, lassitude, weakness, malaise, and even nausea or vomiting. Severe hypotension and/or metabolic acidosis in central adrenal insufficiency develop only under exceptional circumstances such as the extreme stress of delivery, surgery, sepsis, or trauma. Nonetheless, untreated isolated glucocorticoid deficiency can present as a medical emergency.

ACTH deficiency is usually associated with other anterior pituitary hormone deficiencies such as deficiencies of gonadotropins, thyroid-stimulating hormone (TSH; thyrotropin), and/or growth hormone. CRH and ACTH deficiencies with consequent adrenal atrophy results from the use of exogenous glucocorticoids that suppress CRH and consequently lead to suppressed ACTH. Acute glucocorticoid withdrawal in patients treated with high-dose or suppressive doses of glucocorticoids can induce acute glucocorticoid insufficiency. Such situations can be life-threatening even in the absence of mineralocorticoid insufficiency.

The patient described above presented with modest symptoms and laboratory findings that reflected glucocorticoid and mineralocorticoid deficiencies. However, primary adrenal insufficiency can present acutely in "Addisonian crisis." Addisonian crisis is the condition where patients present to a medical professional with hypotension or frank shock (and all its descriptors), decreased mentation or coma, and severe hyponatremia, hyperkalemia (with possible cardiac arrhthymias), hypoglycemia, and metabolic acidosis. While the acidosis of "chronic" primary adrenal insufficiency is usually a hyperchloremic, normal anion gap metabolic acidosis because of a type IV renal tubular acidosis, with hypotension and hypovolemia (especially from Addison-disease-induced vomiting and/or diarrhea), a lactic acidosis (normochloremic, positive anion gap metabolic acidosis) can ensue. Untreated or undertreated. Addisonian crisis can be fatal. Crisis can also develop in treated patients previously diagnosed with primary adrenal insufficiency who experience severe illness such as gastroenteritis, pneumonia, sepsis, surgery, or trauma and do not increase their dose of glucocorticoids.

Differential Diagnosis

Because of its protean manifestations that include tiredness, weakness, dehydration, nausea, vomiting, and diarrhea. Addison disease can be confused with many other conditions such as primary anemias, gastrointestinal disorders, cancer, psychiatric disease, and even malingering. However, the laboratory findings of hyponatremia, hyperkalemia, acidosis, and/or hypoglycemia should raise the specter of adrenal insufficiency in the clinician's differential diagnosis of the patient's problems.

While the 1-hour cosyntropin test was used in this patient to diagnose glucocorticoid insufficiency, other tests are available such as the cortisol response to insulin-induced hypoglycemia, prolonged cosyntropin stimulation test, and the metyrapone test. Because of its diurnal variation, measurements of ACTH are of limited value in differentiating primary from central adrenal insufficiency. If the physician wants to directly measure aldosterone, it can be measured in blood or in a timed urine collection. In timed urine collections, sodium excretion should also be measured with creatinine measured as an index of the completeness of the collection. If measured in blood, a renin measurement should be paired with the aldosterone measurement. Isolated mineralocorticoid insufficiency is a rare inborn error. Renin deficiency can occur in cases of longstanding diabetes but is otherwise uncommon.

The major causes of primary adrenal insufficiency include autoimmune destruction of the adrenal cortex ($\sim$70% of cases) and infection ($\sim$20% of cases). A minority of cases ($\sim$10%) result from: coagulopathy, trauma (with or without hemorrhage), adrenalectomy (e.g., postsurgical), cancer (e.g., infiltrative or metastatic disease), inborn errors, drugs (e.g., mitotane, aminoglutethimide, trilostane, ketoconazole, metyrapone, and RU-486), amyloidosis, and congenital adrenal aplasia.

Autoimmune destruction of the adrenal cortex is histologically recognized by a lymphocytic infiltration of the cortex (e.g., "adrenalitis") with consequent endocrine cell death and gland atrophy. Autoimmune Addison disease can exist as an isolated condition or can exist as part of an autoimmune polyglandular (e.g., "polyendocrine") syndrome (APS). Two types of APS have been recognized: APS type 1 and APS type 2.

The diagnosis of APS type 1 is established when at least two of the following three findings are identified in a patient: mucocutaneous candidiasis, hypoparathyroidism, and Addison disease/adrenal autoantibodies. APS type 1 has also been termed the *autoimmune polyendocrinopathy–candidiasis–ectodermal dystrophy* (APECED) syndrome because associated disorders include dental enamel hypoplasia and nail dystrophy. Other associated diseases in APS type 1 patients include gonaditis (producing primary gonadal failure in women) and autoimmune hepatitis. Less commonly associated conditions are type 1 diabetes mellitus, autoimmune thyroid disease, vitiligo, alopecia, fat malabsorption, IgA deficiency, pernicious anemia, red cell aplasia, and progressive myopathy.

The diagnosis of APS type 2 is confirmed when Addison disease (or adrenal autoantibodies) is associated with type 1 diabetes mellitus and/or autoimmune thyroid disease. Less often associated disorders include gonaditis, hypophysitis, autoimmune hepatitis, vitiligo, alopecia, dermatitis herpetiformis, IgA deficiency, celiac disease, pernicious anemia, immune thrombocytopenia, myasthenia gravis, stiffman syndrome, and Parkinson disease. Because this patient had Addison disease and TPOA, he likely has APS type 2.

APS type 1 is an autosomal recessive disease resulting from mutations in a transcription factor named the *autoimmune regulator* (AIRE). By its nature, APS type 1 is equally common in males and females. Also as an inborn error, it presents in childhood. APS type 2 is more typical of traditional autoimmune diseases being more common in women than in men that presents in later childhood or early adulthood. APS type 2 is polygenic with an HLA influence on its development.

The differential diagnosis of central adrenal insufficiency includes suppression of the hypothalamic–pituitary–adrenal axis by exogenous glucocorticoids, destructive pituitary tumors and their treatment, destructive hypothalamic tumors and their treatment, cerebral trauma, irradiation, infection, bleeding, congenital malformations of the pituitary gland or hypothalamus, and idiopathic hypopituitarism.

Diagnosis

Hyponatremia, hyperkalemia, metabolic acidosis, and prerenal azotemia all supported the diagnosis of mineralocorticoid deficiency. Glucocorticoid deficiency can be confirmed by a deficient cortisol response to the parenteral injection of cosyntropin (Cortrosyn). Cosyntropin is composed of amino acids 1–24 of ACTH. The injection can be intravenous or intramuscular. In the fasting state, a sample for baseline cortisol is drawn, 250 μg of cosyntropin is injected intravenously, and cortisol measurements are taken at +30 and +60 minutes. A baseline plasma renin activity can also be measured, with the patient supine, in order to support or refute the suspected diagnosis of mineralocorticoid deficiency. With primary adrenal insufficiency, renin activity is expected to be elevated.

The serologic diagnosis of autoimmune Addison disease is established by autoantibody testing. An indirect immunofluorescent assay for adrenal cell cytoplasmic autoantibodies (ACA) is available from reference laboratories as was done in the present case. Adrenal enzymes have been shown to be target autoantigens in Addison disease: 21-hydroxylase, 17-hydroxylase, and the P450 sidechain cleavage enzyme. Autoantibody immunoassays have been described for each of these enzymes. Autoantibodies to the P450 sidechain cleavage enzyme occur in autoimmune polyglandular syndromes (see below) but do not occur in isolated Addison disease. Both in reference laboratories and as a kit for purchase, 21-hydroxylase autoantibodies can be determined.

Treatment

Addison disease is treated using replacement doses of glucocorticoids and an oral mineralocorticoid (9-α-fludrocortisone, Florinef). The glucocorticoid replacement should provide the equivalent of ~12 mg of cortisol/m^2 per day in two or three divided doses, with the largest dose in the morning to mimic the normal am rise in cortisol.

Adults usually require 20–30 mg per day of cortisol (e.g., hydrocortisone in pharmacologic parlance). Prednisone and prednisolone have 4 times the potency of cortisol on a mg-for-mg comparison. Dexamethasone has potency 25 times that of cortisol on a mg-for-mg comparison. Because of the longer durations of action of prednisone and dexamethasone (each of which might be used daily) compared with cortisol (duration of action 6–8 hours), some physicians treat adults with these medications in place of cortisol. Children with Addison disease are usually treated 3 times daily with oral hydrocortisone. Salt intake should be liberal.

Addisonian crisis is aggressively treated with intravenous fluid replacement, glucose administration, and stress doses of parental glucocorticoids. In adults, a 100-mg bolus of intravenous hydrocortisone is employed initially. Alternative glucocorticoids include dexamethasone (4-mg doses) and methylprednisolone (20-mg doses). One advantage of dexamethasone is that adrenal function testing can be carried out during treatment because dexamethasone does not cross-react in cortisol immunoassays. This is important if the patient has not previously been diagnosed with Addison disease. Once the patient is weaned to an oral glucocorticoid, oral mineralocorticoid replacement can begin. Overtreatment with glucocorticoids can produce Cushing syndrome, whereas overtreatment with mineralocorticoid can induce hypertension.

Additional Reading

SCHATZ, D. A. AND WINTER, W. E.: Autoimmune polyglandular syndromes. In *Pediatric Endocrinology*, 2nd ed., M. SPERLING, ed., Saunders, Philadelphia, 2002, pp. 671–88.

WINTER, W. E.: Autoimmune endocrinopathies. In *Pediatric Endocrinology*, 4th ed., F. LIFSHITZ, ed., Marcel Dekker, New York, 2003, pp. 683–720.

DEMERS, L. M. AND WHITLEY, R. J.: Function of the adrenal cortex. In *Tietz Textbook of Clinical Chemistry*, 3rd ed., C. A. BURTIS AND E. R. ASHWOOD, eds., Saunders, Philadelphia, 1999, pp. 1530–69.

WINTER, W. E. AND SIGNORINO, M. R.: Immunologic disorders in infants and children. In *Autoimmune Endocrinopathies*, 5th ed., E. R. STIEHM, ed., Saunders, Philadelphia, 2004, pp. 1179–221.

WINTER, W. E.: Laboratory approaches to diseases of the adrenal cortex and adrenal medulla. In *Handbook of Diagnostic Endocrinology*, I. JIALAL, D. W. CHAN, AND W. E. WINTER, eds., American Association of Clinical Chemistry, 1999, pp. 49–88.

LORIAUX, D. L.: Adrenocortical insufficiency. In *Principles and Practice of Endocrinology and Metabolism*, 3rd ed., K. L. BECKER, J. P. BILEZIKIAN, W. J. BREMNER ET AL., eds., Lippincott Williams & Wilkins, Philadelphia, 2001, pp. 739–43.

ORTH, D. N. AND KOVACS, W. J.: The adrenal cortex. In *Williams Textbook of Endocrinology*, 9th ed., J. D. WILSON, D. W. FOSTER, H. M. KRONENBERG ET AL., eds., Saunders, Philadelphia, 1998, pp. 517–664.

TEN, S., NEW, M. AND MACLAREN, N.: Clinical review 130: Addison's disease, 2001. *J. Clin. Endocrinol. Metab.* 86:2909–22, 2001.

TORREY, S. P.: Recognition and management of adrenal emergencies. *Emerg. Med. Clin. North Am.* 23:687–702, 2005.

Case 23

The Hypertensive Accountant

Michael Stowasser and Richard D. Gordon

A 45-year-old accountant was, at his request, referred by his general practitioner to a hypertension unit for investigation because recent need for additional medications had caused unwanted side effects. Diagnosed approximately 10 years previously, his hypertension was, until the past 12 months, under good control [blood pressure (BP) approximately 140/90 mm Hg] with the angiotensin-converting enzyme inhibitor ramipril 5 mg daily. His BP had recently risen to 150/100–170/110 mm Hg. Following addition of the β-adrenoceptor blocker atenolol 50 mg daily, the BP normalized, but the patient now felt lethargic.

He denied headaches, palpitations, sweating episodes, muscle weakness, paresthesia, urinary tract symptoms, or any past history of renal or other cardiovascular disease. He was a nonsmoker, drank little alcohol, tried to follow a no-added-salt diet, and had noticed no recent weight change. There was no family history of hypertension. Physical examination revealed a patient of normal weight for height (72 kg and 175 cm) who did not appear Cushingoid. Heart rate was 84 bpm and BP 144/96 lying down and 148/100 standing. Respiratory and abdominal examinations were unremarkable. The apex beat was not thrusting or displaced, there were no signs of congestive cardiac failure, no radiofemoral pulse delay, no renal or carotid bruits, and no abdominal masses, and peripheral pulses were normal. An echocardiogram was consistent with mild left ventricular hypertrophy and early diastolic dysfunction. A chest x-ray was normal.

Blood was collected for estimation of electrolytes, urea, and creatinine. Sample collection was specifically requested "without stasis" and with the analytes to be measured in plasma (rather than serum), in order to avoid false elevations of potassium. Findings were as follows:

Analyte	Value, Conventional Units	Reference Interval, Conventional Units	Value, SI Units	Reference Interval, SI Units
Sodium (P)	140 mmol/L	135–145	Same	
Potassium (P)	3.6 mmol/L	3.5–5.0	Same	
Chloride (P)	105 mmol/L	100–110	Same	
Bicarbonate (P)	29 mmol/L	22–33	Same	
Urea (P)	13 mg/dL	8–22	4.6 mmol/L	3.0–8.0
Creatinine (P)	0.9 mg/dL	0.6–1.5	0.08 mmol/L	0.05–0.13

Tietz's Applied Laboratory Medicine, Second Edition. Edited by Mitchell G. Scott, Ann M. Gronowski, and Charles S. Eby
Copyright © 2007 John Wiley & Sons, Inc.

Twenty-four hour urinary excretion of norepinephrine and epinephrine was normal. There was no evidence of renal artery stenosis on renal artery duplex ultrasound and renal DTPA isotope scanning. Microscopy of urine was normal with no growth on culture, and no protein was detected.

Primary aldosteronism (PAL) is at present the most common form of specifically treatable and potentially curable hypertension. The diagnosis of PAL depends critically on laboratory testing since it is usually indistinguishable from undifferentiated "essential" hypertension except in instances of advanced disease, when hypokalemia has been allowed to develop. In order to screen for PAL, measurement of the plasma aldosterone/renin ratio was arranged. To facilitate interpretation of the results, ramipril was ceased and atenolol first reduced and then gradually withdrawn, while verapamil slow release 120 mg twice daily and hydralazine 12.5 mg twice daily were introduced. The patient was taught to measure his BP at home using a reliable machine in order to monitor response to the changeover of his medications. The physician requested the blood be collected at least 4 weeks after ceasing atenolol, at approximately 9:00 am (0900h), with the patient seated and having been out of bed for at least 2 hours before collection.

Analyte	Value, Conventional Units	Reference Interval, Conventional Units	Value, SI Units	Reference Interval, SI Units
Aldosterone (P)	14.8 ng/dL	5–30	410 pmol/L	140–830
Renin (P)	0.2 ng mL h^{-1}	1–4	2 mU/L	8–34
Aldosterone/renin ratio (P)	74	<30	205	<100

Renin is expressed here as plasma renin activity (PRA) for conventional units and as active renin concentration (ARC) for SI units. PRA measures generated angiotensin I, is influenced by substrate concentration, and is a radioimmunoassay, while ARC is measured by radioimmunoassay or immunometric assay. Since renin doesn't affect blood pressure directly, but only through angiotensin produced by the action of renin on its substrate, produced by the liver, PRA better reflects angiotensin concentrations. Renin enzyme concentration, on the other hand, can be influenced by substrate concentrations. Thus, if substrate is elevated because of estrogen administration for contraception or postmenopausal treatment, renin concentration falls in an attempt to keep angiotensin concentrations normal.

The patient underwent two further blood collections that again showed elevated aldosterone/renin ratios, consistent with PAL. In order to definitively confirm or exclude PAL, he was admitted to the hypertension unit ward to undergo a fludrocortisone suppression test, which involved measurement of plasma aldosterone during 4 days administration of fludrocortisone acetate (0.1 mg 6 hourly), slow-release sodium chloride (1800 mg thrice daily with meals), a high-salt diet, and sufficient oral slow-release potassium chloride supplements (given 6 hourly) to maintain plasma potassium concentrations in the normal range. The following results were obtained:

Day	Time; Posture	Aldosterone (P) (pmol/L)	Renin (P) (mU/L)	Potassium (mmol/L)	Cortisol (P) (nmol/L)
Basal	0700h; recumbent	250	<2	3.6	368
	1000h; upright	422	2	3.8	276
Day 4	0700h; recumbent	272	<2	3.9	410
	1000h; upright	460	<2	4.0	324

By the last day, the patient required seven slow-release KCl tablets every 6 hours (q6h) to maintain normokalemia. Failure of upright plasma aldosterone to suppress to <165 pmol/L by day 4, despite suppression of renin, and in the absence of a rise in ACTH (inferred from cortisol) between 0700h and 1000h which may have prevented aldosterone suppression, confirmed PAL.

Genetic testing ruled out the presence of the "hybrid" gene abnormality responsible for the rare, glucocorticoid-remediable form of inherited PAL. Computed tomography (CT) scanning of the adrenal glands, using fine (2.5-mm) cuts before and after intravenous contrast enhancement, showed mild thickening of both glands, but with no obvious mass lesions.

The patient then underwent adrenal venous sampling (performed between 0700h and 1000h after overnight recumbency) in order to determine whether aldosterone overproduction was confined to one adrenal [consistent with aldosterone-producing adenoma (APA)] or occurring in both [consistent with bilateral adrenal hyperplasia (BAH)]. Samples were collected from each adrenal vein in turn, and from a peripheral vein (simultaneously with each adrenal venous sample). The procedure yielded the following results:

Site	Aldosterone (P) (pmol/L)	Cortisol (P) (nmol/L)	Aldosterone/Cortisol Ratio
Left adrenal vein	1420	1520	0.9
Peripheral vein	352	310	1.1
Right adrenal vein	13,650	1870	7.3
Peripheral vein	360	322	1.1

Comparison of adrenal with peripheral venous aldosterone/cortisol ratios (rightmost column) revealed definite production of aldosterone by the right adrenal gland, but suppression of aldosterone production by the left, consistent with right adrenal APA.

The patient underwent right-sided laparoscopic adrenalectomy, which resulted in cure of his hypertension. Pathological examination of the removed adrenal revealed a 6-mm cortical adenoma composed predominantly of cells resembling those of zona glomerulosa.

Definition of the Disease

By definition, PAL is characterized by aldosterone production that is excessive to the body's requirements and autonomous with regard to its normal chronic regulator, the renin–angiotensin II (AII) system. This results in excessive sodium reabsorption via amiloride-sensitive epithelial sodium channels within the distal nephron, leading to hypertension and suppression of renin–AII. Urinary loss of potassium, exchanged for sodium at the distal nephron, will result in hypokalemia only if severe and prolonged enough. Once thought to be rare, this condition is now known to be the most common specifically treatable and potentially curable form of hypertension, and may be present in up to 10% of hypertensives. The large majority of patients with PAL are not hypokalemic unless diagnosis is unnecessarily delayed through lack of screening.

The most common pathological subtype of PAL is bilateral adrenal cortical hyperplasia, followed by unilateral adenoma, and adrenocortical carcinoma, which is (fortunately) very rare. Cells contained in APAs may resemble those of zona fasciculata (ZF), zona glomerulosa (ZG), or zona reticularis, or may have cytological features of both ZF and ZG (small, clear, "hybrid cells"). The presence of at least 80% non-ZF (ZG, reticularis, or hybrid) type cells is associated with responsiveness of the tumor to AII, indicated by a rise in aldosterone in response to upright posture (as was seen in this patient) or to low-dose AII infusion. By contrast, unresponsiveness is usually observed in tumors in which 50–100% of the cells are ZF-like.

Unresponsiveness of aldosterone to upright posture is also seen in a rare, dominantly inherited variety of PAL (familial hyperaldosteronism type I, FH-I) which is caused by a "hybrid gene" mutation composed of 11β-hydroxylase gene (*CYP11B1*) sequences at its 5' end and aldosterone synthase gene (*CYP11B2*) sequences at its 3' end. Aldosterone production in FH-I is regulated by ACTH (by virtue of the gene's ACTH-regulated *CYP11B1* regulatory sequences) rather than by AII, and can therefore be suppressed by administering glucocorticoids such as dexamethasone. This mutant gene can be detected by examining peripheral blood DNA.

A second, significantly more common familial variety of PAL (FH-II) is neither glucocorticoid-remediable nor associated with the "hybrid gene" mutation. Both APA and BAH are represented, often within the same family. The search for the genetic mutations causing this form of PAL is currently under way.

Differential Diagnosis and Screening

While the most common cause of hypokalemia in the patient with hypertension is the use of thiazide diuretics, the presence of unprovoked hypokalemia is a valuable clue to the diagnosis of PAL, but is lacking in most cases. Recent studies that have used the aldosterone/renin ratio (rather than relying on plasma potassium concentrations) to screen for PAL among hypertensive populations have shown that most patients with this condition (including the patient described here) are normokalemic, and can masquerade as "essential hypertension." Precautions must be taken to avoid false elevations of plasma potassium leading to masking of hypokalemia by (1) ceasing fist clenching and releasing the tourniquet after venipuncture has been achieve; (2) waiting for at least 10 seconds before gently withdrawing blood; (3) using a syringe and needle rather than a vacutainer, so that blood can be withdrawn in a slow and careful manner, and then gently discharged down the side of the opened sample tube; and (4) separating the plasma from the cells within 30 minutes of collection. In patients who are confirmed as being hypokalemic, the demonstration of significant urinary potassium excretion rates (>20 mmol/day) is indicative of urinary potassium wasting, and therefore serves as further evidence for the presence of PAL. This may occasionally provide some useful additional information (e.g., when medications that interfere with interpretation of renin measurement cannot be ceased) but generally lacks sufficient specificity to be of diagnostic value.

Demonstration of frankly elevated plasma aldosterone concentrations also lacks sensitivity for PAL, since many patients exhibit concentrations that lie within the wide normal range. Such "normal" concentrations could be viewed as "inappropriately normal" in the face of suppression of renin–AII, which, in individuals *without* PAL, would result in suppression of aldosterone.

Provided that patients are not habitually ingesting a low-sodium diet or receiving medications that block aldosterone action or stimulate renin production, or have malignant or concomitant renovascular hypertension, renin is consistently suppressed in PAL. However, while highly sensitive, documentation of suppressed renin lacks specificity (Table 23.1). Treatment with β-blockers, clonidine, or α-methyldopa (all of which reduce β-sympathetic stimulation of renin release), or nonsteroidal antiinflammatory agents (NSAIDs, which promote salt retention and also inhibit renal prostaglandin

Table 23.1   Other Factors and Conditions that Suppress Plasma Renin Activity or
Active Renin Concentration

β-Adrenoceptor blockers
Clonidine
α-Methyldopa
Nonsteroidal antiinflammatory drugs
Oral contraceptive agents (active renin concentration only)
High-salt diet
Advancing age
Chronic renal failure
Other salt-dependent low-renin hypertensive conditions
    Liddle's syndrome
    11β-Hydroxysteroid dehydrogenase type 2 deficiency
    Congenital adrenal hyperplasia due to 11β-hydroxylase or 17 α-hydroxylase deficiency
    Primary glucocorticoid resistance
    Ectopic ACTH syndrome
    Deoxycorticosterone-secreting tumor
    Mineralocorticoid receptor gene mutations
    Pseudohypoaldosteronism type 2

production), consumption of a high-salt diet, advancing age (during which renin levels gradually fall as renal function declines), chronic renal impairment (in which renal renin-producing capacity is reduced and salt retention contributes to renin suppression) and the presence of other salt-dependent, low-renin forms of hypertension may all be associated with renin suppression. The latter group includes (1) Liddle's syndrome, in which genetic mutations of the epithelial sodium channel (ENaC) lead to constitutive channel activation causing salt retention and potassium loss; (2) congenital or acquired (e.g., through ingestion of licorice) deficiency of 11β-hydroxysteroid dehydrogenase type 2 (11βHSD2), an enzyme that normally prevents cortisol from gaining access to and causing excessive stimulation of the mineralocorticoid receptor by converting it to inactive cortisone; (3) hypertensive forms of congenital adrenal hyperplasia caused by mutations in either the 11β-hydroxylase or 17α-hydroxylase genes, which are associated with increased production of the mineralocorticoid 11-deoxycorticosterone (DOC) due to increased circulating ACTH concentrations in response to reduced cortisol concentrations; (4) primary glucocorticoid resistance, which is again associated with ACTH simulation and excessive DOC production; (5) ectopic ACTH syndrome (ACTH produced by extra-pituitary tumors, most commonly lung carcinomas), in which mineralocorticoid hypertension is thought to result from a combination of DOC excess and "overload" of the 11βHSD2 enzyme by very high concentrations of cortisol; (6) DOC-secreting tumors; (7) mutations of the mineralocorticoid receptor gene, which cause a modest constitutive activation of the receptor and also permit progesterone and spironolactone to act as agonists rather than antagonists; and (8) the syndrome of hypertension and hyperkalemia with normal glomerular filtration rate (pseudohypoaldosteronism type 2, PHA-2), which is associated with sodium retention due to defects in genes encoding serine–threonine kinases (WNK) expressed in the distal nephron.

Unlike PAL, aldosterone concentrations are chronically suppressed (as a result of chronic suppression of renin/AII) in all of these salt-dependent, low-renin forms of hypertension with the exception of PHA-2, in which chronically elevated plasma potassium concentrations limit suppression of aldosterone.

The aldosterone/renin ratio is more specific than renin measurement, and is not raised in the first seven of the eight disorders described above. It is also more sensitive for detection of PAL than plasma potassium or aldosterone measurement, becoming raised well before either of these analytes leave their normal ranges. However, it is not without false positives and negatives. Dietary salt restriction, concomitant malignant or renovascular hypertension, pregnancy (in which high concentrations of progesterone antagonizes aldosterone action at the mineralocorticoid receptor) and treatment with diuretics (including spironolactone), dihydropyridine calcium channel antagonists, angiotensin-converting enzyme (ACE) inhibitors, and AII receptor antagonists can all lead to false-negative ratios by stimulation of renin secretion. Because potassium is a powerful chronic regulator of aldosterone secretion, hypokalemia may also be associated with false-negative ratios. As noted above, β-blockers, α-methyldopa, clonidine, and NSAIDs can all suppress renin and produce false positive ratios. False positives may also be seen in patients with impaired renal function (reduced renin production as discussed above, while any associated hyperkalemia tends to elevate aldosterone), advancing age (during which production of renin falls more quickly than that of aldosterone) and in PHA2.

Diuretics should be ceased for at least 6 weeks and other interfering medications for at least 2 (and preferably 4) weeks before measuring the ratio, substituting other medications that have a lesser effect on results, such as verapamil slow-release (plus or minus hydralazine) and prazosin in order to maintain hypertension control. Hypokalemia must be corrected, and the patient should be encouraged to follow a liberal salt diet before ratio measurement. Because of the effects of posture and time of day, sensitivity of the ratio is maximized by collecting blood midmorning from seated patients who have been upright (sitting, standing, or walking) for 2–4 hours. The ratio should be regarded as a screening test only, and should be measured more than once (serially if conditions of sampling, including medications, are being altered) before deciding whether to go on to a suppression test in order to definitively confirm or exclude the diagnosis.

Confirmation of Diagnosis and Subtype Differentiation

Fludrocortisone suppression testing is widely regarded as the most reliable means of confirming or excluding PAL. If this test is positive, further investigations are directed toward determining the subtype of PAL, as the treatment of first choice for each subtype differs (see text below). Genetic testing of peripheral blood for the "hybrid gene" is diagnostic for FH-I, and has virtually supplanted biochemical methods (e.g., demonstration of marked, persistent suppression of plasma aldosterone during several days of dexamethasone administration) of diagnosing this subtype. The great majority of patients with PAL, however, will test negative for the hybrid gene, leaving the more difficult task of separating the unilateral tumorous varieties from BAH. Adrenal CT scanning is usually able to detect aldosterone-producing carcinomas because of their relatively large size (usually >3 cm) but frequently misses APAs (which have an average size of approximately 1 cm) and may be frankly misleading as it cannot distinguish these from nonfunctioning nodules. Similar limitations apply to adrenal magnetic resonance imaging, and adrenal selenocholesterol scanning fails to detect most small tumors. Responsiveness (defined as a rise of at least 50% over basal) of plasma aldosterone during 2 or 3 hours of upright posture following overnight recumbency or during AII infusion was once considered specific for BAH among patients with PAL. However, similar responsiveness is also observed in the AII-responsive variety of APA, which accounts for over 50% of APAs in some series. "Hybrid steroid" concentrations (18-hydroxy- and 18-oxo-cortisol), elevated in FH-I and AII-unresponsive APA, are normal in both BAH and AII-responsive APA, and are therefore of only limited value in differentiating BAH from APA.

For these reasons, adrenal venous sampling is the only dependable way to differentiate bilateral from unilateral PAL. Some centers therefore perform this procedure in all patients with PAL (other than those with FH-I). To avoid effects of posture and diurnal variation on steroid concentrations, sampling should be performed in the morning after overnight recumbency, and stress should be avoided, with any venous cannulation delayed until the start of the procedure. An adrenal to peripheral venous cortisol gradient of at least 3.0 indicates successful cannulation. Calculation of the aldosterone/cortisol ratio for each adrenal and peripheral venous sample corrects for differences in "dilution" of adrenal with nonadrenal venous blood and is essential for interpretation. If the aldosterone/cortisol ratio on one side is significantly (>2 times) higher than the simultaneous peripheral venous ratio, *with a ratio no higher than peripheral on the other side*, the study is considered to show lateralization, indicating that unilateral adrenalectomy should cure or significantly improve the hypertension. Aldosterone concentrations (uncorrected for cortisol) measured on the side of the suppressed, "normal" gland are always higher than peripheral due to effects of ACTH and potassium, and can thereby give the mistaken impression of bilateral adrenal autonomous aldosterone production, or of unilateral, left-sided production when there has been failure to obtain a satisfactory right-sided sample.

Treatment

There is recent evidence that excessive aldosterone has deleterious effects on the heart, blood vessels and kidneys independently of effects on BP. Hence, excess aldosterone must be reduced or its effects adequately blocked at the mineralocorticoid receptor or antagonized at the sodium channel that it activates. Unilateral laparoscopic adrenalectomy for unilateral PAL results in cure of hypertension in 50–60% of patients and improvement in all the remainder. For other patients with PAL, treatment with mineralocorticoid receptor blockade (spironolactone 12.5–50 mg/day or eplerenone 25–100 mg/day) or with antagonism at the sodium channel (amiloride 2.5–20 mg/day) is usually effective, but regular monitoring of electrolyte concentrations and renal function is required to avoid potentially dangerous side effects of hyperkalemia and azotemia due to overtreatment and volume contraction. Spironolactone, through blockade of androgen receptors, can cause gynecomastia and reduced libido in males and painful, lumpy breasts and menstrual irregularities in females, side effects that should be absent with the new, more specific mineralocorticoid receptor antagonist, eplerenone. Patients with the rare FH-I usually show excellent blood pressure responses to glucocorticoids given in low doses (e.g., dexamethasone 0.25–0.5 mg/day) that do not cause Cushingoid side effects, and can also be treated by aldosterone blockade.

Additional Reading

YOUNG, W. F., JR.: Primary aldosteronism: Update on diagnosis and treatment. *Endocrinologist* 7:213–21, 1997.

GORDON, R. D.: Diagnostic investigations in primary aldosteronism. In *Clinical Medicine Series on Hypertension*, A. ZANCHETTI, ed., McGraw-Hill International (UK) Ltd., Maidenhead, 2001, pp. 101–14.

MULATERO, P., RABBIA, F., MILAN, A. ET AL.: Drug effects on aldosterone/plasma renin activity ratio in primary aldosteronism. *Hypertension* 40:897–902, 2002.

STOWASSER, M. AND GORDON, R. D.: The aldosterone-renin ratio for screening for primary aldosteronism. *Endocrinologist* 14:267–76, 2004.

Case 24

Don't "Take Two Aspirin and Call Me in the Morning"

Jacqueline E. Payton

A 13-year-old girl presented to the emergency department of a tertiary medical center complaining of a severe headache and her "heart beating too fast." Her mother reported a 3-month history of headaches occurring 2–3 times per week, bilateral in nature, occurring with sudden onset at any time of day, and lasting less than one hour. The headaches had been increasing in severity. The patient denied nausea, vomiting, photophobia, paresthesias, and aura. She was sleeping 8–10 hours each night and was not allowed any caffeinated beverages. She had not begun menses. Over-the-counter analgesics were ineffective and used only a few times. The patient had no history of upper respiratory infection, seasonal allergies, or sinusitis during the previous 3 months. She had no significant past medical history; she had received all her immunizations. Family history included hypertension, coronary artery disease, and thyroid cancer in her deceased paternal grandfather, migraine headaches in her mother, and hypertension in her father.

Physical evaluation revealed a well-developed, well-nourished child, alert and oriented, in obvious pain. She was diaphoretic and appeared anxious. Vital signs were as follows: temperature 37°C, heart rate 120, respiratory rate 28, blood pressure 180/102 (normal 120/80), height 150 cm, weight 35 kg. Her skin was warm, damp, and without nevi or freckles. Ophthalmic examination revealed pupils equal, round, and reactive to light and accommodation; extraocular muscles intact; retinal vasculature normal; fundi visualized, no papilledema; visual acuity 20/20 bilaterally. Mucous membranes appeared dry; examination of head, ears, nose, and throat was otherwise unremarkable. Neck examination revealed a normal thyroid and no lymphadenopathy. Except for tachycardia, examination of the lungs, heart, and abdomen were within normal limits. Neurological exam demonstrated no focal deficits.

Tietz's Applied Laboratory Medicine, Second Edition. Edited by Mitchell G. Scott, Ann M. Gronowski, and Charles S. Eby
Copyright © 2007 John Wiley & Sons, Inc.

The patient was sent for chest x-ray and CT without contrast of head and abdomen, and blood and urine were collected. Complete blood count was within normal limits. Other remarkable laboratory results were as follows:

Analyte	Value, Conventional Units	Reference Interval, Conventional Units	Value, SI Units	Reference Interval, SI Units
Plasma free metanephrine	413.7 pg/mL	<98.5	2.1 nmol/L	<0.5
Plasma free normetanephrine	603.9 pg/mL	<164.7	3.3 nmol/L	<0.9
24-hour urinary metanephrine	578 μg/day	33–185[a,b] <400[a,c]	2930 nmol/day	167–838[a,b] <2028[a,c]
24-hour urinary normetanephrine	984 μg/day	57–286[a,b] <900[a,c]	5373 nmol/day	311–1562[a,b] <4914[a,c]
24-hour urinary creatinine	0.7 g/day	0.6–1.8[d]	62 mmol/day	5.3–15.9[d]
Calcium, total	8.4 mg/dL	8.6–10.3	2.3 mmol/L	2.15–2.58
Calcium, ionized	4.5 mg/dL	4.5–5.1	1.18 mmol/L	1.13–1.28
Calcitonin, basal	25 pg/mL	≤8[c,d]	25 ng/L	≤8[c,d]
Calcitonin, stimulated	200 pg/mL	≤90[c,d]	200 ng/L	≤90[c,d]

[a]Reference interval is dependent on age and gender.
[b]Normotensive.
[c]Hypertensive.
[d]Reference range for females.

The chest x-ray and head CT revealed no abnormalities. Abdominal CT demonstrated bilateral intraadrenal masses. Thyroid scanning demonstrated increased uptake of radioactive iodine in the left lobe.

The patient was diagnosed with MEN2A. Her clinical symptoms were suggestive of pheochromocytoma. Her abnormal laboratory values include elevated metanephrines and normetanephrines, which were suggestive of pheochromocytoma, and elevated calcitonin, which was suggestive of medullary thyroid carcinoma. Increased uptake of radioactive iodine in the thyroid confirmed the presence of a neoplasm. Her family history of thyroid cancer and hypertension also support the diagnosis. The patient was taken to surgery the next day. Under appropriate α-receptor blockade, the adrenal tumors were removed. Total thyroidectomy was then performed.

Definition of the Disease

Pheochromocytoma is a tumor of neuroectodermal origin arising from chromaffin cells. In these tumors, catecholamine synthesis is elevated and degradation is decreased, leading to an excess of epinephrine and/or norepinephrine. These hormones are then released into the circulation, causing symptoms and signs that include headaches, palpitations, diaphoresis (the classic triad), hypertension, anxiety, tremor, angina, nausea, Raynaud's phenomenon, and livedo reticularis.

Of all pheochromocytomas, 90% are isolated tumors; however, they may occur as part of the genetic multiple endocrine neoplasia (MEN) syndrome. There are two categories of MEN: MEN type 1 (MEN1) and MEN type 2 (MEN2), the latter of which is subcategorized into MEN2A and MEN2B. The MEN syndromes are characterized by the development of multiple endocrine tumors that retain the ability to secrete one or more hormones; clinical symptoms and consequent morbidity are caused by hormone hypersecretion. Although the tumors are often benign, malignant transformation and metastasis does occur. The genetic changes that cause MEN have been determined and will be discussed later.

The majority of pheochromocytomas are sporadic. However, approximately 10% of cases occur in association with a hereditary neoplastic disorder, such as MEN2A or MEN2B, von Hippel–Lindau, or neurofibromatosis. Clinically diagnosed of MEN syndrome may be based on the presence of tumors in two or more endocrine glands. Alternatively, a patient with one tumor and coexisting symptoms may be diagnosed by laboratory testing. MEN types 1 and 2 may be distinguished by the endocrine organs involved and by the genetic mutations present. Recent advances in molecular diagnostics have made early diagnosis possible (before tumors develop) in relatives of MEN patients.

Differential Diagnosis

In a healthy pediatric patient, the most common causes of headache are caffeine withdrawal, stress/tension, sleep deprivation, sinusitis, cluster headache, and migraine. Several of these etiologies were ruled out by taking a careful history. Physical exam and CT of the head demonstrated no hemorrhage, tumor, or other structural malformation.

Of great concern are the symptoms that accompany the headaches in this patient: anxiety, palpitations, and sweating. While these symptoms could be explained by a psychiatric illness, such as an anxiety disorder, the extremely elevated blood pressure observed in the emergency department would not be consistent with a psychiatric cause. In children, hypertension is unusual, and almost always secondary to underlying disease or congenital malformation. The signs and symptoms coincident with headache in this patient are classically associated with pheochromocytoma.

Diagnosis

Unlike most other cancers, pheochromocytomas and other endocrine neoplasias may be diagnosed by the detection of elevations of specific hormones and perturbations of electrolytes. In addition, recurrence or metastatic disease may be detected at an earlier stage by periodic laboratory testing. It is essential that these laboratory tests be highly sensitive and specific because the low incidence of disease will limit the positive predictive value of a diagnostic laboratory test. In a study of patients with MEN2, measurement of plasma metanephrines and normetanephrines had a sensitivity of 97% and specificity of 96%.[1] Thus, measurement of these catecholamine metabolites is *the* recommended diagnostic laboratory test for pheochromocytoma.

Diagnosis of other endocrine tumors may be made by measurement of their corresponding hormones. In the case presented, elevated calcitonin concentrations indicated medullary thyroid carcinoma (MTC), a neoplasm of the C cells of the thyroid. Testing for other MEN tumors includes measurement of electrolytes and other hormones, such as calcium and parathyroid hormone (PTH) in parathyroid gland tumors. Table 24.1 indicates abnormal laboratory tests for other endocrine tumors.

Multiple Endocrine Neoplasia

MEN type 1 (Wermer's syndrome) is characterized by the development of benign and malignant tumors of the *p*arathyroid, entero*p*ancreatic, and *p*ituitary glands ("the 3 Ps").

Table 24.1   Lab Tests for Endocrine Tumors

Type	Tumors (Penetrance)	Abnormalities in Lab Tests[a]	Sensitivity (Specificity)
MEN 1	Parathyroid (95–100%)	↑ Calcium and ↑ PTH	Tx based on clinical picture
	Enteropancreatic (65%)		
	Gastrinoma	↑ Gastrin, ↑ basal gastric acid	20%
	Insulinoma	↑ Insulin	56%
	Glucagonoma	↑ Glucagon	33–59%
	VIPoma	↑ VIP	33–59%
	PPoma	↑ PP and/or ↑ chromogranin A	95% (88%); 70% (55%); combined ↑ sensitivity by 25%
	Pituitary (anterior) (45%)		
	Prolactinoma	↑ Prolactin	
	GH secreting	↑ Growth hormone	
	ACTH secreting	↑ Cortisol and ↑ ACTH	
	Nonfunctioning	None or α subunit	
	Associated tumors		
	Adrenal cortical	↑ Cortisol or ↑ aldosterone	
	Carcinoid	↑ 5-HIAA	
MEN 2A	MTC (95%)	↑ Calcitonin	40–100% (100%)
	Pheochromocytoma (50%)	↑ Normetanephrine/metanephrine	97% (96%)
	Parathyroid (20–30%)	↑ Calcium and ↑ PTH	Tx based on clinical picture
MEN 2B	MTC (100%)	↑ Calcitonin	40–100% (100%)
	Pheochromocytoma	↑ Normetanephrine/metanephrine	97% (96%)
	Associated tumors		
	Mucosal neuromas		
	Medulated corneal nerve fibers		

[a]In plasma; many tests are complimented by imaging (e.g., CT, MRI, radionucleotide uptake).
Key: Tx—therapy; MTC—medullary thyroid carcinoma; PP—pancreatic polypeptide; ACTH—adrenocorticotropic hormone; VIP—vasoactive intestinal peptide; HIAA—5-hydroxyindole acetic acid.
Sources: Data obtained from References 1, 2, 3, 4, 6, 8, 9, and 10.

This autosomal dominant disorder has a population prevalence of approximately 1 in 30,000. Clinical expression of the disease occurs most commonly in the third or fourth decade, when tumor-derived hormonal secretions cause overt illness, such as severe ulcer disease. The average penetrance of each tumor type is listed in Table 24.1. Patients are evaluated regularly with laboratory studies and imaging for signs of disease. The tumors are managed surgically if possible. Hypersecretion of hormones by unresectable tumors is managed medically.[2]

Most MEN1 patients are now identified early in life by genetic testing of relatives of known MEN1 patients. More than 300 germline mutations in the MEN1 tumor suppressor gene have been determined to cause MEN1 syndrome.[3] The MEN1 gene is located at chromosome 11q13, and codes for a 610 amino acid protein called *menin*. MEN1 mutations are found throughout the open reading frame and are of diverse types; mutations cause absence or truncation of the protein. Because there are so many mutations, the first patient identified in a family (index case) must have their MEN1 gene sequenced. Once the mutation is identified, directed genetic testing may be used to identify other affected relatives.

MEN type 2 (Sipple syndrome) is quite similar to MEN1. However, MEN2 may be differentiated from MEN type 1 by the tumors involved, namely, medullary thyroid carcinoma (MTC), pheochromocytoma and in MEN2A, parathyroid tumors, or in MEN2B, mucosal neuromas, and other associated signs (see Table 24.1). MEN2 often presents clinically at an earlier age than MEN1; several cases of MTC have been reported in very young children, especially in MEN2B. MEN2B represents only 5% of MEN2 cases.[2]

As in MEN1, patients are evaluated regularly with laboratory studies and imaging for signs of disease. However, given the high penetrance and aggressive metastatic nature of MTC, the 2001 MEN Consensus Committee recommends thyroidectomy by age 5 years in MEN2A, and by age 6 months in MEN2B.[4] Follow-up calcitonin measurements are used to monitor for MTC recurrence after resection. Morbidity and mortality are more often related to metastatic disease than in MEN1, but may also be secondary to hormonal excess.

Mutations in the RET protooncogene are associated with MEN2. The gene is located on chromosome 10q11.2 and encodes an 1114 amino acid transmembrane tyrosine kinase receptor protein called *ret*. Point mutations cause ligand-independent RET dimerization and constitutive activation of the kinase.[5,6] Recent studies have demonstrated a genotype/phenotype association in MEN2. Specific mutations are associated with earlier onset of MTC, earlier metastasis, and higher mortality (due to delayed treatment). Thus, the Seventh International Workshop on MEN and EUROMEN (2004) recommend that age at thyroidectomy be based on the codon mutated.[7] Early genetic testing of all at-risk family members is highly recommended given the aggressive nature and early development of MTC in MEN2. Because there are fewer than 20 mutations, direct genetic testing is used to diagnose the index case as well as relatives.

References

1. EISENHOFER, G., LENDERS, J. W., LINEHAN, W. M. ET AL.: Plasma normetanephrine and metanephrine for detecting pheochromocytoma in Von Hippel-Lindau disease and multiple endocrine neoplasia type 2. *N. Engl. J. Med. 340*:1872–9, 1999.

2. LARSEN, P. R., AND WILLIAMS, R. H., eds.: *William's Textbook of Endocrinology*, 10th ed., Saunders, Philadelphia, 2003.

3. AGARWAL, S. K., LEE BURNS, A., SUKHODOLETS, K. E. ET AL.: Molecular pathology of the MEN1 gene. *Ann. NY Acad. Sci. 1014*:189–98, 2004.

4. BRANDI, M. L., GAGEL, R. F., ANGELI, A. ET AL.: Guidelines for diagnosis and therapy of MEN type 1 and type 2. *J. Clin. Endocrinol. Metab. 86*:5658–71, 2001.

5. MACHENS, A., NICCOLI-SIRE, P., HOEGEL, J. ET AL.: Early malignant progression of hereditary medullary thyroid cancer. *N. Engl. J. Med. 349*:1517–25, 2003.

6. THAKKER, R. V.: Multiple endocrine neoplasia. *Hormone Res. 56*:S67–72, 2001.

7. MASSOLL, N. AND MAZZAFERRI, E. L.: Diagnosis and management of MTC. *Clin. Lab. Med. 24*:49–83, 2004.

8. GRANBERG, D., STRIDSBERG, M., SEENSALU, R. ET AL.: Plasma chromogranin A in patients with multiple endocrine neoplasia type 1. *J. Clin. Endocrinol. Metab. 84*:2712–17, 1999.

9. LAIRMORE, T. C., PIERSALL, L. D., DEBENEDETTI, M. K. ET AL.: Clinical genetic testing and early surgical intervention in patients with multiple endocrine neoplasia type 1 (MEN1). *Ann. Surg. 239*:637–47, 2004.

10. MUTCH, M. G., FRISELLA, M. M., DEBENEDETTI, M. K. ET AL.: Pancreatic polypeptide is a useful plasma marker for radiographically evident pancreatic islet cell tumors in patients with multiple endocrine neoplasia type 1. *Surgery 122*:1012–19, 1997.

Case 25

Unpleasant Spells

Les G. K. Q. Burke and Ravinder J. Singh

A 22-year-old woman returned to her physician with a one-year history of hypertension. Despite treatment, her blood pressure was still elevated. Six months after the onset of her hypertension she began to experience strange "spells." The spells consisted of palpitations, sweating, and lightheadedness. They usually lasted 5–10 minutes, occurring about twice a day, especially at bedtime. She had been taking her blood pressure medication (phenoxybenzamine 10 mg, two capsules twice daily) regularly. She was on no other medication except Depo-Provera (medroxyprogesterone) every 3 months. The patient denied any family history of hypertension or thyroid tumors, specifically medullary cancer. The patient was referred to an endocrinologist.

On physical examination the patient appeared well and was in no distress. Her blood pressure was elevated at 165/100 mm Hg while medicated. No thyroid nodules were found on palpation. Heart sounds were normal, without murmurs. Lungs were clear to auscultation. No masses were found on palpation, although deep palpation was not performed.

Major endocrine causes of hypertension have been reported to be primary hyperaldosteronism, Cushing syndrome, and pheochromocytoma. Thus, her laboratory test evaluation included plasma aldosterone, 24-hour urine cortisol, and ruled out the possibility of primary aldosteronism and Cushing syndrome. Results for these tests were within normal reference intervals.

Results of testing for pheochromocytoma are shown below:

Analyte/Test	Value, Conventional Units	Reference Interval, Conventional Units	Value, SI Units	Reference Interval, SI Units
Urine-fractionated metanephrines				
Metanephrine	86 μg/day	30–180	436 nmol/day	152–913
Normetanephrine	4256 μg/day	111–419	23,238 nmol/day	606–2288
Plasma-fractionated metanephrines				
Metanephrine, free	62 pg/mL	<100	0.31 nmol/L	<0.50
Normetanephrine	2703 pg/mL	<167	14.6 nmol/L	<0.90

Tietz's Applied Laboratory Medicine, Second Edition. Edited by Mitchell G. Scott, Ann M. Gronowski, and Charles S. Eby

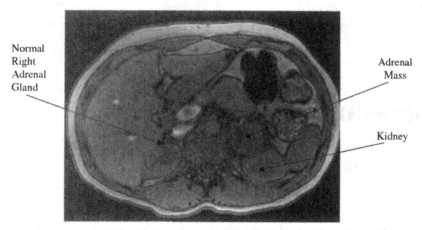

Figure 25.1 MRI examination of the abdomen without and with IV gadolinium demonstrated a 4.8 × 4 × 0.2 × 6.4-cm (AP × trans × CC) enhancing mass in the left adrenal gland. Central portion of this mass demonstrates no contrast enhancement (which may represent an area of central necrosis). Right adrenal gland was observed to be normal.

The results provide strong biochemical evidence for the presence of pheochromocytoma, and no additional biochemical testing was required. These results prompted a CT scan of the patient's abdomen. Imaging showed an ~6.5 cm vascular left adrenal mass. Subsequent ^{131}I-metaiodobenzylguanidine nuclear scan showed radioactive uptake on the left and some mild uptake on the right, leading to a possibility of bilateral process. With the idea of possible bilateral pheochromocytoma, RET protooncogene screening was performed and was negative. The patient's phenoxybenzamine was increased to 40 mg daily. With this treatment, her blood pressure decreased to 133/80 mm Hg.

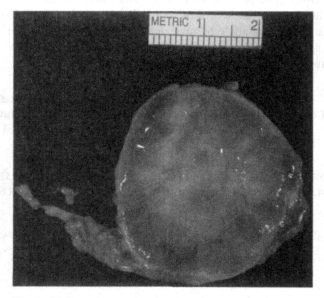

Figure 25.2 Left adrenalectomy was performed, and pheochromocytoma tumor of 8.0 cm with central degenerative changes was resected. The pathologists saw no tumor necrosis and no angiolymphatic invasion.

Abdominal MRI with gadolinium was performed to clarify whether the tumor was indeed bilateral. It showed the disease to be confined to the left adrenal gland (Fig. 25.1). A laparoscopic left total adrenalectomy was planned. The patient was started on a low-salt diet and propranolol 40 mg daily. Her blood pressure decreased to 120/70 with heart rate in the 60s–70s. The day prior to surgery, phenoxybenzamine was increased to 60 mg daily total and propranolol to 60 mg daily. The patient's surgery went well. Her left adrenal gland contained an 8.0 cm well-circumscribed pheochromocytoma with central degenerative changes (Fig. 25.2). No coagulative tumor necrosis or angiolymphatic invasion was seen. The patient was discharged 2 days after surgery.

At discharge, the patient's fractionated metanephrines were normal with free plasma metanephrine 40 pg/mL (0.2 nmol/L) and normetanephrine 152 pg/mL (0.82 nmol/L). The patient was considered to be cured of pheochromocytoma and was advised that her metanephrines would need to be rechecked yearly. With this impressive outcome, the patient was able to celebrate her upcoming college graduation ceremony.

Definition of the Disease

Pheochromocytoma is a lethal tumor of chromaffin cells of the adrenal medulla, which produces "spells" or episodes of hypertension with heart palpitations, severe headaches, anxiety, and sweating. Together, these symptoms are classic for the disease; however, pheochromocytoma can present with multiple other symptoms that can make diagnosis difficult (Table 25.1).[1-3] It is important to remember that among patients with hypertension, pheochromocytomas are present in only ~0.3% of patients.

Pheochromocytoma tumors differ considerably in their rates of catecholamine synthesis, release, and the types of catecholamine produced.[4] Pheochromocytomas secrete mostly catecholamines (epinephrine and norepinephrine), which are preferentially metabolized to metanephrines by the pheochromocytes of the tumor cells that have high concentrations of membrane-bound catechol-O-methyl transferase (COMT). The COMT enzyme preferentially converts catecholamines to metanephrines.[4] Adrenal tumors can produce both norepinephrine and epinephrine, while extra adrenal pheochromocytoma tumors produce exclusively norepinephrine. Therefore, patients with elevated concentrations of plasma metanephrines (metabolite of epinephrine) are likely to have an adrenal tumor, while patients with elevated concentrations of normetanephrine (metabolite of norepinephrine), without metanephrines, could have tumors with an adrenal or extra-adrenal location.

Pheochromocytoma and paraganglioma are primarily sporadic tumors, but up to 20% are associated with rare hereditary endocrine syndromes, such as multiple endocrine neoplasia type 2, von Hippel–Lindau syndrome, neurofibromatosis type 1, and familial paraganglioma syndromes. Such tumors may be detected at a presymptomatic phase on screening members of an affected kindred or as an incidental finding on imaging.[5,6] Recently paraganglioma tumors have been associated with germline mutations in the succinate–ubiquinone oxidoreductase subunit D gene (SDHD). This gene belongs to the mitochondrial complex II family. To confirm familial pheochromocytoma, mutation analysis of VHL, MEN2, RET, and SDH family of genes is generally recommended.[7] Pheochromocytoma in MEN2 patients produces both epinephrine and norepinephrine, whereas tumors in VHL patients produce almost exclusively norepinephrine. MEN2 tumors express more tyrosine hydroxylase, the rate-limiting enzyme in catecholamine synthesis, and thus produce larger amounts of catecholamines and are more likely to produce signs and symptoms than tumors in VHL patients.

Table 25.1 Symptoms and Their Frequency in Patients with Pheochromocytoma

Symptoms	Patients, %
Severe headache	82
Perspiration	67
Palpitations, tachycardia	60
Anxiety	45
Tremulousness	38
Chest, abdominal pain	38
Nausea, vomiting	35
Weakness, fatigue	26
Weight loss	15
Dyspnea	15
Warmth, heat intolerance	15
Visual disturbances	12
Dizziness, faintness	7
Constipation	7
Hypertension	
Sustained	61
Paroxysmal	24
Pallor	44
Retinopathy	
Grades I and II	40
Grades III and IV	53
Abdominal mass	9
Associated multiple endocrine adenomatosis	6

Differential Diagnosis

The diagnosis of pheochromocytoma has been challenging, and numerous cases have been reported, illustrating that the diagnosis can be easily missed. Autopsy series suggest that the undiagnosed tumor can be associated with morbid consequences.[8,9]

Since hypertension is a primary symptom, ruling out other causes of hypertension such as Cushing and primary aldosteronism is an important part of the differential diagnosis. Cushing can be ruled out with normal 24-hour urine cortisol or normal overnight dexamathasone suppression. Primary aldosteronism can be ruled out with normal urine potassium, and a normal plasma aldosterone. Hypertension in pheochromocytoma patients is usually associated with heart palpitations, headache, and sweating and is confirmed with the biochemical evidence of catecholamine/metabolite secretion.

Diagnosis of pheochromocytoma can be challenging as there are a variety of biochemical tests to choose from, including (1) plasma catecholamines (PCAT), (2) urinary catecholamines (UCAT), (3) urinary fractionated metanephrines (UMET), (4) plasma free metanephrines (PMET), and (5) urinary vanillylmandelic acid (VMA).[4,10] Missing a pheochromocytoma may have catastrophic consequences; therefore, in the investigation of suspected tumors, tests with a high level of sensitivity must be employed. Various studies have recently reported that compared to catecholamines and VMA, metanephrines in plasma and urine have the highest sensitivity for the diagnosis of pheochromocytoma. In addition, there have been evidence-based recommendations for limiting the number of tests ordered for the diagnosis of pheochromocytoma.[4,10–12] Since norepinephrine and epinephrine are metabolized to free normetanephrine and metanephrines, respectively, by the pheochromocytoma tumor cells, the sensitivity and specificity has been found to be higher for metanephrines testing compared to catecholamines and VMA.[10]

Historically these tests have been performed by fluorometric, radioenzymatic, and colorimetric methodologies. Now these tests are being performed using chromatographic separation techniques with electrochemical detection in most of the laboratories. With these methodologies, catecholamines are fractionated into epinephrine, norepinephrine, and dopamine and are reported individually. Recently, liquid chromatography tandem mass spectrometry (LC-MS/MS) methodology has been implemented in various clinical laboratories for plasma and urine matanephrines which has proven to be rapid, specific, and cost effective.[13,14] The metanephrine testing involves fractionation into metanephrines and normetanephrines and measures only free unconjugated metanephrines in plasma, while urine measurements involve both free and conjugated metanephrines.

Methods for the analysis of metanephrines have recently improved and as a result are now very sensitive and specific.[4,11] Cutoff values for metanephrines have been calculated (significantly above the 95% reference limits) where the disease can be ruled in with 100% specificity (Tables 25.2–25.4). Normal reference intervals as a function of age and gender are shown in Table 25.4.

Prior to undergoing biochemical testing, patients with a strong clinical suspicion for pheochromocytoma should be taken off medications that may have physiological or analytical interferences.[15] Tricyclic antidepressants (TCAs), levodopa, and significant physical stress (e.g., hypertensive stroke) may elevate concentrations of metanephrines. If clinically feasible, these medications should be discontinued at least 1 week before collection. The LC-MS/MS method is not affected by the interfering substances that affected the previously utilized spectrophotometric (Pisano reaction) method (i.e., diatrizoate, chlorpromazine, hydrazine derivatives, imipramine, MAO inhibitors, methyldopa, phenacetin, ephedrine, or epinephrine). This method is also not subject to the known interference of acetaminophen (seen with the plasma metanephrine high-performance liquid chromatography HPLC-EC method).

Most patients with pheochromocytoma, particularly those who are symptomatic, have increases in plasma or urinary catecholamines or metanephrines well in excess ($2-3\times$) of the normal reference intervals. False-positive results of metanephrines are possible, due to

Table 25.2 Sensitivity and Specificity of Plasma Free Metanephrines at Various Cutoff Values for Diagnosis of Pheochromocytoma

MN[a] cutoff nmol/L (pg/mL)	NMN[b] cutoff nmol/L (pg/mL)	Sensitivity (95% confidence intervals)	Specificity (95% confidence intervals)	References
0.6 (120)	0.9 (172)	96 (80–99)	85 (79–89)	12
0.3 (60)	0.5 (96)	99 (96–100)	89 (87–92)	10
1.2 (240)	2.2 (420)	79	100	10

[a]Metanephrines.

[b]Normetanephrine.

Table 25.3 Sensitivity and Specificity of Urine Metanephrines at Various Cutoff Values for Diagnosis of Pheochromocytoma

MN[a] Cutoff µg/24 hours (nmol/24 hours)	NMN[b] cutoff µg/24 hours (nmol/24 hours)	% Sensitivity (95% confidence intervals)	% Specificity (95% confidence intervals)	References
138 (690) for females 236 (1180) for males	311 (1710) for females 549 (3020) for males	97 (92–99)	69 (64–72)	10
Reference intervals in Table 25.4	Reference intervals in Table 25.4	97 (81–100)	81 (73–88)	11
400 (2000)	900 (4950)	97 (92–99)	95 (93–97)	11

[a]Metanephrines.
[b]Normetanephrine.

Table 25.4 The 95th Percentile Reference Intervals and Clinical Cutoff Values for Urine Metanephrines

	Reference intervals		
Age	Males	Females	Cutoff[a]
Metanephrine µg/24 hours[b]			
3–8	29–92	18–144	≤400
9–12	59–188	43–122	≤400
13–17	69–221	33–185	≤400
18–70	44–261	30–180	≤400
Normetanephrine µg/24 hours[b]			
3–8	34–169	29–145	≤900
9–12	84–422	55–277	≤900
13–17	91–456	57–286	≤900
18–29	103–390	103–390	≤900
30–39	111–419	111–419	≤900
40–49	119–451	119–451	≤900
50–59	128–484	128–484	≤900
60–69	138–521	138–521	≤900
70+	148–560	148–560	≤900
Total Metanephrines µg/24 hours[b]			
3–8	47–223	57–210	≤1300
9–12	201–528	107–394	≤1300
13–17	120–603	113–414	≤1300
18–29	190–583	142–510	≤1300
30–39	200–614	149–535	≤1300
40–49	211–646	156–561	≤1300
50–59	222–680	164–588	≤1300
60–69	233–716	171–616	≤1300
70+	246–753	180–646	≤1300

[a]Concentrations greater than clinical cutoff values rule in pheochromocytoma with 100% specificity.

[b]Conversion factors: metanephrine µg/24 hours × 5.07 = nmol/24 hours; normetanephrine µg/24 hours × 5.46 = nmol/24 hours; total metanephrines µg/24 hours × 5.23 = nmol/24 hours.

accompanying medical conditions, medications, inappropriate sampling conditions, and dietary influences. To achieve maximum specificity, higher cutoff values have been suggested for both the plasma and urine metanephrine tests.

Concentrations of plasma free normetanephrine above 2.2 nmol/L (420 pg/mL) or of metanephrine above 1.2 nmol/L (240 pg/mL) are rarely if ever found in patients without pheochromocytoma, (Table 25.2). Similarly, with a higher cutoff for urine normetanephrines concentrations above 900 μg/24 hours and metanephrines above 400 μg/24 hours reduces the number of false positives from 19% to 5% (Table 25.3). In patients with such elevated concentrations, the tumor should be located by imaging studies followed immediately by the treatment.

It is an exciting period in the history of the biochemical diagnosis of pheochromocytoma when such a lethal disease can be ruled in or out on the basis of a simple test of urine and/or plasma metanephrines. In conclusion, metanephrine measurements are sensitive and specific markers for pheochromocytoma and biochemical evidence of excessive production should be confirmed in both urine and plasma.

References

1. GANGULY, A., HENRY, D. P., YUNE, H. Y., ET AL.: Diagnosis and localization of pheochromocytoma. Detection by measurement of urinary norepinephrine excretion during sleep, plasma norepinephrine concentration, and computerized axial tomography (CT-scan). *Am. J. Med.* 67:21–6, 1979.

2. BRAVO, E. L.: Pheochromocytoma. *Curr. Ther. Endocrinol. & Metab.* 6:195–7, 1997.

3. BRAVO, E. L.: Pheochromocytoma. *Cardiol. Rev.* 10:44–50, 2002.

4. EISENHOFER, G., LENDERS, J. W., AND PACAK, K.: Biochemical diagnosis of pheochromocytoma. *Frontiers Hormone Res.* 31:76–106, 2004.

5. NEUMANN, H. P. AND Freiburg-Warsaw-Columbus Pheochromocytoma Study Group: Germline mutations in nonsyndromic pheochromocytoma. *N. Engl. J. Med.* 346:1459–66, 2002.

6. KUDVA, Y. C., YOUNG, W. F., JR., THOMPSON, G. B., GRANT, C. S., AND VAN HEERDEN, J. A.: Adrenal incidentaloma: An important component of the clinical presentation spectrum of benign sporadic adrenal pheochromocytoma. *Endocrinologist* 9:77–80, 1999.

7. GIMM, O., KOCH, C. A., JANUSZEWICZ, A., OPOCHER, G., AND NEUMANN, H. P.: The genetic basis of pheochromocytoma. *Frontiers Hormone Res.* 31:45–60, 2004.

8. WALTHER, M. M., KEISER, H. R., AND LINEHAN, W. M.: Pheochromocytoma: Evaluation, diagnosis, and treatment. *World J. Urol.* 17:35–9, 1999.

9. Beatty, O. L., Russell, C. F., Kennedy, L., Hadden, D. R., Kennedy, T. L., AND ATKINSON, A. B.: Phaeochromocytoma in Northern Ireland: A 21 year review. *Euro. J. Surg.* 162:695–702, 1996.

10. LENDERS, J. W., PACAK, K., WALTHER, M. M. ET AL.: Biochemical diagnosis of pheochromocytoma: Which test is best? *JAMA* 287:1427–34, 2002.

11. SINGH, R. J.: Advances in metanephrine testing for the diagnosis of pheochromocytoma. *Clin. Lab. Med.* 24:85–103, 2004.

12. SAWKA, A. M. JAESCHKE, R., SINGH, R. J., AND YOUNG, W. F., JR.: A comparison of biochemical tests for pheochromocytoma: Measurement of fractionated plasma metanephrines compared with the combination of 24-hour urinary metanephrines and catecholamines. *J. Clin. Endocrinol. Metab.* 88:553–8, 2003.

13. LAGERSTEDT, S. A., O'KANE, D. J., AND SINGH, R. J.: Measurement of plasma free metanephrine and normetanephrine by liquid chromatography-tandem mass spectrometry for diagnosis of pheochromocytoma. *Clin. Chem.* 50:603–11, 2004.

14. TAYLOR, R. L. AND SINGH, R. J.: Validation of liquid chromatography-tandem mass spectrometry method for analysis of urinary conjugated metanephrine and normetanephrine for screening of pheochromocytoma. *Clin. Chem.* 48:533–9, 2002.

15. EISENHOFER, G., GOLDSTEIN, D. S., WALTHER, M. M., FRIBERG, P., LENDERS, J. W., KEISER, H. R., AND PACAK, K.: Biochemical diagnosis of pheochromocytoma: how to distinguish true- from false-positive test results. *J. Clin. Endocrinol. Metab.* 88:2656–66, 2003.

Part Seven

Diabetes

Cases of diabetes management and complications, ketoacidosis, and hypoglycemia are presented and discussed in Cases 26, 27, and 28, respectively (all edited by MGS).

Tietz's Applied Laboratory Medicine, Second Edition. Edited by Mitchell G. Scott, Ann M. Gronowski, and Charles S. Eby
Copyright © 2007 John Wiley & Sons, Inc.

Case 26

Recent Weight Loss and Polyuria in a 52-Year-Old Man

Anders H. Berg and David B. Sacks

A 52-year-old man with a history of hypertriglyceridemia and a recent toenail infection came to his primary care physician's office complaining of recent onset of nocturia, polyuria, and a 10-lb weight loss. His family history revealed that his father had developed diabetes mellitus at age 60. A limited physical examination revealed normal vital signs, normal fundi (by ophthalmoscopy), and no detectable peripheral neuropathy.

Laboratory data at initial visit were as follows:

Analyte	Value, Conventional Units	Reference Interval, Conventional Units	Value, SI Units	Reference Interval, SI Units
Sodium (B)	139 mmol/L	136–142	Same	
Potassium (B)	3.6 mmol/L	3.5–5.0	Same	
Chloride (B)	98 mmol/L	98–108	Same	
CO_2, total (B)	28 mmol/L	23–32	Same	
Urea nitrogen (B)	13 mg/dL	9–25	12.1 mmol/L	3.2–8.9
Creatinine (B)	0.9 mg/dL	0.7–1.3	310 μmol/L	62–115
Glucose (B)	420 mg/dL	54–99	23.3 mmol/L	3.0–5.5
Anion gap (B)	13 mmol/L	3–15	Same	
Calcium (B)	10.5 mg/dL	8.8–10.5	2.4 mmol/L	2.15–2.5
Insulin (B)	3.2 μU/mL	2–18	22 pmol/L	14–125
HbA_{1c} (B)	10.3%	4.2–5.8	Same	
TSH (B)	1.28 μU/mL	0.5–5.0	1.28 mU/L	0.5–5.0
T4 (B)	10.5 μg/dL	5–11	135 nmol/L	65–142
Glucose (U)	3+	0–0	N/A	
Ketones (U)	1+	Negative	N/A	
Specific gravity (U)	1.040	1.003–1.035	Same	
pH (U)	7.0	4.5–8.0	Same	
Albumin (U)	Negative	Negative		
Urine blood (U)	Negative	Negative		

Tietz's Applied Laboratory Medicine, Second Edition. Edited by Mitchell G. Scott, Ann M. Gronowski, and Charles S. Eby
Copyright © 2007 John Wiley & Sons, Inc.

The markedly increased random serum glucose concentration suggested diabetes mellitus, and after considering the history and presentation, the physician thought that it was most likely type 2 diabetes. The increased HbA_{1c} concentration indicated that the hyperglycemia had been present for some time.[1] Measurement of plasma glucose on a subsequent day gave a value of 300 mg/dL (16.7 mmol/L), establishing the diagnosis of diabetes mellitus.[2] The patient was counseled regarding changes in diet and exercise, and was started on 850 mg oral metformin twice daily (bid). On a follow-up visit one week later his casual (nonfasting) capillary blood glucose concentration obtained by finger stick was 230 mg/dL (12.8 mmol/L). The physician prescribed self-monitoring of blood glucose (SMBG) twice a day. Within a few months the patient gained 6 lb and his HbA_{1c} had dropped to 6.1%. He returned to the clinic after 6 months for a follow-up visit to monitor his glycemic control. He admitted to having increased his consumption of carbohydrates and was exercising less. He denied polyuria or nocturia, visual disturbance, or neuropathic symptoms, and felt well.

Physical examination revealed a blood pressure of 122/72 mm Hg, a regular pulse rate of 64 bpm, and a respiratory rate of 12/minute. Heart sounds were normal with no murmurs, and the lungs were clear to auscultation. Examination of the abdomen revealed no masses or hepatomegaly, and bowel sounds were normal. Ophthalmologic examination showed normal fundi. There was no pedal edema, dorsalis pedis pulses were normal bilaterally, and toes and feet were sensitive to light touch and position.

Laboratory data from a fasting blood sample and urine collected the previous day:

Analyte	Value, Conventional Units	Reference Interval, Conventional Units	Value, SI Units	Reference Interval, SI Units
Glucose (B)	134 mg/dL	54–99	7.4 mmol/L	3.0–5.5
HbA_{1c} (B)	8.0%	4.2–5.8%	Same	
Albumin (B)	1.2 mg/dL	0.0–2.0	12 mg/L	0–20
Microalbumin (U)	9.2 mg Alb/g Cre	0.0–30	1.0 mg/mmol	0.0–3.4

Despite only a relatively mild increase in fasting glucose concentration, the physician was concerned by the increased HbA_{1c}. Although the patient showed no obvious signs of diabetic microvascular complications, the earlier infection raised the possibility of peripheral vascular insufficiency and the resulting susceptibility to infection associated with diabetes.[3] The patient was again counseled firmly to resume his exercise and control his diet, and the physician increased the metformin to 1000 mg bid. Another appointment was made for the patient to see the nutritionist and ophthalmologist, and a follow-up appointment was scheduled in 3 months to consider adding a sulfonylurea to the patient's therapy if no improvement was seen.

Definition of the Disease

Diabetes mellitus is a group of metabolic disorders of carbohydrate metabolism that result in hyperglycemia. The disease is classified into several categories.[4] Type 1 diabetes [formerly known as *insulin-dependent diabetes mellitus* (IDDM)] usually has onset in childhood, frequently presents with an acute episode of severe hyperglycemia often progressing to ketoacidosis, and produces sudden weight loss. Type 2 diabetes [formerly known as *non-insulin-dependent diabetes mellitus* (NIDDM)] is commonly associated with obesity, and hyperglycemic episodes usually occur without ketoacidosis. Although onset is more common in adulthood, the frequency of type 2 diabetes in children is increasing as a result of the rising prevalence of childhood obesity.[2] Other forms of diabetes are rare. These include endocrinopathies such as Cushing's syndrome, reactive diabetes due to pancreatic insult by drugs or infection, and rare genetic/congenital causes, including maturity-onset diabetes of the young (MODY). The fourth category is gestational diabetes mellitus (GDM), which is diabetes first diagnosed during pregnancy; thus, a woman with diabetes who becomes pregnant is not classified as GDM.[2] Hyperglycemia not sufficient to meet the criteria for diabetes is categorized as "prediabetes." Impaired fasting glucose (IFG) is present when fasting plasma glucose concentrations exceed the limits of healthy individuals but fail to meet the criteria for overt diabetes (i.e., 100–125 mg/dL; 5.6–6.9 mmol/L).[2] If diagnosed by an oral glucose tolerance test (OGTT), this is categorized as impaired glucose tolerance (IGT), with a 2-hour plasma glucose ranging within 140–199 mg/dL (7.8–11.0 mmol/L). Both IFG and IGT are termed "prediabetes" and are risk factors for progression to diabetes and cardiovascular disease.[2]

Differential Diagnosis

The diagnosis of diabetes is based solely on documenting an increased concentration of glucose in the blood. There are three ways to diagnose diabetes in a nonpregnant individual, and each must be confirmed on a subsequent day (unless there are unequivocal symptoms of hyperglycemia). The diagnostic criteria of the American Diabetes Association (ADA) are (1) symptoms of diabetes and a casual* plasma glucose concentration ≥200 mg/dL (11.1 mmol/L), (2) fasting* plasma glucose (FPG) ≥126 mg/dL (7.0 mmol/L), or (3) plasma glucose ≥200 mg/dL (11.1 mmol/L) 2 hours after a 75-g oral glucose load.[2] FPG is the recommended diagnostic test because of simplicity, acceptability to patients, and low cost. OGTT is more sensitive than FPG, but suffers from a lack of reproducibility. In addition to measurement of FPG, initial laboratory evaluation should include a fasting lipid profile to monitor for dyslipidemia and urine analysis for ketones and protein.[2,5] Adults should furthermore have measurement of urine microalbumin[4] (to detect early stages of diabetic nephropathy) and serum creatinine (to determine whether overt renal failure has developed).[2] In addition, both SMBG and hemoglobin A_{1c} (HbA$_{1c}$) are used to monitor intraday and longer-term glycemic control, respectively (see Treatment section below).[1,2]

Pathogenesis

The two major forms of diabetes have different underlying molecular defects. Type 1 diabetes results from autoimmune destruction of the β-cells of the pancreas. The consequence is a marked reduction or absence of insulin secretion, and the patients are dependent on an exogenous source of insulin to maintain life. Type 2 diabetes results from a combination of insulin resistance and inadequate insulin secretion. Insulin resistance is a state where target tissues are less responsive to normal insulin concentrations. Unlike glucose or cholesterol,

---

*"Casual" is defined as any time of day without regard to time since last meal. "Fasting" is no intake of calories for at least 8 hours.

insulin resistance is difficult to measure in routine clinical practice. Insulin resistance is relatively common, particularly in obese and pregnant individuals. Initially, the β-cells of the pancreas compensate by increasing glucose-stimulated insulin production, thereby maintaining euglycemia. The increased demand on the β cells by the insulin resistance may result in a progressive loss of β-cell function. If the pancreas is unable to produce adequate insulin to overcome the insulin resistance, the patient progresses to diabetes.

Patients with diabetes are at high risk for the development of complications.[3,6] It is believed that most of the pathologic sequelae of diabetes are caused by hyperglycemia. High glucose concentrations damage tissues through protein glycation and generation of reactive oxygen species (free radicals). Hyperglycemia is particularly damaging to the vascular endothelium. The microvascular damage from chronic hyperglycemia results in diabetic neuropathy, nephropathy, and retinopathy, while macrovascular complications include myocardial infarction, stroke, and peripheral vascular insufficiency. The consequence of these complications is that patients with diabetes have a high rate of blindness, renal failure requiring dialysis, and limb amputations.

Treatment

The first component of the management of diabetes is early detection. Guidelines set forth by the ADA recommend screening to identify asymptomatic individuals who are likely to have diabetes.[2] The rationale for screening is that approximately one-third of people with type 2 diabetes have not been diagnosed. Screening should be performed by FPG, but the OGTT can also be used. The ADA guidelines suggest that screening should be considered every 3 years starting at 45 years of age, but should be commenced at an earlier age or performed more frequently if risk factors for type 2 diabetes are present. Pregnant women should be screened for GDM at 24–28 weeks of gestation with a glucose challenge test. If the serum glucose concentration is ≥ 130 mg/dL (7.2 mmol/L) 1 hour after 50 g of oral glucose is given, an OGTT is performed. (Note that the OGTT for pregnant women is different from that for nonpregnant individuals.) For GDM, 100 g of glucose is ingested and plasma glucose values are measured immediately before the test (fasting) and at 1, 2, and 3 hours after the oral load. Plasma glucose concentrations should be <95, 180, 155, and 140 mg/dL (5.3, 10.0, 8.6, and 7.8 mmol/L) at each of these respective timepoints. If any two values exceed these thresholds, the woman is diagnosed with GDM. Obese children should be screened starting at age 10 if they have affected family members or have signs of insulin resistance.

Patients with IGT or IFG should be encouraged to lose weight and increase physical activity as these factors have been shown to reduce the progression to overt diabetes.[2] Patients with type 1 diabetes require insulin and a diet that restricts intake of simple sugars. Type 2 diabetes is treated according to severity. If the diabetes is mild, diet, exercise, and weight loss may suffice. If these strategies fail, oral hypoglycemic agents (sulfonylureas, metformin, or thiazolidinediones) are added. Insulin is necessary when other interventions are inadequate to maintain glycemic control.

Glycemic control is assessed by both SMBG and measurement of HbA_{1c}.[1,2,5] Patients who require insulin monitor their blood glucose to regulate their insulin doses. SMBG is performed several times a day on a capillary blood sample using a portable meter. (Note that these meters lack adequate precision to permit their use in screening or diagnosis of diabetes.[4]) The value of SMBG in patients with type 2 diabetes who do not require insulin is controversial.

HbA$_{1c}$ is the other measure of glycemic control.[1,2] Glucose reacts with the amino groups on proteins by a nonenzymatic chemical condensation, a reaction termed *glycation*. HbA$_{1c}$ is the fraction of HbA that has been glycated at the *N*-terminal valine of the β chain. The amount of HbA$_{1c}$ is proportional to the glucose concentration to which erythrocytes are exposed. HbA$_{1c}$ is a useful index of mean glycemia over the life of an erythrocyte, which averages 120 days. Therefore, HbA$_{1c}$ reflects average glycemia over the preceding 2–3 months. HbA$_{1c}$ should be measured routinely in all patients with diabetes. The frequency of testing depends on adequacy of glycemic control and recommendations range within every 3–6 months.

Glycemic goals are based on large, prospective, randomized, multicenter studies. The Diabetes Control and Complications Trial (DCCT)[6] examined patients with type 1 diabetes, while patients with type 2 diabetes were enrolled in the United Kingdom Prospective Diabetes Study (UKPDS).[3] The studies were designed to evaluate the effects of intensive plasma glucose control on the development of chronic complications. In both of these trials, improved glycemic control was associated with significantly decreased rates of progression of microvascular complications. The outcomes were linked to HbA$_{1c}$, which was used to evaluate glycemic control. The reference range for HbA$_{1c}$ is 4.0–6.0%, and most organizations recommend a target of 6.5–7.0% for treatment of diabetes.

References

1. BENJAMIN, R. J., AND SACKS, D. B.: Glycated protein update: Implications of recent studies, including the diabetes control and complications trial. *Clin. Chem.* *40*:683–7, 1994.
2. American Diabetes Association. Standards of medical care in diabetes. *Diabetes Care* 28:S4–36, 2005.
3. U.K. Prospective Diabetes Study (UKPDS) Group. Intensive blood-glucose control with sulphonylureas or insulin compared with conventional treatment and risk of complications in patients with type 2 diabetes (UKPDS 33). *Lancet* 352:837–53, 1998.
4. SACKS, D. B., BRUNS, D. E., GOLDSTEIN, D. E., MACLAREN, N. K., McDONALD, J. M., AND PARROTT, M.: Guidelines and recommendations for laboratory analysis in the diagnosis and management of diabetes mellitus. *Clin. Chem.* 48:436–72, 2002.
5. GOLDSTEIN, D. E., LITTLE, R. R., LORENZ, R. A. ET AL.: An overview of the different tests of glycemia in diabetes. *Diabetes Care* 27:1761–73, 2004.
6. The Diabetes Control and Complications Trial Research Group. The effect of intensive treatment of diabetes on the development and progression of long-term complications in insulin-dependent diabetes mellitus. *N. Engl. J. Med.* 329:977–86, 1993.

Case 27

An Unconscious Diabetic Male

Anders H. Berg and David B. Sacks

A 30-year-old man with a 5-year history of type 1 diabetes mellitus was brought by ambulance to the emergency department (ED). He had received 1 L of normal saline intravenously en route. He was unconscious but responsive to painful stimuli. Earlier that week he had a fever and cough associated with excessive thirst. His fever and cough resolved after a few days without the use of antibiotics, but the thirst continued and he developed nausea, vomiting, abdominal pain, and increasing lethargy until the morning of admission, when he could not be roused by a family member. In the ED his mother related that he had never previously been hospitalized for his diabetes. He used 40 units of NPH insulin and 10 units of regular insulin before breakfast and 10 units NPH and 5 units of regular insulin before dinner.

In addition to a decreased level of consciousness, physical examination in the ED was remarkable for round and reactive pupillary reflexes and normal deep tendon reflexes. Vital signs included a heart rate of 140 bpm, blood pressure of 80/50 mm Hg, respiratory rate of 33/min, and oral temperature of 36°C (96.7°F), and a fruity odor was noted on his breath. His abdomen was nontender and bowel sounds were normal. He had poor skin turgor and dry mucous membranes. EKG showed sinus tachycardia with peaked T waves. Laboratory data while in the ED included

Analyte	Value, Conventional Units	Reference Interval, Conventional Units	Value, SI Units	Reference Interval, SI Units
Sodium (B)	140 mmol/L	136–142	Same	
Potassium (B)	5.8 mmol/L	3.5–5.0	Same	
Chloride (B)	97 mmol/L	98–108	Same	
CO_2, total (B)	6 mmol/L	23–32	Same	
Urea nitrogen (B)	27 mg/dL	9–25	9.6 mmol/L	3.2–8.9
Creatinine (B)	2.8 mg/dL	0.7–1.3	248 μmol/L	62–115
Phosphorous (B)	5.0 mg/L	2.4–5.0	1.6 mmol/L	0.8–1.6
Glucose (B)	581 mg/dL	54–99 mg/dL	32 mmol/L	3.0–5.5
pH (WB, art)	6.89	7.35–7.5	Same	
pCO_2 (WB, art)	13 mmHg	35–48	1.7 kPa	4.7–6.4

Analyte	Value, Conventional Units	Reference Interval, Conventional Units
Glucose (U)	4+	Negative
Ketones (U) (nitroprusside dipstick)	Weakly positive	Negative

The combination of increased blood glucose concentrations (hyperglycemia), very low pH (acidemia), low serum bicarbonate, and positive serum ketones at admission establishes the diagnosis of diabetic ketoacidosis (DKA). The history of type 1 diabetes and recent illness support this diagnosis. Despite only a weakly positive ketone assay, the calculated anion gap [Na − (Cl + HCO$_3$) = 37 mmol/L, reference interval 3–15] indicates the presence of unmeasured anions. His history and physical signs indicated that there was also severe intravascular volume depletion. Therapy was initiated in the ED with 20 units of regular insulin IM, followed by continuous IV insulin at 10 units/hour. Within the first 10 hours he was also given 3 L of normal saline and 60 mEq potassium chloride. His vital signs improved, plasma glucose concentrations decreased to 250 mg/dL (13.9 mmol/L), serum creatinine dropped to 2.0 mg/dL (177 μmol/L), and the nitroprusside test for serum ketones became strongly positive. IV fluids and insulin were titrated accordingly, and his blood glucose and pH returned to normal over the next 16 hours.

Definition of the Disease

There is no consensus for definitive criteria to diagnose DKA. The most widely used criteria are plasma glucose above 200–250 mg/dL (11.1–13.9 mmol/L; cutoff varies depending on recommendation followed), serum bicarbonate ≤15 mEq/L, arterial blood pH ≤7.30, and ketones in the urine or blood.[1] Plasma glucose concentrations rarely exceed 800 mg/dL in DKA, although they may be higher in hyperosmolar hyperglycemic states (HHSs).[2] Although it may seem counterintuitive, increased serum ketone concentrations are not always detected in DKA by routine assays.[3] However, patients almost always have an increased anion gap, which provides indirect evidence that ketoacids are present (see section on pathogenesis for further discussion). Hyperosmolar hyperglycemic states (HHS), in contrast, is more common among type 2 diabetic patients and rarely results in ketonemia or an increased anion gap.[4] The incidence of DKA is greatest in children with type 1 diabetes, followed by adults with type 1 diabetes, and is least common in patients with type 2 diabetes.[1] Although a history of type 1 diabetes raises the suspicion of DKA, it is not required because DKA is present in 15–67% of children at the time of initial diagnosis of type 1 diabetes.[1] DKA is sometimes further classified as mild, moderate, and severe according to arterial blood pH, plasma bicarbonate concentration, and CNS symptoms and signs.[2]

Differential Diagnosis

DKA involves hyperglycemia, ketonemia, and acidemia. Each of these can be caused by other metabolic conditions.[5] Nevertheless, relatively few conditions can be mistaken for DKA when criteria are strictly followed. Patients with chronic ethanol abuse, who have an acute episode of nausea, vomiting, and starvation, may develop alcoholic ketoacidosis. These individuals have ketoacidosis, but plasma glucose concentrations are not increased and may be low (hypoglycemia).[6] Starvation ketosis, due to reduced food intake for several days, manifests with mild acidosis (serum bicarbonate >18 mEq/L),[3] and hyperglycemia is not present.[5] Other causes of metabolic acidosis, including methanol,[3] ethylene glycol, or paraldehyde intoxication, lactic acidosis; and chronic renal failure can also have an increased anion gap, but do not exhibit hyperglycemia. Polyuria and polydipsia with dehydration and ketoacidosis can be found with diabetes insipidus, but hyperglycemia is not present.[5]

Pathogenesis

The most common precipitating events for DKA are infection and omission of, or undertreatment with, insulin.[2] Other causes include sudden pancreatic failure (acute pancreatitis or new-onset type 1 diabetes), myocardial infarction, trauma, stroke, or alcohol abuse. The pathophysiology of DKA is a deficiency of insulin signaling with a concomitant increase in counterregulatory hormones, such as glucagon, cortisol, catecholamines, and growth hormone. These changes induce a shift from carbohydrate to lipid catabolism.[3] Without sufficient insulin, glucose cannot be transported into skeletal muscle and fat, and gluconeogenesis and glycogen breakdown (glycogenolysis) are enhanced in the liver. Together these factors dramatically increase blood glucose concentrations. Without insulin-stimulated uptake of glucose (which is mediated by the Glut[4] glucose transporter) into skeletal muscle and adipose tissue, these tissues become relatively starved for intracellular glucose despite the extracellular hyperglycemia. At the same time, triglyceride catabolism (lipolysis) is increased, enhancing fatty acid oxidation and production of acetyl-CoA. Without intracellular glycolysis, the citric acid cycle intermediate oxaloacetate cannot be regenerated from pyruvate. Without oxaloacetate, acetyl-CoA cannot enter the citric acid cycle and is diverted to ketone body formation. There are three ketone bodies, namely, acetoacetate, β-hydroxybutyrate, and acetone. Attenuation of the citric acid cycle also blocks oxidative phosphorylation, resulting in accumulation of NADH. These factors drive "anaerobic" catabolism with production of intracellular H^+ and lactic acid, resulting in the striking ketoacidosis and lactic acidosis.[2] As mentioned above, we see evidence of this in our patient from his blood pH, bicarbonate concentration, and increased anion gap.

Accumulation of ketones and lactate in the blood may be measured directly or indirectly estimated by calculating the anion gap.[5] Routine qualitative tests for ketones are based on nitroprusside, which produces a purple color with acetoacetate on a test strip or tablet. It is important to realize that this semiquantitative test detects predominantly acetoacetate and does not react with β-hydroxybutyrate. In severe DKA, the increased NADH promotes the conversion of acetoacetate to β-hydroxybutyrate, which becomes the predominant ketone species. Thus, routine ketone testing will not detect the majority of ketones present and may be weak or even negative in severe DKA.[3] If DKA is suspected under these circumstances, β-hydroxybutyrate may be measured directly. As seen in our patient, the ketones measured by a nitroprusside-based dipstick may actually increase as the acidemia is resolved due to conversion back to acetoacetate.

The marked hyperglycemia that can occur in DKA or HHS substantially increases plasma osmolality (ketoacids also contribute). Hyperosmolality results in passive extracellular transport of water and a significant osmotic diuresis, resulting in intravascular volume depletion, polyuria, polydipsia, and nocturia.[1] The osmotic diuresis results in loss of water, sodium, potassium, and other electrolytes. Hyperosmolality and acidosis also contribute to worsening mental status changes, starting with blurred vision, lethargy, and obtundation, and eventually progressing to coma. In addition to direct measurement, plasma osmolality can be estimated using the following equation:

$$2[NA+] + \frac{\text{glucose mg/dL}}{18} + \frac{\text{BUN mg/dL}}{2.8} = \text{calculated mOsm/kg } H_2O;$$

Neurologic symptoms usually develop at values >320 mOsm/kg H_2O. In our patient, the estimated osmolality was 323 mOsm/kg H_2O.

Hyperkalemia and hyperphosphatemia are other frequent findings in DKA.[4] Hyperkalemia is a consequence of translocation of potassium from inside cells mediated by buffering of acids, fluid shifts, and the cessation of insulin-stimulated uptake of potassium into cells.[5] Despite increased concentrations of potassium and phosphate in the blood, it is important to appreciate that diuresis results in total body deficits of both electrolytes. Osmotic extracellular shifts and diuresis may also produce significant total-body hyponatremia, although dehydration with hypernatremia may be found.

Treatment

Treatment of DKA involves ensuring hemodynamic stability, restoring intravascular volume, and correcting hyperglycemia and electrolyte disturbances.[2] Frequent monitoring is necessary because glucose and electrolyte concentrations can change precipitously when insulin and IV fluids are given. Electrolytes, BUN, creatinine, and glucose should be monitored every 2–4 hours until the patient is stable.[1] The first defect to address is hemodynamic instability. If there are signs of significant intravascular volume depletion, replacement is initiated with isotonic fluids (usually normal saline) to expand the intravascular volume. Subsequently, isotonic or hypotonic fluids should be infused to correct the patient's dehydration based on sodium measurement and estimated water deficit [estimated water deficit in liters = 0.6 × weight in kg × ([Na+]/140 − 1)].[5] The total water deficit should be replaced gradually (typically over 48 hours) because rapid changes in extracellular osmolality may induce cerebral edema.[1] After initiation of insulin infusion, blood glucose concentration may drop precipitously and cause hypoglycemia, so it is recommended that 5% dextrose be added to IV fluids when blood glucose concentration is below 250 mg/dL (13.9 mmol/L).[5] Insulin therapy is initiated using continuous infusion of regular insulin. The rate of infusion of insulin is based on the glucose concentration, with a target of 150–200 mg/dL (8.3–11.1 mmol/L).[5] Although hyperkalemia is often present in DKA, total body stores of potassium are depleted. Insulin will rapidly reduce serum potassium concentration, and potassium should be supplemented even if serum concentrations are as high as 5.0 mEq/L.[5] Bicarbonate should be replaced only when arterial blood pH <6.9. The reason for this recommendation is that restoration of the tricarboxylic acid cycle by insulin replacement and glucose uptake will result in a much more rapid increase of bicarbonate than can be delivered by intravenous fluid. In addition, there is little evidence that IV bicarbonate improves clinical outcomes.[5] After resolution of the DKA and resumption of oral feeding, transition to an outpatient insulin regimen that maintains normal glycemic targets is made.

References

1. DUNGER, D. B., SPERLING, M. A., ACERINI, C. L. ET AL.: European Society for Paediatric Endocrinology/Lawson Wilkins Pediatric Endocrine Society consensus statement on diabetic ketoacidosis in children and adolescents. *Pediatrics 113*:e133–40, 2004.

2. KITABCHI, A. E., UMPIERREZ, G. E., MURPHY, M. B. ET AL.: Management of hyperglycemic crises in patients with diabetes. *Diabetes Care 24*:131–53, 2001.

3. WALLACE, T. M. AND MATTHEWS, D. R.: Recent advances in the monitoring and management of diabetic ketoacidosis. *Quart. J. Med. 97*:773–80, 2004.

4. NEWTON, C. A. AND RASKIN, P.: Diabetic ketoacidosis in type 1 and type 2 diabetes mellitus: clinical and biochemical differences. *Arch. Intern. Med. 164*:1925–31, 2004.

5. KITABCHI, A. E., UMPIERREZ, G. E., MURPHY M. B. ET AL.: Hyperglycemic crises in diabetes. *Diabetes Care 27*:S94–102, 2004.

6. WRENN, K. D., SLOVIS, C. M., MINION, G. E., AND RUTKOWSKI, R.: The syndrome of alcoholic ketoacidosis. *Am. J. Med. 91*:119–28, 1991.

Case 28

A Diabetic Woman's "Episode"

Anders H. Berg and David B. Sacks

A 55-year-old woman with a 4-year history of type 2 diabetes mellitus was brought to the hospital emergency department (ED) by ambulance at 1:30 pm after she was found unconscious at home. At the scene her blood glucose concentration (measured on capillary blood with a portable glucose meter) was 17 mg/dL (0.9 mmol/L). She was given 50 mL of 50% dextrose (D50) intravenously in the ambulance before arrival at the ED and immediately awoke. In the ED she stated that she took her regular morning insulin dose at 11:30 am, but missed her usual lunch and ate only a peach. She began to feel weak in the shower, called her brother, and told him she was having another "episode," and then passed out; he immediately called emergency medical services. It was estimated she had been unconscious for 45 minutes. She denied recent fever, chills, nausea, vomiting, cough, chest pain, shortness of breath, or dysuria. She admitted to prior episodes of hypoglycemia, but never with loss of consciousness. Her past medical history was significant for hypertension, chronic renal insufficiency, retinopathy, neuropathy, and depression. Her medications included insulin (regular and long-acting NPH), furosemide, metoprolol, generic lisinopril, aspirin, folate, mirtazapine, and atorvastatin.

Physical examination at the hospital revealed an alert woman in no apparent distress. Her heart rate was 77 bpm and blood pressure was 132/78 mm Hg. She was alert and oriented. Her chest was clear to auscultation, heart sounds were normal, and no masses were detected in the abdomen. She had normal strength and brisk peripheral pulses. Neurologic exam was significant for loss of both position sense and light touch up to the midcalf bilaterally.

Laboratory data from the patient's blood while in the ED were as follows:

Analyte	Value, Conventional Units	Reference Interval, Conventional Units	Value, SI Units	Reference Interval, SI Units
Sodium	140 mmol/L	136–142	Same	
Potassium	3.7 mmol/L	3.5–5.0	Same	
Chloride	109 mmol/L	98–108	Same	
CO$_2$, total	21 mmol/L	23–32	Same	
Urea nitrogen	21 mg/dL	9–25	7.5 mmol/L	3.2–8.9
Creatinine	1.4 mg/dL	0.7–1.3	124 µmol/L	62–115

Tietz's Applied Laboratory Medicine, Second Edition. Edited by Mitchell G. Scott, Ann M. Gronowski, and Charles S. Eby

Analyte	Value, Conventional Units	Reference Interval, Conventional Units	Value, SI Units	Reference Interval, SI Units
Glucose	49 mg/dL	54–99	2.7 mmol/L	3.0–5.5
Anion gap	10 mmol/L	3–15	Same	
Calcium	8.8 mg/dL	8.8–10.5	2.2 mmol/L	2.15–2.5
Hemoglobin	12.0 g/dL	13.5–18.0	120 g/L	135–180
Hematocrit	35.4%	40–54	0.354 volume Fraction	0.40–0.54
WBC	8.6×10^6/mL	4–10	Same	
Platelets	234×10^6/mL	150–450	Same	

The patient was diagnosed with hypoglycemia secondary to her missed meal, was fed, and was observed for the rest of the afternoon. She was subsequently discharged home in satisfactory condition with an appointment to follow up with her primary care physician.

At the follow-up visit with her physician she admitted that she had not been monitoring her glucose very often. She also stated that she had been varying the time of her morning insulin injections between 9 and 12 am, and she often did not eat until she "feels an episode coming on." Although she performed self-monitoring of blood glucose (SMBG), she had never used an insulin sliding scale. In addition, she admitted to more episodes of hypoglycemia lately on her SMBG. Her physician had previously recommended the oral hypoglycemic agent thiazolidinedione, but she deferred taking it. A blood sample from the visit revealed a hemoglobin (Hb) A_{1c} of 10.0% (reference range 4–6%) and a casual (nonfasting) blood glucose concentration of 287 mg/dL (15.9 mmol/L). Her glucose meter internal history showed values ranging from 59 mg/dL (3.3 mmol/L) to concentrations above the upper limit of the measurement range of the glucose meter. Averaging daily glucose meter values revealed a mean glucose concentration of 221 mg/dL (12.3 mmol/L). Her physician explained to her that her glycemic control had been extremely poor, and that her risks of both dangerous hypoglycemic and hyperglycemic episodes were significant. He counseled her regarding the importance of regular eating, and injecting her insulin at the same time every day. He adjusted her insulin regimen from NPH insulin to long-acting insulin glargine, and urged her to use a sliding scale to determine her insulin doses. He also scheduled a visit in 3 months and told her to call if she experienced any problems before then.

Definition of the Disease

Hypoglycemia is a blood glucose concentration below the fasting value. However, it is difficult to define a specific limit. The physiologic response to low blood glucose concentrations varies among individuals. Some people do not develop symptoms until very low glucose concentrations are reached. For this reason a clinical diagnosis of hypoglycemia is based on both laboratory values and clinical signs and symptoms. Furthermore, the symptoms of hypoglycemia are common to many disorders, and glucose concentrations below the reference range are not uncommon.[1] A definitive diagnosis of hypoglycemia should be based on Whipple's triad: (1) laboratory evidence of very low blood glucose concentrations (<70 mg/dL or 3.9 mmol/L), (2) symptoms of hypoglycemia, and (3) clinical improvement upon administration of glucose.[2] In most patients, symptoms of hypoglycemia usually begin at glucose concentrations <55 mg/dL (3.0 mmol/L) with sympathoadrenal symptoms such as sweating, tremulousness, nausea, and tachycardia.[3] When glucose is <45 mg/dL (2.5 mmol/L), neuroglycopenic symptoms are common, progressing through fatigue/drowsiness, dizziness, headache, blurry vision, difficulty in speaking, and inability to concentrate, to confusion, loss of consciousness, seizures, and death. Sympathoadrenal symptoms are not always present or may not be noticed (hypoglycemia unawareness).[3]

If a patient is suspected of suffering from recurring hypoglycemia but Whipple's triad has not been fulfilled, a 72-hour supervised fast can be performed.[1] Samples are drawn for analysis of plasma glucose, insulin, C-peptide, and proinsulin every 6 hours. The fast is stopped if the plasma glucose falls below 45 mg/dL (2.5 mmol/L) and the patient develops neuroglycopenic signs or symptoms. A low plasma glucose value alone is inadequate to establish the diagnosis. The absence of signs or symptoms of hypoglycemia during the fast excludes the diagnosis of a hypoglycemic disorder.

Differential Diagnosis

Before evaluating a patient for hypoglycemia, artifactual causes of low glucose values should be excluded. For example, if the blood was collected in a tube without an inhibitor of glycolysis (e.g., sodium fluoride) and more than 1 hour elapsed before glucose was measured, values may be decreased because of red cell glycolysis. Glucose decreases by approximately 5–7% per hour in whole blood at room temperature.[4] Very high hematocrit or increased numbers of WBCs in the specimen increase the rate of glycolysis and decrease glucose concentrations at an even faster rate. Reflectance glucose meters are unreliable at glucose concentrations <60 mg/dL (<3.3 mmol/L), so a diagnosis of hypoglycemia should not be based exclusively on a glucose meter measurement.[4]

The etiologies of hypoglycemia are numerous, with >100 reported causes.[1] A convenient way to classify the disorder is by the age of onset and general health of the individual. Common causes in neonates include prematurity, maternal diabetes mellitus, sepsis, or respiratory distress syndrome. In infants and children unexplained hypoglycemia evokes consideration of Reye's syndrome, congenital hyperinsulinism (also called "persistent hyperinsulinemic hypoglycemia of infancy," caused by mutations in an ATP-dependent potassium channel resulting in alterations of the β-cell glucose-sensor and unrestrained insulin release even at very low glucose levels), and inborn errors of metabolism. The last category includes disorders of glycogenolysis, gluconeogenic defects, hereditary fructose intolerance, organic acidemias, or defects in amino acid and fatty acid metabolism. Common causes of hypoglycemia in a healthy-appearing adult without known coexisting disease include insulinoma, factitious hypoglycemia, ketotic (idiopathic) hypoglycemia, anorexia/starvation, and drugs (e.g., ethanol, salicylates, sulfonylureas, propranolol, haloperidol). A condition that was commonly diagnosed in the past is reactive (postprandial) hypoglycemia, in which patients developed sympathoadrenal symptoms of hypoglycemia 1–3 hours after eating a meal. Although low glucose concentrations could be found in some of these individuals, this syndrome has been largely debunked. In most cases the symptoms did not correlate with low blood glucose concentrations, and underlying psychoneuroses could explain the symptoms for many of the patients. As a result, testing for reactive hypoglycemia is discouraged when patients exhibit only sympathoadrenal symptoms. Nevertheless, a full diagnostic workup for clinically significant hypoglycemia should be conducted for individuals who experience reproducible signs and symptoms of neuroglycopenia. Postprandial hypoglycemia is infrequent, and the demonstration of hypoglycemia (by measuring blood glucose concentrations) during spontaneously occurring symptomatic episodes is necessary to establish the diagnosis. A diagnosis of hypoglycemia should not be made unless a patient meets the criteria of low blood glucose concentration with typical symptoms alleviated by administration of glucose. The OGTT should not be used in the diagnosis of reactive hypoglycemia. For healthy individuals prescribed medication, dispensing errors where patients are accidentally given hypoglycemic agents are a possibility; β-adrenergic blocking agents or sulfhydryl drugs can also sometimes produce hypoglycemia as an unwanted side effect. In individuals who appear ill, ingestion of medications or toxins should be considered. Causes in hospitalized patients with new-onset hypoglycemia include errors with their inpatient nutrition and insulin therapy regimen. Illnesses that predispose to or cause hypoglycemia include panhypopituitarism, liver failure, adrenal failure (Addison's disease), renal failure, congestive heart failure, and sepsis.

Insulinoma can usually be detected using a 72-hour fast (which needs to be conducted in the hospital) with detection of inappropriately increased insulin and C-peptide concentrations. Accidental insulin overdose or missed meals are the most common causes of hypoglycemia in patients with diabetes who require insulin. Factitious hypoglycemia due to inappropriate administration of insulin can be determined by detecting increased serum insulin concentrations without a concomitant increase in C-peptide concentrations.

Pathogenesis

Hypoglycemia can be caused by interference with any stage in the cycle of glucose flux and metabolism. Decreased food intake is an intuitively obvious but uncommon cause in otherwise healthy patients with intact counterregulatory mechanisms. Inappropriately increased insulin (insulinoma, insulin or sulfonylurea overdose) results in rapid uptake of absorbed sugars, as well as suppressed hepatic glucose production and decreased catabolism of fats and amino acids. Interference with liver glucose production (gluconeogenesis) because of intrinsic defects (liver failure, glycogen storage defects, gluconeogenic defects) or insufficient gluconeogenesis (adrenal insufficiency, hypopituitarism) results in fasting hypoglycemia, particularly during periods of stress. Inborn errors of metabolism can interfere with glucose homeostasis by interfering directly with gluconeogenesis (fructose-1,6-diphosphatase deficiency and hereditary fructose intolerance), blocking the supply of gluconeogenic precursors (pyruvate carboxylase deficiency), blocking glycogenolysis (glucose-6-phosphatase deficiency), or dramatically increasing glycolysis because of defects in catabolism of other calorie sources (decreased fatty acid oxidation caused by carnitine or medium-chain acyl-CoA dehydrogenase deficiency).

In patients with diabetes mellitus, hypoglycemia is usually due to excess insulin with compromised glucose counterregulation. All three defenses against falling plasma glucose are impaired; specifically, insulin concentration does not decrease, glucagon does not increase, and the increase in epinephrine is attenuated. The reduced sympathoadrenal response also causes hypoglycemia unawareness, which is an absence of the symptoms that allow an individual to recognize hypoglycemia. This condition, which occurs in type 1 and advanced type 2 diabetes,[3] has a profound effect on the lives of people with diabetes. As one would predict, intensive therapy to decrease diabetic complications and its lower HbA_{1c} targets significantly increases the risk of severe hypoglycemic episodes.

Treatment

Treatment of an acute hypoglycemic episode typically involves little more than oral or intravenous glucose. Restoration of blood glucose usually produces rapid recovery. Immediate treatment is often achieved with an intravenous bolus of 50% dextrose in water, followed by saline drip with 5–20% dextrose, if needed.

In alcoholic patients, in addition to glucose, thiamine should be administered to prevent precipitating Wernicke–Korsakoff syndrome. Management of recurrent hypoglycemic episodes relies primarily on identifying and treating the underlying cause. Insulinomas can be excised, adrenal insufficiency is treated with corticosteroids, and patients with some inborn errors of metabolism can be treated with special dietary supplements. In patients with diabetes mellitus, treatment consists of reevaluation and adjustment of therapy. If the patient is not performing SMBG frequently, the physician should initiate or increase their daily home monitoring and schedule appointments for follow-up.

References

1. SERVICE, F. J.: Hypoglycemic disorders. *N. Engl. J. Med. 332*:1144–52, 1995.
2. American Diabetes Association: Defining and reporting hypoglycemia in diabetes: A report from the American Diabetes Association Workgroup on Hypoglycemia. *Diabetes Care 28*:1245–9, 2005.
3. CRYER, P. E.: Diverse causes of hypoglycemia-associated autonomic failure in diabetes. *N. Engl. J. Med. 350*:2272–9, 2004.
4. SACKS, D. B.: Carbohydrates. In *Tietz Textbook of Clinical Chemistry and Molecular Diagnostics*, 4th ed., C. A. BURTIS, E. R. ASHWOOD, AND D. E. BRUNS, eds., Elsevier Saunders, St. Louis, 2006, pp. 837–902.

Part Eight

Calcium and Parathyroid Hormone (PTH)

Cases of renal osteodystrophy, osteoporosis, and hyperparathyroidism are reported and discussed in Cases 29 (edited by AMG), 30 (edited by CSE), and 31 (edited by MGS), respectively.

Tietz's Applied Laboratory Medicine, Second Edition. Edited by Mitchell G. Scott, Ann M. Gronowski, and Charles S. Eby

Case 29

Bad to the Bone

Chelsea A. Sheppard and Corinne R. Fantz

A 26-year-old woman with a history of end-stage renal disease (ESRD) and congestive heart failure (CHF) secondary to Goodpasture's syndrome that was diagnosed 6 years ago, presented to her physician with a 6 week history of worsening skin problems. The patient had been receiving dialysis 3 times per week for 3 years. Additionally, she had been on vitamin D therapy for the past 6 months for suspected renal osteodystrophy. For the past 6 weeks the patient described induration and darkening of the skin on her inner thighs and abdomen, which had progressed. She now had necrotic tissue and decomposition of the eschar of both inner thighs and her abdomen, which were intensely painful. The patient denied any recent fever.

On physical examination, the patient's vital signs were stable and she was in no acute distress. On cardiac examination, she was tachycardic with a laterally displaced point of maximum impulse (PMI) and a 3/6 holosystolic murmur in the apex. Her lungs were clear to auscultation. Her abdomen was almost entirely indurated with small ulcerations on the left lateral aspect of the abdominal wall, and was rigid and tender. Bowel sounds, however, were present. Additionally, the patient had an enlarging 10 × 8-cm necrotic plaque with surrounding stellate purpuric morphology on the inner thighs bilaterally. Other features of the examination disclosed no abnormalities.

Laboratory tests, including a complete blood count and iron studies, demonstrated leukocytosis with an absolute neutrophilia and anemia of chronic disease. Wound cultures from the leg and abdomen grew *Pseudomonas aerginosa* and methicillin-resistant *Staphylococcus aureus* (MRSA).

Laboratory results are shown below:

Analyte	Value, Conventional Units	Reference Interval, Conventional Units	Value, SI Units	Reference Interval, SI Units
Sodium	131 mEq/L	135–145	131 mmol/L	135–145
Potassium	3.2 mEq/L	3.5–5.0	3.2 mmol/L	3.5–5.0
Chloride	96 mEq/L	100–110	96 mmol/L	100–110
CO_2, total	23 mEq/L	20–32	23 mmol/L	20–32
Calcium	8.8 mg/dL	8.5–10.5	2.2 mmol/L	2.13–2.63
Urea nitrogen	49 mg/dL	7.0–25.0	17 mmol/L	2.5–14.3
Creatinine	6.3 mg/dL	0.6–1.4	557 μmol/L	53–124

Tietz's Applied Laboratory Medicine, Second Edition. Edited by Mitchell G. Scott, Ann M. Gronowski, and Charles S. Eby

Analyte	Value, Conventional Units	Reference Interval, Conventional Units	Value, SI Units	Reference Interval, SI Units
Glucose, random	124 mg/dL	65–100	6.9 mmol/L	3.6–5.6
Protein, total	6.9 g/dL	6.4–8.4	69 g/L	64–84
Albumin	1.2 g/dL	3.5–4.8	12 g/L	35–48
AST	27 U/L	7.0–40.0	27 U/L	7.0–40.0
ALT	21 U/L	17–63	21 U/L	17–63
ALP	317 U/L	30–110	317 U/L	30–110
PTH	127 pg/mL	14–66	127 ng/L	14–66
Iron	31 μg/dL	53–167	5.6 μmol/L	9.5–29.8
TIBC	167 μg/dL	161–497	29.4 μmol/L	28.8–89
% Saturation	19		0.19	
Ferritin	667 ng/mL	7–283	1499 pmol/L	15.7–636

At this time, due to her elevated serum parathyroid hormone (PTH) concentration, a therapeutic parathyroidectomy was contemplated. However, because of the classic skin changes, which were consistent with calciphylaxsis, a known complication of excess vitamin D therapy, the clinician suspected that the parathyroid concentration was falsely elevated and consulted the laboratory about ordering biologically active PTH. Results were as follows on repeat analysis:

Analyte	Value, Conventional Units	Reference Interval, Conventional Units	Value, SI Units	Reference Interval, SI Units
Total ("intact") PTH	127 pg/mL	14–66 pg/mL	127 ng/L	14–66 ng/L
CAP (1-84) PTH[a]	40.8 pg/mL	5.0–39.0 pg/mL	40.8 ng/L	5.0–39.0 ng/L
CIP (7-84) PTH[b]	86.2 pg/mL	2.5–29 pg/mL	86.2 ng/L	2.5–29 ng/L
CAP/CIP	0.5	1.1–6.9	—	—

[a]CAP = cyclase-activating PTH.
[b]CIP = cyclase-inhibiting PTH.

A diagnosis of low-turnover osteodystrophy and excessive vitamin D replacement was supported by the laboratory results; however, a bone biopsy to confirm the suspected diagnosis was not performed. The patient was evaluated for wound treatment with hyperbaric oxygen therapy, but was not a candidate because of the severity of her CHF. The areas of necrosis were extensively debrided. The patient was treated with broad-spectrum antibiotics and sent home with a wound vacuum. Additionally, treatment of adynamic osteodystrophy including a reduction in vitamin D therapy was initiated. At her 6-month follow-up, her calciphylaxis had resolved.

Definition of the Disease

Patients with ESRD, especially those on dialysis, can develop osteodystrophy with vastly differing histopathologic changes despite an initially common pathogenic pathway.[1] Glomerular damage leads to retention of phosphate, while tubular injury reduces the production of $1,25(OH)_2D_3$. Hyperphosphatemia further suppresses the production of $1,25(OH)_2D_3$ and inhibits reabsorption in the kidney as well as absorption of calcium in the gut. Osteodystrophy is a result of the disruption and imbalance of complex mechanisms that regulate the secretion and absorbance of calcium, phosphorus, PTH, and vitamin D. Chronic renal insufficiency (CRI) commonly causes excess secretion of PTH due to long-term low circulating concentrations of ionized calcium. This results in secondary hypertension HPT. The severity of secondary hyperparathyroidism (HPT), with or without mineralization defect, may result in bone lesions, characterized as one of three types: high or normal turnover, low turnover, or adynamic bone disease. These different types are due to variable deposition of collagen and rate of bone formation. The therapeutic approach (i.e., the use of vitamin D, calcium vs. non-calcium-containing phosphate binders, and choice of calcium dialysate concentration) will vary depending on the type of bone disease.

High-turnover disease occurs as a result of decreased urine phosphate excretion secondary to renal insufficiency. Decreased excretion without decreased absorption ultimately results in hyperphosphatemia. This begins a cascade of events culminating in increased synthesis and release of PTH. Increased serum phosphate inhibits the activity of 1-α-hydroxylase, resulting in a decrease in $1,25(OH)_2D_3$. $1,25(OH)_2D_3$ stimulates intestinal absorption of biologically active ionized calcium. Decreased serum calcium ultimately stimulates the release and synthesis of PTH. Ionized calcium is also deposited in soft tissues, contributing to the loss of serum calcium. Additionally, the negative feed back on PTH from $1,25(OH)_2D_3$ is compromised not only by the decreased concentrations of $1,25(OH)_2D_3$ but also by decreased binding of $1,25(OH)_2D_3$ to specific receptors on parathyroid cells during renal failure. Thus, the administration of $1,25(OH)_2D_3$ or the non-calcemic analogue of vitamin D is therapeutic in this setting.[2]

Low-turnover osteodystrophy is characterized as either osteomalacia or adynamic or aplastic bone disease. The pathogenesis of osteomalacia is associated with aluminum toxicity. Aluminum contamination of the dialysate water used in dialysis was the historical source. However, direct ingestion of aluminum, utilized for its phosphate binding properties, is the more commonly implicated source. Regardless, aluminum adversely affects mineralization, decreases osteoblastic bone formation, and increases osteoclastic bone resorption. Patients without excessive aluminum deposition and extremely low PTH concentrations may have aplastic bone disease, which is associated with high peritoneal dialysate calcium concentrations and the use of oral calcium carbonate.

Pathogenesis

PTH is an 84-amino-acid, linear polypeptide, secreted by the parathyroid glands, which acts through a G-protein-coupled receptor (PTHR) located on renal tubular cells and osteoblasts.[3] This hormone regulates bone and mineral ion homeostasis but also is centrally responsible for the osteodystrophy of primary and secondary hyperparathyroidism including chronic renal insufficiency. Only the most N-terminal portion, not the entire hormone, is required for PTH receptor activation and is therefore may be referred to as "1-84 PTH" or the "biologically active PTH." A series of N-truncated, carboxy-terminal fragments, or non-(1-84)-PTH, are generated through metabolism of whole PTH in the liver.[4] However, they are also generated and secreted by the parathyroid glands. These fragments can reenter the circulation and are excreted mainly by the kidneys.[5] Normally, the ratio of whole PTH to that of the fragments is approximately 3–4 : 1; however, several situations can cause this ratio to increase substantially, such as decreased blood calcium and ESRD.[6,7]

Unlike 1-84 PTH, non-(1-84)-PTH is not suppressible with calcium. Additionally, non-(1-84)-PTH has been shown to inhibit bone turnover, formation, resorption, and osteoclast formation. There is some evidence to suggest that non-(1-84)-PTH binds to a different receptor than whole PTH altogether. It has been hypothesized that these fragments have an inhibitory effect on bone remodeling and that they antagonize the calcemic effects of 1-84-PTH. In fact, experiments in animal models and in vitro have confirmed that when these fragments are coinfused with PTH, they prevent the expected increase in bone formation and serum calcium concentrations.

In dialysis patients, serum calcium is lowered and the ratio of 1-84 PTH to non-(1-84)-PTH increases. The converse is also true when the serum calcium is increased. Furthermore, non-(1-84)-PTH fragments, which are increased in primary and secondary hyperparathyroidism, have been found in vitro to inhibit osteoclast formation and to bind a novel class of PTH receptor, distinct from PTHR.[8,9] Additionally, Langub and coworkers have shown that these fragments antagonize the effect of co-infused PTH (i.e., increasing bone formation and serum calcium), suggesting that even when vitamin D is excessively administered, the serum calcium may be normal because of the actions of 7-84 PTH, a specific fragment frequently measured by older assays leading to overestimation of the concentration of 1-84 PTH in circulation.[10] Interestingly, this physiologic response may itself become pathologic when the predominant 7-84 PTH action causes adynamic bone disease, with the potential complication of extensive vascular calcification, or calciphylaxis.

Differential Diagnosis

At this time, bone biopsy for histologic diagnosis of osteodystrophy remains the gold standard; however, development of noninvasive laboratory tests to distinguish between these entities is highly desirable. Measurement of serum concentrations of PTH should theoretically distinguish high bone turnover from adynamic bone disease. In high-turnover bone disease, one expects serum PTH concentration to be elevated, while an extremely low serum concentration of PTH is expected in adynamic bone disease. Unfortunately, immunoassays designed to specifically measure PTH have been shown to cross-react with a number of inactive PTH fragments. Recently, second-generation PTH assays have claimed to measure the 1-84 PTH, with no reported cross-reactivity from PTH fragments. This case report reviews the complexity of PTH testing in the setting of ESRD, the current PTH assays available, and the ability of the second-generation PTH assays to distinguish between different etiologies of renal osteodystrophy.

The first assays to measure PTH were radioimmunoassays (RIAs), which used single antibodies directed against the C-terminal portion of the hormone and thus could not distinguish between whole PTH and the variable amount of reactive fragments. This was especially confounding in ESRD when the amount of circulating fragments could be very high. Predictably, bone histology correlated poorly to the calculated PTH.[11] With the advent of two-site immunoradiometric assays (IRMAs), which used both a solid-phase capture antibody to the C-terminus and a labeled detection antibody to the N terminus, it was believed that only the "intact PTH" molecule (1-84 PTH and not the fragments) would be measured.[12] These are referred to as *first-generation IRMAs*. However, again, with relation to bone histology, the measured PTH seemed to overestimate the severity of disease.[13] Furthermore, when these measurements were used to direct therapy, there was a tendency to overcorrect, leading to iatrogenic adynamic bone disease.[14] This and the trend to treat patients with higher doses of vitamin D may explain the increase in prevalence of adynamic bone disease in recent years.

Second-generation PTH IRMAs have recently emerged. Currently, there are two assays commercially available, namely, the Nichols Advantage Bio-Intact PTH (San Clemente, CA) and the Scantibodies, CAP assay (Santee, CA). These assays have been shown to have no cross-reactivity with any of the known inactive PTH fragments. Thus, it was hypothesized that an accurate approximation of circulating antagonist fragments (CIPs) could be made by subtracting the value of the biologically active PTH, which is measured by second-generation IRMA, from the value of the first-generation IRMA, "intact PTH" assays (the intact assays measure both the whole molecule and the N terminal truncated, inactive PTH fragments). There is some evidence that the ratio of the active PTH (CAP) to inactive PTH fragments (CIP) is lower in adynamic bone disease than in high- or normal-bone-turnover osteodystrophy.[1] Monier-Faugere et al.[1] have claimed success in identifying patients with high bone turnover versus adynamic bone disease using the ratio of active to inactive PTH fragments. However, in their study the reference ranges for normal controls and patients with adynamic bone disease overlap too much to distinguish between them. Additionally, others have not found this value to correlate well with bone histology or other markers of bone metabolism.[15–17] Even supporters of using the ratio state that alone it is not diagnostic of adynamic bone disease.[1] It has been suggested, however, that the accumulation of these fragments in plasma may have an inhibitory effect on bone remodeling and could account for the adynamic bone disease seen with aggressive treatment of high-turnover bone disease.[10]

The utility of second-generation PTH IRMAs and the calculation of a ratio remain controversial in the evaluation of renal osteodystrophy because of the lack of consensus with bone histology. However, as more is understood about the role of PTH and its fragments, the opportunity for noninvasive laboratory diagnosis may become reality. Until that time, it is important to know which assay your laboratory is using and to understand its performance characteristics in the clinical setting in which it is being used.

Treatment

The treatment of hyperparathyroidism is etiology-dependent. A parathyroidectomy can be curative in a patient with a solitary parathyroid adenoma causing primary hyperparathyroidism, while vitamin D therapy is reserved for secondary hyperparathyroidism leading to high turnover bone disease. Of note, a more recent study demonstrated that lowering parathyroid activity therapeutically in patients with ESRD on hemodialysis favors the development of adynamic bone disease and may affect the development and progression of arterial calacification.[18] Adynamic bone disease, on the other hand, is treated by increasing bone turnover, which is accomplished by increasing serum PTH. Thus, lowering the dose of or eliminating altogether the use of vitamin D and calcium-based phosphate binders is more appropriate. Also being investigated is the use of calcilytics and calcimimetics and lowering of dialysate calcium. For more detailed treatment guidelines, the reader should refer to the National Kidney Foundation kidney disease outcome quality initiative (K/DOQI) clinical practice guidelines for bone metabolism and disease in chronic kidney disease.[19]

References

1. MONIER-FAUGERE, M. C., GENG, Z., MAWAD, H. ET AL.: Improved assessment of bone turnover by the PTH-(1-84)/large C-PTH fragments ratio in ESRD. *Kidney Int.* 60:1460–8, 2001.

2. BUSHINSKY, D. A.: Bone disease in moderate renal failure: Cause, nature, and prevention. *Ann. Med. Rev.* 1948:167–76, 1997.

3. BRINGHURST, F. R.: Circulating forms of parathyroid hormone: Peeling back the onion. *Clin. Chem.* 49:1973–5, 2003.

4. SEGRE, V. E., PERKINS, A. S., WITTERS, L. A., AND POTTS, J. JR.: Metabolism of parathyroid hormone by isolated rat Kupffer cells and hepatocytes. *J. Clin. Invest.* 67:449–57, 1981.

5. HILPERT, J., NYKJAER, A., JACOBSEN, C. ET AL.: Megalin antagonizes activation of parathyroid hormone receptor. *J. Biol. Chem.* 274:5620–5, 1999.

6. MAYER, G. P., KEATON, J. A., HURST, J. G., AND HEBENER, J. F.: Effects of plasma calcium concentration on the relative proportion of hormone and carboxyl fragments in parathyroid venous blood. *Endocrinology* 104:1778–84, 1979.

7. FREITAG, J., MARTIN, K. J., HRUSKA, K. A., ANDERSON, C. ET AL.: Impaired parathyroid hormone metabolism in patients with chronic renal failure. *N. Engl. J. Med.* 298:29–32, 1978.

8. DIVETI, P., INOMATA, N., CHAPIN, K., SINGH, R., JUPPNER, H., AND BRINGHURST, F. R.: Receptors for the carboxy-terminal region of PTH (1-84) are highly expressed in osteocytic cells. *Endocrinology* 142:916–25, 2001.

9. DIVETI, P., JOHN, M. R., JUPPNER, H., AND BRING-HURST, F. R.: Human PTH-(7-84) inhibits bone resorption in vitro via actions independent of the type 1 PTH/PTHrP receptor. *Endocrinology* 143:171–6, 2002.

10. LANGUB, M. C., MONIER-FUGERE, M. C., WANG, G., WILLIAMS, J. P., KOSZEWSKI, N. J., AND MALLUCHE, H. H.: Administration of PTH-(7-84) antagonizes the effects of PTH-(1-84) on bone in rats with moderate renal failure. *Endocrinology* 144:1135–8, 2003.

11. ANDRESS, D. L., ENDRES, D. B., MALONEY, N. A., KOPP, J. B., COBURN, J. W., AND SHERRARD, D. J.: Comparison of parathyroid hormone assays with bone histomorphometry in renal osteodystrophy. *J. Clin. Endocrinol. Metab.* 63:1163–9, 1986.

12. NUSSBAUM, S. R., ZAHRADNIK, R. J., LAVIGNE, J. R. ET AL.: Highly sensitive two-site immunoradiometric assay of parathyrin, and its clinical utility in evaluating patients with hypercalcemia. *Clin. Chem.* 33:1364–7, 1987.

13. QUARLES, L. D., LOBAUGH, B., AND MURPHY, G.: Intact parathyroid hormone overestimates the presence and severity of parathyroid-mediated osseous abnormalities in uremia. *J. Clin. Endocrinol. Metab.* 75: 145–50, 1992.

14. ELDER, G.: Pathophysiology and recent advances in the management of renal osteodystrophy. *J. Bone Miner. Res.* 1:2094–105, 2002.

15. REICHEL, H., ESSER, A., ROTH, H., AND SCHMIDT-GAYK, H.: Influence of PTH assay methodology on the differential diagnosis of renal bone disease. *Nephrol. Dial. Transplant.* 18:759–68, 2003.

16. NAKINISHI, S., KAZAMA, J. J., SHIGEMATSU, T. ET AL.: Comparison of intact PTH assay and whole PTH assay in long-term dialysis patients. *Am. J. Kidney Dis.* 38:S172–4, 2001.

17. GODBER, I. M., PARKER, C. R., LAWSON, N. ET AL.: Comparison of intact and "whole molecule" parathyroid hormone assays in patients with histologically confirmed post-renal transplant osteodystrophy. *Ann. Clin. Biochem.* 39:314–17, 2002.

18. LONDON, G. M., MARTY, C., MARCHIAS, S. J., GUERIN, A. P., METIVIER, F., AND DE VERNEJOUL, M.: Arterial calcifications and bone histomorphometry in end-stage renal disease. *J. Am. Soc. Nephrol.* 15:1943–51, 2004.

19. National Kidney Foundation: K/DOQI clinical practice guidelines for chronic kidney disease: Evaluation, classification, and stratification. Kidney disease outcome quality initiative. *Am. J. Kidney Dis.* 39:S1–246, 2002.

Case 30

A Middle-Aged Woman with Colle's Fracture

Catherine A. Hammett-Stabler, Ph.D.

A 59-year-old Caucasian female was referred to an endocrinologist following treatment for a fracture to her left wrist. She reports that the fracture occurred approximately 2 months earlier when she tripped on a rough sidewalk and fell while walking her dog. She is otherwise in good health.

On physical examination, the patient is a 5-ft-tall, 94-lb middle-aged woman who describes herself as physically fit and in good health. She reports running 3–4 miles 3 times per week and participating in additional physical exercise that includes weight and resistance training. Her past medical history includes two full-term, uneventful pregnancies, menopause at age 41, but no history of thyroid disease, diabetes, or Cushing syndrome. A daily multivitamin supplement is her only current medication. She has never received hormone replacement therapy. She has no documented family history of osteoporosis, although she recalls her grandmother losing height as she aged and developing a dowager's hump, and notes that her 80-year-old mother appears to be losing height as well. The following laboratory results were obtained:

Analyte	Value, Conventional Units	Reference Interval, Conventional Units	Value, SI Units	Reference Interval, SI Units
Hemoglobin	13.9 g/dL	12–16	139 g/L	120–160
Hematocrit	40%	36–46	0.40 volume	0.36–0.46
Glucose	110 mg/dL	65–110	6.11 mmol/L	3.61–11.05
Creatinine	0.8 mg/dL	0.4–1.1	70.7 μmol/L	61.9–97.2
Urea nitrogen	14 mg/dL	7–21	5.0 mmol/L	2.5–7.5
Sodium	141 mmol/L	135–145	Same	
Potassium	4.0 mmol/L	3.5–5.0	Same	
Bilirubin, total	0.9 mg/dL	0–1.2	15.39 μmol/L	0–20.5
Calcium	9.1 mg/dL	8.5–10.2	2.28 mmol/L	2.12–2.55
Alkaline phosphatase	287 U/L	30–120	4.88 μkat/L	0.51–2.04
TSH	2.9 IU/mL	0.1–4.6	Same	

Tietz's Applied Laboratory Medicine, Second Edition. Edited by Mitchell G. Scott, Ann M. Gronowski, and Charles S. Eby
Copyright © 2007 John Wiley & Sons, Inc.

Analyte	Value, Conventional Units	Reference Interval, Conventional Units	Value, SI Units	Reference Interval, SI Units
PTH	62 pg/mL	12–72	62 ng/L	12–72
25-Hydroxyvitamin D	39.6 ng/mL	25–80	99 nmol/L	62.5–200
Urine free cortisol	30 μg/24 h	3.5–45	82.8 nmol/24 h	9.66–124.2
Urine NTx	178 mmol BCE/mmol creatinine	19–63	Same	

At this time a dual-energy x-ray absorptimetry (DEXA) scan was performed to determine bone density:

Anatomic site	BMD (g/cm^2)	Z-Score	T-Score
Spine, L2–4	0.877	−2.1	−2.54
Femoral neck, L	0.956	−0.4	−0.79

On the basis of the bone density report and the clinical laboratory data, a diagnosis of primary osteoporosis was made. The patient was counseled to continue her current exercise program. Calcium citrate with vitamin D and a bisphosphanate, alendronate, was initiated. The patient was scheduled to return to the clinic in 3 months for a follow-up urine NTx.

Definition of the Disease

Today, we recognize that osteoporosis occurs across all age groups and affects both genders. Osteoporosis is recognized as a disorder of bone remodeling that leads to deformations in the bone micro/macroarchitecture, and a decrease in, or loss of, bone mass and density. With these events bone loses strength, becomes fragile, and as a consequence, is prone to fracture.

Bone turnover or remodeling is a finely orchestrated process involving interactions between osteoblasts, osteoclasts, and osteocytes. By some estimates, the skeleton is completely remodeled every 10 years. For a healthy individual, more bone is formed during the first three decades of life than is lost, with peak bone mass and density occurring between ages 30 and 36. After this, more bone is lost on an annual basis than formed, although the rate of loss is hardly noticeable for most (<1% each year in both genders). When a woman enters menopause, the rate of loss accelerates and as much as 2% is lost each year for about 5 years or so.

Accelerated bone turnover is problematic because the bone formed is often of poor quality. Cortical bone becomes more porous. Trabeculae become thin, and gaps are often found between neighboring trabeculae where connections should be. As a result, bones become weak and less able to endure "normal" stresses. For many women, some, as yet undetermined, process causes the rate of turnover to slow down after about 5 years and bone continues to be lost but at a slower rate. For others, as in the case of our patient, bone turnover continues at an accelerated rate and leads to osteoporosis.

Generally, estrogen deficiency is thought to be the dominant factor leading to osteoporosis regardless of gender. It is clear, however, that other hormones and local factors contribute to bone health and disease, including androgens, calcitonin, parathyroid hormone, thyroxin, vitamin D, vitamin K, ionized calcium, insulinlike growth factors (IGFs), transforming growth factors (TGFs), platelet-derived growth factors (PDGFs), and interleukins (ILs).

Type 1 osteoporosis is characterized by an accelerated rate of bone resorption—in other words, high bone turnover—in response to declining estrogen concentrations. Calcium concentrations increase, leading to suppression of parathyroid hormone (PTH) secretion. This form of the disease occurs at a greater frequency in women and typically has the greatest impact on trabecular bone. As mentioned previously, all women undergo an accelerated loss of bone mass with menopause. In type 1, the rate of loss does not diminish after a few years but continues at an accelerated rate for another 10–20 years if left untreated.

In type 2 osteoporosis bone loss occurs slowly, beginning as early as age 40, continues over several decades, and may not be recognized before the individual has reached age 70. The disturbance in bone remodeling appears to be more osteoblast-related; osteoclasts create a resorption cavity of normal or even less-than-normal depth, but impaired osteoblast activity leads to less matrix formation. As a result, both trabecular and cortical bone are affected.

Although some suggest that the type of osteoporosis isn't important since the treatment is the same, the facts remain that there are differences between types 1 and 2 in the onset, severity, and which type of bone is most involved. These make a difference in terms of the fractures encountered. In type 1, fractures of the vertebrae, wrist, and ankle are more common. The vertebral fractures are usually the crush types that cause deformation and pain. As these occur, patients lose up to 25% of their vertebral height. Another indicator may be new onset of tooth loss despite good oral hygiene because the jaw, mandible, and maxilla contain significant amounts of trabecular bone. In type 2, fractures occur most commonly at the hip, proximal humerus, proximal tibia, and pelvis. The vertebral fractures that these patients experience occur typically in the mid-thoracic area, cause less pain, occur gradually, and lead to the formation of a deformation known as *dorsal kyphosis*, or "dowager's hump."

The relationship between osteoporosis and estrogen deficiency in women was first suggested by Albright in 1941. More recently, decreased estrogen and testosterone have been implicated in the development of the disease in men. Estrogens exert a beneficial effect on bone through two primary mechanisms: (1) they hold bone resorption in check by inhibiting synthesis of specific cytokines (particularly IL-1 and IL-6) that are known to stimulate bone resorption; and (2) they enhance local synthesis of growth factors such as TGF-β and TGF-1 that stimulate PTH-mediated bone formation.

Abnormalities in bone turnover also occur secondarily to a number of other diseases and medications (see Table 30.1). Since the resulting bone loss can be slowed or stopped if the primary disorder is treated, it is important that the workup of these patients also include evaluation of the more common disorders and a review of medications.

The thyroid hormones, T3 and T4, contribute to normal bone development and metabolism. Increasing concentrations of these hormones stimulate osteoclast activity and consequently bone resorption by activating receptors on osteoblasts. Although formation is also stimulated, the rate of resorption is greater. Parathyroid hormone (PTH) also plays key roles in both formation and resorption. Osteoblasts, but not osteoclasts, have receptors for the hormone, so both actions appear to be mediated through the osteoblasts. Continuous, high-dose exposure to PTH (as occurs in primary hyperparathyroidism) inhibits bone collagen synthesis and increases bone resorption, whereas collagen synthesis and bone formation are stimulated with intermittent, low-dose exposure

Table 30.1   Causes of Secondary Osteoporosis

Endocrine and metabolic diseases	Hyperthyroidism, Cushing syndrome, hypogonadism, hyperparathyroidism, Turner syndrome, panhypopituitarism
Renal diseases	Renal failure, renal insufficiency, vitamin D deficiency, renal tubular acidosis
Connective tissue diseases	Osteogenesis imperfecta, glycogen storage diseases, homocystinuria, Marfan syndrome, amyloidosis, rheumatoid arthritis
Others	Malignancies, microgravity, prolonged bed rest, chronic liver diseases, chronic obstructive pulmonary disease, amyloidosis, malabsorption
Medications	Glucocorticoids, thyroxine, heparin, cyclosporine, tacrolimus, aromatase inhibitors, LH-RH agonists, diuretics, ethanol, neuroleptics, aluminum, antacids (phosphate binders), methotrexate, anticonvulsant drugs, lithium, cholestyramine

of bone to PTH. These two paradoxical events relate to production and stimulation of local factors like macrophage-colony-stimulating factor (m-CSF), nuclear factor-$\kappa\beta$ ligand (RANKL), and osteoprotegerin.

Excess glucocorticoids regardless of the cause (tumor, hyperplasia, or ingestion), has a negative impact on bone. Through their effects on growth factors, carrier proteins, and cytokines, the hormones stimulate proliferation of osteoclasts while inhibiting maturation of osteoblasts. Glucocorticoids also directly inhibit intestinal transport and renal reabsorption of calcium leading to secondary hyperparathyroidism, as well as stimulating the parathyroids to increase PTH secretion.

Diagnosis

The diagnosis of osteoporosis requires a thorough review of the medical history, evaluation of bone mineral density (BMD), and investigation for secondary causes. Currently, dual-energy x-ray absorptimetry (DEXA) is the imaging technique most commonly used to assess BMD. DEXA scans involve minimal radiation exposure and are completed within a few minutes. Compact instruments, suitable for screening extremities, such as the hand, ankle, wrist, or forearm, are found in many clinics. Larger instruments, used to measure BMD in the hip, spine, or whole body, are found in most hospitals and freestanding radiology centers.

Bone mineral density is defined as the average mineral content per unit volume of bone scanned. This measurement is reported along with Z- and T-scores that compare the patient to defined controls and reflect the deviation of the patient's BMD from the control. The Z-score normalizes the patient's data to that of age- and gender-matched controls, while the T-score compares the patient to a healthy 35-year-old who is presumably at peak bone mass. The patient, such as our case, who has a DEXA T-score of more than -2.5 SD (standard deviations) is considered to have osteoporosis. Additional imaging techniques, including computed tomography, quantitative ultrasound, and magnetic resonance imaging, are evolving and may replace DEXA in the future.

Initially the laboratory's role is in the evaluation of the patient's adrenal, thyroid, renal, and hepatic function to identify, or exclude, any secondary causes and to identify nutritional deficiencies in vitamin D and calcium.

Treatment and Monitoring

Treating the patient diagnosed with osteoporosis takes a multipronged approach that includes an assessment of additional risk factors that the patient can control or modify. Unless the patient has a history of renal stones or hypercalcemia, one of the first steps is to encourage increased calcium and vitamin D intake through diet or supplementation. Habits that are known to correlate with increased bone loss, such as smoking or excessive alcohol consumption, are discouraged. Exercise, particularly weight-bearing exercise, improves bone density and is encouraged.

One of the most important aspects of treatment is fracture prevention. By some estimates, osteoporosis leads to more than 1.5 million fractures annually, including 300,000 fractures of the hip, 250,000 of the wrist, and about 700,000 fractures of the vertebra. For many patients, a fracture is more than an inconvenience; it is a serious, potentially life-threatening event. The risk of mortality following a fracture increases with age, particularly for men. Surviving the event does not mean a return to normalcy. About a quarter of patients who were independent and ambulatory before sustaining a hip fracture require long-term care afterward. Patients who have severe osteoporosis experience fractures with minimal trauma; but for most, the fracture occurs as the result of an accidental fall. Therefore, preventing falls is a primary goal for many patients. A home visit by an occupational therapist may identify the need to improve lighting, secure rugs, or for the use of supports or handrails.

Currently available drug therapy focuses on suppression of bone resorption. Because of the relationship between estrogen and bone resorption, hormone replacement therapy was for many years the first therapeutic option. But this changed in 2002 when data from the Women's Health Initiative suggested increased risks of breast cancer, coronary artery disease, stroke, and pulmonary embolism with a combined estrogen–progesterone formula. Although these risks were not found with other estrogen therapies, there was concern that for many women the risks outweighed the bone benefits. For these women, and when hormone therapy is contraindicated, there are other options. The bisphosphonates are probably the most frequently prescribed drugs for the treatment of osteoporosis and osteopenia. Alendronate, the most widely used of the class, acts by inhibiting farnesyl diphosphate synthase within the osteoclast, causing the cell to undergo premature apoptosis. Second- and third-generation bisphosphonates are thought to also induce osteoclast death but by inhibiting mitochondrial respiration. Selective estrogen receptor modulators (SERMs) have been developed specifically to target the estrogen receptors of bone yet have minimal activity to the estrogen receptors in reproductive tissue. Calcitonin may be administered parenterally via intramuscular or subcutaneous injection, or intranasally, and acts by inhibiting osteoclasts.

One of the most promising therapeutic interventions is the use of parathyroid hormone fragments and analogs. Teriparatide is a biosynthetic PTH fragment containing the biologically active region of the molecule. A small dose is given once daily as a subcutaneous injection to mimic the conditions under which PTH stimulates bone formation. At this writing, teriparatide is the only drug available to increase bone formation.

Role of Bone Markers

Bone is a complex tissue, so it is not surprising that a number of biochemical compounds are involved in bone turnover. These include enzymes, collagen precursors, byproducts of bone formation, and bone degradation products. Unfortunately, none is sufficiently specific to be diagnostic for osteoporosis. They do, however, have roles in the evaluation and treatment of these patients, especially in assessing fracture risk and in monitoring treatment. The analytes associated with bone resorption include urinary calcium, tartrate-resistant acid phosphatase, bone sialoprotein, type 1 collagen crosslinked telopeptides, and pyridinium derivatives; those reflecting bone formation include bone alkaline phosphatase, osteocalcin, and the type 1 collagen propeptides:

> *Collagen crosslinks.* Type I collagen is stabilized and strengthened by crosslinking between amino acids of the chains forming the triple helix. During bone resorption portions of these crosslinks are released into the circulation and subsequently excreted into the urine. The smaller fragments include pyridinoline (Pyr) and deoxypyridinoline (D-Pyr), which are found as peptide-bound forms and as free crosslinks. Bone is the primary source, but a small amount does originate from other sources. The development of antibodies specific to sequences of the amino- and the carboxy-terminal telopeptide regions of type 1 collagen have allowed for the development of assays known as NTx and CTx. Neither NTx nor CTx is recycled or metabolized after release into the circulation, and both are excreted into the urine.

> *Tartrate-resistant acid phosphatase* (TRAP). Osteoclasts, hepatic Kupffer's cells, and macrophages express an acid phosphatase resistant to inhibition by tartrate ions. Unfortunately, the inability to distinguish between TRAP originating from osteoclasts versus other cells hindered the use of this enzyme as a bone marker. Recently an isoform, designated as TRAP 5b because of its electrophoretic migration, was found to have slightly different chemical properties that allow its distinction from TRAP originating from other cells. Several immunoassays specific to this bone-specific form are under evaluation.

> *Bone alkaline phosphatase isoenzyme.* Alkaline phosphatase is a membrane-associated glycoprotein originating from many cells. Synthesis of the bone, liver, and kidney isoenzymes is regulated by the same gene, but afterward the bone and liver isoenzymes undergo posttranslational modification. The two isoenzymes retain enough structural similarity so that separation even using monoclonal antibody–based immunoassays is often difficult.

> *Osteocalcin.* Both osteoblasts and otodontoblasts synthesize osteocalcin, but since osteoblasts greatly outnumber otodontoblasts, most of the protein in the circulation reflects osteoblast activity. The protein originates as a 75-amino-acid propeptide that is first carboxylated before further posttranslational processing. The degree of carboxylation determines the protein's affinity for calcium and calcium-containing proteins and minerals and is directly influenced by vitamin K. Some studies suggest that patients with type II osteoporosis have a higher ratio of undercarboxylated to fully carboxylated OC and that a higher serum concentration of the undercarboxylated form correlates with an increased risk of fracture.

When using bone markers, several points should be remembered. First, resorption and formation are not independent, but closely linked processes. As a result, in active osteoporosis and during drug therapy, both are usually affected. Trends are often similar; however, since bone markers originate from or act at difference points within resorption or formation, one marker should not be expected to behave identically to another. All markers exhibit a circadian pattern in which highest concentrations are usually observed in the early-morning hours. Concentrations vary seasonally with higher levels observed in winter months and in northern latitudes. Intraindividual variation within a given day can be high, especially for those measured in urine. These factors complicate the use of the bone markers and require that collection be standardized in much the same way that we have standardized collection of cortisol or microalbumin.

One of the best uses of bone markers is in the assessment of the effectiveness of drug therapy. Although BMD measurements are used in the diagnosis, 1–2 years of drug therapy may be necessary before significant changes can be detected. Prolonged use of these drugs during this time, if little or no benefit is being achieved, is undesirable because of the expense and potential for adverse events. Fortunately, the bone markers respond quite rapidly if therapy is working. Markers should decline in response to anti-resorptive drug therapy. A significant decrease will be seen with the resorption markers within 1–3 months and within 3–6 months for the formation markers. Increased concentrations of the markers related to formation will be seen with treatment with drugs that stimulate formation, as in the case of the PTH analogs.

Bone markers are also useful in the initial assessment of patients to identify patients who have accelerated bone turnover before the loss is detected by DEXA. A 4-year follow-up study of postmenopausal women found that those whose bone markers were increased above the reference range at menopause lost 3–5 times more bone compared to those whose markers were within the premenopausal ranges. Other studies have shown that high bone turnover reflected by increased bone marker concentrations is associated with increased fracture risk. Following changes in the concentrations of the bone markers is useful in assessing the patient's risk of fracture, particularly after therapy is initiated. Finally, with the availability of PTH, another potential role for bone markers has been proposed: guiding the choice of therapy. Some investigators suggest that the antiresorptive agents (such as the bisphosphonates) are more useful in treating patients with type 1 osteoporosis, whereas those with type 2 are better treated using anabolic therapy (PTH, at this time). The use of bone markers can aid in this distinction. Currently, the expense of PTH is seen as a limitation, but as other anabolic agents become available, this may become a reasonable approach.

For this particular patient, the initial evaluation did not reveal a secondary cause of her low BMD. As indicated, a diagnosis of primary osteoporosis was determined and a bisphosphonate initiated. On her return visit to the clinic her urine NTx was found to have decreased to 100 mmol BCE/mmol creatinine, indicating effective drug therapy and compliance.

Additional Reading

EPSTEIN, S.: The roles of bone mineral density, bone turnover, and other properties in reducing fracture risk during antiresorptive therapy. *Mayo Clin Proc.* 80: 379–88, 2005.

FITZPATRICK, L. A.: Secondary causes of osteoporosis. *Mayo Clin Proc.* 77:453–68, 2002.

GARNERO, P., AND DELMAS, P. D.: Contribution of bone mineral density and bone turnover markers to the estimation of risk of osteoporotic fracture in postmenopausal women. *J. Musculoskelet. Neuronal. Interact.* 4:50–63, 2004.

HAMMETT-STABLER, C. A.: The use of biochemical markers in osteoporosis. *Clin. Lab. Med.* 24:175–97, 2004.

MAHAKALA, A., THOUTREDDY, S., AND KLEEREKOPER, M.: Prevention and treatment of postmenopausal osteoporosis. *Treat. Endocrinol.* 2:331–45, 2003.

Case 31

A 10-Year-Old Boy with Pain-Induced Seizures

Lorin M. Henrich, Alan D. Rogol, and David E. Bruns

A 10-year-old male with a history of learning disabilities, developmental delay, and attention deficit hyperactivity disorder (ADHD) suffered a nonfebrile seizure after he hit his knee while getting into the shower. The patient had no prior history of seizure, but his mother had experienced multiple "pain-induced" seizures. The patient was in no apparent distress and his respiration, pulse, and blood pressure were normal. He denied headaches or visual problems and had no evidence of a head injury. An EEG and head CT were normal. STAT serum chemistry tests revealed hypercalcemia (Table 31.1). The following values were found:

Analyte	Concentration, Conventional Units	Reference Interval, Conventional Units	Concentration, SI Units	Reference Interval, SI Units
Sodium	138 mmol/L	137–145	Same	
Potassium	4.6 mmol/L	3.6–5.0	Same	
Chloride	104 mmol/L	98–107	Same	
CO_2	23 mmol/L	18–27	Same	
Glucose	87 mg/dL	65–110	4.8 mmol/L	3.6–6.1
Total calcium	12.0 mg/dL	8.5–10.5	3.1 mmol/L	2.2–2.7
Phosphorus	3.1 mg/dL	4.0–7.0	1.0 mmol/L	1.3–2.3
Creatinine	0.6 mg/dL	0.7–1.3	53 mol/L	62–115

On evaluation by a pediatric endocrinologist, the patient denied symptoms of hypercalcemia, including abdominal pain, constipation, muscle pain, or tiredness. A soft right parasternal murmur was noted. The finding of hypercalcemia in combination with arrhythmia was suggestive of Williams syndrome, but an EKG was normal and echocardiography revealed no evidence of supravalvular aortic stenosis or any cardiac abnormality. Additional laboratory studies were obtained:

Tietz's Applied Laboratory Medicine, Second Edition. Edited by Mitchell G. Scott, Ann M. Gronowski, and Charles S. Eby
Copyright © 2007 John Wiley & Sons, Inc.

Analyte	Value, Conventional Units	Reference Range, Conventional Units	Value, SI Units	Reference Range, SI Units
Albumin	4.7 g/dL	3.5–5.0	47 g/L	35–50
Total calcium	12.2 mg/dL	8.5–10.5	3.2 mmol/L	2.2–2.7
Ionized calcium	7.0 mg/dL	4.5–5.6	1.7 mmol/L	1.1–1.4
Phosphorus	3.1 mg/dL	4.0–7.0	1.0 mmol/L	1.3–2.3
Creatinine	0.9 mg/dL	0.7–1.3	80 mol/L	62–115
Magnesium	2.4 mg/dL	1.6–2.3	1 mmol/L	0.66–0.95
Anion gap	14 mmol/L	12–20	Same	
ALP	215 U/L	50–380	Same	
Intact PTH	60.3 pg/mL	10.0–65.0	6.6 pmol/L	1.1–7.1
T4	6.3 μg/dL	5–12	81 nmol/L	64–154
TSH	1.73 μU/mL	0.7–7.0	1.73 mU/L	0.7–7.0
Urine calcium	237 mg/24 hours	42–353	5.9 mmol/day	1.0–8.8
Urine phosphorus	842 mg/24 hours	400–1300	27 mmol/day	13–42
Urine creatinine	903 mg/24 hours	600–2500	8 mmol/day	5–22
Total urine volume	1220 mL			

The patient's hypercalcemia was accompanied by hypophosphatemia and normo-calciuria. The thyroid function tests did not suggest hyperthyroidism, and the anion gap showed no evidence of metabolic acidosis. Plasma PTH was within the reference interval, but inappropriately high for the calcium concentration. On the basis of these results, a diagnosis of mild primary hyperparathyroidism was reached. Because the patient's mother had a history of seizures, familial hypocalciuric hyperparathyroidism (FHH) was included in the differential. Both parents were evaluated for hypercalcemia and hypo-phosphatemia, and were found to be normal. A 99*m*-technetium sestamibi scan of the patient's parathyroid region demonstrated no evidence of adenoma or ectopic tissue. Because the patient was asymptomatic, no immediate action was taken.

Over the next few years, the patient's calcium remained between 11.0 and 12.2 mg/dL. His plasma PTH was stable, and he remained asymptomatic. Five years after the initial diagnosis, the patient developed dysuria and symptoms consistent with nephrolithiasis, and he thus underwent parathyroidectomy. Immediately before removal of any glands, the plasma PTH was 260 pg/mL. Three and one-half enlarged-appearing glands were then removed. Intraoperative PTH values of 50 pg/mL and 56 pg/mL were obtained at 25 and 45 minutes after gland removal. The observed decline in PTH indicated that the bulk of the hyperfunctioning tissue had been removed, and the surgery was completed. Histologic evaluation of the resected parathyroid tissue indicated diffuse hyperplasia of all four glands.

Definition of the Disease

In primary hyperparathyroidism (HPT), a primary abnormality in one or multiple para-thyroid glands results in inappropriate secretion of parathyroid hormone (PTH). Primary HPT is most common in postmenopausal women and is rarely found in patients under 15 years of age. The majority of cases (70–80%) are due to a single parathyroid adenoma that arises sporadically. The remaining cases are due to diffuse parathyroid hyperplasia (15–20%) or, rarely, parathyroid carcinoma (1–2%). Most patients with primary HPT are asymptomatic, and the diagnosis is made on the incidental finding of hypercalcemia. Patients with mild primary HPT typically experience relatively small, intermittent elevations in plasma calcium concentrations, and exhibit symptoms such as fatigue, muscle weakness, constipation, and depression. In more severe cases, hypercalcemia is prolonged and patients may develop cognitive dysfunction, chondrocalcinosis, osteopenia, and hypertension. Approximately 15–20% of patients develop hypercalciuria-induced nephrolithiasis that may progress to renal insufficiency.

Maintenance of an appropriate extracellular calcium concentration is critical for many physiological processes, and therefore the concentration of circulating calcium is tightly regulated. PTH, a peptide hormone secreted by the parathyroid chief cells, is the primary hormonal regulator of plasma calcium homeostasis. There is a steep, inverse sigmoidal relationship between PTH and calcium such that a small decrease in plasma free calcium elicits a larger increase in PTH secretion.

PTH acts on bone, kidney, and intestine to increase plasma calcium concentrations and enhance urinary phosphate excretion. PTH increases plasma calcium concentrations by acting directly on kidney and bone through type 1 PTH receptors (PTH1R). In the distal nephron, PTH increases calcium reabsorption by enhancing voltage-sensitive calcium channel conductance. In the proximal tubule, PTH strongly induces transcription of the 25-hydroxyvitamin D 1α-hydroxylase gene. The hydroxylase catalyzes production of the active form of vitamin D, 1,25-dihydroxyvitamin D, which acts on intestinal enterocytes to enhance absorption of calcium and phosphate. In bone, PTH induces osteoblast-mediated differentiation of osteoclasts, resulting in enhanced bone reabsorption and release of calcium and phosphate into the extracellular fluid. PTH also strongly inhibits phosphate reabsorption in the proximal tubules.

PTH secretion is negatively controlled by a feedback loop in which increased calcium activates the calcium-sensing receptor (CaSR) in the parathyroid gland, resulting in inhibition of PTH secretion. Thus, normal PTH secretion is suppressed under hypercalcemic conditions.

Measurements of plasma calcium and PTH are critical for the diagnosis of primary HPT. Approximately 40% of total calcium is bound to circulating proteins and is physiologically inactive. Perturbations in plasma protein concentrations or alterations in the calcium–protein binding equilibrium (due to pH or temperature) can alter total calcium concentrations in plasma. Therefore, total calcium should be interpreted in the context of plasma albumin and total protein. Measurement of free ("ionized") calcium provides a more accurate indication of the concentration of biologically active calcium.

The biologically active, full-length PTH peptide (PTH 1–84) consists of 84 amino acids and is able to bind and activate PTH1R. Once secreted, the PTH (1–84) undergoes metabolism in the liver and kidneys, resulting in the release PTH fragments consisting of both amino-terminal (N-terminal) and carboxyl-terminal (C-terminal) fragments. The majority of PTH fragments in circulation consist of C-terminal fragments lacking the first 34 amino acids that are unable to interact with the classical PTH1R. Because C-terminal PTH fragments are cleared primarily by glomerular filtration, their concentrations are significantly increased in renal failure.

The measured concentration of PTH depends on the type of assay used. This becomes especially important during long-term patient monitoring when new assay methods may be implemented and reference intervals may change markedly. Early PTH assays were radioimmunoassays that employed single antibodies directed against epitopes located in the C-terminal region of the peptide. These assays could not distinguish PTH (1–84) from C-terminal fragments, and thus PTH (1–84) was overestimated by 40–50% or more, particularly in the context of renal failure. Two-site immunometric (sandwich) assays were developed to circumvent this problem. Initial immunometric assays utilized one antibody directed against an N-terminal region of PTH and another directed against the C-terminal region. These "intact PTH" assays were thought to specifically recognize PTH (1-84). However, HPLC analysis of circulating PTH fragments revealed that intact PTH assays detect a peak of immunoreactivity consistent with synthetic PTH (7-84). Newer "biointact" (biologically intact) immunometric assays employ an antibody specific for the first four amino acids of PTH (1-84) and a second antibody directed toward the C-terminal region. These assays specifically detect PTH (1-84) and not PTH (7-84) or other C-terminal fragments. Biointact PTH is typically 40–50% lower than intact PTH, and there is a linear correlation between measurements obtained by the two assays. Measurement of biointact PTH may be preferred in the context of renal failure due to accumulation of non-PTH (1-84) fragments. However, both assay types have been shown to predict bone turnover in patients with secondary hyperparathyroidism resulting from end-stage renal disease (ESRD).

PTH is undetectable or below the lower limit of the reference interval in the setting of hypercalcemia that is not induced by HPT. Failure to suppress circulating PTH concentrations in response to increased calcium confirms the diagnosis of HPT. Patients with severe primary HPT typically exhibit plasma calcium values above the reference interval concurrent with elevations in plasma PTH. In contrast, patients with mild primary HPT may have normal to slightly increased calcium (<11 mg/dL) and PTH within the reference interval. However, a value of PTH within the reference interval is inappropriate in the context of hypercalcemia and is therefore highly suggestive of primary HPT. Approximately one-third of primary HPT patients are hypophosphatemic and exhibit mild hyperphosphaturia. Although PTH induces reabsorption of calcium in the kidney, elevations in plasma calcium stimulate PTH-independent glomerular filtration of calcium. Therefore, 40–50% of patients also have hypercalciuria. Patients with mild primary HPT may exhibit normal urinary excretion of calcium and phosphorus. Thus, demonstration of inappropriate circulating concentrations of PTH in the presence of normal to increased calcium is crucial for the diagnosis of primary HPT.

At least 30–40% of patients with primary HPT have increased serum concentrations of 1,25-dihydroxyvitamin D, which is associated with hypercalciuria and subsequent nephrolithiasis. Because PTH also inhibits reabsorption of bicarbonate in the kidney, patients with primary HPT may also have a mild metabolic acidosis. Hypomagnesemia is not uncommon, and markedly increased bone-specific ALP may indicate bone involvement.

Differential Diagnosis

In the setting of an increased calcium concentration, primary HPT must be distinguished from other causes of hypercalcemia. Primary HPT is responsible for $>90\%$ of hypercalcemia cases in outpatients. The most frequent cause of hypercalcemia in the inpatient setting is malignancy. Low serum albumin and increased free calcium are characteristic findings for metastatic bone disease. Hypercalcemia can also result from tumor-mediated secretion of PTH-related peptide (PTHrP), a peptide hormone that binds and activates the PTH1 receptor in bone and kidney. Increased PTHrP frequently coexists with bone metastases and may be the primary cause of hypercalcemia in such patients. PTHrP can be quantified by immunometric assays, but the diagnosis of cancer-related hypercalcemias is usually made without use of the assays.

Vitamin D intoxication is responsible for a number of non-parathyroid-dependent hypercalcemic disorders. In granulomatous diseases such as sarcoidosis, unregulated 1,25-dihydroxyvitamin D 1α-hydroxylase activity results in greatly increased synthesis of 1,25-dihydroxyvitamin D and subsequent hypercalcemia. Hypercalcemia due to increased 1,25-dihyroxyvitamin D can also occur during the first 4 years of life in Williams's syndrome, a developmental disorder in which patients present with mental retardation, "elfin" facies, and supravalvular aortic stenosis. Approximately 10% of patients with thyrotoxicosis have mild hypercalcemia with low 1,25-dihydroxyvitamin D. Milk-alkali syndrome and adrenal insufficiency can also induce hypercalcemia.

Nonparathyroid causes of hypercalcemia are usually easily distinguished from primary HPT. Malignancy-induced hypercalcemia is rarely seen without advanced disease that is clinically apparent. Hypocalciuria rather than hypercalciuria is typical of granulomatous disease, and thyrotoxicosis can be diagnosed by thyroid function tests. Moderate primary HPT may produce hyperchloremic acidosis, whereas other causes of hypercalcemia such as the milk-alkali syndrome are more often associated with metabolic alkalosis. The most important laboratory value for the differential diagnosis of hyper-calcemia is PTH. PTH will be low or undetectable in non-parathyroid-dependent hypercalcemia, and inappropriately nonsupressed in the face of increased calcium in primary HPT.

Secondary and tertiary forms of HPT also exist. Secondary HPT, a common complication of renal failure, is associated with inadequate production of 1,25-dihydroxyvitamin D. Unlike patients with primary HPT, secondary/tertiary HPT patients have normal or low serum calcium. Almost all patients with secondary HPT have increased ALP, whereas ALP is increased in only 10% of patients with primary HPT. In tertiary HPT, chronic secondary HPT results in hyperplasia of the parathyroids. These patients, like those with primary HPT, have increased PTH and hypercalcemia. However, differentiation of primary HPT from secondary or tertiary HPT is rarely a problem because most patients with secondary or tertiary HPT will have clinically appa-rent symptoms of underlying renal disease.

Because treatment strategies depend on the etiology of the disease, it is important to determine whether primary HPT is due to a parathyroid adenoma or diffuse hyperplasia and whether the hyperparathyroidism is sporadic or inherited. Ultrasonography, MRI, and 99m-technetium (radionuclide) sestamibi scintigraphy can be used for detection of adenomas or ectopic glands. Sestamibi scintigraphy is the preferred method for detection of parathyroid adenomas or diffuse hyperplasia. Its sensitivity for detection of parathyroid adenomas is 85–100%. Reported sensitivities for detection of parathyroid hyperplasia vary (45–83%), and surgical exploration may be necessary.

Among patients with diffuse parathyroid hyperplasia, approximately 20% of cases are associated with inherited germline mutations. Inherited forms of primary HPT tend to manifest earlier in life than does sporadic HPT and should be considered in young patients and those with a family history of hypercalcemia.

The inherited MEN (multiple exdocrine neoplasia) syndromes are autosomal domi-nant disorders that are characterized by the development of multiple endocrine neoplasms, including parathyroid tumors. MEN1 is associated with inactivating mutations in *MEN1*, a putative tumor suppressor gene located on chromosome 11q13. Primary HPT occurs in nearly all cases of MEN1 and is often the first manifestation of the disease. Mutations in the protooncogene *RET* (located on chromosome 10q11.2) are found in the majority of cases of MEN2A, primary HPT occurs less frequently (5–20%) in MEN2A and often presents late in disease. However, thyroid carcinomas are frequent, and therefore the presence of an elevated calcitonin favors MEN2A. DNA sequencing can be used to detect mutations in *MEN1* or *RET*.

FHH is an autosomal dominant disorder caused by a mutation in the calcium-sensing receptor (CaSR) that results in a shift of the setpoint of the parathyroid gland for calcium. Heterozygotes for CaSR mutations often present in childhood with mild hypercalcemia, hypophosphatemia, and inappropriately increased PTH. Unlike primary HPT, the disease is considered benign and is not associated with osteopenia, nephrolithiasis, or cognitive dysfunction. One distinguishing feature of FHH is the presence of hypocalciuria due to increased PTH-independent renal calcium reabsorption. In patients with a family history of hypercalcemia, a total urinary calcium excretion of less than 100 mg/day, or a ratio of calcium clearance to creatinine clearance below 0.01, favors a diagnosis of FHH over sporadic primary HPT. Homozygotes for the CaSR mutation present with severe neonatal HPT and often have serum calcium concentrations greater than 15 mg/dL.

Treatment

A 1990 NIH Consensus Conference (updated in 2002) recommended parathyroidectomy as the treatment of choice for all symptomatic patients with primary HPT. Removal of the abnormal parathyroid gland corrects calcium and PTH concentrations in virtually all cases with parathyroid adenomas. In patients with diffuse parathyroid hyperplasia, removal of three and one-half glands or removal of all glands with autotransplantation of a parathyroid fragment into the forearm can prevent permanent hypoparathyroidism. Failure of return to normocalcemia occurs in 2–16% of cases. Surgical intervention is contraindicated in patients with FHH because hypercalcemia reoccurs after parathyroidectomy unless all glands are removed.

The success of parathyroidectomy can be monitored by intraoperative measurement of PTH. Since the half-life of full-length PTH is less than 2 minutes, a decrease in plasma PTH to less than 50% of the initial concentration within 10–20 minutes of gland removal indicates successful removal of hyperfunctioning parathyroid tissue.

In asymptomatic patients, surgery is not required if the following criteria are met: age >50 years, serum calcium <11.4 mg/dL, urinary calcium excretion <400 mg/day, reduction in creatinine clearance no greater than 30% of normal, and bone mineral density no less than 2 SDs below age- and sex-matched controls. Asymptomatic patients should be monitored semiannually for changes in serum calcium, creatinine, and PTH. Routine evaluation for cardiac abnormalities, bone density changes, and neuromuscular deficiencies should be included. The new calcimimetic agents that activate the CaSR and decrease plasma PTH offer a nonsurgical option for selected patients. Calcimimetic agents act as allosteric activators of the CaSR and act to lower plasma PTH.

References

1. BRINGHURST, F. R., DEMAY, M. B., AND KRONENBERG, H. M.: Hormones and disorders of mineral metabolism. In *Williams Textbook of Endocrinology*, 10th ed., P. R. LARSEN, H. M. KRONENBERG, S. MELMED, AND K. S. POLONSKY, eds., Saunders, Philadelphia, 2003, pp. 1303–71.

2. DAVIES, M., FRASER, W. D., AND HOSKING, D. J.: The management of primary hyperparathyroidism. *Clin. Endocrinol. 57*:145–55, 2002.

3. ENDRES, D. B. AND RUDE, R. K.: Mineral and bone metabolism. In *Tietz Textbook of Clinical Chemistry and Molecular Diagnostics*, 4th ed., C. A. BURTIS,

E. A. ASHWOOD, AND D. E. BRUNS, eds., Saunders, Philadelphia, 2005, pp. 1891–1965.

4. INABNET, W. B.: Intraoperative parathyroid hormone monitoring. *World J. Surg. 28*: 1212–15, 2004.

5. MARTIN, K. J., JUPPNER, H., SHERRARD, D. J. ET AL.: First- and second-generation immunometric PTH assays during treatment of hyperparathyroidism with cinacalcet HCl. *Kidney Int. 68*:1236–43, 2005.

6. MARX, S. J.: Hyperparathyroid and hypoparathyroid disorders. *N. Engl. J. Med. 343*:1863–75, 2001.

7. YOUNES, N. A., SHAFAGOI, Y., KHATIB, F., AND ABABNEH, M.: Laboratory screening for hyperparathyroidism. *Clin. Chim. Acta 353*:1–12, 2005.

Part Nine

Miscellaneous Endocrine Diseases

Cases of Zollinger–Ellison disease and carcinoid syndrome are presented in Cases 32 and 33, respectively (both edited by AMG).

Tietz's Applied Laboratory Medicine, Second Edition. Edited by Mitchell G. Scott, Ann M. Gronowski, and Charles S. Eby

Case 32

Laboratory Tests Ignored

Oren Zinder

A 75-year-old white female with a past medical history significant for hypertension, Alzheimer's disease, and chronic diarrhea presented to the emergency department (ED) with a complaint of 5 days of watery diarrhea (four to five stools per day), fever, and weakness. She reported that a week ago she had attended a funeral where she had some Lebanese food, and 4 days prior to arrival at the ED she began having loose bowel movements, some with bright red blood in them. The patient denied vomiting, but reported some nausea. The patient denied having shortness of breath or chest pain, but did admit to some diffuse abdominal pain associated with the diarrhea. She has had a fever of 100.9°F, generalized weakness, anorexia, and malaise, and her diarrhea has been sporadic over the past few months. This complaint had been extensively worked up in two previous admissions to the ED, but besides mild chronic inflammation seen on biopsy, no other cause for the symptoms was determined.

The past medical history showed COPD with a mild restrictive and obstructive pattern, peptic ulcer disease, hiatal hernia, esophageal dysmotility, hypothyroidism, and hypertension, with a recent hospitalization for diarrhea and hypertensive urgency. The patient has no alcohol or smoking history, is married, and has five children.

Physical examination showed that the patient was uncomfortable, avoided movement, and kept her legs pulled up close to her abdomen. Temperature, heart rate, respiratory rate, and blood pressure were all normal. The lungs were clear to bilateral auscultation, the heart sounds were regular, and an ejection murmur was best heard at the right upper sternal border, radiating to both carotids. There was no peripheral edema, and adequate perfusion was seen. The patient was alert, awake, and well oriented, and sensation was grossly intact. Strength was 5/5 throughout. A full range of motion was seen in all extremities. Bowel sounds were present and increased in frequency. Abdomen was distended, and was tender to superficial and deep palpitations, with some voluntary guarding. A positive guaiac stool was obtained.

An abdominal CT scan showed signs of mucosal thickening on the ascending colon and transverse colon, extending to the splenic flexure. Sigmoidoscopy performed on the day of admission to the ED showed some edema and erythema in the sigmoidal mucosa. Laboratory results are shown below:

Tietz's Applied Laboratory Medicine, Second Edition. Edited by Mitchell G. Scott, Ann M. Gronowski, and Charles S. Eby
Copyright © 2007 John Wiley & Sons, Inc.

Analyte	Value, Conventional Units	Reference Interval, Conventional Units	Value, SI Units	Reference Interval, SI Units
Hemoglobin	11.8 g/dL	11.7–16.0	118 g/L	117–160
Hematocrit	33.8%	35–47	0.338 v/v	0.35–0.47
WBC	24,000 cells/μL	4.5–11.0 × 10^3	Same	Same
Platelets	195,000 cells/μL	140–440 × 10^3	Same	Same
INR	1.23	0.54	Same	Same
Sodium	139 mmol/L	135–148	Same	Same
Potassium	4.7 mmol/L	3.5–5.0	Same	Same
Chloride	108 mmol/L	95–107	Same	Same
Bicarbonate	23 mmol/L	22–26	Same	Same
BUN	46 mg/dL	7–18	16.4 mmol urea/L	2.5–6.4
Creatinine	2.7 mg/dL	0.6–1.1	238.7 μmol/L	53–97
Glucose	174 mg/dL	70–105	9.66 mmol/L	3.9–5.8
Calcium	9.0 mg/dL	8.5–10.3	2.25 mmol/L	2.15–2.50
Total protein	7.3 g/dL	6.1–8.0	73 g/L	61–80
Albumin	3.5 g/dL	3.5–5.0	35 g/L	35–50
AST	24 U/L	8–25	0.41 μkat/L	0.17–0.58
ALT	12 U/L	10–28	0.20 μkat/L	0.12–0.60
ALP	71 U/L	53–141	1.21 μkat/L	0.9–2.4
Total bilirubin	1.1 mg/dL	0.3–1.2	18.8 mmol/L	5.0–21

Follow-up

The patient was discharged from the ED in a stable state, but without a definitive diagnosis. Some weeks after her discharge, a laboratory technician was summarizing data and came across the following elevated results for this patient: gastrin 2590 pg/mL (reference interval 0–130 pg/mL) at second admission to the ED and 2750 pg/mL at the most recent (third) ED admission 2 months afterward. Concerned that these elevated results may have been overlooked by the attending physician, the laboratory contacted him. The physician was not aware of the results and was surprised as they had not considered Zollinger–Ellison syndrome (ZES) in their differential diagnosis.

On further investigation of this case, the patient had been subsequently readmitted to the ED and seen by a different physician, one month after the abovementioned (third) admission, with a similar presentation, and with even more severe diarrhea and cramps. The patient expired 6 days later.

It is clear that the patient described above suffered from multiple afflictions, but even after the laboratory notified the attending physician of the extremely high gastrin concentrations, in the expiration summary only the presence of diarrhea, cramps, and peptic ulcer disease are noted. No mention is made of the possible presence of ZES. The rarity of this disease was probably the reason for this oversight by the physicians. Yet, all the important signs and symptoms were present, in both the clinical presentation and the laboratory results. The consequences of this disease are severe and may be fatal, as is the case for many rare diseases, but when considered as part of the differential diagnosis, this fatal cascade can be arrested.

Definition of the Disease

Zollinger–Ellison syndrome (ZES) is characterized by severe hypersecretion of gastric acid, refractory peptic ulcer disease localized to the stomach and the upper gastrointestinal tract, malabsorption, and diarrhea, which is sometimes severe. Nausea, vomiting, and heartburn are present in about 35% of the cases. Approximately 25% of ZES patients present with bleeding. These are primarily patients with the sporadic form of the disease and not those with multiple endocrine neoplasia type 1 (MEN1). ZES is often associated with MEN1, a genetic dominant autosomal disorder due to mutations (over 25 have been documented) in the MEN1 gene on exon 10 of chromosome 11q13. The syndrome involves neoplasia in the parathyroid, pancreatic islet endocrine tumors, pituitary adenomas, and adrenal adenomas. The main pancreatic manifestation of MEN1 is a gastrinoma leading to hypersecretion of gastrin and its physiological consequences. ZES is the major cause of morbidity and mortality in MEN1. The ZES tumors are usually multicentric, making surgical treatment inefficient; however, pharmacologic gastrectomy is possible using H_2 receptor antagonists (cimetidine or ranitidine) and proton pump inhibitors such as omeprazole.

This disease was first described by Zollinger and Ellison in 1955, and is quite rare, with an incidence of approximately one in a million in the general population of the United States, and up to one in a hundred in patients with peptic ulcers. Diagnosis is usually between the ages of 30 and 50, and is further delayed when the patient is taking proton pump inhibitors (e.g., omeprazole). In ZES, there is no discrimination between males and females, and its presentation is sporadic, with symptoms ebbing and flowing at intervals.

Gastrin is found in multiple forms, but the major forms found in the circulation are G34 ("big" gastrin) and G17 ("little" gastrin). An additional form, G14 ("mini" gastrin), is also found but in much smaller concentrations. The 17 C-terminal amino acids are required for maximal physiological activity, namely, the activation of gastric acid secretion from the gastric parietal cells. G17 is much more potent than G34 in stimulating acid secretion following meals, and their half-lives in blood are 6 and 36 minutes, respectively. Gastrin is secreted by the G cells of the antral mucosa of the stomach, by G cells in the proximal duodenum, and by delta cells of the pancreas. It is transported in blood via the liver to the parietal cells of the stomach fundus, where it stimulates the secretion of acid following its binding to the gastrin/CCK receptor. In the presence of a gastrinoma, the parietal cell mass increases, resulting in hypersecretion of gastric acids and acidemia. Normally, the acid inhibits further secretion of gastrin in a feedback mechanism aimed at limiting prolonged acid secretion, but in ZES this feedback effect is overridden.

Gastrin also has a trophic effect on enterochromaffin-like cells in the gastric mucosa, which may result in gastric carcinoid tumors. Approximately 35% of MEN1 patients develop gastric carcinoid tumors.

The periodic, and excessive, hypersecretion of gastric acid results in malabsorption via activation of pepsinogens. This can cause severe damage to the gastric mucosa, by acid inactivation of pancreatic enzyme activity, and by corrosion of the enterocytes by the high H^+ concentration. The damaged gastric mucosa results in the main presenting symptom of diarrhea in ZES. This may be combined with steatorrhea, due mainly to the insolubility of some of the bile acids in the low-pH environment, and acid inactivation of the pancreatic lipase. All of the abovementioned factors contribute to the presence of severe cramps. Finally, the low pH in the upper intestinal tract may result in vitamin

B_{12} malabsorption, since it interferes with the facilitative role of intrinsic factor on the absorption of vitamin B_{12} in the ileum.

Differential Diagnosis

The differential diagnosis of Zollinger–Ellison syndrome is complicated by a number of factors. Patients usually present with bouts of diarrhea (sometimes bloody), cramps, and weight loss. These may also be attributed to other diseases involving malabsorption such as celiac disease, Crohn's syndrome, pancreatic insufficiency, and bacterial over-growth syndrome (which results in bile acid loss). In addition, in peptic ulcer patients the use of proton pump inhibitors substantially delays the diagnosis as gastric acid secretion is inhibited and thus many of the identifying symptoms of ZES become muted.

Initially, the diagnosis of ZES was made on clinical grounds, confirmed by surgical exploration, and treated by total surgical resection of the stomach to control the gastric acid hypersecretion. The only biochemical assay used at the time was the measurement of gastric acidity by aspiration of fasting gastric fluid and by H^+ titration. Since then, there have been substantial changes in the diagnosis of gastrinomas, due mainly to the determination of gastrin by immunoassays. At present, the diagnosis is based on a combination of criteria, including clinical presentation, gastrin radioimmunoassay results, gastric fluid testing for acidity, and some diagnostic imaging evaluations, which, because of the relatively small tumor size, have not been very effective.

In addition to the exclusion of other malabsorption syndromes that present with symptoms similar to those due to ZES, the diagnosis of ZES must differentiate it from other conditions in which there is an elevation of gastrin, such as achlorhydria or hypochlorhydria, which could be a consequence of autoimmune atrophic gastritis. This latter disease entity is one of the more common causes of hypergastrinemia, and can be attributed to the presence of antiparietal cell antibodies. In addition, the use of proton pump inhibitors must be addressed, as they might hide the presence of the gastrinoma by inhibiting acid secretion. Another possible interference in the diagnosis is the presence of *Helicobacter pylori*, which might also cause moderate gastrin hypersecretion due to decreased acid secretion following the induction of the infection, and the activity of proinflammatory cytokines. It is rare, however, for a patient to have both ZES and *H. pylori*, as the acidity due to ZES may in fact eradicate the *H. pylori*.

Basal acid output is probably the best single test for ZES, and the upper limit of normal is 15 mEq/h. This test may not be easily available, so the measurement of gastric fluid pH on fluid aspirated by nasal tube is a reasonable alternative, using a pH of 2 as the cutoff. Below this pH, ZES must be seriously considered, while a pH >2, having excluded the use of antisecretory agents, is indicative of hypochlorhydria and not ZES.

Determination of plasma gastrin concentration is a required test in the diagnosis of Zollinger–Ellison syndrome. Patient preparation for the plasma gastrin test must be carefully adhered to. Food ingestion has a significant effect on plasma gastrin concentration, and therefore the sample must be obtained in the fasting condition. Serum and heparinized or EDTA plasma give similar results; however, in order to avoid any enzymatic digestion, the blood should be centrifuged at 4°C within 30 minutes following collection. A fasting plasma concentration of gastrin in excess of 1000 g/L is very suggestive of ZES, and in conjunction with a gastric fluid pH of <2, establishes a firm diagnosis of the disease. Elevated serum gastrin concentration may also be due to the absence of the acid feedback control on the gastrin secretion control mechanism found in chronic atrophic gastritis, or occasionally in patients on long-term proton pump inhibitors. Both these entities exhibit very little acid secretion, and this possibility must be taken into account in evaluating the plasma gastrin results.

When gastrin concentrations are between 50 and 1000 pg/mL, the diagnosis of ZES cannot be ruled out, and a secretin challenge test is suggested. The procedure for this test is as follows. A test dose of secretin (SecreFlo) 0.2 μg (0.1 mL) is given IV to test for possible allergies. If no untoward reactions occur, 0.4 μg/kg of SecreFlo is administered IV over one minute (bolus). Blood samples are collected at 2, 5, 10, and 20 minutes after the injection. A second type of confirmatory test is the calcium gluconate challenge (4 mg elemental calcium/kg body weight for 3 hours); however, there have been conflicting reports about its efficacy. In gastrinoma patients, these challenges should result in the elevation of plasma gastrin by at least 200 ng/L above the basal level. In nongastrinoma states of hypergastrinemia such as peptic ulcer disease, hypercalcemia, obstructed gastric outlet, or retained gastric antrum, the rise in plasma gastrin following these challenges should not be more than 50 ng/L.

Treatment

Surgical cure of Zollinger–Ellison syndrome has, in the past, been the first choice of treatment for patients with ZES. This treatment has, however, been ineffective because of the multiple loci of the gastrinoma tumor cells. Treatment of ZES is aimed at diminution of the hyperacidity, and control of the tumor growth. The very effective use of the proton pump inhibitors available today (e.g., omeprazole) makes it possible to reach the goal of reducing the hyperacidity. H_2 antagonist inhibitors, which were in use prior to the introduction of proton pump inhibitors, were also quite effective in reducing the deleterious effects of the hyperacidity, such as ulcers, diarrhea, and dehydration. Ranitidine would probably be the first choice among these agents because of the very low incidence of adverse effects and minimal interactions with other drugs. The goal of all these treatments is to reduce acid output to less than 10 mEq/h in uncomplicated ZES, and to less than 5 mEq/h in those patients suffering from both ZES and MEN1. The reduction of acid secretion below these rates will almost always result in healing of the ulcerations and substantial reduction of the other manifestations of hyperacidity.

With respect to control of tumor growth, there is no consensus. Surgical ablation is difficult, and at best it will be possible to entirely remove the primary tumor, but not the metastases. Chemotherapy has been tried and has been found to involve deleterious side effects in these patients.

Additional Reading

GIBRIL, F. AND JENSON, R. T.: Zollinger-Ellison syndrome revisited: Diagnosis, biologic markers, associated inherited disorders, and acid hypersecretion (review). *Curr. Gastroenterol. Rep.* 6:454–63, 2004.

HENDERSON, A. R. AND RINKER, A. D.: Gastric, pancreatic, and intestinal function. In *Tietz Textbook of Clinical Chemistry*, 3rd ed., C. A. BURTIS and E. R. ASHWOOD, eds., Saunders, Philadelphia, 1999, pp. 1274–8, 1307–9.

ROY, P. K., VENZON, D. J., SHOJAMANESH, H. ET AL.: Zollinger-Ellison syndrome. Clinical presentation in 261 patients. *Medicine* 79:379–411, 2000.

THAKKER, R. V.: Multiple endocrine neoplasia type I. *Endocrinol. Metab. Clin. North Am.* 29:541–67, 2000.

TOMASSETTI, P., SALOMONE, T., MIGLIORE, M., CAMPANA, D., AND CORINALDESI, R.: Optimal treatment of

Zollinger-Ellison syndrome and related conditions in elderly patients (review) *Drugs Aging 20*:1019–34, 2003.

VARRO, A., AND ARDILL, J. E. S.: Gastrin: An analytical review. *Ann. Clin. Biochem. 40*:472–80, 2003.

EDKINS, J. S.: On the chemical mechanism of gastric secretion. *Proc. Roy. Soc. B 76*:376, 1905.

ZOLLINGER, R. M. AND ELLISON, E. H.: Primary peptic ulcerations of the jejunum associated with islet cell tumors of the pancreas. *Ann. Surg. 142*:709–28, 1955.

Hot Flashes and Abdominal Pain

Jennifer Snyder

During a routine physical examination, a 45-year-old woman complained to her gynecologist of a 3-month history of transient burning sensations in her face and chest that would last for a few minutes, and then pass. She stated that she experienced these "hot flashes" between 7 and 8 times per day, and often they disrupted her sleep. She had no other physical complaints, and she denied any menstrual cycle irregularities. To determine whether she was menopausal, the physician ordered a serum follicle stimulating hormone (FSH) test which was 10.9 IU/L (premenopausal reference interval: 1–10 IU/L) on day three of the patient's menstrual cycle. Suspecting the woman's symptoms were due to perimenopausal transition, her doctor prescribed venlafaxine (a selective serotonin reuptake inhibitor), to minimize her hot flashes.

Despite treatment, the patient continued to have hot flashes, and one month later developed postprandial upper right quadrant pain, occasionally accompanied by abdominal distension and what she referred to as "excessive flatulence." She was referred to a gastroenterologist, who performed an abdominal ultrasound that revealed a 5-mm mass embedded in the wall of the gallbladder, thought to represent either a polyp or a gallstone. Despite normal liver function tests, the patient elected to undergo a laparoscopic cholecystectomy. Pathology on the gallbladder revealed a 3-mm stone.

One month after the surgery, the patient reported she was feeling much better; however, 4 months after surgery, she returned again to the gastroenterologist with stomach complaints. This time, she stated that she was having intermittent "episodes" where she became disoriented, then experienced hot flashes, right upper quadrant pain, vomiting, and diarrhea. These episodes began approximately one month after the cholecystectomy, but had recently become more frequent. She had lost 15 lb because of a decrease in appetite during and after these attacks.

Laboratory data included the following:

Analyte	Value, Conventional Units	Reference Range, Conventional Units	Value, SI Units	Reference Range, SI Units
AST	40 U/L	14–38	0.68 μkat/dL	0.24–0.65
ALT	61 U/L	15–48	1.04 μkat/dL	0.26–0.82
ALP	133 U/L	38–126	2.26 μkat/dL	0.65–2.14

Analyte	Value, Conventional Units	Reference Range, Conventional Units	Value, SI Units	Reference Range, SI Units
Bilirubin, total	0.3 mg/dL	0.0–1.2	5.1 μmol/L	0.0–20.5
Amylase	32 U/L	30–110	0.54 μkat/dL	0.51–1.87
Lipase	107 U/L	44–232	1.82 μkat/dL	0.75–3.94
Carcinoembryonic antigen	0.9 ng/mL	<5	0.9 μg/L	<5
CA 19-9	8 U/mL	<37	8 kU/L	<37

To rule out a bowel obstruction, radiographic examination included an upright chest, plus supine and upright abdominal films. These revealed multiple air fluid levels with dilated loops of small bowel. As these results indicated a possible small bowel obstruction, a small bowel follow-through with barium contrast was done that showed evidence of a circumferential smooth-walled narrowing in the mid-to-distal ileum. A laparoscopic small bowel exploration was performed, and a 5-cm mass was removed from the ileum along with five mesenteric lymph nodes. These specimens were sent to pathology for immunohistochemistry, which demonstrated reactivity with chromogranin A and synaptophysin, two markers for neuroendocrine tumors. On the basis of this result, the physician ordered serum chromogranin A and 24-hour urine 5-hydroxyindoleacetic acid (5-HIAA) measurements one week after the surgery. The results were

Chromogranin A	150 ng/mL (normal = 0–51 ng/mL)
5-HIAA (24-hour urine)	161.4 mg/24 hours (normal = 2–8 mg/24 hours)

Additionally, an Octreoscan using radiolabeled octreotide (a somatostatin analog that binds to somatostatin receptors expressed on the surface of carcinoid tumors) and abdominal computed tomography (CT) were performed that revealed lesions in the liver compatible with metastatic disease.

On the basis of these findings, the patient was diagnosed with carcinoid syndrome due to metastatic carcinoid tumor. She was placed on octreotide therapy, and her 5-HIAA concentrations decreased, as did her "episodes," now noted to be consistent with carcinoid syndrome.

Carcinoid Syndrome and Carcinoid Tumors

Carcinoids are rare neuroendocrine tumors with features of both benign and malignant cancers. The term *carcinoid* was first used in 1907 by S. Oberndorfer to designate these tumors as having characteristics of both carcinomas and adenomas.[1] Carcinoid tumors resemble carcinoma morphologically, but their growth is less aggressive, similar to adenomas. The incidence of clinically recognized carcinoid tumors in the United States is about 1–2 per 100,000 people; however, many instances of carcinoid tumor are found incidentally during surgery or at autopsy.[2]

Carcinoid tumors arise from enterochromaffin (EC) cells, glandular endocrine-hormone-producing cells found throughout the body. The highest proportion of EC cells are located in the small intestine, followed by the appendix, rectum, lung, and pancreas, and occasionally other locations.[3] EC cells were named for their ability to "silver-stain" with potassium chromate (chromaffin); silver staining is due to EC cell production of the paracrine hormone serotonin.[4]

Carcinoid tumors are subdivided into foregut, midgut, and hindgut tumors based on tissue of origin, silver stain patterns, and clinical features.[5] Foregut tumors arise in the stomach, duodenum, pancreas, or lungs; midgut tumors, from the jejunum, ileum, appendix, or ascending colon; and hindgut tumors, from the transverse descending and sigmoid colon or rectum. Foregut carcinoids produce the serotonin precursor 5-hydroxytryptophan (5-HTP) and take up silver stain only after treatment with reducing agent (termed *agyrophil*). Midgut carcinoids produce serotonin [5-hydroxytryptamine (5-HT)] and take up silver stain without the presence of a reducing agent (termed *argentaffin*). Hindgut carcinoids seldom produce either 5-HTP or 5-HT, or react with silver stain. Tumors found in the midgut are most often associated with the liver metastases that can cause the classical "carcinoid syndrome," found in the patient described above.[5]

Carcinoid syndrome is a rare complication of carcinoid tumors found in <10% of patients.[6] The syndrome is most commonly characterized by hot red flushing of the face and diarrhea, but additional symptoms may include abdominal pain (longstanding), sweating, wheezing, pellagra, telangiectasia, right-sided heart failure, and hypotension.[1] Flushing has been attributed to tumor production of kallikreins, proteins that cleave plasma kininogens and activate the strong vasodilator bradykinin.[7] Diarrhea is likely due to increased 5-HT, which stimulates intestinal motility and inhibits intestinal absorption.[7] EC cells in the midgut normally convert small amounts of the amino acid tryptophan into 5-HT (<1% of bioavailable); however, in the case of a patient with carcinoid syndome, as much of 60% of the total bioavailable tryptophan may be converted to 5-HT.[8] This overproduction of 5-HT causes diarrhea when released locally by tumors in the midgut, but can also be responsible for other symptoms of carcinoid syndrome when released into systemic circulation by liver metastases. As carcinoid tumors have been known to produce other amines, proteins, and prostaglandins, some of these molecules may also account for symptoms found in patients with carcinoid syndrome.

Diagnosis

Macroscopically, carcinoid tumors are solid and yellow-tan in color, due to high lipid content. Histologically, carcinoid tumors are composed of small cells with regular, round nuclei, and their growth patterns may be described as insular, trabecular (ribbonlike), glandular, mixed (trabecular and glandular), or undifferentiated.[4] Carcinoid tumors react with neuron-specific enolase (NSE), chromogranin A, and synaptophysin on immunohistochemistry, which are not specific for carcinoid, but indicate cells of neuroendocrine origin.[9] Serum chromogranin A concentrations can also be useful as a predictor of disease prognosis; one study demonstrated poor survival rates in carcinoid patients with chromogranin A concentrations above 5000 ng/mL.[10]

Laboratory analysis of the patient with suspected carcinoid almost always involves measurement of 24-hour urine 5-hydroxyindoleacetic acid (5-HIAA). 5-HT is metabolized to 5-HIAA by monoamine oxidase in the liver, and 5-HIAA is then excreted in the urine.[5]

Normal 24-hour excretion of 5-HIAA is 2–8 mg/day. Urinary 5-HIAA concentrations greater than 100 mg/day are highly specific for carcinoid tumors, and repeated measurements can be useful in determining the success of therapy.[10]

However, ingestion of many foods and drugs may interfere with measurement of 5-HIAA, including pineapples, walnuts, bananas, chocolate, kiwi, avocado, acetaminophen, aspirin, and ephedrine. Additionally, patients with malabsorption syndromes (i.e., Whipple's disease or nontropical sprue) and some types of cancer may have elevated 5-HIAA.[10]

5-HIAA is most useful as a diagnostic marker for midgut carcinoids with high tumor load; 5-HIAA measurements usually cannot detect foregut or hindgut carcinoid tumors that do not produce large amounts of 5-HT, and 5-HIAA may be only slightly elevated in patients with midgut carcinoid without metastasis.[11]

It is important to note that for cases of carcinoid syndrome, patients seldom experience symptoms until they have liver metastases. Although the surgery removed the original tumor in this patient, the liver metastases were still producing serotonin, and thus these analytes were still elevated.

5-HT in the circulation is actively absorbed by platelets; thus platelet 5-HT can also be used for diagnosis of carcinoids. Platelet 5-HT is a more sensitive diagnostic marker for carcinoid than is 5-HIAA and thus may be useful in detecting foregut and hindgut carcinoids. Additionally, platelet 5-HT concentrations are unaffected by consumption of serotonin-rich foods.[11] However, since concentrations of 5-HT in platelets are low (normal $= 125-500$ ng$/10^9$ platelets) and quantification can be technically challenging, most clinical laboratories routinely use urine 5-HIAA for diagnosis of carcinoid tumors.[8]

Abdominal computed tomography (CT) and Octreoscan imaging techniques are helpful in determining the location of carcinoid tumors and the extent of metastasis once diagnosis has been made biochemically.[10] Abdominal CT with radiographic contrast is a highly sensitive method for identifying carcinoid metastases to liver. Octreoscan involves ingestion of a radiolabeled octreotide (a somatostatin homolog). Since almost all neuroendocrine tumors have somatostatin receptors, the radiolabeled octreotide is taken up by the carcinoid tumor, and the tumor may then be visualized using scintigraphy. Octreoscan is more sensitive than CT in determining the location of the primary tumor.

Treatment and Prognosis

When possible, surgical removal of carcinoid tumors is the best therapy.[3,5] When complete removal of the tumor is impossible, debulking can help relieve symptoms of carcinoid syndrome. Frequently liver metastases are debulked using ablation therapy, either cryoablation or radiofrequency ablation. Another debulking technique is hepatic artery embolization (stopping blood flow to tumor), either alone or in combination with chemotherapeutic agents.

The most helpful pharmacotherapeutic agent for patients with carcinoid syndrome is the somastatin analog, octreotide, which is sold under the brand name Sandostatin (Novartis Pharmaceuticals Corp., East Hanover, NJ).[3,12] Octreotide controls the symptoms of carcinoid syndrome in most patients, and may prevent tumor growth or even destroy existing tumor in some patients. Octreotide is available in either a short-acting (given by injection 3–4 times per day) or long-acting (taken every 10–14 days) formulation.

Since carcinoid tumor growth is very slow, the prognosis for most patients is encouraging.[3] When tumors have not metastasized, complete surgical removal of the tumor usually cures the patient. Survival rates are not quite so high for patients with metastasis, especially those exhibiting the carcinoid syndrome, but with new treatments most patients can expect to live more than 5 years after diagnosis.

References

1. CAPLIN, M. E., BUSCOMBE, J. R., HILSON, A. J. ET AL.: Carcinoid tumour. *Lancet 352*:799–805, 1998.
2. KULKE, M. H. AND MAYER, R. J.: Carcinoid tumors. *N. Engl. J. Med. 340*:858–68, 1999.
3. WARNER, R. P.: *Review of Carcinoid Disease*, The Carcinoid Cancer Foundation, Inc., 2003.
4. SITARAMAN, S. V. AND GOLDFINGER, S. E.: Carcinoid tumors. *Up-to-Date Online* [12.3] 8/25/2004.
5. LIPS, C. J., LENTJES, E. G., AND HOPPENER, J. W.: The spectrum of carcinoid tumours and carcinoid syndromes. *Ann. Clin. Biochem. 40*:612–27, 2003.
6. VINIK, A. Carcinoid tumors, *Endotext. org.* 8/2/2004.
7. SITARAMAN, S. V. AND GOLDFINGER, S. E. The carcinoid syndrome. *Up-to-Date Online* [12.3] 7/30/2002.
8. KEMA, I. P., DE VRIES, E. G., AND MUSKIET, F. A.: Clinical chemistry of serotonin and metabolites. *J. Chromatogr. B, Biomed. Sci. Appl. 747*:33–48, 2000.
9. HENSON, D. E. AND ALBORES-SAAVEDRA, J., eds.: *Pathology of Incipient Neoplasia*, 3rd ed., Oxford University Press, Oxford, UK, 2001.
10. SITARAMAN, S. V. AND GOLDFINGER, S. E.: Diagnosis of the carcinoid syndrome. *Up-to-Date Online* [12.3] 8/31/2001.
11. MEIJER, W. G., KEMA, I. P., VOLMER, M. ET AL.: Discriminating capacity of indole markers in the diagnosis of carcinoid tumors. *Clin. Chem. 46*:1588–96, 2000.
12. SITARAMAN, S. V. AND GOLDFINGER, S. E.: Treatment of carcinoid tumors and the carcinoid syndrome. *Up-to-Date Online* [12.3] 3/24/2003.

Part Ten

Genetically Inherited Disorders

Cases of medium-chain acyl CoA dehydrogenase (MCAD), methylmalonic acidemia, ornithine transcarbamylase deficiency, "Maple syrup" urine disease (MSLID), and isovaleric acidemia are presented and discussed in Cases 34, 35, 36, 37, and 38, respectively (all edited by AMG); cases of Angelman syndrome and hemochromatosis are reported in Cases 39 (edited by MGS) and 40 (edited by CSE), respectively.

Tietz's Applied Laboratory Medicine, Second Edition. Edited by Mitchell G. Scott, Ann M. Gronowski, and Charles S. Eby
Copyright © 2007 John Wiley & Sons, Inc.

Case 34

Feed a Cold

Dennis Dietzen

A 19-month-old male was taken to a local emergency department after being found unresponsive in his crib at 10:00 am (1000 h). The child had been well until the previous day, when he was noted to be sleepy and went to bed earlier than usual at 4:00 pm (1600 h). Initial blood chemistry analysis revealed a glucose of 12 mg/dL (0.67 mmol/L), total CO_2 of 18 mmol/L (normal 20–28 mmoL/L), normal electrolytes, and an anion gap of 17 (normal 4–14) with a normal lactate concentration. The elevated anion gap prompted toxicologic analysis for illicit drugs of abuse, salicylates, acetaminophen, and ethanol. These analyses were negative. Urinalysis revealed trace ketones and calcium oxalate crytstals. The patient was immediately started on IV glucose for profound hypoglycemia and adminstered 4-methylpyrazole (Fomepazole), a synthetic inhibitor of alcohol dehydrogenase for suspected ethylene glycol poisoning. En route to a tertiary care pediatric hospital he developed generalized seizure activity requiring lorazepam, phenobarbital, and phenytoin for control.

On arrival at the pediatric hospital, physical exam was remarkable for a decreased temperature of 94°F (34.4°C), heart rate of 113, respiratory rate of 30, and blood pressure of 103/50. The heart rate and rhythm were regular, and the lungs were normal. The extremities were cool distally but well perfused. Neurologically, the child had diffusely decreased tone and did not withdraw his extremities in response to noxious stimuli, or exhibit spontaneous movement. Because of a possible infectious cause for the encephalopathy, the child was empirically treated with cefotaxime, acyclovir, and doxycycline pending the results of serology and spinal fluid studies. Both culture and PCR analyses for herpes simplex virus and Epstein–Barr virus were negative. Bartonella serology was also negative.

An examination of the family history revealed that the patient was the product of nonconsanguineous parents and had three healthy siblings, 9- and 13-year-old brothers, and a 15-year-old sister. A paternal uncle and multiple children in the maternal lineage died in infancy of unknown causes. This family history prompted submission of serum samples for amino acid and acylcarnitine analysis and urine for organic acid analysis. Serum amino acid analysis was unremarkable, but urine organic acid analysis (see Fig. 34.1) showed elevated concentrations of adipic, suberic, and 5-OH hexanoic acids, in addition to hexanoylglycine. Hexanoyl, octanoyl, and decanoylcarnitine were present in plasma at concentrations 10,000, 25, and 2 times the upper limit of normal, respectively. These findings were consistent with the diagnosis of medium-chain acyl

Tietz's Applied Laboratory Medicine, Second Edition. Edited by Mitchell G. Scott, Ann M. Gronowski, and Charles S. Eby
Copyright © 2007 John Wiley & Sons, Inc.

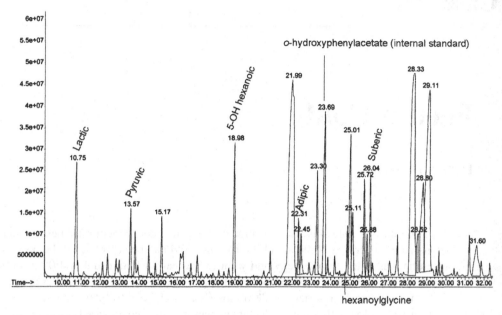

Figure 34.1   Chromatogram of urinary organic acid analysis for potential MCAD deficiency.

CoA dehydrogenase (MCAD) deficiency. The diagnosis was confirmed by genetic testing that revealed a homozygous A→ G mutation at nucleotide 985.

Definition of the Disease

MCAD deficiency (reviewed in 1,2) was first described in 1982 and is now recognized as one of the most common inborn metabolic disorders predominantly affecting Caucasians of northern European descent. The MCAD gene has been localized to chromosome 1, and defects are inherited in an autosomal recessive pattern. MCAD deficiency leads to an inability to completely oxidize fatty acids, impairing the supply of respiratory substrates to multiple tissues during times of prolonged fasting. The condition is commonly unknown until a period of decreased oral intake occurs in conjunction with an intercurrent illness as simple as a cold or the flu. The main clinical features of the disease include vomiting, lethargy, coma, and seizures. During acute episodes, common laboratory findings include hypoglycemia, mild hyperammonemia, mild acidosis, and increased circulating liver enzyme activities. The severity of the disorder may vary widely even in the same family ranging from complete lack of symptoms to sudden death from a single episode.

Pathogenesis

During periods of fasting, circulating glucose concentration is normally maintained by glycogenolysis and gluconeogenesis. When glucose stores are exhausted, nonesterified fatty acids are mobilized from adipose tissue and become the major oxidative substrate for a number of tissues, including the liver and both cardiac and skeletal muscle. The brain does not oxidize fatty acid directly but instead relies on acetoacetate and β-OH butyrate, products of the acetyl CoA derived from β-oxidation.[3]

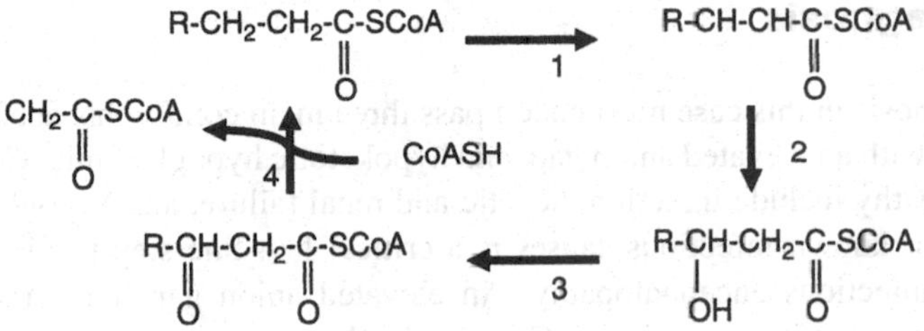

R-CH$_2$-CH$_2$-C-SCoA $\xrightarrow{\quad 1 \quad}$ R-CH-CH-C-SCoA
║ O ║ O

CH$_2$-C-SCoA $\xleftarrow{\quad 4 \quad}$ CoASH

║ O

R-CH-CH$_2$-C-SCoA $\xleftarrow{\quad 3 \quad}$ R-CH-CH$_2$-C-SCoA
║ O ║ O   OH ║ O

Figure 34.2   β-Oxidation cycle.

Fatty acids are transported in blood bound to albumin and enter cells by both diffusion and carrier-mediated pathways. The oxidation of long-chain fatty acids begins with transport through the mitochondrial membrane system in the form of carnitine esters and delivery to the mitochondrial matrix as coenzyme A thioesters. The β-oxidation spiral consists of the ordered activity of four enzymes (see Fig. 34.2): (1) acyl CoA dehyrodgenase, (2) enoyl CoA hydratase, (3) 3-hydroxylacyl CoA dehydrogenase, and (4) 3-ketoacylthiolase. Each successive turn of the cycle results in the formation of one molecule of acetyl CoA and a fatty acid that is two carbon atoms shorter than when it entered the β-oxidation cycle.

Long-chain fatty acyl CoA esters are initially oxidized by an acyl CoA dehyrogenase specific for chain lengths of 14–20 carbon atoms. When shortened to less than 14 carbons, the acyl CoA esters become substrates for another dehydrogenase specific for chain lengths ranging from 4 to 12 carbon atoms. There is an additional acyl CoA dehydrogenase activity in the mitochondrial matrix with specifity toward carbon chains that are 4 and 6 carbons in length.

The metabolic consequences associated with decreased activity of medium-chain acyl CoA dehydrogenase can be traced directly to diminished synthesis of acetyl CoA. Inadequate substrate acetyl CoA first prevents citrate formation. In the mitochondrial matrix, citrate is necessary for the continued operation of the Krebs cycle and adequate generation of ATP. Inadequate supplies of cytosolic acetyl CoA prevent the formation of N-acetylglutamate and malonyl CoA. The former is required for carbamylphosphate synthase activity, the initial step in urea synthesis. The latter is a potent inhibitor of mitochondrial fatty acid uptake. The net effect of diminished acetyl CoA, then, is decreased ATP production, hyperammonemia, and uncontrolled accumulation of fatty acyl CoA intermediates leading to a restricted pool of free CoA. Without an adequate pool of free CoA, propionyl carboxylase is also inhibited. This enzyme begins the process of pyruvate conversion to glucose (gluconeogenesis) and contributes to the profound hypoglycemia associated with MCAD deficiency.

The accumulated fatty acyl CoA intermediates have two potential metabolic fates:

1. They may become substrates for microsomal ω-oxidation, a process resulting in the formation of dicarboxylic fatty acids. These dicarboxylic acids (adipic, suberic, and sebacic) are readily excreted in the urine and are a sensitive indicator of disturbances in medium-chain fatty acid oxidation. These compounds lack specificity, however, as they are also detected during fasting uncomplicated by metabolic disease.

2. The excess fatty acyl CoA species shift the acyl CoA ↔ acylcarnitine equilibrium in the direction of acylcarnitine formation. These resulting medium-chain acylcarnitine species circulate in blood in abnormally high concentration. The presence of elevated C6–C10 carnitine esters in blood is both a sensitive and specific indicator of MCAD deficiency.

Differential Diagnosis

The differential diagnosis in this case must encompass three main conditions: acute encephalopathy, acidosis with an elevated anion gap, and hypoketotic hypoglycemia. Common causes of encephalopathy include infection, hepatic and renal failure, and hypoglycemia. Laboratory testing for known infectious causes is a critical first-line step to distinguish infectious from noninfectious encephalopathy. An elevated anion gap may arise from an endogenous or exogenous source of acid. Common endogenous acids that potentially elevate the anion gap are L-lactic acid, D-lactic acid, β-hydroxybutyric acid, and acetoacetic acid. Ingestion of a variety of common substances may also precipitate an elevated anion gap. The presence of oxalate crystals in the urine of the infant in this case suggested ingestion of ethylene glycol, which is oxidized to glycolic and oxalic acids. Comprehensive toxicology screening is necessary to rule out accidental or intentional ingestion. Finally, hypoketotic hypoglycemia in a child may arise from hyperinsulemic states (hypersecretion or criminal administration), growth hormone deficiency, or disorders of fatty acid oxidation or ketogenesis. The clinical context is key to delineating the cause for the hypoglycemia. Hypoglycemia that occurs postprandially or following a short fast suggests endocrine causes, while longer fasts (>12 hours) suggest a disorder in fatty acid oxidation or ketogenesis.

Guided by early laboratory studies that did not support an infectious or toxicologic etiology for the encephalopathy and a family history significant for sudden death in infancy, the acidosis and hypoglycemia pointed to an inborn error of metabolism. The specific enzyme defect can often be isolated by biochemical analyses. In MCAD deficiency, medium-chain dicarboxylic acids (e.g., adipic, suberic, sebacic), hexanoylglycine, 3-phenylpropionylglycine, and suberylglycine may all be detected during acute illness. In between episodes, however, organic acid excretion may be normal. Analysis of serum acylcarnitines suffers less from limitations due to episodic excretion. Abnormal organic acids that accumulate in cells circulate in blood as carnitine esters that are analyzed by tandem mass spectrometry in centers specializing in inborn metabolic disease. As in this case, specific acylcarnitine patterns can establish a diagnosis with high probability. Genetic analyses play a limited role in the diagnosis of fatty acid oxidation disorders, except in the case of MCAD deficiency. In MCAD deficiency, A → G substitution at nucleotide 985 results in a missense mutation (Lys → Asp) and accounts for 90% of disease-causing mutations. In other disorders, when acylcarnitine analysis and genetic testing cannot provide a definitive diagnosis, enzymatic activity studies in cultured fibroblasts are required to establish a specific diagnosis.

Prognosis and Treatment

The prognosis for undiagnosed MCAD deficiency is poor. The initial presentation is fatal in 20–25% of the cases, and many more cases of sudden death in infants due to MCAD deficiency may go undiagnosed. One postmortem analysis of blood from 7000 cases of sudden death in infants uncovered 23 cases of MCAD deficiency.[4] Children who do survive the initial episode have a high probability for permanent cognitive impairment.

The treatment for MCAD deficiency is two-pronged and highly effective. The two mainstays of treatment are avoidance of fasting and supplementation with carnitine. The former prevents mobilization and oxidation of fatty acids. Particular attention to caloric requirements must be paid during periods of illness that precipitate long periods of fasting. Carnitine serves as a detoxifying agent to remove toxic medium-chain fatty acyl intermediates. In one 3-year follow-up study of MCAD-deficient patients, 71% did not have a recurrence of symptoms after initiation of such treatment.[5]

Because of its sudden and unsuspected onset, high mortality and morbidity, and effective treatment, MCAD deficiency is an attractive candidate for newborn screening programs. At least 26 states currently carry out screening for this disorder using tandem mass spectrometry. Continued expansion of newborn screening will prevent the development of catastrophic illness, permanent neurologic damage, and death due to MCAD deficiency.

References

1. ROE, C. R. AND DING, J.: Mitochondrial fatty acid oxidation disorders. In *The Metabolic and Molecular Bases of Inherited Disease*, 8th ed., D. R. SCRIVER, A. L. BEAUDET, W. S. SLY, AND D. VALLE, eds., McGraw-Hill, New York, 2001, pp. 2297–326.

2. WANDERS, R. J. A., VREKEN, P., DEN BOER, M. E. J., WIJBURG, F. A., VAN GENNIP, A. H., AND IJLST, L.: Disorders of mitochondrial fatty acyl CoA β-oxidation. *J. Inher. Metab. Dis. 22:*442–87, 1999.

3. WOLFE, R. R.: Metabolic Interactions between glucose and fatty acids in humans. *Am. J. Clin. Nutr. 67:* 519S–26S, 1998.

4. CHACE, D. H., DIPERNA, J. C., MITCHELL, B. L., SGROI, B., HOFMAN, L. F., AND NAYLOR, E. W.: Electrospray tandem mass spectrometry for analysis of acylcarnitines in dried postmortem blood specimens collected at autopsy from infants with unexplained cause of death. *Clin. Chem. 47:*1166–82, 2001.

5. IAFOLLA AK, THOMPSON RJ, ROE CR. Medium-chainacyl CoA dehydrogenase deficiency: clinical course in 120 affected children. J. Pediatr. 124:409–15, 1994.

Case 35

Acute Neonatal Ammonia Intoxication

Dennis Dietzen

An 8-day-old infant presented to the emergency unit of an outside hospital with a 2-day history of decreased responsiveness, decreased urine output, and grunting. The patient was the product of a full-term pregnancy and was delivered vaginally without complications. On presentation his vital signs were significant for temperature of 94.6°F (34.8°C), pulse of 120, respiratory rate of 40, and blood pressure of 80/45. Physical exam revealed a soft, nontender abdomen without hepatosplenomegaly. Urine ketones were strongly positive, and remarkable blood chemistry values are shown below:

Analyte	Value, Conventional Units	Reference Interval, Conventional Units	Value, SI Units	Reference Interval, SI Units
Glucose	6 mg/dL	40–100	0.33 mmol/L	2.2–5.5
Total CO$_2$	8 mmol/L	20–28	Same	
Ammonia	3128 μmol/L	0–40	Same	
Total calcium	5 mg/dL	8.0–11.5	1.25 mmol/L	2.0–2.9
pH	7.23	7.35–7.45	Same	
Anion gap	25 mmol/L	4–14	Same	
Creatinine	1.4 mg/dL	0.1–0.5	124 μmol/L	8.9–44

The patient was started on intravenous glucose and calcium gluconate. Due to serum ammonia concentration, bolus doses of arginine, phenylacetate, and benzoic acid were administered for a presumptive urea cycle disorder. Following transport to a tertiary pediatric medical center, hemodialysis was initiated to achieve a rapid decrease of plasma ammonia to 127 μmol/L. CBC was notable for severe leukopenia (1200/μL, normal 5000–20,000/μL) and ampicillin, gentamicin, and fluconazole were administered because of the subsequent risk for infection. Liver enzyme studies revealed no abnormalities. Total bilirubin was slightly elevated at 3.6 mg/dL (61.6 μmol/L) for a child of his age (normal: 0.1–1.3 mg/dL, 1.7–22.2 μmol/L). Blood, urine, and spinal fluid were

Tietz's Applied Laboratory Medicine, Second Edition. Edited by Mitchell G. Scott, Ann M. Gronowski, and Charles S. Eby

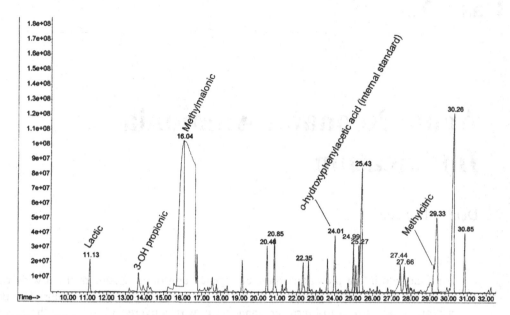

Figure 35.1 Chromatogram of urinary organic acid analysis from patient with methylmalonic acidemia.

collected for culture. Blood and urine samples were submitted for amino acid and organic acid analysis.

Serum and urine amino acid analysis did not reveal any abnormalities. This finding effectively excluded most urea cycle disorders. However, urine organic acid analysis (see Fig. 35.1) was notable for a methylmalonic acid concentration of 8200 μg/mg creatinine (normal: <5 μg/mg creatinine) and detection of methylcitric acid and 3-OH propionic acid (normal: undetectable). Serum volatile analysis was notable for a propionic acid concentration of 5200 μmol/L (normal: <5 μmol/L). On the basis of these laboratory tests, a diagnosis of methylmalonic acidemia was made. Phenylacetate, benzoic acid, and arginine were discontinued in favor of carnitine and vitamin B_{12} administration. Subsequent complementation analysis of dermal fibroblasts indicated that the mutation in this infant was of the mut^0 type.

Definition of the Disease

Methylmalonyl CoA mutase catalyzes the conversion of L-methylmalonyl CoA to succinyl CoA and has an absolute requirement for the cofactor, adenosylcobalamin. Methylmalonic acidemia (reviewed in 1), a deficiency of methylmalonyl CoA mutase activity, was first reported in the late 1960s. Mutase deficiency occurs in 1:50,000–1:80,000 births and is caused by a variety of mutations that affect either the mutase apoenzyme (mut^0, mut^- subtypes)[2] or the transport and synthesis of adenosylcobalamin (*cblA and cblB* subtypes).[3,4] The gene encoding the apoenzyme has been localized to chromosome 6. Mutations causing the mut^0 phenotype are associated with little or no detectable mutase activity or immunologically reactive protein. In the mut^- phenotype, an abnormal mutase is formed that exhibits a normal K_m for methylmalonyl CoA but a K_m for adenosylcobalamin that is elevated 200–5000 fold. The *cblA* subtype is caused by mutation in the MMAA gene on chromosome 4 that encodes a product putatively thought to mediate cobalamin transport into mitochondria. The *cblB* subtype has been traced to mutations in the MMAB gene on chromosome 12 that may play a role in the transfer of the adenosyl moiety to cobalamin.

The disease subtypes are indistinguishable at presentation, but the *mut*⁻, *cblA*, and *cblB* subtypes are generally responsive to cobalamin supplementation. All forms of the disease are inherited in an autosomal recessive fashion and characterized clinically by neonatal or infantile onset of lethargy, failure to thrive, recurrent vomiting, hypotonia, dehydration, and respiratory distress. Laboratory presentation includes severe metabolic ketoacidosis with an elevated anion gap and normal serum cobalamin concentrations. Other laboratory findings often include hypoglycemia, hyperammonemia, hyperglycinemia/glycinuria, leukopenia, and thrombocytopenia. Classic methylmalonyl CoA mutase deficiency is distinct from other disorders of cobalamin metabolism (*cblC*, *cblD*, *and CblF* subtypes) that cause a combined methylmalonic aciduria and homocystinuria. Methylmalonic acidemia should likewise not be confused with uncomplicated cobalamin deficiency that results in mild secondary elevations of circulating methylmalonic acid and megaloblastic anemia.

Pathogenesis

Like many other inborn errors of metabolism, clinical symptoms of methylmalonic acidemia are more likely to occur during a catabolic state. This state is induced when glucose/glycogen stores are depleted (e.g., during a long fast or minor illness). Tissue energy requirements are met by oxidation of fatty acids and ketones. During catabolism, Krebs cycle intermediates are utilized for the synthesis of glucose and fatty acids and replenishment of Krebs cycle carbon, a process termed *anaplerosis*, is achieved by mobilization of amino acids from muscle tissue. In particular, the carbon skeletons of valine, isoleucine, methionine, and threonine enter the citric acid cycle as succinyl CoA through a common three-carbon intermediate, propionyl CoA. Propionyl CoA carboxylase converts propionyl CoA to D-methylmalonyl CoA. Methylmalonyl CoA racemase then catalyzes isomerization of the D-methylmalonyl CoA to its L stereoisomer. Finally, branched-chain methylmalonyl CoA is linearized to succinyl CoA by methylmalonyl CoA mutase for entry into the citric acid cycle. Deficiency of propionyl CoA carboxylase has also been reported in this pathway (see Fig. 35.2). No cases of methylmalonyl CoA racemase deficiency have been documented.

Methylmalonyl CoA mutase deficiency leads to abnormal accumulation of other organic acids derived from propionyl CoA. Excessive propionyl CoA may become a

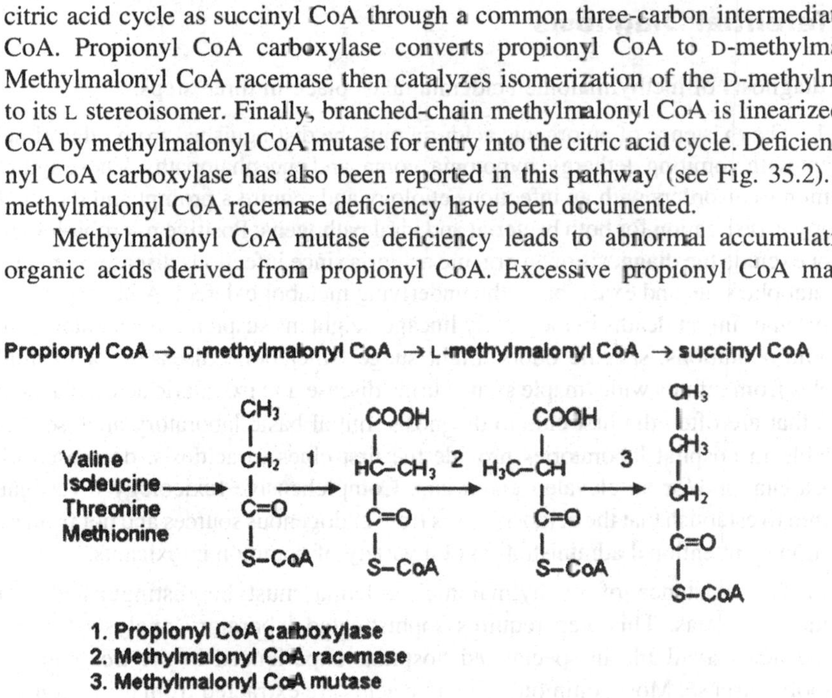

Propionyl CoA → D-methylmalonyl CoA → L-methylmalonyl CoA → succinyl CoA

1. Propionyl CoA carboxylase
2. Methylmalonyl CoA racemase
3. Methylmalonyl CoA mutase

Figure 35.2   Summary of pathway leading to succinyl CoA formation and entry into citric acid cycle.

substrate for citrate synthase and condense with oxaloacetate to form the seven carbon tricarboxylic acid, methylcitrate. Propionic acid itself is too volatile to be detected by standard urine organic acid analysis but a polar metabolite, 3-OH propionic acid, is also formed via mitochondrial β-oxidation or microsomal ω-oxidation. This compound along with malonic and tiglic acids are often detected in the urine of affected individuals.

The pathologic manifestations of methylmalonic acidemia are thought to arise by at least two mechanisms. The first is restriction of the intracellular CoA pool. As in many inborn metabolic errors, the accumulation of CoA intermediates reduces free CoA concentrations and restricts many mitochondrial processes. For example, low free CoA concentrations inhibit propionyl CoA carboxylase, thereby retarding gluconeogenesis and exacerbating hypoglycemia. In addition, low free CoA prevents proper operation of carbamyl phosphate synthase, the first step in urea synthesis, contributing to the hyperammonemia observed in affected individuals. As in the case presented here, hyperammonemia can be severe.

The organic acids that accumulate in methylmalonic aciduria may also directly poison mitochondrial metabolism. Intracellular methylmalonic acid concentrations in affected individuals may reach millimolar concentrations, and other metabolites such as methylcitric acid continue to accumulate over time. It has been hypothesized that methylmalonic acid directly inhibits the mitochondrial respiratory chain at complex II (succinate dehydrogenase), but there is little evidence to support this. It appears more likely that these acids act as competitive inhibitors of Krebs cycle operation. Methylmalonic acid inhibits generation of oxaloacetate by pyruvate carboxylase, a key anaplerotic enzyme, leading to depletion of Krebs cycle intermediates. Methylcitrate is a potent inhibitor of citrate synthase, aconitase, and isocitrate dehydrogenase activities leading to reduced flux through the cycle and reduced ATP synthesis.

Differential Diagnosis

The diagnosis of methylmalonic acidemia takes place in three steps:

1. The existence of an organic aciduria must be distinguished from other illnesses that present with vomiting, lethargy, hypotonia, coma, and encephalopathy. These symptoms are common to disorders with an infectious etiology and require a prompt and thorough microbiology investigation for both bacterial and viral pathogens. Positive microbiological studies do not exclude the diagnosis of an organic aciduria since infectious disease often precipitates the catabolic state and exacerbates the underlying metabolic defect. A history of consanguinity or other infant deaths in the family lineage heightens suspicion for metabolic disorders. In some conditions, specific odors might suggest metabolic disease. For example, urine samples from infants with "maple syrup" urine disease and isovaleric acidemia have distinct odors that are often the first clue to diagnosis. Initial basic laboratory analyses commonly available in hospital laboratories provide the first clues to acidosis: decreased blood pH, hypocapnia, and/or an elevated anion gap. Comprehensive toxicology investigations are required to establish that the acidosis arises from endogenous sources and not from accidental ingestion or intentional administration of a variety of common intoxicants.

2. The existence of methylmalonic acidemia must be distinguished from other organic acidemias. This step requires sophisticated laboratory analysis for amino and organic acids available in specialized hospitals experienced in the treatment of inborn metabolic disease. Most commonly, organic acids are extracted from urine, rendered volatile by derivatization, and then analyzed by gas chromatography/mass spectrometry. Metabolite identification is made on the basis of retention time and mass spectrum.

Severe deficiencies of methylmalonyl CoA mutase are accompanied by excessive excretion of methylmalonic acid and other upstream metabolites already mentioned such as methylcitrate and 3-OH propionate.

3. The subtype of methylmalonic aciduria must be identified for both therapeutic and prognostic purposes. These studies require cultures of dermal fibroblasts from the patient, which are examined for propionate uptake following fusion with cell lines of known phenotype. In the patient reported above, fibroblasts with the *cblA* and *cblB* phenotypes corrected deficient propionate uptake but cells with the *mut* phenotype did not. High doses of cobalamin were unable to restore propionate metabolism in the patient fibroblasts, indicating that the methylmalonyl CoA mutase deficiency in this patient was of the mut^0 variety and therefore unlikely to be responsive to vitamin B_{12} therapy.

Prognosis and Treatment

Four basic regimens are employed in the treatment of patients with methylmalonic academia: (1) supplementary vitamin B_{12} is utilized when indicated, (2) the diet is restricted in precursors of methylmalonic acid (valine, isoleucine, threonine, and methionine) and frequent feedings are used to avoid development of a catabolic state, (3) L-carnitine is administered under the premise that excretion of accumulated metabolites of methylmalonic acid is enhanced, and (4) chronic oral antibiotic therapy has been utilized in some cases to decrease the generation of propionic acid by gut bacteria.

Better recognition and earlier treatment have led to dramatic improvements in long-term survival.[5] Survival rates of the initial metabolic crisis improved from 30% in the 1970s to better than 90% in the 1990s. The clinical course of the disease correlates mainly with response to vitamin B_{12}. Patients with the mut^0 phenotype are not responsive to vitamin B_{12} and have the worst prognosis. Nearly all of these patients suffer early death and severe developmental impairment. Patients with the mut^- or *cblB* phenotypes have an intermediate prognosis, with about half remaining well through their early teens. Patients with the *cblA* phenotype are very responsive to vitamin B_{12}, and about 70% remain well into their teens. With increased survival, however, has come recognition of the long-term complications of the disease. The most common of these include growth and mental retardation, movement disorders related to the destruction of the basal ganglia, and chronic renal failure.[6] Screening for methylmalonic acidemia is included in the expanded newborn screening programs of many states and might be expected to further enhance the survival and delay onset of the complications of this disorder.

References

1. FENTON, W. A., GRAVEL, R. A., AND ROSENBLATT, D. S.: Disorders of propionate and methylmalonate metabolism. In *The Metabolic and Molecular Bases of Inherited Disease*, 8th ed., D. R. SCRIVER, A. L. BEAUDET, W. S. SLY, AND D. VALLE, eds., McGraw-Hill, New York, 2001, pp. 2165–93.

2. LEDLEY, F. D. AND ROSENBLATT, D. S.: Mutations in *mut* methylmalonic acidemia: Clinical and enzymatic correlations. *Hum. Mutat.* 9:1–6, 1997.

3. DOBSON, C. M., WAI, T., LECLERC, D. ET AL.: Identification of the gene responsible for the cblA complementation group of vitamin B_{12}-responsive methylmalonic acidemia based on analysis of prokaryotic gene

rearrangements. *Proc. Natl. Acad. Sci. USA* 99: 15554–9, 2002.

4. DOBSON, C. M., WAI, T., LECLERC, D. ET AL.: Identification of the gene responsible for the cblB complementation group of vitamin B_{12}-dependent methylmalonic aciduria. *Hum. Mol. Gen.* 11:3361–9, 2002.

5. HÖRSTER, F. AND HOFFMANN, G. F.: Pathophysiology, diagnosis, and treatment of methylmalonic aciduria-recent advances and new challenges. *Pediatr. Nephrol.* 19:1071–4, 2004.

6. BAUMGARTER, E. R. AND VIARDOT, C.: Long-term follow-up of 77 patients with isolated methylmalonic acidemia. *J. Inher. Metab. Dis.* 18:138–42, 1995.

Case 36

Not Just a Picky Eater

Douglas F. Stickle and Richard E. Lutz

An 18-month-old white female was transferred from an outside hospital for further evaluation of possible liver failure. Three weeks earlier, her parents noted repeated episodes of a decreased energy level and lethargy with tremors and shaking when the child was eating. Initial laboratory results ordered by the primary care physician were as follows:

Analyte	Value, Conventional Units	Reference Interval, Conventional Units	Value, SI Units	Reference Interval, SI Units
Na	141 mM	137–145	Same	
K	4.3 mM	3.6–5.0	Same	
Cl	101mM	98–107	Same	
CO_2	24 mM	15–35	Same	
BUN	2 mg/dL	4–20	0.71 mM	1.4–7.1
Cr	0.6 mg/dL	0.4–1.0	53 μM	35–88
ALKP	141 U/L	25–500	Same	
ALT	2494 U/L	3–45	Same	
AST	1344 U/L	20–60	Same	

The patient was referred to a secondary-level hospital where coagulopathy and hyperammonemia were also identified. Urine organic acids were sent to a reference laboratory. Results were as follows:

Analyte	Value, Conventional Units	Reference Interval, Conventional Units	Value, SI Units	Reference Interval, SI Units
NH_3, venous	356 μM	12–46	Same	
PT	24 s	11–15	Same	
PTT	67 s	22–36	Same	

The patient was then transferred to a tertiary care center and received fresh-frozen plasma transfusions and lactulose for elevated ammonia concentrations. EBV and hepatitis panels were negative. An ultrasound of the liver showed no lesions or abnormalities.

Tietz's Applied Laboratory Medicine, Second Edition. Edited by Mitchell G. Scott, Ann M. Gronowski, and Charles S. Eby
Copyright © 2007 John Wiley & Sons, Inc.

On physical exam the patient was a well-developed $1\frac{1}{2}$-year-old female who was awake but appeared lethargic. No scleral icterus was noted. The patient had been born at term by cesarean-section and has previously been healthy. Her immunizations were up-to-date. There were no known medical allergies. The patient's parents and a 4-year-old brother were apparently healthy. There was no family history of liver disease, including α1 antitrypsin deficiency or Wilson's disease. There was no family history of sudden infant death, hyperammonemia, or unexplained encephalopathy.

While the child was being evaluated at the tertiary care center, urine organic acid results were forwarded from the reference lab:

Analyte	Value, Conventional Units	Reference Interval, Conventional Units	Value, SI Units	Reference Interval, SI Units
Orotic acid	35 mmol/mol creatinine	<6	Same	

Elevated urine orotic acid, in combination with elevated ammonia, and the absence of other organic acid anomalies strongly suggested ornithine transcarbamylase (OTC) deficiency. Plasma amino acids obtained at the tertiary care center showed undetectable citrulline, ornithine at the upper limits of normal, and a relatively low arginine:

Analyte	Value, Conventional Units	Reference Interval, Conventional Units	Value, SI Units	Reference Interval, SI Units
Alanine	599 μM	152–459	Same	
Arginine	31 μM	32–153	Same	
Citrulline	0 μM	0–57	Same	
Glutamine	1327 μM	353–883	Same	
Methionine	65 μM	9–45	Same	
Ornithine	128 μM	18–136	Same	

The overall findings were consistent with a diagnosis of partial OTC deficiency. As urea is the end product of human nitrogen disposal, the relatively low BUN in the original laboratory findings was consistent with inadequate urea generation by the urea cycle.

Patient Outcome

The patient was placed on a protein-restricted diet (10 g/kg per day) and sodium phenylbutyrate (Buphenyl, 2 g per day). Liver function tests and ammonia improved dramatically over the course of 2 days of hospitalization. DNA studies for detection of mutations in the OTC gene are pending.

The patient's mother is expecting a male child in 3 months. Because of the possible X-linked hereditary nature of the patient's condition, the male fetus is at risk for a more severe form of OTC deficiency, which may present early in life with life-threatening hyperammonemia and hyperglutaminemia that can cause permanent brain damage and a high risk of neonatal death or long-term complications. Although prenatal diagnosis by mutation analysis for the fetus is available, this option was not chosen because of the late stage of the pregnancy. In addition, the patient's mother is at risk for postdelivery decompensation, if she is a partial OTC carrier who has not manifested the disease as yet. Because of these circumstances, it was recommended that the mother plan to deliver in a medical center that is equipped to deal with the possibility of severe neonatal illness, with neonatal ICU monitoring, monitoring of ammonia, and assessment of plasma amino acids recommended within the first day of life, as well as maternal observation in the postpartum period.

Definition of the Disease

Ornithine transcarbamylase (OTC) deficiency is an X-linked disorder that disables the entry of nitrogen into the urea cycle. Ornithine transcarbamylase catalyzes the condensation of ornithine with carbamyl phosphate derived from ammonia to form citrulline. The urea cycle, functioning primarily in liver cells, acts to eliminate nitrogen via the formation of urea, which is subsequently excreted in urine. Ammonia is derived primarily from amino acid catabolism; as proteins are constantly being both produced and degraded in normal metabolism, nitrogen disposal via the activity of the urea cycle is essential to prevent hyperammonemia. Deficiency of any of the five enzymes associated with the urea cycle is life-threatening because of the toxicity of high concentrations of ammonia, which can cause encephalopathy and death. Ammonia toxicity is the primary mode of presentation of cases of urea cycle defects, with symptoms of lethargy, vomiting, and coma. Because OTC deficiency is X-linked, severe neonatal cases are more likely in male than in female infants. Correspondingly, partial deficiency may exist in females, may go unrecognized or may have a delayed presentation that may be clinically less severe.

Differential Diagnosis

Hyperammonemia with encephalopathy is a central finding in clinical presentation of urea cycle defects. Hyperammonemia is, however, not a specific finding. The differential diagnosis from hyperammonemia is a long list of possible disorders, including renal disease, liver dysfunction of any etiology, and numerous specific inborn errors of metabolism that are not directly associated with the urea cycle (e.g., methylmalonic acidemia, pyruvate carboxylase deficiency), as well as deficiency of any one of the five central enzymes of the urea cycle. In the absence of patent liver or kidney dysfunction, it is essential to investigate such findings with both plasma amino acid and urine organic acid profiles. OTC deficiency will likely be characterized by elevated glycine, glutamine, and ornithine concentrations, with an unmeasurable concentration of citrulline, and a large elevation in urine orotic acid concentrations. Orotic acid is derived from the condensation of carbamyl phosphate with aspartate, and the large excess of orotate found in OTC deficiency is readily detected in urine. In complete OTC deficiency, with neonatal onset of symptoms, such a combination of findings would be regarded as diagnostic; in cases of later onset of symptoms, such findings (albeit potentially with comparatively lesser degrees of departure of analyte concentrations from their reference intervals) are strongly suggestive of partial OTC deficiency. In both cases, a definitive diagnosis can be obtained by enzymatic activity measurement from liver biopsy and/or genetic analysis for OTC mutations. Genetic analysis involves PCR amplification of DNA, single-strand conformational polymorphism (SSCP) analysis of the resulting fragments, and sequence analysis of any abnormal exon fragments. Approximately 75% of mutations are detectable by such an approach. Successful detection of a mutation makes possible carrier testing and allele tracking analysis. More than 240 mutations distributed throughout the OTC gene have been described, with 21% of those found in patients with late-onset disease.

It is essential in the initial stages of clinical management that ammonia measurements be made with careful adherence to specimen collection and handling requirements so as to avoid obtaining inaccurate and potentially misleading measurements due to preanalytical factors. Note also that plasma amino acids and urine organic acid analyses are not typically available with a rapid turnaround time, and symptomatic treatment must ensue on an emergent basis without a definitive diagnosis. However, it is possible that results of a large-panel metabolic profile from newborn screening by tandem mass spectrometry may be available, and this can be of some assistance in severe neonatal cases. In particular, tandem mass spectrometry for newborn screening samples can, in principle, detect profiles suggestive of deficiencies of the urea cycle other than OTC deficiency [specifically; citrullinemia, argininemia, and carbamyl phosphate synthetase (CPS) deficiency]. Late-onset or acquired forms of OTC deficiency in males is not unknown. In females, partial OTC deficiency may go undiagnosed, but may involve protein avoidance and sporadic or episodic sickness associated with food intake.

Treatment

Short-term emergency treatment of OTC deficiency involves management of hyperammonemia, which in severe cases can involve both dialysis and drug treatment to enhance nitrogen excretion. Pharmacologic intervention is to provide substrates (benzoate, phenylacetate) that can combine nitrogen from precursors to the urea cycle for subsequent elimination by excretion. Administration of sodium benzoate allows formation of excretable hippuric acid by combination with glycine. Administration of sodium phenylacetate allows formation of excretable phenylacetylglutamine by combination with glutamine.

Long-term treatment of OTC deficiency involves protein restriction as well as drug treatment. Long-term drug treatment utilizes oral phenylbutyrate, which is metabolized to phenylacetate. Because both citrulline and arginine are distal to OTC in the urea cycle, these are given as supplements in treatment of OTC deficiency. Vigilance must be maintained for hyperammonemia. Monitoring of plasma amino acids at regular intervals is recommended to detect any progressive change in effectiveness of treatment. Liver transplant has been utilized in some cases of complete OTC deficiency. Although treatment of OTC deficiency can prevent life-threatening hyperammonemia, the brain damage of toxic hyperammonemia that may have occurred during presentation of undiagnosed cases is not reversible. Nonetheless, treatment can prevent further cognitive decline. As is the case with all metabolic disorders, professional intervention should probably also extend beyond the patient to the realm of family studies and genetic counseling as appropriate.

Additional Reading

BACHMANN, C.: Inherited hyperammonemias. In *Physician's Guide to the Laboratory Diagnosis of Metabolic Diseases*, 2nd ed., N. BLAU, M. DURAN, M. E. BLASKOVICS, AND K. M. GIBSON, eds., Springer, Berlin, 2003.

LEONARD, J. V.: Disorders of the urea cycle. In *Inborn Metabolic Diseases*, 3rd ed., J. FERNANDES, J. M. SAUDUBRAY, AND G. VAN DEN BERGHE, eds., Springer-Verlag, Berlin, 2000.

MAESTRI, N. E., BRUSILOW, S. W., CLISSOLD, D. B., AND BASSETT, S. S.: Long-term treatment of girls with ornithine transcarbamylase deficiency. *N. Engl. J. Med.* 335:855–60, 1996.

Ornithine transcarbamylase deficiency (#311250): Online Mendelian inheritance in man [http://www. ncbi.nlm.nih. gov/entrez/dispomim.cgi?id = 311250 (accessed Oct. 2005)]. [Further information on laboratory practice in molecular analysis of ornithine transcarbamylase deficiency is available from the Biochemical Genetics and Metabolism Laboratory, Children's National Medical Center, Washington, DC: http://www.cnmcresearch.org/ testing/OTC_ FAX_ package.pdf (accessed Oct. 2005)].

SCAGLIE, F., ZHENG, Q., O'BRIEN, W. E. ET AL.: An integrated approach to the diagnosis and prospective management of partial ornithine transcarbamylase deficiency. *Pediatrics* 109:150–2, 2002.

TUCHMAN, M. AND BATSHAW, M. L.: Management of inherited disorders of ureagenesis. *Endocrinologist, 12*:99–109, 2002.

TUCHMAN, M., JALEEL, N., MORIZONO, H., SHEEHY, L., AND LYNCH, M. G.: Mutations and polymorphisms in the human ornithine transcarbamylase gene. *Hum. Mutat. 19*:93–107, 2002.

Case 37

The "Fussy" Neonate

Patricia M. Jones and Dinesh Rakheja

On day of life (DOL) 4, a Hispanic female infant presented to the emergency department (ED) with fussiness and crying. She was the second child of a 26-year-old mother. She was born at term via normal vaginal delivery and weighed 7 lb 5 oz at birth. The placental examination showed acute chorioamnionitis. Examination in the ED revealed bilateral corneal abrasions. Blood was collected for a sepsis workup, and she was sent home on antibiotics and eyedrops. On DOL 9 she was brought to the ED with complaints of decreased oral intake and increasing lethargy. Her breathing appeared labored. During examination in the ED, she became nonresponsive and required tracheal intubation and assisted ventilation; subsequently she was admitted to the intensive care unit.

Laboratory data were as follows:

Analyte	Value, Conventional Units	Reference Interval, Conventional Units	Value, SI Units	Reference Interval, SI Units
Sodium	136 mmol/L	135–146	Same	Same
Potassium	4.9 mmol/L	3.5–6.0	Same	Same
Chloride	108 mmol/L	98–106	Same	Same
CO_2	11 mmol/L	18–31	Same	Same
AGAP	17	7–16	Same	Same
Glucose	24 mg/dL	74–127	1.3 mmol/L	4.1–7.0
pH	7.23	7.35–7.45	Same	Same
pCO_2	24 mm Hg	35–48	3.19 kPa	4.66–6.38
pO_2	84 mm Hg	83–108	11.17 kPa	11.04–14.36
HCO_3	11 mmol/L	17–24	Same	Same
Base excess	−18 mEq/L	−7 to −1	−18 mmol/L	−7 to −1
Ammonia	50 μmol/L	56–92	Same	Same
ALT	10 U/L	6–50	Same	Same
AST	59 U/L	10–80	Same	Same

Blood cultures were negative.

The initial laboratory results for this infant showed severe hypoglycemia. There was a metabolic acidosis accompanied by an elevated anion gap and a base deficit of 18. These

Tietz's Applied Laboratory Medicine, Second Edition. Edited by Mitchell G. Scott, Ann M. Gronowski, and Charles S. Eby

results are suggestive of an inborn error of metabolism (IEM). Liver enzymes and ammonia were normal, essentially ruling out a urea cycle defect. A serum amino acid and urine organic acid were ordered immediately at the time of her second ED visit, and the results of those tests are as follows:

Analyte	Value, Conventional Units	Reference Interval, Conventional Units	Value, SI Units	Reference Interval, SI Units
Amino acid analysis, serum				
Leucine	4375 μmol/L	47–160 μmol/L	Same	Same
Isoleucine	588 μmol/L	26–91 μmol/L	Same	Same
Valine	1155 μmol/L	64–336 μmol/L	Same	Same
Organic acid analysis, urine (see also Fig. 37.1)	Presence of 2-hydroxyisovaleric acid, 2-hydroxyisocaproic acid, and 2-hydroxy-3-methylvaleric acid			

These results, along with the presence of alloisoleucine, are diagnostic for maple syrup urine disease (MSUD). Alloisoleucine is difficult to separate from other amino acids in a standard amino acid HPLC program. It usually coelutes with methionine, and so an

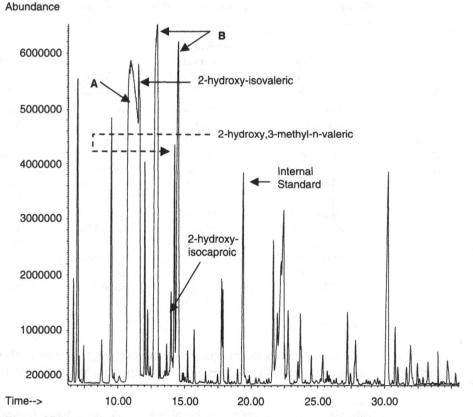

Figure 37.1   Organic acid profile showing the three diagnostic peaks (2-hydroxyisovaleric acid, 2-hydroxy, 3-methyl-*n*-valeric, 2-hydroxy-isocaproic) amid large peaks of 3-hydroxybutyric acid (A) and acetoacetate (B).

elevated methionine concentration in these patients may actually be alloisoleucine. In the organic acid analysis, the hydroxy analogs of the ketoacid forms result from the trimethylsilyl derivatization of the compounds when prepared for GC/MS analysis.

Definition of the Disease

Maple syrup urine disease (MSUD, Online Mendelian Inheritance in Man #248600; http://www.ncbi.nlm.nih.gov/entrez/dispomim.cgi?id = 248600) is a disorder of branched chain amino acid metabolism that is pan-ethnic and occurs in the general population at a frequency of about 1 : 185,000. In the Older Order Mennonite population in Pennsylvania, it occurs in approximately 1 in 176 newborns.

In the second step in catabolism of these amino acids, branched-chain α-keto acid dehydrogenase (BCKD, Enzyme Commission Number EC 1.2.4.4; http://www.expasy.ch/cgi-bin/nicezyme.pl?1.2.4.4) converts the α-keto acid form of leucine, isoleucine, and valine to the next step (Fig. 37.2). When BCKD is deficient, a buildup of the branched-chain amino acids and their corresponding branched-chain α-keto acids occurs.

MSUD patients can be divided into five phenotypes: classic, intermediate, intermittent, thiamine-responsive and dihydrolipoyl dehydrogenase (E3)–deficient. Classic MSUD is the most severe, with generally less than 2% of normal enzymatic activity. It presents with a neonatal onset of encephalopathy. The variant forms may have as much as 30% of normal enzymatic activity and generally present before 2 years of age.

Branched-chain amino acids constitute about 35% of the indispensable amino acids in muscle. They are both ketogenic and glucogenic, and are precursors for fatty acid and cholesterol synthesis, and substrates for energy production. The BCKD necessary for their metabolism is a multienzyme complex that contains three catalytic enzymes—a decarboxylase, a transacylase, and a dehydrogenase—and two regulatory enzymes—a phosphatase and a kinase—that control the BCKD complex activities. Because of this complexity, there is considerable genetic heterogeneity associated with MSUD. The genes for the catalytic enzymes have been assigned to four different chromosomes, and 63 mutations have currently been identified. Work is ongoing to correlate clinical phenotypes with genetic mutations.[1]

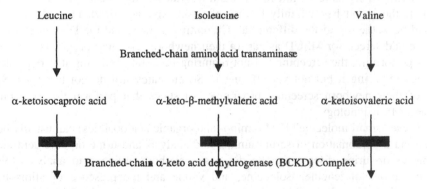

Figure 37.2   Initial steps in catabolism of the branched-chain amino acids. In MSUD the α-ketoacid dehydrogenase is deficient, resulting in the accumulation of the amino acids leucine, isoleucine, and valine, and their α-ketoacid transaminated forms.

Pathogenesis

The buildup of the branched-chain amino acids and their α-ketoacids, especially leucine, is toxic and has been implicated in affecting the biosynthesis of serotonin and catecholamines. The excess amino acids and ketoacids also interfere with neuronal and astrocyte metabolism. MSUD causes spongy changes in white matter and delayed myelination. Most untreated patients with the classic form of MSUD die in the early months of life from neurological deterioration and recurrent clinical crisis. Normal intellect is generally not seen in patients whose treatment is delayed until after 14 days of life. Rapid diagnosis and prompt treatment is essential for a positive long-term outcome.

Differential Diagnosis

The differential diagnosis in this infant at the time of her second ED visit included an IEM, sepsis, severe dehydration, and liver dysfunction, with IEM at the top of the list. Many IEM cases classically present a few days after birth with increasing lethargy and decreasing food intake or food intolerance. In utero these infants are well because of the normal functioning of the maternal enzymes to perform the reactions that are deficient in the fetus. Depending on the specific IEM in question, pregnancies are often uncomplicated, and weight and health status of the infant at birth are normal. After birth, the infant's own enzymes are required for metabolizing ingested nutrients, and complications ensue where a metabolic block exists. Classically these infants present with a variety of general symptoms that may include lethargy, hypotonia, hypoglycemia, acidemia, elevated liver enzymes, and hyperammonemia. Although not noted in this case, in some cases the urine may have an odor. For MSUD the odor would be sweet. The symptoms are similar to those that can be seen with an array of other disorders. Diagnosis is often compounded by the fact that an intercurrent infection may be present. In many cases the intercurrent infection may have actually precipitated the clinical crisis by requiring the neonate's body to utilize the deficient pathway, and thus exacerbating the effects of the deficiency.

While symptoms of inborn metabolism error are nonspecific, IEM should be ruled out in any infant who presents with these general symptoms, or a "failure to thrive" syndrome. The finding of sepsis or an infection should not rule out the possibility of a concomitant IEM. If the infant has a family history of an unexplained death in a sibling, an IEM should be at the top of the differential. Currently 36 states and the District of Columbia require and screen for MSUD as part of their newborn screening programs, with 3 more states performing the screening but not requiring it, 2 states offering it if requested, and 2 states requiring it but not yet offering it. Seven states still do not test for MSUD as part of their newborn screening programs. All states that perform this screening use tandem MS technology.

These "small molecule" IEM (amino- and organic acidopathies) can usually be diagnosed via a combination of serum amino acid analysis and urine organic acid analysis. Maple syrup urine disease can be diagnosed by both amino acid analysis (elevated concentrations of leucine, isoleucine, and valine and the presence of alloisoleucine) and organic acid analysis (the presence of 2-hydroxyisovaleric acid, 2-hydroxyisocaproic acid, and 2-hydroxy-3-methyl-N-valeric acid in the urine). Amino acid analysis is generally performed by ion exchange high-performance liquid chromatography (HPLC) coupled to a postcolumn addition of a colorimetric agent (frequently ninhydrin) and detection of the amino acids photometrically at 570 nm, or a combination of 570 nm and 440 nm. Organic acid analysis most commonly utilizes gas chromatography/mass spectrometry (GC/MS), in which the sample is extracted and then derivatized with trimethylsilane. Trimethylsilyl derivatives are fragmented by electron impact ionization in the mass spectrometer and identified by comparison to a library of mass spectra. Newborn screening methods generally identify a combination of amino acid and organic acid masses and retention times using liquid chromatography–tandem mass spectrometry (LC-MS/MS) methods in the multiple reaction monitoring (MRM) mode.

Treatment

The branched-chain amino acids leucine, isoleucine, and valine are essential amino acids. They are not produced in the body, but must be obtained in the diet, and are necessary for proper growth and development. Like many IEM forms of treatment, MSUD treatment requires a careful balancing act between supplying too few of the amino acids for proper growth, and supplying too many of the amino acids and causing a buildup of toxic concentrations of the amino acids or their metabolites.

Figure 37.3 shows the concentration of leucine present in this infant's blood from the date of diagnosis through the first year of life. The infant was on a restricted diet, and the difficulty in regulating this amino acid in the blood is clearly demonstrated. Valine and isoleucine concentrations showed similar results. Treatment for MSUD is essentially twofold: long-term dietary intervention to control the concentrations of the branched-chain amino acids and aggressive intervention during clinical crisis and periods of acute metabolic decompensation. Prognosis is much better for the variant forms than for classic MSUD; however, treatment regimens for the classic form continue to be improved.[2]

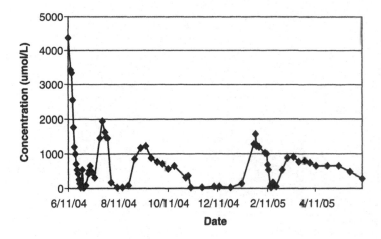

Figure 37.3   Leucine concentrations over the course of the first year of life.

References

1. NELLIS, M. M., KASINSKI, A., CARLSON, M. ET AL.: Relationship of causative genetic mutations in maple syrup urine disease with their clinical expression. *Mol. Genet. Metab. 80*:189–95, 2003.

2. MORTON, D. H., STRAUSS, K. A., ROBINSON, D. L., PUFFENBERGER, E. G., AND KELLEY, R. I.: Diagnosis and treatment of maple syrup disease: A study of 36 patients. *Pediatrics 109*:999–1008, 2002.

Additional Reading

CHUANG, D. T., AND SHIH, V. E.: Maple syrup urine disease (branched-chain ketoaciduria). In *The Metabolic and Molecular Bases of Inherited Disease*, 8th ed., C. R. SCRIVER, A. L. BEAUDET, W. S. SLY, ET AL., eds., McGraw-Hill, New York, 2001, pp. 1971–2005.

OGIER DE BAULNY, H. AND SAUDUBRAY, J. M.: Branched-chain organic acidurias. *Semin. Neonatol. 7*:65–74, 2002.

PEINEMANN, F. AND DANNER, D. J.: Maple syrup urine disease 1954 to 1993. *J. Inherit. Metab. Dis. 17*:3–15, 1994.

Case 38

The "Sleepy" Neonate

Dinesh Rakheja and Patricia M. Jones

A 9-day-old Hispanic boy was brought to the emergency room by his mother. Since his birth, his mother had noted that he was excessively sleepy, so much so that he would take a long time to feed because of his inability to stay awake. When he was brought to medical attention, the infant had not passed stool for the last 3 days. He had been delivered vaginally at 37 weeks after an uncomplicated pregnancy and weighed 7 lb 8 oz at birth. Examination in the emergency department showed an emaciated infant with a strong odor. The child was asleep during examination but could easily be awakened. There was no organomegaly, the abdomen was soft and nondistended, and bowel sounds were present. The clinical differential diagnostic considerations included sepsis and inborn errors of metabolism.

Initial laboratory results were as follows:

Analyte	Value, Conventional Units	Reference Interval, Conventional Units	Value, SI Units	Reference Interval, SI Units
Sodium	144 mmol/L	139–146	Same	Same
Potassium	4.8 mmol/L	3.0–7.0	Same	Same
Chloride	109 mmol/L	98–106	Same	Same
CO_2	15 mmol/L	18–31	Same	Same
AGAP	20	5–14	Same	Same
pH	7.43	7.35–7.45	Same	Same
pCO_2	22 mm Hg	41–54	2.93 kPa	5.47–7.20
pO_2	56 mm Hg	30–50	7.47 kPa	4.00–6.67
HCO_3	15 mmol/L	17–24	Same	Same
Base excess	−9 mEq/L	−7 to −1	−9 mmol/L	−7 to −1
Ammonia	179 μmol/L	56–92	Same	Same
ALT	12 U/L	5–45	Same	Same
AST	116 U/L	9–80	Same	Same
Glucose	57 mg/dL	74–127	3.17 mmol/L	4.1–7.1
Creatinine	0.9 mg/dL	0.2–0.6	79.56 μmol/L	17.68–53.04
Urea nitrogen	27 mg/dL	2–19	9.64 mmol/L	0.71–6.78

Tietz's Applied Laboratory Medicine, Second Edition. Edited by Mitchell G. Scott, Ann M. Gronowski, and Charles S. Eby

The normal pH with low serum bicarbonate and pCO_2 suggest respiratory compensation for a metabolic acidosis. The anion gap further points to the accumulation in the serum of an acidic anion, either exogenous or endogenous. In a neonate, with no history of exogenously administered substance, an inborn error of metabolism should be ruled out. Although the infant has hyperammonemia, a disorder of urea cycle is unlikely because those disorders are not associated with acidosis and usually result in much higher ammonia concentrations, often in the range of >1000 μmol/L. In fact, hyperammonemia may be found in other metabolic disorders including organic acidemias, congenital lactic acidosis, dibasic amino acid transport disorders, and fatty acid oxidation disorders. The hypoglycemia in this infant is probably secondary to poor oral intake. The mildly elevated serum creatinine and blood urea nitrogen are also likely due to poor oral intake and represent prerenal azotemia secondary to dehydration. In summary, the initial laboratory investigations suggest an inborn error of metabolism. With this in mind, further testing was performed to screen for a metabolic disorder including urine organic acid and serum acylcarnitine analyses (see also Figs 38.1 and 38.2):

Analyte	Value, Conventional Units	Reference Interval, Conventional Units	Value, SI Units	Reference Interval, SI Units
Organic acid analysis, urine	Massive excretion of isovalerylglycine and 3-hydroxyisovaleric acid			
Acylcarnitine analysis, serum				
Total acylcarnitine	98 μmol/L	0–26	Same	Same
Isovalerylcarnitine	16.8 μmol/L	0–0.7	Same	Same

While performing the urine organic acid profile, the metabolic laboratory technician noted that the urine had a distinctly strong odor that reminded her of the "rotten cheese"

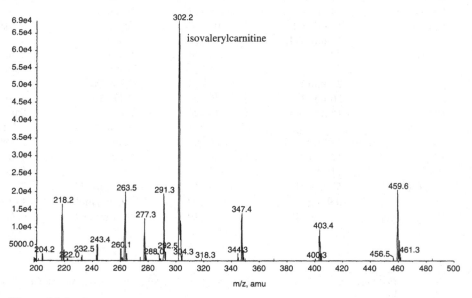

Figure 38.1   Serum acylcarnitine profile showing a large peak of isovalerylcarnitine.

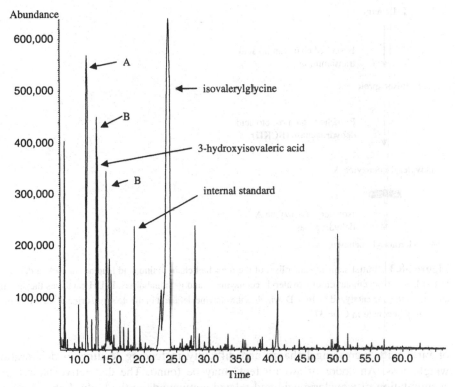

Figure 38.2   Urine organic acid profile showing large peaks of isovalerylglycine and 3-hydroxyisovaleric acid along with marked ketonuria (A—3-hydroxybutyrate; B—acetoacetate).

smell that emanates from poorly aereted feet after prolonged sweating. The marked elevations of serum isovalerylcarnitine and urine isovalerylglycine and 3-hydroxyiso valeric acid are diagnostic for isovaleric acidemia.

Definition of the Disease

Isovaleric acidemia (IVA, Online Mendelian Inheritance in Man #243500; http://www.ncbi.nlm.nih.gov/entrez/dispomim.cgi?id = 243500) is an inborn error of metabolism caused by a deficiency of the enzyme isovaleryl–coenzyme A dehydrogenase (IVDH, Enzyme Commission EC 1.3.99.10; http://www.expasy.ch/cgi-bin/nicezyme.pl?1.3.99.10). The disorder is not rare, and newborn screening programs have established the prevalence of IVA to be 1 in 62,500 newborns in Germany and 1 in 250,000 in United States.[1,2] It is inherited as an autosomal recessive disease, and the gene that encodes IVDH resides on chromosome 15q14-q15. IVDH is a mitochondrial enzyme that catalyzes the oxidation of isovaleryl–coenzyme A to 3-methylcrotonyl–coenzyme A, a step in the catabolic pathway of the ketogenic branched-chain amino acid leucine (Fig. 38.3).

With respect to clinical presentation, we can classify patients with IVA into two broad categories: those who present in early neonatal life with a sudden-onset severe illness and those who have chronic intermittent disease and present later in infancy. Our patient had the classic features of neonatal-onset IVA. Typically, the illness begins within a few days

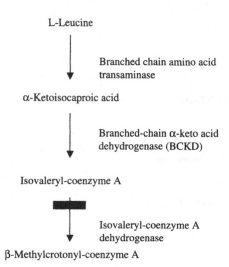

L-Leucine

Branched chain amino acid
transaminase

α-Ketoisocaproic acid

Branched-chain α-keto acid
dehydrogenase (BCKD)

Isovaleryl-coenzyme A

Isovaleryl-coenzyme A
dehydrogenase

β-Methylcrotonyl-coenzyme A

Figure 38.3   Initial steps in catabolism of the branched-chain-amino acid leucine. In IVA, a deficiency of IVDH leads to accumulation of isovaleryl–coenzyme A and its metabolites. IVDH catalyzes the step immediately after the one catalyzed by BCKD, which is the enzyme deficient in maple syrup urine disease (see the case of the "fussy" neonate in Case 37).

of birth with increasing lethargy and difficulty in feeding leading to dehydration and weight loss. An "odor of sweaty feet" may be found. The distinctive odor represents accumulation of isovaleric acid and related compounds in the body. Laboratory investigation typically shows metabolic acidosis with mild lactic acidemia and ketosis. There may be pancytopenia, hypocalcemia, and hyperammonemia. Many neonates do not survive the acute illness and die of acidosis, cerebral edema, infections, and/or bleeding. Those who do survive the initial acute phase go on to follow a chronic intermittent course. Patients with the chronic intermittent form of the disease typically have had their first episode of acute illness by the time they are one year old. The acute episodes usually follow a minor stress such as an upper respiratory infection and sometimes increased intake of protein-rich foods. The usual symptoms include lethargy, vomiting, and "sweaty feet odor," with laboratory evidence of acidosis and pancytopenia. Some of these patients may have hyperglycemia, which along with ketosis can lead to a misdiagnosis of diabetic ketoacidosis. The acute symptoms resolve with protein-restricted diet, and these children may learn to avoid protein-rich foods. This dietary strategy and fewer numbers of infections lead to fewer acute episodes, as the child grows older. Some children may have developmental delay and mental retardation, probably a result of untreated acute events.

Pathogenesis

IVDH is a homotetramer; it is composed of four identical peptides. It is initially synthesized in the cytoplasm as a 45 kDa precursor peptide. The precursor protein undergoes posttranslational processing, during its transport into the mitochondria, to form the mature 43 kDa peptide. Four of these mature peptides form a homotetramer with the dehydrogenase activity. Six classes of variant enzymes are recognized on the basis of molecular heterogeneity. Class I mutant alleles show point mutations and normal processing, so that the molecular weights of the precursor and mature peptides are normal. Classes II, III, and IV mutant alleles show point mutations or small deletions that lead to the formation of smaller precursor peptides and/or smaller mature peptides. Classes V and VI mutant alleles form no protein product at all. Class V mutant alleles form an apparently normal mRNA that is not further translated into the precursor peptide. On the other hand, class VI mutant alleles form unstable mRNA or have defective transcription so that no mRNA is formed. With the wider use of expanded neonatal screening programs, a relatively common mutation (932C > T) has been identified that is associated with a mild IVA phenotype, suggesting a genotype–phenotype correlation.[3]

A deficiency of IVDH leads to a block in the conversion of isovaleryl–coenzyme A to 3-methylcrotonyl–coenzyme A and an excessive accumulation of isovaleryl–coenzyme A. The body tries to rid itself of the toxic isovaleryl–coenzyme A by conjugating it with glycine and carnitine to form isovalerylglycine and isovalerylcarnitine. These compounds are relatively nontoxic, water-soluble, and readily excreted in urine. Other metabolites of isovaleric acid include 3-hydroxyisovaleric acid and 4-hydroxyvaleric acid; the latter is further oxidized to methylsuccinic acid, which is then dehydrogenated to methylfumaric acid. Methylsuccinic and methylfumaric acids may also be detected in the urine as may some other minor metabolites such as 3-hydroxyisoheptanoic acid, isovalerylglutamic acid, isovalerylglucuronide, isovalerylalanine, and isovalerylsarcosine. The pathophysiologic basis of the toxicity of isovaleric acid and its metabolites is not completely elucidated. In high concentrations seen in symptomatic patients, isovaleric acid inhibits succinate–coenzyme A ligase in the tricarboxylic acid cycle and is also toxic to granulopoietic precursors in bone marrow cultures. Isovaleryl coenzyme A inhibits the urea cycle enzyme, N-acetylglutamate synthetase, explaining the occurrence of hyperammonemia.

Differential Diagnosis

Failure to thrive with increasing lethargy in infants may occur as a result of sepsis, but should always raise the possibility of an underlying inborn error of metabolism. In fact, sepsis may unmask an underlying metabolic disorder and be the first presentation of an inborn error of metabolism. The initial laboratory workup, in a symptomatic child, will provide clues for more definitive tests. The "sweaty feet" odor of IVA may occur in patients with other branched-chain organic acidemias, most notably glutaric aciduria type II or multiple coenzyme A carboxylase deficiency that lead to the accumulation of metabolic intermediates with similar odor. However, urine organic acid profile of markedly elevated isovalerylglycine and 3-hydroxyisovaleric acid are characteristic for IVA. Other organic acidemias have different and characteristic combinations of organic acid excretion patterns.

The diagnosis of IVA can be made by gas chromatography/mass spectrometry (GC/MS) analysis of urine for organic acids, which shows the typical profile of elevated isovalerylglycine and 3-hydroxyisovaleric acid. Other intermediates of this pathway may also be excreted in the urine. Column chromatography is the method of separation of substances in a mixture based on the relative affinity of the substances for stationary phase (chromatography column) and mobile phase (carrier gas or liquid in which the mixture is carried through the chromatography column). For GC, the relevant substances (organic acids) in the mixture (urine) are first extracted (with organic solvents) and chemically modified (by making trimethylsilyl derivatives) so that they are easily volatilized and carried by the mobile gaseous phase (nitrogen gas). As the purified organic acids elute out of the chromatography column, they are presented to the mass spectrometer coupled to the chromatograph. Here the purified organic acids are bombarded by electrons and fragmented into ions (electrospray inonization). Each organic acid has a characteristic ion spectrum (mass spectrum) that can then be used in its identification. Liquid chromatography/tandem mass spectrometry (LC/MS/MS) works on principles similar to those of GC/MS. LC utilizes a liquid mobile phase (acetonitrile) and the substances of interest do not have to be volatilized. Coupling of two mass spectrometers in "tandem" (MS/MS) allows a greater degree of specificity and sensitivity in identification of substances. LC/MS/MS has revolutionized newborn screening for metabolic disorders and can detect elevated concentrations of isovalerylcarnitine in microliter quantities of blood. Similarly, LC/MS/MS can help in prenatal diagnosis by detecting isovalerylcarnitine in amniotic fluid. If required, IVDH deficiency may be demonstrated by in vitro enzyme assay in fibroblasts grown from a patient's skin biopsy. Currently 25 states require and screen for IVA as part of their newborn screening programs, with 6 more states performing the screening but not requiring it, 2 states offering it if requested, and 3 states requiring it but not yet offering it. Fourteen states and District of Columbia do not test for IVA as part of their newborn screening programs. All states that perform this screening use LC/MS/MS technology.

Treatment

Since IVA occurs as a result of a block in leucine catabolism, the basics of treatment for these patients revolve around prevention of leucine flux through its catabolic pathway and detoxification of accumulating branched-chain organic acid intermediates. The first goal is achieved by restriction of leucine in the diets of these patients and maintaining euglycemia. During an acute episode, rapid intravenous glucose administration provides substrate for energy production, thereby shutting down ketogenic pathways such as leucine catabolism. Administration of carnitine and/or glycine is the second arm of treatment; these compounds conjugate with isovaleric acid to form nontoxic, water-soluble, and easily excreted products: isovalerylcarnitine and isovalerylglycine.

References

1. SCHULZE, A., LINDNER, M., KOHLMULLER, D., OLGEMOLLER, K., MAYATEPEK, E., AND HOFFMANN, G. F.: Expanded newborn screening for inborn errors of metabolism by electrospray ionization-tandem mass spectrometry: Results, outcome, and implications. *Pediatrics 111*:1399–406, 2003.
2. CHACE, D. H., KALAS, T. A., AND NAYLOR, E. W.: Use of tandem mass spectrometry for multianalyte screening of dried blood specimens from newborns. *Clin. Chem. 49*:1797–817, 2003.
3. ENSENAUER, R., VOCKLEY, J., WILLARD, J. M. ET AL.: A common mutation is associated with a mild, potentially asymptomatic phenotype in patients with isovaleric acidemia diagnosed by newborn screening. *Am. J. Hum. Genet. 75*:1136–42, 2004.

Additional Reading

SWEETMAN, L. AND WILLIAMS, J. C.: Branched chain organic acidemias. In *The Metabolic and Molecular Bases of Inherited Disease*, 8th ed. C. R. SCRIVER, A. L. BEAUDET, W. S. SLY, AND D. VALLE, eds, McGraw-Hill, New York, 2001, pp. 2131–5.

OGIER DE BAULNY, H. AND SAUDUBRAY, J. M.: Branched-chain organic acidurias. *Semin. Neonatol.* 7:65–74, 2002.

Case 39

A Happy but Developmentally Delayed 5-Year-Old Boy

Alison E. Presley and David E. Bruns

A pediatrician in a rural community referred a 5-year-old child to a large pediatric center for workup of developmental delay. The child had missed major developmental milestones, did not speak at all, and had experienced three seizurelike episodes in the last 3 years. Additional history elicited from the mother regarding her son's skill set revealed that balancing and sitting were achieved late for age, and walking was mastered just last year. In addition to his mental retardation, heat intolerance often provoked self-removal of garments in public, and he exhibited a habitual stereotypic "hand-flapping" motion. Behaviorally, the child was not withdrawn, but instead seemed to be perpetually happy and affectionate. At the referral institution, a workup to find the cause of the patient's developmental delay was begun.

Physical examination revealed a well-nourished, alert child with normal vital signs. Slight microcephaly, microbrachycephaly (flattened occiput), and prominent prognathia were noted. Associated features also included deeply set (yet properly spaced) eyes, a large protruding tongue, and a pointed chin. Verbal communication was absent; however, nonverbal/receptive communication and object usage skills were adequate. Cranial nerves were intact, and occasional tongue-thrusting repetitive motions were observed. Abnormal hypotonicity was noted in the trunk, while hyperreflexia was noted in the limbs. Gait dysfunction (ataxia combined with uplifted, flexed hands and arms) with jerky movements was observed.

Blood and urine collected for extensive biochemical organic and amino acid profiling revealed no evidence of inborn errors of metabolism. Cytogenetic karyotyping showed 46 XY chromosomes, effectively ruling out trisomy 21 (Down's syndrome). PCR (polymerase chain reaction) testing for fragile X syndrome showed a normal number of CGG repeats. To investigate the possible presence of Angelman syndrome, molecular cytogenetic region probes for *SNRPN* (small nuclear ribonucleoprotein polypeptide N, a promoter that lies in a CpG island of 15q11-13) and D15S10 (molecular designation for a region of chromosome 15q11-13) were utilized. Probe hybridization to both chromosome 15 s was observed; thus no deletions were detected. Southern blot analysis was performed on *Xba*- and *Not* I-digested DNA with the *SNRPN* exon α probe, and normal methylation

Tietz's Applied Laboratory Medicine, Second Edition. Edited by Mitchell G. Scott, Ann M. Gronowski, and Charles S. Eby
Copyright © 2007 John Wiley & Sons, Inc.

pattern was discovered. Finally, PCR amplification of 10 exons within the *UBE3A* gene (ubiquitin protein ligase E3A) on chromosome 15q11-13 was performed. A four-nucleotide insertion mutation in one copy of the child's *UBE3A* gene was identified, which resulted in a frameshift, a predicted premature translational stop, and an ultimate truncating mutation. The clinical features along with the *UBE3A* mutation led to the diagnosis of Angelman syndrome.

Definition of Disease

In 1965, English pediatrician Dr. Harry Angelman entitled a paper "Puppet Children: a report of three cases." Others reported additional cases that resembled his description of patients with jerky movements and laughing faces, and the syndrome has since been renamed after Dr. Angelman.

The spectrum of Angelman syndrome (AS) possesses a wider range of phenotypes than originally appreciated. A summary of AS by Clayton-Smith and Lean[1] delineates the clinical aspects of the disorder. Observation reveals certain *consistent* clinical features, which include severe developmental delay, absence of speech, gait ataxia, and uniqueness of behavior. *Frequently* observed features include microcephaly before age 2, seizures before age 3, or characteristic EEG patterns that may be intermittently documented such as large-amplitude slow spike waves and triphasic delta waves. *Associated* features sometimes observed in AS children include a flat occiput, prognathia, wide mouth with widely spaced teeth, hyperactive reflexes, uplifted flexed upper extremities, heat intolerance, sleep disturbance, and fascination with water or shiny objects.

The unique behavior of AS patients is arguably the most specific and recognizable diagnostic clue, and served as the strong unifier in the diagnosis of AS before the pathogenesis of the syndrome was understood. Frequent bouts of easily provoked (or unprovoked) laughter, incessant smiling, quick excitability, and a short attention span are elements of the typical AS demeanor.

Pathogenesis

AS is caused by dysfunction of the *UBE3A* gene on chromosome 15q11-13. The gene encodes a ubiquitin protein ligase, E3A, which marks (via the enzymatic ubiquitinase activity) certain proteins for cellular degradation. The *UBE3A* gene region possesses brain-specific imprinting, meaning that neural cells preferentially express the gene from only one of the two parental alleles. The *UBE3A* imprinting is termed "brain-specific" because imprinting of this region is noted only in neural tissue, and not in other tissues of the body. However, *UBE3A* expression is also thought to be almost exclusively limited to the brain. An imprinting center (IC) on chromosome 15 controls molecular marking of the gene region as "maternal" or "paternal" via methylation of specific loci. This epigenetic (a level of genetic coding overlying the actual DNA sequence information) molecular marking method encodes paternal DNA as unmethylated loci on chromosome 15q11-13 and maternal DNA as methylated loci. In the neural cells of normal individuals, the *SNRPN* gene locus is a paternally imprinted (unmethylated) region that contains the complex IC, and expression of this paternal region is "turned on" by the coded methylation pattern and "turns off" the methylated maternal region. A complementary inverse occurs in gene *UBE3A* within the neural cells of normal individuals, where methylation of chromosome 15 "turns on" expression of the maternal *UBE3A* copy and unmethylation

Table 39.1 Summary of Molecular Disease Mechanisms and Detection Methods for As and PWS

Major molecular mechanism	Frequency in Angelman syndrome	Frequency in Prader–Willi syndrome	Possible detection method	Methylation-specific PCR result
Deletion (~4 Mb) of chromosome 15q11-13	70–75% (maternal)	75% (paternal)	Cytogenetics FISH	Abnormal
Uniparental disomy (UPD)	2–3% (paternal)	22% (maternal)	RFLP analysis	Abnormal
Imprinting center (IC) defect	3–5%	3%	IC sequence screening	Abnormal
UBE3A mutation (specific to AS)	5–10%	N/A	UBE3A gene sequencing	Normal
Chromosomal rearrangement in chromosome 15q11-13 region	<1% (maternal)	<1% (paternal)	Cytogenetics FISH	Normal
No (or other) detectable abnormality	~10–15%	Very few cases	N/A	Normal

"turns off" expression of the paternal *UBE3A* copy. This differential expression of maternal and paternal genes within neural cells, regulated by epigenetic molecular marking in the form of methylation pattern, is seen in the setting of normal neural development. In two disorders, AS and Prader–Willi syndrome (PWS), this intricate mechanism of differential expression of genes is upset, as discussed below.

In AS, there are four major mechanisms by which the expression of the maternal copy of the *UBE3A* gene is compromised. The most common mechanism (~75% of cases) is deletion of the maternal chromosome 15q11-13 region. Alternatively (~3% of cases), paternal uniparental disomy (UPD) may be present, resulting in two inherited paternal copies of an unmethylated ("turned off") *UBE3A* gene. A less common pathology (~5%) leading to AS is an imprinting center (IC) defect resulting in abnormal methylation. An imprinting center defect usually stems from a mutation within the center itself, or less often from a translocation within this region, and is inherited in an autosomal dominant fashion. The defect impairs the proper functions of the imprinting center, such as "erasing" and "resetting" of methylation patterns within the chromosomes of gametes that are passed on during reproduction. Depending on which parent possessed the inherited defect, the offspring could receive two chromosomes that both possess the same imprinting pattern. For example, if the mother has an IC mutation that she passes to her son, the son could inherit an abnormally unmethylated ("turned off") maternal chromosome 15 and a paternal unmethylated chromosome 15, resulting in no expression of the *UBE3A* gene, producing AS. The final molecular mechanism (~10%) involves a mutation within the *UBE3A* gene (see Table 39.1).

Diagnosis

Several diagnostic tests are used to detect the different classes of abnormalities found within AS. DNA methylation analysis can be performed to examine the status of the chromosome 15q11-13 region. For this testing, patient DNA is digested by *Xba* and *Not*I methylation-sensitive restriction enzymes, which cannot cut the maternal, methylated sites. The reproducible result of this digestion in a normal chromosome 15 is to create shorter, fragmented pieces of paternal DNA, and longer, methylation-protected lengths of maternal DNA. Southern blot with a *SNRPN* probe (a locus within the 15q11-13 region) to highlight the region of interest can then be performed. A normal control should possess both a maternal methylated 4.2-kb (kilobase) band and a paternal unmethy-lated 0.9-kb band. An abnormal methylation result, meaning a single unmethylated 0.9 kb band, would be observed in cases of AS caused by either a 15q11-13 deletion (no maternal *SNRPN* locus for the probe to highlight), UPD (no maternal *SNRPN* locus for the probe to highlight), or an IC defect (abnormally unmethylated maternal DNA digested and maternal *SNRPN* locus highlighted as 0.9-kb band).

Most investigations performed to confirm a clinical suspicion of AS commence with methylation analysis (see Fig. 39.1). If an abnormal methylation result is obtained (as it is in the great majority of AS cases), further categorization of the molecular defect can be achieved by using a cytogenetic fluorescence in situ hybridization (FISH) probe specific to the D15S10 locus that lies next to the *UBE3A* gene. An absence of the hybridization signal on one of the two chromosome 15 s in a cell would indicate 15q11-13 deletion, the most common genetic cause of AS. If FISH is negative, proceeding to restriction length fragment polymorphism analysis (RLFP) may be warranted to investigate the presence of UPD. If RLFP is normal, an IC defect may be the cause.

A mutation within the *UBE3A* gene itself is the only major genetic mechanism of AS that will yield a normal methylation pattern. As in the case presented above, PCR sequen-cing of the *UBE3A* gene region can be requested, although many laboratories require a negative methylation analysis result before performing mutation analysis. Many different kinds of mutations within the gene have been identified to date, including nucleotide inser-tions and deletions of small numbers of bases that may be undetectable at the cytogenetic level, and therefore are detected only at the molecular level. The predicted encoding defects include frameshifts, early stop codons, and missense mutations, most of which probably cause early protein truncation.

A different clinical syndrome, Prader–Willi syndrome (PWS), is closely related to AS by a similar genetic mechanism, and shares the features of developmental delay with mild to moderate mental retardation. Children with PWS exhibit a phenotype characterized by central obesity, almond-shaped eyes with a downturned mouth, hypogenitalism with infer-tility, and short stature. PWS is caused by three major genetic mechanisms that inversely

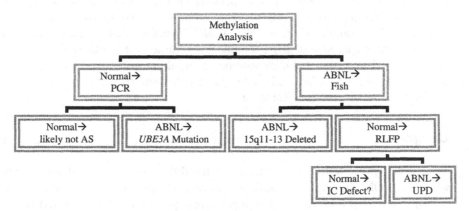

Figure 39.1 Angelman syndrome (AS) testing algorithm.

parallel the mechanisms underlying AS, and all result in the absence of expression of normally active paternally inherited genes in the same chromosome 15q11-13 region. Whereas AS is connected to a single gene, the pathogenesis of PWS seems to involve two or more genes. The first genetic mechanism is deletion of the paternal chromosome 15q11-13 region ($\sim$75% of cases). In the second mechanism, PWS can be caused by maternal UPD in which two maternal copies of chromosome 15 are inherited ($\sim$20% of cases). Finally, an IC microdeletion has been found in a minority of PWS ($\sim$3% of cases) (see Table 39.1).

Prognosis

No known treatments or cures for Angelman syndrome are available. Expected lifespan is not shortened, and some of the behavioral traits wane with age. Attention span may increase, sleep may improve, and excitability may decrease with adulthood. Scoliosis and contractures may occur secondary to hypertonicity of limbs. Special services for the neurologic, educational, and physical aspects of the disorder are necessary. Patients generally cannot live independently, and require supervision.

Documentation of the molecular genetic defect underlying the particular patient's cause of AS can be important for genetic counseling of the parents. AS mechanisms such as deletion of the chromosome 15q11-13 region and UPD carry a low recurrence risk for a subsequent pregnancy. By contrast, AS mechanisms such as a *UBE3A* mutation and IC defects can carry either a low recurrence risk *or* a 50% chance of having a second AS child, depending on whether the defect was sporadic or inherited.

References

1. CLAYTON-SMITH, J. AND LAAN, L.: Angelman syndrome: A review of the clinical and genetic aspects. *J. Med. Genet.* 40:87–95, 2003.
2. CASSIDY, S. B., DYKENS, E., AND WILLIAMS, C. A.: Prader–Willi and Angelman syndromes: Sister imprinted disorders. *Am. J. Med. Genet. (Semin. Med. Genet.)* 97:136–46, 2000.
3. GOLDSTONE, A. P.: Prader–Willi syndrome: Advances in genetics, pathophysiology and treatment. *Trends Endocrin. Metab.* 15:12–20, 2000.
4. MALZAC, P. ET AL.: Mutation analysis of UBE3A in Angelman syndrome patients. *Am. J. Hum. Genet.* 62:1353–60, 1998.

Additional Reading

BURTIS, C. A., ASHWOOD, E., AND BRUNS, D. E., eds.: *Tietz Textbook of Clinical Chemistry and Molecular Diagnostics*, 4th ed., Saunders Elsevier, Philadelphia, 2006.

Online Mendelian Inheritance in Man, OMIM (TM): Entry 601623 UBE3A. McKusick-Nathans Institute for Genetic Medicine, Johns Hopkins Univ (Baltimore, MD) and National Center for Biotechnology Information, National Library of Medicine (Bethesda, MD), 2000. World Wide Web URL: http://www.ncbi.nlm.nih.gov/omim/.

WALTER, J. AND PAULSEN, M.: Imprinting and disease. *Semin. Cell Devel. Biol.* 14:101–10, 2000.

Case 40

The Asymptomatic Iron Man

Elise Krejci

A 65-year-old Caucasian male presented to his primary care physician for a routine physical exam prior to retiring. He had enjoyed excellent health throughout his life, and did not
report any new symptoms at the time. His past medical history included elevated prostate-
specific antigens that had been evaluated with multiple negative prostate needle biopsies,
and hypercholesterolemia treated with diet and medication. Family history was notable for
cardiovascular disease, hypertension, and breast cancer. He did not smoke, and consumed
less than one beer or glass of wine per week. On direct questioning, he did not acknowledge chest pain, shortness of breath, arthralgias, fatigue, cold intolerance, or decreased
libido.

Physical exam showed a healthy-appearing white male weighing 208 lb with a blood
pressure of 147/81 and a regular pulse of 72 bpm. Head, eye, ear, nose, throat (HEENT)
exam was unremarkable. Heart and lung exams were normal. The abdominal exam was
unremarkable with no evidence of hepatosplenomegaly. Scrotal exam showed normal
testes. Skin exam showed normal distribution of a summer tan and male pattern facial
and body hair.

His internist ordered the following laboratory studies as part of a general health
screening:

Analyte	Value, Conventional Units	Reference Interval, Conventional Units	Value, SI Units	Reference Interval, Conventional Units
WBC	$8.2 \times 10^3/\mu L$	4–11	$8.2 \times 10^9/L$	4–11
Hemoglobin	15.2 g/dL	13.5–16.5	152 g/L	135–165
Platelet count	$297 \times 10^3/\mu L$	140–400	$297 \times 10^9/L$	140–400
aPTT	28 s	23–36	Same	
Prothrombin time	13.2 s	11–15.5	Same	
Glucose	119 mg/dL	70–110	6.6 mmol/L	3.9–6.1
Creatinine	0.7 mg/dL	0.7–1.2	62 μmol/L	62–106
Protein, total	7.9 g/dL	6–8	79 g/L	60–80
Albumin	3.8 g/dL	3.5–5.0	30 g/L	35–50 g/L
Bilirubin, total	0.5 mg/dL	0.2–1.2	8.6 μmol/L	3–21
Alkaline phosphatase	42 U/L	35–120	0.71 μkat/L	0.60–2.04

Tietz's Applied Laboratory Medicine, Second Edition. Edited by Mitchell G. Scott, Ann M. Gronowski, and
Charles S. Eby
Copyright © 2007 John Wiley & Sons, Inc.

Analyte	Value, Conventional Units	Reference Interval, Conventional Units	Value, SI Units	Reference Interval, Conventional Units
ALT	72 U/L	8–47	1.22 μkat/L	0.14–0.80
AST	60 U/L	10–42	1.02 μkat/L	0.17–0.71
Serum iron	240 μg/dL	45–160	43.0 μmol/L	8.1–28.6
Total iron binding capacity	287 μg/dL	220–420	51.4 μmol/L	39.8–75.2
Transferrin saturation	71%	21–50	0.71 fraction	0.21–0.50
Ferritin	450 ng/mL	20–323	450 μg/L	20–323

Serum iron and total iron binding capacity (TIBC) were repeated on a morning blood specimen after overnight fasting: iron 194 μg/mL, TIBC 298 μg/mL, and transferrin saturation 65%. Hepatitis B and C serologies were negative.

The patient was referred to a hematologist, who recommended a liver biopsy to confirm and quantify excess tissue iron deposition and to assess liver damage due to mildly elevated transaminases. Steatosis and mild portal inflammation, but no fibrosis or architectural abnormalities were seen on trichrome and reticulin stains. In addition, there was moderate periportal and pericanalicular iron deposition, primarily in the hepatocytes. The total liver iron was reported as 4896 units (normal = 200–2400) and the hepatic iron index was 1.3. Molecular diagnostic testing for the two most common HFE gene mutations associated with hereditary hemochromatosis was performed, and the patient was compound heterozygous for a mutation that coded for substitution of tyrosine for cysteine at amino acid 282 (C282Y), and a second mutation that coded for substitution of aspartate for histidine at amino acid 63 (H63D).

Treatment

The patient began weekly therapeutic phlebotomies. A fingerstick whole-blood hemoglobin determination was done prior to each collection to ensure that he was not anemic (threshold 12.0 mg/dL), and CBC and ferritin were repeated after every four procedures. After 12 phlebotomies, his ferritin was 48 ng/mL, and his hemoglobin was 13.1 g/dL. He continues to have a therapeutic phlebotomy every 2–3 months to maintain his ferritin <100 ng/mL.

Definition of the Disease

Hereditary hemochromatosis (HH) is an autosomal recessive disease with incomplete penetrance due to multiple disease modifying genetic and acquired factors that causes excessive absorption of dietary iron and subsequent iron deposition primarily affecting the liver, endocrine organs, heart, and skin. HH is particularly prominent in persons of northern European descent with an incidence of approximately 1 in 200 based on genetic testing, but with variable penetrance. The classic triad associated with hemochromatosis, first described in the nineteenth century, is diabetes, a result of iron deposition in the pancreas; grayish hyperpigmentation, due to iron deposition in the skin; and cirrhosis, a result of iron deposition in the liver leading to fibrosis. Additional symptoms of advanced iron overload include congestive heart failure, hypogonadism, and arthritis. Patients presenting with multiorgan failure due to iron overload from HH are rarely encountered today. Instead, symptomatic hereditary hemochromatosis usually manifests as malaise, fatigue, arthrlagias, and impotence in the fourth and fifth decades in men. Onset of symptoms is delayed in women due to chronic, increased physiologic iron loss prior to menopause.

Pathogenesis

Excess iron is hazardous because it produces free-radical formation. Oxidative injury causes DNA cleavage, impaired protein synthesis, and impairment of cell integrity and cell proliferation, leading to cell injury, fibrosis, mutagenesis, and cancer.

Normal iron homeostasis involves recycling of iron from erythrocytes; loss of iron through shedding of epithelia cells and intestinal enterocytes; blood loss due to trauma, menses, and pregnancy; and tightly regulated absorption of dietary iron. Daily replacement requirements are approximately 1.0 mg for men and 2.0 mg for menstruating women. Dietary iron is absorbed through the gastrointestinal tract after binding to transferrin and undergoing receptor-mediated endocytosis. Within the enterocyte, the iron dissociates from transferrin, binds to ferritin, and is subsequently released and transported out of the enterocyte in response to increased erythropoietic demands for iron.

While substantial progress has been achieved in identifying the proteins that regulate iron absorption, our understanding of both physiologic and pathologic processes is incomplete. "Classic hemochromatosis" is associated with mutations in the HFE gene located on chromosome 6. One function of the HFE protein is to interact with cell membrane transferrin receptor and facilitate iron uptake. The most common HFE mutation substitutes tyrosine for cysteine at position 282, and results in a protein with decreased affinity for the transferrin receptor, and decreased iron uptake. Based on the crypt-programming model of HH, undifferentiated HFE mutation immature enterocytes cannot take up plasma iron and mature into iron-starved enterocytes that avidly absorb dietary iron and transport it into the blood.

HFE also appears to be involved in regulation of hepcidin, a protein synthesized in hepatocytes that controls release of intracellular storage iron. Normally, hepcidin concentrations are low, when plasma iron is low, facilitating intracellular iron release; and hepcidin concentrations are elevated when plasma iron concentration is high, inhibiting release of storage iron. Low hepcidin levels have been reported in iron-overloaded HH patients, but the details of HFE–hepcidin regulation are incomplete. Less common forms of hemochromatosis have been linked to mutations in other iron-regulating proteins, including hepcidin, hemojuvelin, ferroportin, and transferrin receptor 2.

Differential Diagnosis

The early symptoms of hemochromatosis, such as fatigue, arthralgias, and malaise, are nonspecific, and primary care physicians should consider iron overload due to hemochromatosis in addition to inflammatory, infectious, autoimmune, malignant, and psychiatric disorders when patients present with these complaints. While hepatomegaly, arthritis, hyperpigmentation of the skin, testicular atrophy, and signs of congestive heart failure are more specific for iron overload, causes other than HH should be considered, including ineffective erythropoiesis due to chronic hemolysis in severe forms of thalassemia, chronic transfusions, excessive dietary or supplement sources of iron and liver disease, including toxic or viral hepatitis, Wilson's disease, α1-antitrypsin deficiency, nonalcoholic fatty liver disease, and primary sclerosing cholangitis.

Diagnosis of Iron Overload

The first step in evaluating a patient suspected of iron overload is measurement of serum iron, transferrin saturation, and ferritin. Transferrin, a B_1 globulin with two Fe^{3+} binding sites, is the plasma iron transport protein. Normally, transferrin saturation is about one-third, and total circulating iron is approximately 2.5 mg. Ferritin is a protein shell composed of 24 subunits, and is the intracellular storage site for Fe^{2+}. Due to chronic leakage form cells, minute amounts of ferritin can be detected in blood, proportional to total body stores. Analytical methods for measuring serum iron typically involve acidifying serum to convert Fe^{3+} to Fe^{2+}, which complexes with a chromagen, and absorption at an appropriate wavelength is proportional to iron concentration. Total iron binding capacity is determined by adding excess Fe^{3+} to a patient's serum to saturate iron binding sites on transferrin, removal of unbound iron, followed by determination of iron content. Transferrin saturation (TS) is calculated: serum Fe/TIBC $\times$ 100. Various immunologic methods are used to measure serum ferritin concentration. Overall, these analytical methods are robust, but physiologic and pathologic variables can have significant impact on results. It is generally accepted that there is a diurnal variation in serum iron concentrations, and that a fasting morning specimen should be ideal. A recent study of normal volunteers[1] compared iron, TIBC, and ferritin results collected at 4-hour intervals (8:00 am, noon, 4:00 pm) on day 1 and the following morning. Their findings confirmed significant variation in serum iron (ranging from 42% lower to 107% higher compared to 8:00 am on day 1) and transferrin saturation, but there was no consistent diurnal pattern. The variation for repeated TIBC and ferritin results was not clinically important.

Transferrin saturation is the most sensitive indicator of iron overload, and screening guidelines recommend a transferrin saturation cutoff of 45%. However, testing should be repeated, by convention on a morning fasting sample, and in the absence of recent ingestion of iron supplements, to improve specificity. If TS is repeatedly elevated, other conditions that can cause increases in serum iron and TS, including oral or parenteral iron supplementation, acute hepatitis, and aplastic anemia, are excluded. While elevated serum ferritin ($>$200 μg/L in premenopausal women and $>$300 μg/L in men and postmenopausal women) is not as sensitive as TS for iron overload, if $>$1000 μg/L, evidence of hepatic injury is more likely to be observed on examination of a liver biopsy. However, ferritin can be elevated in other conditions such as infections, inflammations, and liver disease.

Liver biopsy is the gold standard. The liver biopsy is examined for fibrosis and inflammation using routine hematoxylin and eosin staining. A Prussian blue histochemical stain can be performed to evaluate qualitatively the presence of iron within the tissue. To obtain a more quantitative determination of liver iron, a hepatic iron index is performed on one of the core biopsies using spectroscopy (hepatic iron concentration/56 $\times$ patient's age). The expected value is less than 1.0. Results between 1.0 and 1.9 suggest mild, nonspecific iron accumulation, and may occur in patients who are heterozygous for C282Y, compound heterozygous C282Y/H63D, or homozygous C282Y, as well as in patients with other forms of chronic liver disease or iron overload. An index $>$1.9 is typically obtained in homozygous C282Y homozygous HH patients. While the liver biopsy can give diagnostic as well as prognostic information, it is an invasive procedure and is subject to sampling error, as studies have shown that iron is not distributed evenly through the liver. The patient presented in this case had an index of 1.3 consistent with a mild iron burden and his compound heterozygous HFE mutation status.

Less invasive methods of estimating iron stores include magnetic resonance imaging (MRI) and computerized tomography (CT). Accurate measurement of total body iron can be determined by magnetic susceptometry with a superconducting quantum interference device (SQUID), or repeated phlebotomy until iron deficiency occurs. However, SQUID technology is not available in most communities, and phlebotomy does not provide prognostic information regarding liver injury.

Molecular testing is accomplished by searching for the two most common *HFE* gene mutations, C282Y and H63D. C282Y heterozygosity may contribute to iron overload when combined with other conditions such as chronic alcoholism or hepatitis, but it should not be considered the sole cause of iron overload and should not be considered diagnostic of hereditary hemochromatosis. At present, only homozygosity for C282Y and compound heterozygosity for C282Y/H63D should be considered indicative of hereditary hemochromatosis. Cross-sectional population studies have shown that between 60% and 80% of those at genetic risk will develop biochemical penetrance in the form of abnormal ferritin and transferrin saturation. The use of DNA-based tests alone may fail to identify 20–40% of Caucasian patients and most black patients with clinical evidence of hemochromatosis but without the C282Y mutation. Liver biopsy, to confirm iron overload and to evaluate for other types of hepatic disease, is recommended in this group. As more is learned about the regulation of iron absorption, it is likely that new molecular targets will be added to genetic screening for HH.

Not all patients' diagnosed with HH require a liver biopsy. Current recommendations would defer a liver biopsy in patients who are homozygous for C282Y mutation, have biochemical evidence of iron overload, and have normal liver enzymes. Some experts would also defer a liver biopsy if the ferritin is <1000 µg/L.

Treatment

Treatment is simple, inexpensive, and safe. The first step is to rid the body of excess iron using phlebotomy of 500 mL of whole blood (equivalent to approximately 200–250 mg of iron) approximately once weekly. The patient's hematocrit must be monitored to avoid causing anemia. Ferritin levels are tested periodically to monitor iron levels. Phlebotomy should be continued until transferrin saturation is less than 50% and serum ferritin levels are less than 50 ng/mL. Therapeutic phlebotomy may improve or even cure some of the manifestations and complications of the disease, such as fatigue, elevated liver enzymes, hepatomegaly, early liver fibrosis, arthralgias, and hyperpigmentation, but not cirrhosis or hepatoma. Once iron levels return to normal, maintenance therapy every 2–4 months for life begins. Until recently, blood removed from people diagnosed with hemochromatosis could not be added to the volunteer blood supply, even if the person met all criteria to be a donor. However, in 2000, the FDA released guidelines that permit blood collection centers to collect blood from donors with a diagnosis of HH. One blood center that actively recruited HH donors reported that 76% met eligibility requirements for donation. In addition, HH donors had a lower rate of deferral due to anemia.[2]

Screening for Hereditary Hemochromatosis

Genetic and biochemical screening for hereditary hemochromatosis is controversial. Hereditary hemochromatosis has a long latency period, the complications of iron overload are preventable if treatment is commenced, and the treatment is easy, safe, and inexpensive. However, because not all people with the C282Y mutation will develop laboratory signs of iron overload or damage, or clinical symptoms, genetic-based screening will overestimate disease burden. Genetic screening of selected populations is appropriate, including first-degree relatives of HH patients who are C282Y homozygotes or C282Y/H63D compound heterozygotes.

A recent study compared proband genetic testing and screening of healthy patients in a primary care setting.[3] This study assessed the phenotypic expression of disease through history, examination, serum iron indices, and liver biopsy in 672 asymptomatic C282Y homozygotes identified through either family screening of probands or genetic screening in the family practice setting. There were comparable levels of hepatic iron concentration, hepatic fibrosis, and cirrhosis in subjects from each group.

Of the 672 homozygotes detected, 39.1% had significant hepatic iron loading and were therefore at risk for long-term complications. Cirrhosis was found in 5.6% of male and 1.9% of female asymptomatic homozygotes. Twenty-five patients in the study had repeat liver biopsies. In all cases in which cirrhosis was not present, removal of excess iron by treatment of disease resulted in improvement of the liver fibrosis score. This study shows that genetic-based screening is equally beneficial for the population as a whole and for family members of patients with hereditary hemochromatosis.

References

1. DALE, J. C., BURRITT, M. F., AND ZINSMEISTER, A. R.: Diurnal variation of serum iron, iron-binding capacity, transferrin saturation, and ferritin levels. *Am. J. Clin. Pathol. 117*:802–8, 2002.
2. LEITMAN, S. F.: Hemochromatosis subjects as allogeneic blood donors: A prospective study. *Transfusion 43*:1538–44, 2003.
3. POWELL, L. W., DIXON, J. L., RAMM, G. A. ET AL.: Screening for hemochromatosis in asymptomatic subjects with or without a family history. *Arch. Intern. Med. 166*:294–301, 2006.

Additional Reading

PIETRANGELO, A.: Hereditary hemochromatosis—a new look at an old disease. *N. Engl. J. Med. 350*:2383–97, 2004.
BEUTLER, E., FELITTI, V. J., KOZIOL, J. A., HO, N. J., AND GELBART, T.: Penetrance of 845G → A (C282Y) HFE hereditary haemochromatosis mutation in the USA. *Lancet 359*:211–18, 2002.

ADAMS, P. C., REBOUSSIN, D. M., BARTON, J. C. ET AL.: Hemochromatosis and iron-overload screening in a racially diverse population. *N. Engl. J. Med. 352*:1769–78, 2005.

Part Eleven

Infectious Diseases

Cases of Epstein–Barr virus (EBV), neurosyphilis, Lyme disease, allergic bronchopulmonary aspergillosis, *Helicobacter pylori*, and West Nile virus are reported and discussed in Cases 41, 42, 43, 44, 45, and 46, respectively (all edited by AMG).

Tietz's Applied Laboratory Medicine, Second Edition. Edited by Mitchell G. Scott, Ann M. Gronowski, and Charles S. Eby

Case 41

Tired, Hot, and Lumpy

J. Stacey Klutts

A 13-year-old girl from an affluent neighborhood was taken to her pediatrician because of a one-week history of malaise and loss of appetite associated with a several-pound weight loss. She also complained of a 4-day history of "lumps in her neck" and a fever to 102°F (39°C), as well as a mild sore throat over the previous 24 hours. There had been no associated nausea or vomiting, and the fever had been controlled with acetaminophen. The patient has two siblings and attended a private school where she was in the 8th grade. There were no known contacts with sick people at home or school. She denied sexual activity, but did claim to have a boyfriend. The patient has historically been healthy, presenting to the pediatrician only for well-child checkups and immunizations, which were all up-to-date.

Physical examination revealed a mildly ill-appearing teenager with no evidence of acute distress. Her blood pressure was 119/70, pulse 79, and temperature 100°F (37.8°C). On head and neck exam, bilateral, anterior cervical lymphadenopathy was noted along with tonsilar enlargement and an exudative pharyngitis that was diffuse. No splenomegaly or hepatomegaly were observed. The exam was otherwise unremarkable.

The presence of the triad of fever, lymphadenopathy, and pharyngitis in this teenager suggested that this patient might have infectious mononucleosis (IM). To help confirm this clinical suspicion, the physician obtained a CBC with differential and a heterophile antibody test. The results were available before the patient left the office:

Analyte/Test	Value, Conventional Units	Reference Interval, Conventional Units	Value, SI Units	Reference Interval, SI Units
Hemoglobin	13.5 g/dL	12.0–16.0	2.09 mmol/L	1.86–2.48
Hematocrit	40%	35–45	0.40	0.35–0.45
WBC count	$12.0 \times 10^3/\mu L$	4.5–11.0	$12.0 \times 10^9/L$	4.5–11.0
Platelet count	$210 \times 10^3/\mu L$	150–450	$210 \times 10^9/L$	150–450
Heterophile antibody	Nonreactive	Nonreactive		

These are female-specific reference ranges.

Tietz's Applied Laboratory Medicine, Second Edition. Edited by Mitchell G. Scott, Ann M. Gronowski, and Charles S. Eby
Copyright © 2007 John Wiley & Sons, Inc.

Analyte/Test	Cell Type	Value, Percentage	Reference Interval, Percentage
WBC differential	Neutrophils	38	57–67
	Lymphocytes	48	23–33
	Monocytes	3	3–7
	Eosinophils	1	1–3
	Basophils	0	0–1
	Atypical	9	0
	Lymphocytes	—	—

While the CBC and differential would suggest that this patient does have IM, the heterophile antibody assay was nonreactive. However, the pediatrician still made a presumptive diagnosis of IM and discharged the patient with instructions to take ibuprofen for fever and pain, avoid contact sports, and return to his office in one week for follow-up. In the meantime, the following laboratory studies were performed:

Analyte/Test	Result[a]
EBV viral capsid antigen (VCA), IgG	Positive
EBV viral capsid antigen (VCA), IgM	Positive
EBV early antigen, IgG	Positive
EBV nuclear antigen	Negative

[a]Reference interval/serological profile depends on EBV infection history.

A final diagnosis of EBV-associated IM was made. The patient continued on supportive therapy. The fever and pharyngitis resolved within 1 week and the lymphadenopathy, within 2 weeks. However, she remained fatigued for 4 additional weeks but was able to continue attending school on a regular basis.

Definition of the Disease

Epstein–Barr virus is a human herpesvirus that is cytotropic for B lymphocytes. This virus occurs worldwide, and most people (>90%) become infected at some point during their lifetime.[1] Primary infection tends to occur at an early age, especially in lower socioeconomic groups and developing countries. When infection occurs during early childhood, there are usually only very mild symptoms or no symptoms at all. However, if a primary EBV infection occurs during adolescence or adulthood, then infectious mononucleosis (IM) often arises. In a typical case of IM, a prodromal period consisting of malaise, anorexia, and/or myalgias usually precedes the onset of the syndrome by a few days to a week. The syndrome is typically characterized by fever to 102–104°F (39–40°C) (90% of patients), cervical lymphadenopathy (90%), diffuse and exudative pharyngitis (33%), and/or rash (5%). Splenomegaly is found in about half of IM patients, and usually occurs during the second or third week of illness. Liver involvement can also occur, but more rarely. This syndrome typically resolves within 2–3 weeks, but the malaise may remain for months.

Following the primary infection, EBV persists as a latent infection, likely within memory B cells. Latent virus can reactivate later in life, but this often occurs subclinically. EBV is not highly contagious in that it is spread primarily through saliva. However, because people who are latently infected can potentially shed virus, it is essentially impossible to prevent its transmission. For these reasons, there are no special precautions or isolation procedures recommended for primarily infected patients.

In addition to being the most common cause of IM, EBV has also been associated with a variety of malignancies, including Burkitt's lymphoma, nasopharyngeal carcinoma, primary CNS lymphoma, and posttransplant lymphoproliferative diseases.[2]

Differential Diagnosis

Because most people in the population have been exposed to EBV, direct detection of the virus in the setting of an IM-like syndrome is usually insufficient for diagnosis. Furthermore, culture of EBV is beyond the scope of most hospital or small diagnostic laboratories. For these reasons, serological testing is the primary method for the diagnosis of primary EBV infections.

In patients where classical IM is suspected, the first test that is typically performed is one for heterophile antibodies (also referred to as the "Monospot" test).[3] This tests for antibodies against Paul Bunnell antigens on sheep, horse, or cow erythrocytes that are present in 40% of IM patients during the first week, and in 80–90% during the third week. These antibodies rapidly disappear after the first month, making them a useful marker for acute infection. When this test is positive in the setting of appropriate signs and symptoms, it is highly suggestive of EBV-associated IM (EBV-IM). However, a nonreactive test in this setting cannot rule out EBV-IM, as some patients do not develop these antibodies, and they can be found only after 2–3 weeks in others. This is especially true when testing young children. In addition to heterophile antibodies, the presence of atypical lymphocytes along with an absolute lymphocytosis is also suggestive of EBV-IM. In the majority of patients with uncomplicated IM, a complete blood count with differential and heterophile antibodies is sufficient to make the diagnosis. However, infections with cytomegalovirus (CMV), adenovirus, and *Toxoplasma gondii* have also been shown to cause a similar syndrome. Thus, to confirm EBV as the cause of disease in cases where the heterophile antibody is negative, EBV-specific serologic testing is indicated.

Most laboratories offer tests for antibodies against three specific EBV antigen complexes: the viral capsid antigen (VCA), the nuclear antigen (NA), and the early antigen (EA). When the heterophile antibody test is negative, measurements of four markers are usually performed: IgM and IgG to VCA, and IgG to NA and to EA. Similar to heterophile antibodies, IgM antibodies to VCA appear early in infection and usually disappear within 4–6 weeks. As such, these antibodies are also good markers for acute infection. IgG antibodies to VCA also appear in the acute phase of infection, peak at 2–4 weeks, but persist for life. In most patients, IgG antibodies to EA appear early in infection and become undetectable in 3–6 months. However, this marker fails to rise in a number of patients, and remains elevated for years in others. Antibody (IgG) to NA is the only marker not seen in the acute phase, but is an indicator of past or remote infection. It gradually appears 2–4 months after the onset of illness and persists for life. The interpretation of these serological results can be somewhat complex (see Table 41.1). However, in most situations, patients can be categorized into one of four EBV diagnoses: susceptible to EBV infection, a primary acute infection, past infection, or reactivation.

As mentioned above, EBV has also been associated with a number of malignancies, usually in a setting of immunological deficiency (e.g., posttransplant lymphoproliferative disease or primary CNS lymphoma). While serology might be useful in determining a patient's serological status with respect to EBV prior to a transplant, it is not as useful

Table 41.1   Typical Serological Profiles For Each EBV Diagnostic Category[a]

EBV disease stage	Anti-VCA IgG	Anti-VCA IgM	Anti-EB NA-1 IgG	Anti-EA-D IgG
Susceptible	−	−	−	−
Primary acute	+/−	+	−	+
Past infection	+	−	+	−
Reactivation	+	+/−	+	+/−

[a]*Key:* + = positive; − = negative.

in establishing a link between EBV and a new malignancy. In these situations, quantitative testing is required, and this is typically accomplished by quantitating the EBV DNA in an appropriate clinical sample using real-time PCR. While this molecular testing for EBV is also available for the diagnosis of infectious mononucleosis, it is currently considered investigational and is performed much less often than the typical serology. This is due primarily to cost and concerns over false-positive tests since this virus can be found within B lymphocytes of most healthy people.

Treatment

Treatment for IM is supportive for the vast majority of patients.[4] While corticosteroids have been shown to shorten the duration of fever and pharyngitis, they are not recommended for uncomplicated disease. However, in cases of impending airway obstruction due to tonsillar enlargement, corticosteroids are indicated. Additionally, because of the risk of splenic rupture, contact sports should be avoided for 6–8 weeks in IM patients, especially in those with splenomegaly.

References

1. STRAUS, S. E., COHEN, J. I., TOSATO, G., AND MEIER, J.: NIH conference: Epstein-Barr virus infections: Biology, pathogenesis, and management. *Ann. Intern. Med.* *118*:45–58, 1993.
2. COHEN, J. I.: Epstein-Barr virus infection. *N. Engl. J. Med. 343*:481–92, 2000.
3. STORCH, G. A.: Diagnostic virology. *Clin. Infect. Dis. 31*:739–51, 2000.
4. LINDE, A.: Epstein-Barr virus. In *Manual of Clinical Microbiology*, 8th ed., P. R. MURRAY, E. J. BARON, J. H. JORGENSEN, M. A. PFALLER, AND R. H. YOLKEN, eds., ASM Press, Washington, DC, 2003, pp. 1331–40.

Case 42

A Rash on the Soles of the Feet

Robyn M. Atkinson

A 43-year-old male presented to the infectious disease clinic with a 2-month history of worsening skin rash and lesions. The lesions were not painful and were predominantly on his face and forearms, but also covered the palms of his hands and soles of his feet. He was treated one month prior to this presentation with azithromycin, and the rash had improved slightly. In addition to the worsening rash and skin lesions, he noted the development of painless lesions on his penis that were resolving at the time of presentation. He also reported a history of night sweats, which coincided with the appearance of the rash, a sore throat, mild weight loss, headaches without visual alterations, and mild neck stiffness. The day prior to presentation he noted a single episode of anal discharge that was yellow and nonbloody. He had no history of fever, chills, nausea, vomiting, diarrhea, or penile discharge.

His past medical history is significant for HIV, which was diagnosed 24 years earlier, idiopathic thrombocytopenic purpura resulting in a splenectomy 16 years earlier, and bipolar disorder diagnosed 18 years earlier with a suicide attempt 5 years ago. He has been on intermittent HAART therapy and his infectious disease history is positive for hepatitis B, gonorrhea, HPV (human papilloma virus) with anal warts, and herpes simplex virus 1 and 2. His most recent PPD skin test (purified protein derivative) for tuberculosis was negative.

On physical examination, he was well-appearing and pleasant. His neurological exam was normal; his neck was supple, yet there was decreased range of motion with nontender bilateral submandibular lymphadenopathy. No mucosal lesions were noted; penile lesions were erythematous, approximately 0.5 cm in diameter, and slightly raised. The lesions on the face and forearms were up to 0.7 cm in diameter and appeared excoriated with an eschar. There were two nonerythematous nontender raised ulcerated lesions on his palms and three such lesions on the bottoms of his feet. The clinic was suspicious for secondary syphilis and ordered a serum RPR (rapid plasma reagin), which was positive at 1 : 256. A follow-up FTA-ABS (fluorescent treponemal antibody absorbed test) was also reactive. At this time, the patient reported having sexual contact with a partner about a year ago who initially reported a history of syphilis and then later denied that information.

Given his HIV status and secondary syphilis diagnosis, he was admitted for a lumbar puncture to rule out neurosyphilis. His CSF revealed a total of 93 cells, with two nucleated cells. Glucose was normal at 59 mg/dL, and protein was slightly elevated at 62 mg/dL.

Tietz's Applied Laboratory Medicine, Second Edition. Edited by Mitchell G. Scott, Ann M. Gronowski, and Charles S. Eby

A CSF VDRL (Venereal Disease Research Laboratory test) was reactive at a dilution of 1 : 16. He was diagnosed with secondary syphilis with concurrent neurosyphilis and was treated with intravenous penicillin G for 14 days.

Definition of Disease

Syphilis is an infectious disease caused by the spirochete *Treponema pallidum*. The disease was named for the mythical swine herder Syphilis, who was cursed with disease by Apollo, as described in an Italian tale by physician Girolamo Fracastoro in 1530.[1]

Syphilis has three distinct stages:

1. *Primary syphilis* is characterized by a single, painless sore or chancre, which marks the entry point of the organism into the body. The sore can appear on any exposed surface (most commonly on mucosal surfaces) such as external genitalia, the vagina, the anus or in the rectum, the lips, or inside the mouth. Sores are typically firm, round, and small and usually appear within 21 days of infection.[1] The sores last 3–6 weeks, and because of the painless nature of the sore they often go unnoticed. Therefore, individuals may not recognize that they are infected and may pose a danger to themselves, as they are at risk for latent infection; they can also pass the disease on to others, although transmission rates are higher when an active lesion is present. *Latent infection* is defined as the period of infection with no obvious symptoms of disease, yet the individual will be serologically positive. If serologies are discovered to be positive within one year of infection, the individual is in the early latent phase of disease.[2] An individual who has been infected for over a year is in the late latent phase of disease.[2]

2. *Secondary syphilis* is characterized by systemic manifestations of the disease. The presenting feature is usually a rash and lesions on the mucous membranes. The rash is typically rough, red, or brownish red, and found mainly on the palms of the hands and soles of the feet.[1] Rash may be accompanied by fever, swollen lymph nodes, sore throat, patchy hair loss, headache, weight loss, muscle ache, and fatigue.[1] The rash can appear concurrent with a healing chancre or can appear several weeks to years later. The rash will resolve without treatment, but without treatment the risk of developing late or tertiary disease is greater.

3. *Tertiary disease* (or late disease) is the result of organism dissemination throughout the body. It can affect the brain, nerves, eyes, heart, liver, and joints, resulting in awkward muscle movements, paralysis, gradual blindness, and dementia.[1] Neurosyphilis was once regarded as a phase of disease exclusive to this category of tertiary syphilis, but it has been shown that neurosyphilis can be present at any stage of the disease process.

The diagnosis of the case presented above was secondary syphilis with concurrent neurosyphilis. As mentioned, neurosyphilis is no longer considered to be a distinct phase of disease. It is a manifestation of infection that can occur early with the appearance of the chancre, late in disease when blindness and dementia have set in, or at any point in between. Up to 10% of individuals with neurosyphilis will be asymptomatic, and symptomatology may be different depending on the stage of disease with which it is associated.[1] The possible symptoms of neurosyphilis include cognitive dysfunction, motor or sensory nerve deficits, ocular or auditory deficits, cranial nerve palsies, meningitis, or seizures, although rare.[1] Early neurosyphilis typically presents as meningitis with or without cranial nerve or ocular involvement. Late neurosyphilis involves the brain and spinal cord, leading to general paresis, rapid progressive dementia with episodes of psychosis, bowel and bladder dysfunction, and sensory ataxia. These symptoms should not be confused with those seen in tertiary syphilis; tertiary syphilis and neurosyphilis are two distinct processes.

Evidence has shown that individuals with *T. pallidum* infection are likely to have a 5 times greater chance of acquiring concurrent HIV infection and increased risk for transmission of HIV than are those without syphilis. In the setting of HIV, the course of disease progression for syphilis can be altered and/or accelerated. HIV infection carries an increased risk of developing neurosyphilis as well as an increased risk for treatment failure. One study demonstrated that neurosyphilis is more likely to develop during primary or secondary syphilis when the RPR is $>1:32$, the CD4 count is <250 cells/μL, or viral RNA concentrations are >500 copies/μL.[1]

Differential Diagnosis

The diagnosis of any stage or phase of syphilis can be complicated, especially in the setting of HIV. In primary syphilis, the hallmark symptom is a painless lesion usually on the external genital. The differential diagnosis would include other STDs such as genital herpes, chancroid, or lymphogranuloma venereum (LGV). Most of these diseases create a painful lesion or local lymphandenopathy. The lesions associated with secondary syphilis can be confused with other skin manifestations, such as pityriasis rosea, psoriasis, erythema multiforme, tinea versicolor, viral exanthema, scabies, or even a drug reaction. The simplest test used to diagnosis syphilis at these stages is a dark-field examination and/or direct fluorescent antibody (DFA) stain on lesion exudates or tissue.[2] The spirochetes will be visible on examination.

However, if the initial lesion has healed, a diagnosis can be made using the results of two sets of serological tests. PCR and culture are not helpful in the diagnosis of this disease. First-line testing should include one of the nontreponemal tests. These include the VDRL (Venereal Disease Research Laboratory test) and the RPR (rapid plasma reagin test) performed on serum.[1] These tests look for the production of antibodies to cardiolipin, which is elevated initially in the course of infection but is not specific to the spirochete causing disease. A reactive titer is $>1:32$; titers less than $1:8$ are considered false positives in the presence of a negative FTA-ABS (see discussion below).[1] The nontreponemal tests correlate well with disease activity and eventually become nonreactive after successful treatment or after an extended period of infection. However, some individuals are classified as "serofast" in that their RPR or VDRL results will remain positive for life. The sensitivity for the VDRL is around 80%, and the specificity is around 98% for detecting primary disease.[2] For the RPR, sensitivity is around 86%, and specificity is around 98%.[2] Other medical conditions such as autoimmune disease, pregnancy, mononucleosis, rickettsial infections, or other spirochete infections can create false-positive results. For this reason and especially in low-prevalence populations, any positive result should be followed by confirmatory tests, the treponemal tests.[2] These are the FTA-ABS (fluorescent treponemal antibody absorbed test) and the TP-PA (*T. pallidum* particle agglutination assay). These assays detect antibodies that are specific to the spirochete and once positive, will remain positive for life. The sensitivity and specificity for the FTA-ABS are 84% and 94%, respectively for detecting primary disease.[2] Therefore, in an effort to diagnose syphilis, a positive RPR should be followed by an FTA-ABS. If positive, syphilis is confirmed. However, a negative RPR with a reported history of a documented yet distant (especially untreated) exposure should also be followed by an FTA-ABS to rule out latent infection.

The symptoms associated with neurosyphilis can be attributed to a number of other diseases or manifestations. Often, individuals with neurosyphilis will present with delusions or dementia or other major affective disorders, prompting an evaluation by a psychiatrist rather than an infectious disease specialist. In this instance, the patient is not getting the required treatment. So, it is slowly becoming the standard of care that individuals admitted to the hospital with dementia or delusions be screened for syphilis to rule out this etiology. Other infectious agents such as herpes viruses, Epstein–Barr virus, arboviruses, enteroviruses, and even advanced HIV disease can cause symptoms similar to those seen in neurosyphilis.

Neurosyphilis is diagnosed when the serum RPR and/or FTA-ABS are reactive, the patient's CSF profile is abnormal with an elevated white count (>5 cells/mm^3) or elevated protein, and a CSF VDRL is positive. Neurological symptoms may or may not be present. There are rare occurrences of neurosyphilis with a normal CSF profile, but this is not common, and all three components are needed for a diagnosis. The CSF VDRL (the preferred test for CSF) is highly specific yet only 30–70% sensitive, and the FTA-ABS on the CSF is less specific but highly sensitive. Either test alone is not comprehensive enough for a diagnosis.

CSF invasion by the bacterium can occur in primary and secondary stages of disease, creating an abnormal CSF profile; therefore, CSF analysis is not recommended as part of the routine evaluation during these stages. The CDC criteria for performing a lumbar puncture are (1) neurological or ocular symptoms, (2) late latent syphilis or unknown duration of infection, (3) active tertiary disease, or (4) evidence of treatment failure. Imaging, such as an MRI, can be helpful in demonstrating low-density lesions in the brain and spinal cord that are characteristic of central nervous system (CNS) infection.

When there is concurrent HIV infection, the diagnosis of syphilis can be difficult as there can be an altered serological response. Often, individuals with HIV have a delayed or weak antibody response, so they may not be positive in the expected timeframe. Or the opposite may be the case; they may produce higher than normal levels of antibody, creating false-negative test results due to a prozone effect.[3] The prozone effect occurs when the antibody concentration in the sample is greater than the antigen concentration in the assay, thereby binding all the antigen and preventing the formation of a precipitin, creating what looks like a negative result.[3] However, when the serum is diluted and the antigen and antibody are in the appropriate ratios, a reactive result is seen. To complicate matters, CSF abnormalities are commonly present in the early stages of HIV and can therefore interfere with a diagnosis. The CSF profile in HIV disease with concurrent primary or secondary syphilis is unknown. Therefore, some sources recommend a lumbar puncture on all HIV patients regardless of stage of disease or symptomatology.[1]

Treatment

Penicillin G given parenterally has been the longstanding treatment for all stages of syphilis. For primary or secondary stages, benthazine penicillin G at 2.4 million units given IM in a single dose is recommended if within 1 year of exposure.[1] If a longer course of infection is suspected, multiple rounds of treatment may be needed. For neurosyphilis, the recommended treatment is aqueous crystalline penicillin G at 18–24 million units per day for 10–14 days administered IV at 3–4 million units every 4 hours. Some literature suggests treatment up to 4 weeks in some cases, and ceftriaxone is not an appropriate substitute. Ideally, individuals who are allergic to penicillin should be desensitized prior to treatment, especially for neurosyphilis, yet it has been demonstrated that successful treatment of primary syphilis can be achieved with a single 2-g dose of azithromycin. However, careful and close follow-up is highly recommended with this choice of therapy.

Individuals treated for primary or secondary syphilis should be seen by a physician at 6 months and 12 months following treatment for clinical evaluation as well as serological follow-up. Individuals who are treated successfully will have a negative RPR and a positive FTA-ABS. Also, due to the association of HIV and syphilis, individuals treated for syphilis should also be evaluated for HIV. It should also be stressed that successful treatment and recovery does not preclude an individual from acquiring the disease again.

Follow-up for neurosyphilis is more complex. For otherwise healthy individuals, follow-up should consist of serum and CSF analysis at 6 and 12 months posttreatment. Individuals with HIV should have serum and CSF examined at 3, 6, 9, 12, and 24 months until parameters return to within normal limits and their antibody response indicates treatment success.[1] If CSF cell counts or protein are still abnormal after 2 years, retreatment is recommended.

References

1. BAUGHN, R. AND MUSHER, D.: Secondary syphilitic lesions. *Clin. Microbiol. Rev. 18*:205–16, 2005.
2. FARNES, S. AND SETNESS, P.: Serological test for syphilis. *Postgrad. Med. 87*:37–46, 1990.
3. JURADO, R., CAMPBELL, J. AND MARTIN, P.: Prozone phenomenon in secondary syphilis. *Arch. Intern. Med. 153*:2496–8, 1993.

Additional Reading

GOLDEN, M., MARRA, C., AND HOLMES, K.: Update on syphilis: Resurgence of an old problem. *JAMA 290*: 1510–14, 2003.

LYNN, W. AND LIGHTMAN, S.: Syphilis and HIV: A dangerous combination. *Lancet Infect. Dis. 4*:456–66, 2004.
Syphilis Surveillance Report: www.cdc.gov/std/Syphilis2002.

Case 43

When Life Gives You Lemons

Robert S. Liao

A 22-year-old woman presented to her physician with worsening monthly episodes of arthritis of the knee, without having sustained a previous accident or injury. She had a history of unexplained fevers with myalgias for the past 12 months. Two years ago, the patient was diagnosed with Achilles tendonitis and suffered several ankle sprains. She lived in the state of Wisconsin and was an active cross-country runner and hockey player. The patient had several tick exposures but denied any history of a rash or having been bitten.

Physical examination showed pain and stiffness during active range of motion and a large effusion of the right knee joint. A synovial fluid specimen from the knee showed a leukocyte count of $1.1 \times 10^5/\text{mm}^3$ (72% granulocytes). Joint fluid was sent to the microbiology lab and was negative for Gram's stain and culture. Additional lab testing revealed an ANA titer of only 1 : 40 and a negative rheumatoid factor.

Serology for Lyme borreliosis (Lyme disease) using enzyme-linked immunosorbent assay (ELISA) for IgG was subsequently ordered, and the result was positive. However, indirect immunofluorescence assay (IFA) for IgM was equivocal. The Lyme disease serology results were withheld, and the patient's serum was referred out for additional testing. An IgG immunoblot was strongly positive (greater than 5 bands present) indicating seropositivity for *Borrelia burgdorferi*, the causative agent of Lyme borreliosis. Additionally, synovial fluid from the knee joint aspiration tested positive by PCR for *B. burgdorferi* DNA (OspA).

The patient was diagnosed with stage 3 Lyme disease and treated with oral doxycycline 100 mg BID for 60 days. The case was reported to the state health laboratory, and the patient fully recovered 2 months later without further treatment.

Definition of Disease

Lyme disease is caused by bacteria of the spirochaete family, which are grouped in the *Borrelia burgdorferi* Spirochaetaeae family complex. Lyme disease is one of the most common vectorborne diseases in North America and Europe. The vectors of Lyme disease are several closely related ixodid ticks. In the northeastern and midwestern United States, *Ixodes scapularis* is the vector while *Ixodes pacificus* is the vector in the west.

Tietz's Applied Laboratory Medicine, Second Edition. Edited by Mitchell G. Scott, Ann M. Gronowski, and Charles S. Eby
Copyright © 2007 John Wiley & Sons, Inc.

The clinical features important for diagnosing Lyme disease (or borreliosis) differ somewhat between the United States and Europe because of the different genospecies of *Borrelia* present in the different geographic regions. As a consequence, the large amount of clinical evidence accumulated in the United States might not completely apply to the disease in Europe and elsewhere.[1] In the United States, Lyme disease is localized mostly to states in the northeastern, mid-Atlantic, and upper north-central regions, and to several counties in northwestern California. The majority of Lyme disease cases are reported to the CDC from the states of Connecticut, Rhode Island, New York, Pennsylvania, New Jersey, Maryland, Massachusetts, Minnesota, and Wisconsin.

Similar to other spirochetal infections, Lyme disease is a multisystem and multistage infection with remissions and exacerbations at each stage. A complete presentation of all three stages of Lyme disease is an extremely unusual event in which erythema migrans (EM) skin rash at the site of the tick bite is followed by nervous system and heart involvement, and then later on by arthritis. Early infection consists of stage 1 (localized infection) and stage 2 (disseminated infection). The localized infection of stage 1 consists of a primary EM that may begin days to weeks after a tick bite. Most patients do not remember the tick bite. Skin is the most frequently affected tissue in Lyme disease, and EM is the most important clinical sign.[2]

EM is followed within days by clinical manifestations of hematogenous dissemination (stage 2). In U.S. patients, disseminated infection can result in multiple secondary skin lesions whose appearance is similar to the initial EM. Approximately 18% of patients will present only with malaise, headache, fever and chills, regional lymphadenopathy, and generalized achiness. The early signs and symptoms are typically intermittent and changing. Approximately 15% of untreated patients will develop frank neurologic abnormalities (neuroborreliosis) that may occur alone or in combinations: cranial neuritis (including bilateral facial palsy), meningitis, encephalitis, motor and sensory radiculoneuritis, mononeuritis multiplex, and cerebellar ataxia or myelitis. Usually, pain as a result of radiculoneuritis is the most pronounced clinical symptom. Early neuroborreliosis typically features aseptic meningitis and involvement of cranial and peripheral nerves.

Approximately 5% of untreated patients develop cardiac involvement. Lyme carditis is most commonly characterized by fluctuating degrees of atrioventricular blocks as a result of conduction disturbances. The course is usually favorable.

Stage 3 is late or persistent infection and occurs months to years after initial exposure. Arthritis is the most frequent clinical sign. Approximately 60–70% of untreated patients infected with *B. burgdorferi* will develop intermittent epidsodes of joint swelling and pain that may recur for years. The course of Lyme arthritis is highly variable and can last for several years. Lyme arthritis presents most commonly in large joints, especially the knee, and usually one or two joints at a time (monoarthritis or oligoarthritis). The elbow, ankle, shoulder, hip, and temporomadnibular joints are also less commonly affected. Some patients with pronounced joint effusions have disproportionately mild pain. Joint inflammation usually lasts a few days to weeks or months separated by periods of complete remission.

Persistent infection can also manifest in U.S. patients as a mild, late neurologic syndrome called *Lyme encephalopathy* that manifests primarily by subtle cognitive disturbances. Although there are no inflammatory changes in the CSF, intrathecal antibody production to *B. burgdorferi* is often present. In Europe, a chronic skin manifestation called *acrodermatitis chronica atrophicans* is also sometimes observed.[3]

Differential Diagnosis

Lyme disease is a nationally notifiable disease and is diagnosed using a combination of a history of known exposure in an endemic area, recognition of clinical features, and serologic studies (ELISA and immunoblot). Lyme disease presents with diverse clinical signs and symptoms that can be of low or even no diagnostic value. This diversity can result in delayed clinical diagnosis and the mistaken diagnoses of Lyme disease, often due to erroneous interpretations of serological results. The best clinical marker for the disease is the initial erythema migrans rash (≥ 5 cm).

The differential diagnosis of Lyme arthritis is broad and requires the exclusion of other causes of arthritis. The most common cause of bacterial arthritis is *Neisseria gonorrhoeae*. The diagnosis of Lyme arthritis may be confused with other rheumatic diseases, particularly in the absence of a history of EM. Lyme arthritis is most like pauciarticular juvenile arthritis in children and reactive arthritis in adults. Only 30–50% of the patients with Lyme arthritis may recall having been bitten by a tick or having EM. Lyme arthritis can be mistaken for an acute bacterial septic arthritis or recurrent pauciarticular rheumatoid arthritis.[2]

The test of choice for evaluation of a patient with suspected Lyme arthritis should be serum IgG antibodies since false-negative results of serologic examination are rarely encountered. Many commercial serology tests are available for Lyme disease, including screening tests (immunofluorescence, hemagglutination, and ELISA), and confirmatory immunoblots. For Lyme borreliosis serology testing in the United States, the Centers for Disease Control and Prevention currently recommends a two-test approach to increase specificity. Samples that are first tested by ELISA or indirect immunofluorescence assay (IFA) are followed by immunoblotting (Western blotting) for confirmation of positive or equivocal results. However, it is extremely important to note that serologic testing should be used only to confirm a clinical diagnosis.[4] Hence it is used only in patients with a very high index of suspicion for Lyme disease. Positive *B. burgdorferi* serology without clinical signs and symptoms is widely mistaken as an indication for antibiotic treatment. It is worth noting that the U.S. Food and Drug Administration (FDA) has cleared over 60 immunoserological assays for Lyme disease for blood, plasma, and serum specimens, but none of them have yet been approved for use with CSF or joint fluid.

In general, patients with Lyme arthritis have higher *B. burgdorferi*–specific antibody titers than do patients with any other manifestation of Lyme disease. However, patients in the early stages of Lyme disease may not produce detectable concentrations of antibody. False-negative serology results are also possible if antibiotic therapy, administered early in the disease, prevents antibody production from reaching detectable concentrations. False-positive serology results are possible as a result of cross-reactions with with EBV, *Rickettsia*, and *Treponema pallidum* (syphilis). Furthermore, *B. burgdorferi* IgG and even IgM antibody titers decline slowly after treatment but may remain detectable for many years after infection. Thus, serological testing cannot reliably distinguish between active and inactive disease.[4]

Culture of *B. burgdorferi* on Barbour–Stoenner–Kelly medium (BSK) should be used as the method of choice for skin biopsy specimens of early skin manifestations. However, culture has only rarely been successful from synovial fluid and CSF. The low recovery rate from synovial fluid and CSF probably reflects the small number of viable bacteria in those anatomic sites.

Borrelia burgdorferi DNA has been detected by PCR in the synovial fluid of up to 80% of untreated patients with Lyme arthritis. Most studies of the use of PCR for analysis of synovial fluid or synovial tissue specimens have involved patients who are strongly seropositive for *B. burgdorferi* and who undergo testing for the monitoring of disease activity.[5] PCR testing of synovial fluid samples is of potential value in the treatment of patients with established Lyme arthritis, but should not be used for the diagnosis of seronegative patients with suspected Lyme disease.[6]

Patients with acute neuroborreliosis (stage 2), especially with meningitis, may have intrathecal production of antibody to *B. burgdorferi*. However, intrathecal serology is less frequently positive in patients with the chronic neuroborreliosis (Lyme encephalopathy) that manifests in persistent infections (stage 3). Similarly, culture of CSF can be positive shortly after the onset of clinical signs and symptoms (stage 2) in less than 10% of patients, usually with meningitis. However, *B. burgdorferi* is not culturable from the CSF of patients with chronic neuroborreliosis (stage 3). DNA has been detected by PCR in CSF samples in only a very small number of patients. There have not been any well-documented cases of seronegative Lyme disease with demonstrable Lyme antibodies or *B. burgdorferi* DNA present in the CSF.

Treatment

In the evaluation of patients with suspected Lyme disease, priority should be given to careful clinical assessment and judgment, which can be supplemented by appropriate laboratory testing. Treatment with antibiotics is beneficial for all stages of Lyme disease, but is most successful early in the course of the illness.[3] Prevention relies mainly on avoiding exposure to tick bites. The treatment for Lyme disease depends in large part on the stage of the disease and the complication (erythema chronicum migrans, carditis, neurologic, arthritis).[2] After an appropirate antibiotic therapy (i.e., intravenous ceftriaxone or oral doxycycline), 90% of Lyme arthritis patients will become asymptomatic within 2–3 months. Treatment failures do occur in spite of antibiotic treatment, and a second course of therapy may be necessary; 10% of adults and fewer than 5% of children with Lyme arthritis develop persisting inflammatory joint disease in excess of 1 year, which may eventually result in joint destruction. Lyme arthritis is the only chronic inflammatory arthritis in which the specific cause is known and can be cured. Synovial inflammation may persist in some patients with Lyme arthritis after the apparent eradication of *B. burgdorferi* from the joint with antibiotic therapy.

References

1. REED, K. D.: Laboratory testing for Lyme disease: Possibilities and practicalities. *J. Clin. Microbiol. 40*:319–24, 2002.
2. MANDELL, G. L., BENNETT, J. E., AND DOLIN R., eds.: *Mandell, Douglas, and Bennett's Priniciples and Practice of Infectious Diseases*, 6th ed., Elsevier Churchill Livingstone, Philadelphia, 2005.
3. STANEK, G. AND STRLE, F.: Lyme borreliosis. *Lancet 362*:1639–47, 2003.
4. http://www.fda.gov/medbull/summer99/Lyme.html.
5. CARLSON, D., HERNANDEZ, J., BLOOM, B. J. ET AL.: Lack of *Borrelia burgdorferi* DNA in synovial samples from patients with antibiotic treatment–resistant Lyme arthritis. *Arthritis Rheum. 2*:2705–9, 1999.
6. NOCTON, J. J., DRESSLER, F., RUTLEDGE, B. J., ET AL.: Detection of *Borrelia burgdorferi* DNA by polymerase chain reaction in synovial fluid from patients with Lyme arthritis. *N. Engl. J. Med. 330*:229–34, 1994.

Case 44

The Wheezing Woodsman

Paula Revell

A 29-year-old man presented to his physician with a history of mild asthma since childhood. His asthma had been managed with periodic use of an albuterol inhaler. He had never required admission to a hospital because of wheezing. He had a chronic morning cough. His asthmatic symptoms worsened after he moved to a very old log-cabin house in a wooded area, 8 months ago. Four months prior to admission he reported chest pain and shortness of breath, particularly after working in his yard and laying ground mulch. Three weeks prior to admission he experienced onset of left-sided chest pain with increased productive cough, night sweats, and weight loss of 2.6 kg. At this time he went to his physician and was treated for "pneumonia" with a course of azithromycin. A tuberculin skin test was negative. His symptoms did not improve, and he was admitted to the hospital.

On physical examination the patient appeared well. No lymphadenopathy was found. Scattered crackles were heard over the left upper lobe without signs of consolidation or a pleural friction rub. His temperature was 37.1°C, his pulse was 87, his respirations were 22, and his blood pressure was 115/75. Electrolytes and a comprehensive metabolic panel were normal. Laboratory tests revealed an elevated white blood cell count (14,000/μL; reference interval, 4000–13,000/μL), and eosinophil count [34% (4760/μL); reference interval 1–4%]. The neutrophil count was normal. The total serum IgG and IgE concentrations were 1430 mg/dL (reference interval 600–1400 mg/dL) and 4077 IU/mL (reference interval 0–180 IU/mL), respectively. A chest x-ray showed bronchiectasis in the superior lobe of the left lung and paratracheal and hilar lymphadenopathy. Routine aerobic and fungal cultures of sputum revealed the absence of pathogenic microorganisms. A repeat tuberculin skin test was again negative, but a skin prick test showed an immediate reaction for *Aspergillus*. Additional testing revealed an elevated IgE specific for *A. fumagatis* of 46.5 kU/L.

The patient's symptoms matched the diagnostic criteria for allergic bronchopulmonary aspergillosis (ABPA). Determination of this diagnosis was based on a combination of clinical, laboratory, and radiographic criteria (see Table 44.1).

Tietz's Applied Laboratory Medicine, Second Edition. Edited by Mitchell G. Scott, Ann M. Gronowski, and Charles S. Eby
Copyright © 2007 John Wiley & Sons, Inc.

Table 44.1   Diagnostic Criteria for ABPA

Asthma
Peripheral blood eosinophilia
Immediate cutaneous reactivity to *Aspergillus*
Elevated total serum IgE concentration (>1000 ng/mL or >417 IU/mL)
Elevated serum IgE antibodies specific for *Aspergillus*
Serum precipitating antibodies (IgG) to *Aspergillus*
Current or previous pulmonary infiltrates
Central bronchiectasis

Source: Reference 1.

Definition of the Disease

Allergic bronchopulmonary aspergillosis (ABPA) is a severe pulmonary disease caused by hypersensitivity to *Aspergillus* spp. (primarily *A. fumigatus*, although other species, including *A. niger*, have been implicated).

The genus *Aspergillus* comprises a group of saprophytic, filamentous, spore-forming fungi commonly found in nature; this organism can be isolated from vegetation, decaying organic matter, soil, or air. There are over 185 known species of *Aspergillus*; the three most common human pathogens are *A. fumigatus*, *A. niger*, and *A. flavus*. These organisms can cause disease in both immunocompetent and immunocomprimised individuals; the diseases range from life-threatening invasive pneumonia to subacute infections such as aspergilloma in previously existing pulmonary cavities, to chronic hypersensitivity diseases such as ABPA.

ABPA is an immunologically mediated lung disease that is found primarily in individuals with persistent asthma, cystic fibrosis (CF), or both. In patients with persistent asthma the incidence of ABPA is 1–2%; for patients with CF the incidence is higher, with reports ranging from 2% to 15%.[2,3] This disease also has an increased association with particular HLA genotypes, HLA-DR2 and HLA-DR5.[4] Colonization or infection of the lungs by *Aspergillus* is initiated by inhalation of airborne spores that are small enough to reach the alveoli. Repeated inhalation of these spores leads to colonization of the airway, and the individual becomes sensitized to the organism. Once sensitized, a Th2-type immune response is induced, resulting in an increase in total serum IgE concentration, *Aspergillus*-specific antibodies, and significant eosinophilic infiltration. In addition, fungal proteases may damage the bronchial epithelial cells directly. This exaggerated host response and direct damage due to *Aspergillus* antigens, combined with the repair and remodeling process in the airways, leads to the severe fibrosis and lung damage.

There are five clinical stages of ABPA.[5] These stages do not necessarily occur in sequence. Stage 1 is acute ABPA, with eosinophilia, immediate-type skin reactivity to *Aspergillus* antigens, an elevated serum total IgE concentration, *Aspergillus*-specific IgE and IgG, and pulmonary infiltrates on chest radiograph (this patient is in the acute stage). Stage 2 is the disease in remission, with immediate-type skin reactivity and *Aspergillus*-specific antibodies persisting in the absence of radiographic findings or peripheral eosinophilia. Stage 3 is termed *exacerbation* and by definition occurs only in patients with a previous diagnosis of ABPA; in this stage all the characteristics from stage 1 are present with a twofold increase in serum total IgE concentrations and new pulmonary infiltrates. Stage 4 is characterized by steroid dependence. Stage 5 involves chronic end-stage lung disease with fixed airflow obstruction, bronchiectasis, and fibrosis.

Differential Diagnosis

Patients presenting with peripheral blood eosinophilia, increased wheezing, pulmonary infiltrates, and elevated total serum IgE should be considered for ABPA. The initial skin test screen is highly sensitive but not specific. As a result, this simple test can rule out ABPA, but a positive skin test requires further evaluation.

A variety of pulmonary disorders may present with similar findings, including acute exacerbation of asthma. Patients with steroid-dependent asthma should be evaluated for ABPA. Bacterial, viral, and fungal pneumonia should also be considered in patients with pulmonary infiltrates. Typically these patients are acutely ill with fever, and often have purulent sputum. Importantly, there is radiologic similarity between ABPA and tuberculosis, and patients with ABPA may receive antituberculous therapy for an extended period of time while lung damage due to poorly controlled ABPA continues. The absence of fever and the negative culture results from our patient's sputum sample are two clues that lead away from acute bacterial, viral, or fungal pneumonia. Churg–Strauss syndrome, eosinophilic pneumonia, and hypersensitivity pneumonitis may result in peripheral blood eosinophilia.

ABPA can be a difficult diagnosis and should not be based on a single clinical or laboratory finding. For instance, 25% of asthmatics show an immediate cutaneous reaction to *Aspergillus* antigens, yet the incidence of ABPA in this population is only 1–2%.[2,6] This complexity of diagnosis lead to the establishment of a set of diagnostic criteria in 1977, and is listed in Table 44.1.[1] Beacause of the complexity of laboratory testing required to diagnose ABPA, a stepwise approach aids in proper diagnosis and minimizes unnecessary testing. First, a patient should be given a skin test; a negative result rules out ABPA. This test is sensitive but not specific. Following a positive skin test, the total serum IgE concentration should be measured; if this concentration is >417 IU/mL (>1000 ng/mL), then concentrations of *Aspergillus*-specific IgE should be measured. Additional testing for *Aspergillus*-specific IgG can also be done. Individuals who meet the criteria for diagnosis in the absence of central bronchiectasis (CB) are said to be ABPA-seropositive; these patients are at an earlier stage of the disease and treatment may prevent further lung damage. Patients with CB are classified as ABPA-CB.

Treatment

The goals of ABPA treatment are to prevent or minimize progression of lung damage, and to manage associated asthmas. There are two aspects to treatment of ABPA: (1) a nonspecific attenuation of the massive immune response and resulting inflammation and (2) a decrease in antigen burden associated with colonization of the bronchial tree.

Corticosteroids have long been the cornerstone of treatment for ABPA. Oral corticosteroids are highly antiinflammatory and result in a decrease in serum IgE and eosinophilia, a clearing of pulmonary infiltrates, and a reduction of bronchospasm. There is debate over whether the long-term use of steroids prevents the decline of lung function.

There have been three prospective, randomized, controlled clinical trials addressing the utility of azoles in the treatment of ABPA.[7] The theory behind this treatment is reduction of the colonizing organisms, potentially leading to a decrease in host immune response to the allergens as well as the reduction of direct damage due to fungal proteases. In all the trials the results showed a significant reduction in immunological markers of disease activity; however, none of the trials showed significant improvement of lung function. It is important to note that the majority of patients enrolled in these trials were classified as ABPA-CB and likely had an element of irreversible lung disease. Future studies of patients in earlier stages of the disease (ABPA-S) are needed to assess whether the reduction in the fungal burden early in disease may indeed result in prevention of permanent lung damage.

References

1. ZANDER, D. S.: Allergic bronchopulmonary aspergillosis. *Arch. Pathol. Lab. Med. 129*:924–8, 2005.
2. GREENBERGER, P. A., AND PATTERSON, R.: Allergic bronchopulmonary aspergillosis and the evaluation of the patient with asthma. *J. Allergy Clin. Immunol. 81*:646–50, 1988.
3. STEVENS, D. A., MOSS, R. B., VISWANATH, P. ET AL.: Allergic bronchopulmonary aspergillosis in cystic fibrosis—state of the art: Cystic Fibrosis Foundation Consensus Conference. *Clin. Infect. Dis. 37*:225–64, 2003.
4. CHAUHAN, B., SANTIAGO, L., KIRSCHMANN, D. A. ET AL.: The association of HLA-DR alleles and T cell activation with allergic bronchopulmonary aspergillosis. *J. Immunol. 159*:4072–6, 1997.
5. PATTERSON, R., GREENBERGER, P. A., AND HARRIS, K. E.: Allergic bronchopulmonary aspergillosis. *Chest 118*:7–8, 2000.
6. SHAH, A., AND PANJABI, C.: Allergic bronchopulmonary aspergillosis: A review of a disease with a worldwide distribution. *J. Asthma. 39*:273–89, 2002.
7. WARK, P. A. B., GIBSON, P. G., AND WILSON, A. J.: Azoles for allergic bronchopulmonary aspergillosis associated with asthma (review). *Cochrane Database Syst. Rev. 3*:1–11, 2004.

Case 45

Not Just Heartburn

Ariel Goldschmidt

A 29-year-old woman presented to the emergency department complaining of nausea, vomiting, upper abdominal pain, and an inability to "hold food or water down" for the past 2 days. She denied experiencing fever, chills, or diarrhea. She also denied recent travel, outdoor excursions, or eating anything out of the ordinary. Previous to this, she had been healthy and had been in the hospital only once when she gave birth to a healthy male infant at term.

At the time of presentation, the patient was afebrile, and all other vital signs were normal. Physical examination revealed a woman with her hand on her abdomen in mild distress. There was mild tenderness to palpation over the abdomen, which could not be localized to a particular area. Rebound tenderness was absent. There was no evidence of ascites. All other physical examination findings were within normal limits. On review of systems, the patient admitted to "occasional queasiness" and a 6-lb (2.7 Kg) weight loss over the past year, which she attributed to her once-a-week exercise regimen. She denied having excessive fatigue or poor appetite.

Feeling that the patient's condition did not warrant immediate admission to the hospital, emergency staff instructed the patient to make an appointment at the local gastroenterology clinic within a week. By the time of her clinic appointment, the patient's symptoms had resolved. Bloodwork, including a chemistry profile and complete blood count, were sent to the lab. A urine pregnancy test was negative. The patient was given a prescription for an H2 blocker, and was instructed to begin taking it in the event that she continued to experience symptoms of "heartburn." She was instructed to follow up with another clinic appointment in 2 weeks.

At the follow-up appointment, the patient complained of recurrent episodes of nausea, vomiting, indigestion, and upper abdominal pain. She noted that the abdominal pain became worse several hours after eating a meal. The patient was informed that her complete blood count showed a mild microcytic anemia. Iron studies were consistent with iron deficiency anemia. Fecal occult blood testing (FOBT) was positive. The patient was scheduled for an upper GI endoscopy the following week.

The findings on endoscopy included erythematous gastropathy, a 2-cm clean-based gastric ulcer in the body (Fig. 45.1), and a patulous antrum concerning for prior healed ulcers.

Tietz's Applied Laboratory Medicine, Second Edition. Edited by Mitchell G. Scott, Ann M. Gronowski, and Charles S. Eby

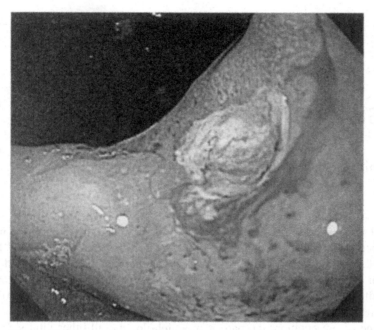

Figure 45.1   Gastric ulcer, as seen during endoscopy. (Courtesy of Dr. Dayna Early.)

The pathology report obtained 2 days later indicated: "Severe chronic active gastritis and ulcer; *Helicobacter pylori* organisms identified" (Fig. 45.2).

The patient was started on an immediate therapy regimen consisting of amoxicillin, clarithromycin, and omeprazole, with gradual improvement in her symptoms. At follow-up endoscopy, her ulcer was nearly healed (Fig. 45.3).

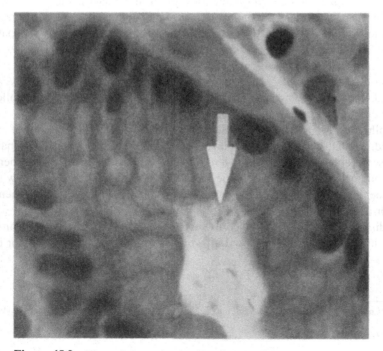

Figure 45.2   Histopathology, showing *H. pylori* organisms (arrow).

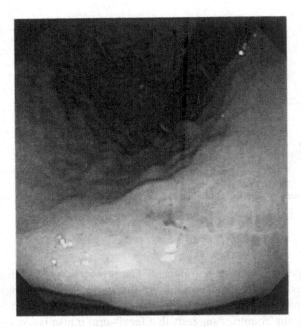

Figure 45.3   Healing gastric ulcer. (Courtesy of Dr. Dayna Early.)

Definition of the Disease

In 1979, spiral bacteria were observed in human stomach biopsy specimens by Australian pathologist J. Robin Warren, who proposed an association between the bacteria and gastritis and ulceration. Warren and his colleague Barry Marshall isolated and cultured the organisms in 1982, naming them *Campylobacter pylori*. Subsequent observation showed significant phenotypic and genotypic differences between the newly isolated organisms and the *Campylobacter* genus, and thus the *Helicobacter* genus was created in 1989. At present, this genus includes the gastric colonizing species *Helicobacter pylori*, and over 20 other gastric and intestinal colonizing species.

   Helicobacter pylori bacteria are microaerophilic, nonsporulating, highly motile, curvilinear gram negative rods, measuring approximately 3.5 × 0.75 μm, with two to seven sheathed flagellae at one end. The species has evolved survival characteristics that enable it to survive and multiply in the gastric environment, which is hostile to most bacteria. These include microaerophilism for survival within the mucus gel, spiral shape and flagella for motility, adhesins for adherence to epithelial cell surfaces, and abundant urease activity, which converts urea to bicarbonate and ammonium ions that buffer gastric acidity. In addition, *H. pylori* organisms produce several virulence factors that interact with host cells, including VacA and CagA. VacA, or vacuolating cytotoxin A, causes endocytotic abnormalities and vacuole formation in epithelial cells and is produced by approximately 50% of all strains. CagA is a pathogenic protein that is phosphorylated in epithelial cells and leads to changes in cell signaling. A high proportion of patients with peptic ulcers in Western countries are infected with CagA-positive strains. However, studies in Japan, where CagA positive strains are highly prevalent, have failed to show a statistical association between CagA strain positivity and peptic ulcer disease in that country.[1]

   Prevalence of *H. pylori* infection is chiefly related to age and geographic location. In young adults in Western countries, the average prevalence is approximately 20%; by age

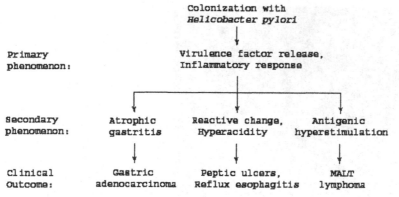

Figure 45.4   Association of *H. pylori* colonization and disease states. (Adapted from Ref. 2.)

50, greater than 50% of individuals have been infected. The prevalence is significantly higher in developing countries. Overall, about one-third of the world's current population has been infected with *H. pylori*. The high prevalence in areas where sanitary conditions are suboptimal and in developing countries suggests that fecal–oral transmission occurs. Although *H. pylori* have been isolated from dental plaque, the existence of oral–oral transmission has not been proved.[2]

Individuals infected with *H. pylori* are at increased risk for atrophic gastritis, reflux esophagitis, gastric and duodenal ulcers, mucosa-associated lymphoid tissue (MALT) lymphoma, and adenocarcinoma (Fig. 45.4). More than 90% of patients in Western countries with duodenal ulcers carry *H. pylori*, since the gastric colonizing *H. pylori* cause gastric hypersecretion of acid and other complex physiologic changes that affect the proximal duodenum. A smaller proportion of patients (50–80%) with gastric ulcers are colonized by *H. pylori*, since many gastric ulcers are due to NSAID (non-steroidal anti-inflammatory drug) or aspirin use.[2]

Symptoms

Most acquisition of *H. pylori* worldwide occurs in children and is clinically silent for decades. Acquisition of *H. pylori* as an adult may cause an acute upper gastrointestinal illness with nausea and upper abdominal pain, lasting from 3 to 14 days. In the long term, infected individuals may experience chronic dyspepsia secondary to atrophic gastritis. Patients with gastric or duodenal ulcers frequently experience gradual onset of a gnawing, burning pain in the midstomach area between meals and in early morning hours. Melena and hematemesis may also occur. Symptoms worrisome for carcinoma/lymphoma include excessive weight loss, fatigue, and dysphagia.[2]

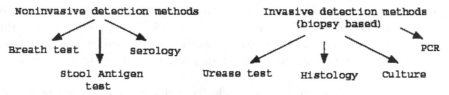

Figure 45.5   Noninvasive and invasive methods for detection of *H. pylori* infection.

Diagnosis

Tests for detection of *H. pylori* infection can be broadly divided into noninvasive tests and invasive tests requiring upper GI endoscopy with biopsy (Fig. 45.5).

No "gold standard" test exists for *H. pylori* detection; however, according to FDA criteria, a patient is considered to be positive for *H. pylori* infection if either culture or a combination of two other biopsy-based tests (i.e., rapid urease test and histology) are positive.[3]

Breath Testing

The characteristic, high urease activity of *H. pylori* can effectively be used for detection of the organism in the laboratory. Urea breath testing involves the administration of a small quantity of carbon isotope–labeled urea orally with subsequent measurement of the level of carbon isotope in CO_2 excreted in the breath. Administration of ^{14}C urea for testing exposes patients to only 1 μCi (one microcurie) of radioactivity; however, concerns about radiation have led to increased research of tests using ^{13}C-labeled urea. Traditionally, this has involved measurement of the $^{13}CO_2/^{12}CO_2$ ratio in breath with a mass spectrometer. Mass spectrometers are very sensitive but have the disadvantage of being large, complex instruments requiring specialized technicians, and have high capital and maintenance costs. Newly developed infrared spectrophotometers can measure the $^{13}CO_2/^{12}CO_2$ ratio as accurately as can mass spectrometers with lower cost and easier operation.

Preliminary studies have shown that breath testing using an infrared spectrophotometer can result in *H. pylori* detection with sensitivity and specificity of ≤98%. Breath testing may be used for initial screening of dyspeptic patients or for follow-up after therapy; however, it is necessary to wait 2 weeks after therapy to test because of the possibility of false negatives from medication (e.g., due to acid suppression from proton pump inhibitors). Additionally, a small number of false positives may occur from other urease positive organisms (e.g., *Proteus* spp., *H. heilmanii*).[4] Currently, urea breath testing is not yet FDA-approved for patients under the age of 18.

Stool Antigen Detection

Stool antigen detection may be used as an alternative to urea breath testing for initial diagnostic screening of patients with dyspepsia or for monitoring the effectiveness of therapy. It is especially appealing as a first-line noninvasive screening test in the pediatric population, because it does not require venipuncture. Importantly, when stool antigen detection is used to ascertain successful eradication of *H. pylori*, patients must be tested at least 4 weeks after completion of therapy.

Certain drawbacks are associated with the traditional stool antigen test, which uses a noncompetitive sandwich immunoassay with polyclonal antibodies to *H. pylori*. Specifically, it has been shown that *Helicobacter* species other than *H. pylori*, some of which have been reported in human disease, react with the commercially available polyclonal test. Recently, a stool antigen test using monoclonal antibodies has been developed that is theoretically more accurate than the polyclonal antibody test because of increased antigenic specificity for *H. pylori*. The key to the development of a monoclonal antibody assay was the use of cells of the coccoid form of *H. pylori* as an immunogen in the process of somatic hybridization, since *H. pylori* is believed to be in the coccoid form outside the stomach.[5] A recent study comparing the commercially available monoclonal test to the traditional polyclonal test showed increased sensitivity and specificity of the monoclonal test (88% and 98%, respectively, vs. 64% and 93%).[6]

Serology

Historically, serologic methods for *H. pylori* detection have had relatively low sensitivity and specificity compared to other methods, although more recent technological advances have improved their utility. IgM, IgG, and/or IgA antibodies can develop in response to *H. pylori* antigens; however, IgG antibodies have the best correlation with *H. pylori* infection and greatest clinical usefulness. IgG antibody concentrations usually fall slowly but significantly after successful treatment of *H. pylori* infection.[2] However, serology test results can be positive in cases of either active or past *H. pylori* infection.

There have been recent advances in the serologic diagnosis of *H. pylori*, including the use of purified and recombinant antigens instead of crude bacterial lysate, a virulence-specific ELISA, the quantitation of virulence-specific antibodies using microparticle immunofluorescence, and new rapid point-of-care devices for serum or whole blood. ELISA is the most common laboratory-based method, and new ELISA assays have sensitivities and specificities >90%. Rapid, point-of-care serologic tests utilize latex agglutination or immunochromatography for qualitative detection of *H. pylori* antibodies in serum or whole blood. These tests generally have lower accuracy compared with laboratory-based tests, but are popular because they are rapid and inexpensive.[7]

Endoscopy

Endoscopy with biopsy permits inspection of pathology and allows detection of ulcers and neoplasms, but is invasive and relatively expensive and time-consuming. Following endoscopy, several modalities for *H. pylori* detection are available (e.g., Table 45.1 lists sensitivities and specificities of biopsy-specimen-based methods for detection of *H. pylori* infection).

Histology

Histology allows direct visualization of *H. pylori* organisms and evaluation of the extent and nature of tissue involvement with detection of potential malignancy. Organisms can be visualized using standard H&E staining, although special stains such as Warthin–Starry silver, Wright–Giemsa, Steiner, or Acridine Orange are typically employed for improved visualization. Rod-shaped organisms are seen along the luminal surfaces of epithelial cells and in the luminal mucus. Drawbacks of histologic examination include the possibility of biopsy being performed in the wrong area in the case of patchy gastritis, insensitivity for detection of small numbers of organisms, and long turnaround time.

Table 45.1 Biopsy-Specimen-Based Methods for Detection of *H. pylori* Infection

Method	Sensitivity, %	Specificity, %	PPV, %	NPV, %
CLOtest	89.0	98.1	96.0	94.4
Culture	89.5	99.1	97.8	94.6
Histology	92.2	99.7	99.3	96.1
PCR	99.4	95.6/99.1	98.2	99.7

Source: Data from Reference 13.
CLOtest is a Urease test

Table 45.2   Biochemical Characteristics of *Helicobacter pylori* and Related Bacteria

Characteristic	*Helicobacter pylori*	*Helicobacter mustelae*	*Helicobacter felis*	*Campylobacter jejuni*
Urease	+	+	+	−
Catalase	+	+	+	+
Oxidase	+	+	+	+
H$_2$S production	−	−	−	+
Nitrate reduction	−	+	+	+
Resistance to nalidixic acid (30-μg disk)	+	−	+	−
Cephalothin (30-μg disk)	−	+	−	+
Growth at 42°C	−	+	+	+
Growth at 37°C	+	+	+	+
Growth at 25°C	−	−	−	−

Source: Data from Reference 2.

Culture

Ground biopsy specimens can be cultured for *H. pylori* on enriched nonselective media (e.g., chocolate agar) or selective antibiotic-containing media such as Skirrow's medium (trimethoprim, vancomycin, polymyxin B) at 37°C (98°F) under moist micro-aerobic conditions (5% oxygen) for 2–5 days. Cultures using noninvasive methods (e.g., aspiration of gastric juice) have been shown to be insufficiently sensitive. Culture of *H. pylori* organisms enables determination of antimicrobial susceptibilities, but it is not optimally sensitive or performed in most laboratories because of the special media and growth requirements needed during transport and incubation. Culture plates typically show small, mucoid colonies that are 1–2 mm thick. *H. pylori* organisms are urease-, catalase-, and oxidase-positive, and resistant to nalidixic acid (Table 45.2).

Urease Testing

Urease testing involves the introduction of a biopsy specimen into a medium containing urea and a pH indicator that changes color at alkaline pH. The most popular commercially available test is the CLOtest, which relies on diffusion of urease into an agar gel and shows average sensitivities and specificities of ~96% after 24 hours. An ultrarapid test with dry urea substrate embedded in filter paper (Pronto Dry) is now commercially available and produces faster results with slightly lower sensitivity (sensitivity ~84%, specificity ~98% at 30 minutes).[8] A recently developed urease test using monoclonal antibodies to capture *H. pylori* urease has failed to show greater accuracy than did CLOtest.[9] Medications for *H. pylori* interfere with all urease-based tests.

PCR Amplification

Original studies with PCR focused on maximizing sensitivity and specificity for detection of *H. pylori* (Table 45.1). New research is focused on real-time PCR for detection of strain-specific virulence or resistance to antibiotics. Recently, promising results were

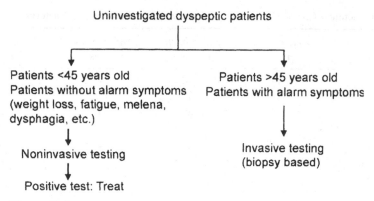

Figure 45.6   Management of uninvestigated dyspepsia. (Adapted from Ref. 14.)

obtained using SYBR® Green biprobe technology and melting curve analysis of probe PCR product duplexes for determination of point mutations in the 23S rRNA gene (clarithromycin resistance is due to single-point mutations in the peptidyltransferase region of the 23S rRNA gene).[10] Improvements in the accuracy of real-time assays and development of PCR tests using stool samples may lead to increased availability of PCR-based tests for *H. pylori.*

Treatment

Treatment of *H. pylori* infection is recommended for patients with concurrent peptic ulcer disease or gastric MALT lymphoma. Successful treatment in these patients can result in healing of ulcers and regression of MALT lymphoma. Treatment of infected individuals with symptoms of dyspepsia (mild stomach upset or indigestion) is controversial. There is increasing evidence to support a "test and treat" strategy in these patients, in which patients are tested noninvasively and treated if positive. A 7-year prospective study of 500 dyspeptic patients in primary care at Odense University Hospital in Denmark found that the test-and-treat strategy was as safe and effective as prompt endoscopy and resulted in less costly use of resources[11,12] (Fig. 45.6).

The noninvasive test-and-treat strategy should be limited to young patients with low risk of cancer. Patients with higher risk of cancer should be evaluated by invasive methods.[11,12]

Helicobacter pylori is susceptible to a variety of antimicrobial agents, but none have proved therapeutic effectiveness when used as a single agent. Effective regimens include two antimicrobial agents (e.g., amoxicillin, clarithromycin, tetracycline, or metronidazole) plus either ranitidine bismuth citrate, bismuth subsalicylate, or a proton pump inhibitor (lansoprazole, omeprazole, esometrazon, or rabeprazole sodium). FDA-approved treatment regimens range from 1 to 4 weeks in length. Resistance of *H. pylori* to antibiotics, especially to imidazoles such as metronidazole and macrolides such as clarithromycin, is increasing.[2]

References

1. KATO, S., SUGIYAMA, T., KUDO, M. ET AL.: CagA antibodies in Japanese children with nodular gastritis or peptic ulcer disease. *J. Clin. Microbiol.* *38*:68–70, 2000.

2. BLASER, M. J.: *Helicobacter pylori* and related organisms. In *Principles and Practice of Infectious Diseases*, 5th ed., G. MANDELL, ed., Churchill Livingstone, 2000.

3. FDA, Division of Anti-Infective Drug Products: *Points to Consider: Clinical Development and Labeling of Anti-infective Drug Products*. March 1995 Addendum. *Helicobacter pylori-Associated Peptic Ulcer Disease*, indication no. 25. Center for Drug Evaluation and Research, 1995.

4. KATO, M., SAITO, M., FUKUDA, S. ET AL.: 13C-Urea breath test, using a new compact nondispersive isotope-selective infrared spectrophotometer: Comparison with mass spectrometry. *J. Gastroenterol.* *39*:629–34, 2004.

5. SUZUKI, N., WAKASUGI, M., NAKAYA, S. ET AL.: Production and application of new monoclonal antibodies specific for a fecal *Helicobacter pylori* antigen. *Clin. Diagn. Lab. Immunol.* *9*:75–8, 2002.

6. ANDREWS, J., MARSDEN, B., BROWN, D. ET AL.: Comparison of three stool antigen tests for *Helicobacter pylori* detection. *J. Clin. Pathol.* *56*:769–71, 2003.

7. VAIRA, D., HOLTON, J., MENEGATTI, M. ET AL.: New immunological assays for the diagnosis of *Helicobacter pylori* infection. Gut 45 (Suppl 1):I23–7, 1999.

8. MORIO, O., RIOUX-LECLERCQ, N., PAGENAULT, M. ET AL.: Prospective evaluation of a new rapid urease test (Pronto Dry) for the diagnosis of *Helicobacter pylori* infection. *Gastroenterol. Clin. Biol.* *28*:569–73, 2004.

9. NAKATA, H., ITOH, H., ISHIGUCHI, T. ET AL.: Immunological rapid urease test using monoclonal antibody for *Helicobacter pylori*. *J. Gastroenterol. Hepatol.* *19*:970–4, 2004.

10. SCHABEREITER-GURTNER, C., HIRSCHL, A. M., DRAGOSICS, B. ET AL.: Novel real-time PCR assay for detection of *Helicobacter pylori* infection and simultaneous clarithromycin susceptibility testing of stool and biopsy specimens. *J. Clin. Microbiol.* *42*:4512–8, 2004.

11. LASSEN, A.T., HALLAS, J., AND SCHAFFALITZKY DE MUCKADELL, O. B.: *Helicobacter pylori* test and eradicate versus prompt endoscopy for management of dyspeptic patients: 6.7 year follow up of a randomised trial. *Gut* *53*:1758–63, 2004.

12. LASSEN, A. T., PEDERSEN, F. M., BYTZER, P. ET AL.: *Helicobacter pylori* test-and-eradicate versus prompt endoscopy for management of dyspeptic patients: A randomised trial. *Lancet* *356*:455–60, 2000.

13. VAN DOORN, L. J., HENSKENS, Y., NOUHAN, N. ET AL.: The efficacy of laboratory diagnosis of *Helicobacter pylori* infections in gastric biopsy specimens is related to bacterial density and vacA, cagA, and iceA genotypes. *J. Clin. Microbiol.* *38*:13–7, 2000.

14. GATTA, L., RICCI, C., TAMPIERI, A., AND VAIRA, D.: Non-invasive techniques for the diagnosis of *Helicobacter pylori* infection. *Clin. Microbiol. Infect.* *9*:489–96, 2003.

Case 46

The Dangers of Yardwork

Nathan A. Ledeboer

In late summer, a 78-year-old male presented to the emergency department (ED) of a Midwestern hospital after a period of shortness of breath, headache, and general malaise. On admission, the patient also complained that he "felt his blood pressure was high." Before the onset of symptoms the patient had spent 2 days working in the yard. Family members accompanying the patient noted changes in mental status with periods of confusion, decreased appetite, and lethargy. The patient denied any specific pain or discomfort, and his previous medical history was unremarkable. He denied any tobacco or alcohol use. His travel and social histories were also unremarkable.

On initial examination, the patient was febrile at 39°C, hypertensive with a blood pressure of 219/93 mm Hg, had a heart rate of 72 beats per minute (bpm), and respiration rate of 20 breaths per minute. On physical examination the patient appeared alert and oriented. He was calm, was cooperative, and spoke clearly. His cardiovascular exam revealed elevated blood pressure. The respiratory, gastrointestinal, integumentary, and muscular/skeletal exams were unremarkable. On admission to the ED the patient was started on ceftriaxone, azithromycin, and several antihypertensive drugs.

Laboratory tests included a basic metabolic panel, complete blood count, urinalysis, and blood cultures (aerobic and mycologic). The results of the basic metabolic panel and urinalysis were within reference intervals. The blood and fungal cultures resulted in no growth leading to discontinuation of the ceftriaxone and azithromycin. The results of the complete blood count are listed below:

Analyte	Value, Conventional Units	Reference Interval, Conventional Units	Value, SI Units	Reference Interval, SI Units
WBCs	11.4×10^3/mcL	3.8–9.8	11.4×10^9/L	5.0–10.0
RBCs	5.31×10^6/mcL	4.5–5.7	5.31×10^{12}/L	4.5–5.7
Hemoglobin	15.4 g/dL	13.8–17.2	10.1 mmol/L	8.7–11.2
Hematocrit	46.10%	40.7–50.3	Same	
Platelets	200×10^3/μL	140–440	200×10^9/L	150–400
Neutrophils	27%	39–74	Same	
Lymphocytes	67%	20–54	Same	
Monocytes	6%	4.0–14.0	Same	
Eosinophils	0%	0–6	Same	
Basophils	0%	0–3	Same	

Tietz's Applied Laboratory Medicine, Second Edition. Edited by Mitchell G. Scott, Ann M. Gronowski, and Charles S. Eby
Copyright © 2007 John Wiley & Sons, Inc.

Because of the febrile illness, combined with the changes in mental status and headache, a lumbar puncture was performed. Results for laboratory tests on the CSF are as follows. The CSF was clear and colorless with 63 cells/μL, including 30 cells/μL nucleated cells (25% neutrophils, 65% lymphocytes, 10% monocytes). The CSF protein was also elevated at 91 mg/dL. CSF glucose was within reference limits, the viral PCRs were negative, and the *Cryptococcus neoformans* antigen was also negative. Arboviral serologies (CSF and serum) were referred to the state public health laboratory.

When the arboviral serologies returned from the state lab, the serologies were negative for Eastern encephalitis virus IgM, Western encephalitis virus IgM, and California encephalitis virus IgM with less than 1:20 titers. Serologies were positive for Saint Louis encephalitis virus IgM and West Nile virus IgM. Because of cross-reactivity between Saint Louis encephalitis IgM and West Nile IgM the serologies will often result in double positives. To determine true positive, titers for each virus are compared and the titer that is twice that of the lower titer is the true positive. In this case the result for Saint Louis encephalitis IgM was positive with a titer of 8.33 (a positive titer is considered greater than 3) and the West Nile IgM was positive with a titer of 29.42. Since the West Nile IgM titer was more than twice that of the Saint Louis encephalitis IgM titer, the patient was considered positive for West Nile virus. Additionally, the CSF serologies were positive for West Nile IgM with titers similar to the serum results.

Convalescent specimens from patients diagnosed with West Nile virus should be submitted to the state public health laboratory 2–3 weeks after the acute specimen is collected.

Definition of the Disease

The West Nile virus is a 10-11 kb (kilobase), positive-sense, single-stranded RNA virus belonging to the family Flaviviridae.[1,2,3] It is an enveloped icosahedral virus with worldwide distribution. West Nile virus is closely related to other members of the Japanese encephalitis virus antigen complex, resulting in serological cross-reactivity.[6]

West Nile virus has emerged as a serious threat to human health within recent years. Most cases of West Nile and other arboviral disease are documented in the months of June through September, when mosquitoes and other arthropods are most active. West Nile emerged in the United States following a 1999 outbreak in New York and became endemic when investigators determined that the virus survived in wintering mosquitoes.[1,2,4–6]

Once transferred to humans, the typical incubation period for the virus ranges from 3 to 14 days. While the most severe cases of West Nile can result in a life-threatening meningoencephalitis, the majority of cases of West Nile are mild and clinically unapparent. In about 20% of cases, infected individuals will develop a 3–6-day febrile illness characterized by headache and general malaise.[4–6]

Approximately 1 in 150 west Nile patients will develop meningoencephalitis manifesting as a febrile illness with severe headaches, neck stiffness, stupor, altered mental status, coma, tremors, convulsions, muscle weakness, and abnormal movements. Replication of the virus in various peripheral sites precedes invasion of the central nervous system (CNS). It is believed that the virus migrates from the peripheral sites through the olfactory system into the CNS. Once inside the CNS, patients can develop encephalitis, meningitis, or a combination of both: meningoencephalitis. This condition typically presents in elderly and immunocomprimised patients.[4–6]

Differential Diagnosis

Infectious causes of altered mental status must be differentiated from those conditions resulting from metabolic changes, exposure to toxins, increased cranial pressure, and physiological changes (e.g., tumors) on the basis of patient history and physical examination. Once other causes of the change in mental status have been ruled out, the infectious causes of neuroinvasive disease can include sepsis, meningitis, and encephalitis. When febrile illness progresses over several days, and neurologic changes are present, especially when the findings are compatible with meningitis and/or encephalitis, the patient's age, comorbid conditions, and exposure history should be considered when undertaking the differential diagnosis.

West Nile encephalitis must be differentiated from other causes of enchepalopathy such as subacute bacterial endocarditis, infectious mononucleosis, Legionnaires' disease, Lyme disease, Rocky Mountain Spotted Fever (RMSF), and herpesvirus infections. While the clinician can differentiate between these etiological agents using laboratory tests, conducting a thorough patient history can eliminate many. Elderly patients are at very low risk for contracting Epstein–Barr virus infectious mononucleosis. Patients who have neither traveled to endemic areas for Lyme disease and RMSF nor have had significant tick exposure are at low risk for contracting these bacterial agents. Additionally, routine blood cultures can assist in assessing bacterial endocarditis provided empiric antibiotic therapy has not been initiated prior to collecting the blood cultures.

More difficult is distinguishing between neuroinvasive disease caused by West Nile virus and those diseases caused by other arthropodborne viral pathogens. Patients infected with other flaviviruses, α-viruses, and bunyaviruses (Japanese equine encephalitis, Saint Louis encephalitis, Powassan fever, Western equine encephalitis, Eastern equine encephalitis, and La Crosse virus) will often require laboratory tests to identify the causative agent. Again, a thorough patient history consisting of a travel history combined with laboratory tests can be of great assistance in arriving at a final diagnosis. For example, Japanese equine encephalitis is found primarily in individuals with travel history to Asia, while Eastern and Western equine encephalitis cases are confined primarily to their respective coasts in the United States. However, West Nile and Saint Louis encephalitis viruses are distributed throughout the continental United States. Additionally CBC and CSF chemistries can be helpful in differentiating between flavivirus infections. Leukocytosis is suggestive of Eastern equine encephalitis, St. Louis encephalitis, and California encephalitis in patients with acute encephalitis. Also, patients presenting with West Nile may exhibit lymphopenia that is especially pronounced in immunocomprimised individuals. West Nile encephalitis also results in moderate pleocytosis of the CSF with elevated protein in the CSF.

Laboratory studies to conclusively determine the infectious agent should include serum serologies, CSF serologies, and CSF PCR. If possible, serum specimens should be obtained within 8 days of the onset of symptoms. CSF samples should also be obtained within 5–10 days of the onset of symptoms. While most clinical laboratories refer suspected West Nile cases to commercial reference laboratories or state public health laboratories for the CDC IgM assay (sensitivity nears 100%, specificity nears 100% with confirmatory testing), several commercial assays are also available. These tests include the PanBio West Nile IgM capture ELISA, immunofluorescence assay, and the Focus Diagnostic West Nile Virus IgM ELISA and can be used in the hospital clinical laboratory. These assays are advantageous because results are available in less than 48 hours and the sensitivity nears 100% for many of the assays. However, because of cross-reactivity between West Nile and other flaviviruses, confirmatory testing such as the plaque reduction neutralization assay is prescribed by CDC guidelines. Viral culture or PCR on specimens (West Nile virus is not readily cultivable on CSF samples) may also be helpful in patients infected for 2 weeks or less. However, these assays have shown only moderate sensitivity in acute illness, likely due to the transient nature of viremia. PCR is most beneficial in immunocomprimised patients who are unable to mount a significant immune response to the virus.[6]

While encephalitis and meningitis are the most serious conditions resulting from West Nile virus, West Nile can also manifest itself as aseptic meningitis and must be differentiated from two other common causes of aseptic meningitis: enterovirus and herpesvirus.

Pathogenesis

A West Nile virus reservoir is maintained in nature between certain bird populations and the mosquito. Susceptible bird populations will maintain an infectious viremia for 1–4 days before dying or developing lifelong immunity. Mosquitoes become infected when they take a blood meal, circulate the virus in their blood, and reinfect natural hosts or incidental host by carrying the virus in their salivary glands.[2,5,6] While susceptible bird species are the natural host of West Nile, humans and horses are incidental hosts. Direct human-to-human or animal-to-human transfer has not been shown.[6] Although animal-to-human transfer is not possible in the absence of the mosquito, it is possible to transfer the virus transplacentally, through breast milk, and through tissue and fluid transplantation.[2,6]

Animal models of West Nile pathogenesis suggest that the virus is inoculated subcutaneously and spread to the draining lymph nodes, spleen, and serum.[1] Replication of the virus in the lymphatic system results in a high-titer viremia that precedes infection of the CNS. Once in the CNS, the virus will preferentially target and invade the cerebellar Purkinje cells and anterior horn cells of the spinal cord as well as the neurons of the thalamus and basal ganglia.[1,3] Why the virus targets these specific cell types remains a mystery, although recent evidence suggests that the viral envelope may target unidentified receptors on these cells. As neuronal degeneration proceeds, a CD8-positive T-cell response is detectable along with induction of host cell apoptosis resulting in further neuronal damage.[1,3]

The CD8-positive T-cell response is followed by the appearance of IgM in the second week of infection. The coordinated response of the CD8-positive T cells, interferon producing γ/δ T cells, B cells, and antibody are critical components of the host response to clear the infection.[1]

Treatment

Treatment for West Nile virus is supportive and dependent on the type of infection. In patients with severe infection, treatment often consists of hospitalization with IV fluids, respiratory care, and suppression of secondary infections. Ribavirin, interferon, gammaglobulin, steroids, antiseizure medications, and osmotic agents have been used to a great degree in managing cases of West Nile virus. However, the efficacy of these treatments has not been assessed in a controlled study. Patients infected with West Nile virus are believed to develop lifelong immunity to the virus due to the absence of recurrent infections. There is no vaccine for humans.[1,4–6]

The best strategy for managing cases of West Nile is prevention and control of the mosquito population. Persons with exposure to mosquitoes should use insect repellants containing diethyltoluamide (DEET) or permethrin. In addition, community mosquito control measures such as spraying and draining standing water will prevent mosquito breeding and will control the population size.[6]

References

1. GRANWEHR, B. P., LILLIBRIDGE, K. M., HIGGS, S. ET AL.: West Nile virus: Where are we now? *Lancet Infect. Dis. 4*:547–56, 2004.

2. GOULD, L. H., AND FIKRIG, E.: West Nile virus: A growing concern? *J. Clin. Invest. 113*:1102–7, 2004.

3. OMALU, B. I., SHAKIR, A. A., WANG, G. ET AL.: Fatal fulminant panmeningopolio-encephalitis due to West Nile Virus. *Brain Pathol. 13*:465–72, 2003.

4. PETERSEN, L. H., MARFIN, A. A., AND GUBLER, D. J.: West Nile virus. *JAMA 290*:524–8, 2003.

5. ZAK, I. T., ALTINOK, D., MERLINE, J. R. ET AL.: West Nile Virus Infection. *Am. J. Roentgenoi. 184*:957–61, 2005.

6. Center for Disease Control, Division of Vector-Borne Infectious Diseases: http://www.cdc.gov/ncidod/dvbid/westnile/index.htm, 2005.

Part Twelve

Nonhematologic Malignancies

Cases of breast cancer, ovarian cancer, prostate cancer, germ cell tumor, and gestational trophoblastic disease are presented and discussed in Cases 47, 48, 49, 50, and 51, respectively (all edited by AMG).

Tietz's Applied Laboratory Medicine, Second Edition. Edited by Mitchell G. Scott, Ann M. Gronowski, and Charles S. Eby
Copyright © 2007 John Wiley & Sons, Inc.

Case 47

An Important Finding on Routine Screening

Joan K. Riley

A 53-year-old female was in excellent health when a mass was found in her right breast on an annual screening mammogram. A breast needle biopsy was performed and demonstrated the presence of an estrogen-receptor-positive ductal carcinoma in situ and an estrogen-receptor-negative invasive carcinoma on multiple margins. The mass was grade 2 out of 3 and measured 1 cm in diameter. The patient underwent a lumpectomy, and at this time the lymph nodes were negative. One month later the margin was positive on one side, and thus a right total mastectomy was performed. The patient was placed on tamoxifen (antiestrogen) and continued taking the drug for 5 years until a CT scan showed liver metastases. Subsequently the patient received chemotherapy with Taxotere (docetaxel; a mitotic inhibitor). It was later determined by immunohistochemistry (IHC) that her cancer overexpressed HER2/*neu*, and the patient began taking Herceptin (trastuzumab). Two years later, a CT scan revealed progression of the disease. She was started on carboplatin (alkylating agent–platinum compound), Taxotere, and Herceptin. CA 15-3 was measured and was 24 U/mL (0–30 U/mL). One month later her CA 15-3 was 40 U/mL and 2 months later, it was 64 U/mL. A CT scan showed an increase in the size of the liver mass. Seven months later she presented for selective internal hepatic radiation therapy. Her CA 15-3 was 189 U/mL at this time. She continues to undergo chemotherapy.

Definition of the Disease

Breast cancer is the most common nondermatologic cancer in the world, and aside from lung cancer, it is the leading cause of cancer-related deaths among American women. It is estimated that over 200,000 new cases of breast cancer are diagnosed in the United States each year. In addition, approximately 40,000 women and 400 men die annually in the United States from this disease. Risk factors associated with the development of breast cancer include increased age, reproductive history (nulliparous, delayed childbearing), early menarche, late menopause, certain genetic mutations (BRCA1 and BRCA2), family history of breast cancer, and exposure to certain carcinogens.[1]

Tietz's Applied Laboratory Medicine, Second Edition. Edited by Mitchell G. Scott, Ann M. Gronowski, and Charles S. Eby

Breast cancers are usually derived from either the epithelial lining of the large or intermediate-size ducts (ductal) or from the epithelium of the terminal ducts of the lobules (lobular). The cancer may be either noninvasive (in situ) or invasive (infiltrating). Noninvasive cancers do not metastasize. Symptomatic women may have a palpable lump with margins that are not well defined. In addition, they may also experience a change in the size or shape of the breast, nipple retraction or discharge, redness, edema, attachment of a mass to the skin, an axillary mass, or swelling of the arm.[1,2]

Many women with breast cancer are asymptomatic; thus regular screening mammography is important for early detection. Mammography is able to detect breast cancer before the mass is palpable, and it is this early detection that improves survival. The American Cancer Society recommends annual screening mammograms in asymptomatic women beginning at age 40. Screen-film mammography is the primary method of breast cancer screening. It is estimated that annual screening mammograms decrease mortality due to breast cancer by 20–35% in women 50–69 years of age and to a lesser extent in women 40–49 years of age.[3] The sensitivity range for of mammography is 60–90%. This variability is due in part to breast density, which is greater in younger women, as well as tumor size and location.[2] The benefit of screening mammography in women less than 50 years of age is equivocal because of its lack of sensitivity and the low incidence of breast cancer in this age group. The benefit of screening mammography in women ages 50–69 is clear. The specificity of mammography in women less than 50 years of age ranges from 30–40% for nonpalpable masses to 85–90% for clinically obvious abnormalities.[2] Although mammography is fallible, it is the main tool for breast cancer screening and is unlikely to be replaced in the near future by new technologies.

Differential Diagnosis

Conditions to be considered in the differential diagnosis of breast cancer include mammary dysplasia, fibroadenoma, intraductal papilloma, lipoma, and fat necrosis.[2] The diagnosis of breast cancer is based on the examination of tissue or cells obtained by biopsy. The gold standard for diagnosis and prognosis in breast cancer is the TNM staging system established by the American Joint Committee on Cancer and the International Union Against Cancer (T = size of the tumor, N = extent of regional lymph node involvement, and M = presence or absence of distant metastases). The degree of axillary lymph node involvement is the major prognostic indicator for later systemic disease.[1] The second factor that predicts disease outcome is tumor size. The majority of breast cancers are histopathologically classified as either (1) ductal, which constitutes approximately 70–80% of breast cancers, or (2) lobular, representing approximately 10% of breast cancers.[4] These classifications are further divided into noninvasive (in situ) or invasive (infiltrating) tumors. Tumor grade should be established for almost all invasive breast carcinomas. The Nottingham combined histologic grade is recommended. Tumor grade is determined by evaluating morphologic features, including tubule formation, nuclear pleomorphism, and mitotic count. Since chemotherapeutic agents are known to inhibit rapidly dividing cells, the mitotic count may be the most important component of the grading system.[1]

Laboratory values that may aid in patient evaluation include a continually elevated sedimentation rate, which may indicate disseminated disease. γ-GT (GGT) and 5' nucleotidase (5' NT) concentrations may be used to distinguish liver versus bone metastases. Advanced breast cancer may also be associated with hypercalcemia. Finally, tumor markers that are secreted by tumor cells can be used to assess prognosis, detect disease recurrence, and monitor therapy, but they are not used to screen or to diagnose breast cancer.[2] Serum marker concentrations mirror tumor load and thus are not sensitive enough to be used for screening and early diagnosis of this disease. In addition, tumor markers display a lack of specificity in early-stage breast cancer. For example, CA 15-3 has been reported to have a sensitivity of 10–15% in patients with stage I disease. In addition, CA 15-3 concentrations may be increased in benign breast or ovarian disease, thus decreasing its specificity.[5]

The CA 15-3 (breast cystic fluid protein or BCFP) assay measures serum concentrations of MUC1, which is seldom elevated early in the course of breast cancer. MUC1 is a large glycoprotein expressed on the apical surface of polarized epithelial cells. Cellular transformation leads to the shedding of MUC1 into the bloodstream.[5] Prior to the initiation of treatment, CA 15-3 concentrations may be used as a prognostic indicator. Concentrations of CA 15-3 greater than 50 U/mL suggest the presence of disseminated disease. Elevations in CA 15-3 concentrations that do not return to the normal range following treatment may indicate that the patient did not respond to treatment and may suggest a poor prognosis.[6] However, the American Society of Clinical Oncology (ASCO) has established guidelines stating that neither CA 15-3 nor CA 27-29 should be used for screening, diagnosis, staging, or surveillance after primary treatment. The guidelines also state that "Low CA 15-3 concentrations do not exclude metastases" and "Routine use of CA 15-3 to monitor the course of therapy cannot be recommended."[7]

CA 27-29, like CA 15-3, measures circulating MUC1 concentrations. As mentioned previously, ASCO has recommended that it also should not be used for screening, diagnosis, or staging; however, CA 27-29 was approved by the U.S. Food and Drug Administration (FDA) to detect recurrent breast cancer in patients with stage II or stage III disease.[5] Similar to CA 15-3, CA 27-29 concentrations may be elevated in noncancerous situations such as first-trimester pregnancy, endometriosis, ovarian cysts, and benign breast disease, to name only a few.[8]

Carcinoembryonic antigen (CEA) was one of the first identified tumor markers. It is largely expressed during fetal development; however, this protein is also expressed in certain adult tissues. Elevated CEA concentrations may indicate the presence of a tumor. However, blood concentrations of CEA may be increased in conditions other than cancer, including cirrhosis, pancreatitis, renal failure, and even heavy smoking, all of which may result in elevated CEA concentrations.[8] Again, ASCO guidelines state "CEA is not recommended for screening, diagnosis, staging, or routine surveillance of breast cancer patients after primary therapy" and also suggest that "Routine use of CEA for monitoring response of metastatic disease to treatment is not recommended. However, in the absence of readily measurable disease, or an elevated MUC-1 marker (CA 15-3 and/or CA 27-29), a rising CEA may be used to suggest treatment failure."[7]

Treatment

Breast cancer treatment may differ depending on the patient's risk profile and the oncologist. Therapy may include breast conservation surgery with radiation or mastectomy. After surgery, chemotherapy or hormone therapy is suggested for patients with potentially curable disease. The combination of anthracycline (antibiotic/intercalating agent) and cyclophosphamide (alkylating agent) may increase survival as compared to the traditional combination of cyclophosphamide, methotrexate (antimetabolite), and fluorouracil (antimetabolite).[1,2] However, morbidity due to chemotherapy is a significant concern. Thus, molecular markers that predict whether a tumor will respond to a specific therapy are important in determining the most optimal treatment regimen. Three commonly used molecular markers for breast cancer are the estrogen receptor (ER), progesterone receptor (PR), and HER2/*neu*.[1] Expression of these proteins on tumor cells is routinely determined by immunohistochemistry (IHC). In addition, HER2/*neu* expression is also established by fluorescent in situ hybridization (FISH), where available. The pattern of expression of these molecular markers forms the basis of a classification system in which tumors are identified as hormone-receptor-positive or HER2/*neu* positive, or tumors that are negative for all three markers. This classification system is employed in the diagnosis and treatment of cancer patients and in addition may help stratify patients as to the risk of recurrence.[9]

Tumors that express the ER are likely to respond to tamoxifen and other antiestrogen agents. Studies have shown that the ER is expressed in 50–70% of invasive breast cancers. It has been estimated that 50–60% of tumors that are ER-positive respond to hormone therapy whereas only 5–10% of ER negative tumors respond to this treatment. Subsequently, it has been shown that approximately 70–80% of breast cancers that express both the ER and PR respond to hormone therapy. To date it is unclear whether PR status increases the predictive power of ER status.[1,2]

HER2/*neu* is a tyrosine kinase that belongs to the epidermal growth factor receptor (EGFR) family. Approximately 20% of all breast cancers have HER2/*neu* gene amplification. It is estimated that 5% of breast cancers have HER2/*neu* overexpression without gene amplification.[1] Overexpression of HER2/*neu* on cancer cells is associated with a poor prognosis, a high risk of relapse, and death. The presence of HER2/*neu* on cancer cells suggests that they will respond to Herceptin, a humanized monoclonal antibody that is specific for the extracellular domain of HER2/*neu*.[9] Studies suggest the use of Herceptin increases survival when combined with anthracycline-containing chemotherapy regimens such as anthracycline and cyclophosphamide or paclitaxel in metastatic breast cancer. In general, tumors that express HER2/*neu* seldom express the ER receptor and thus rarely respond to endocrine therapy.[1]

There is potential clinical utility in measuring serum HER2/*neu* concentrations. The extracellular domain of HER2/*neu* may be cleaved by matrix metalloproteinase, resulting in a 97–115-kDa glycoprotein that is present in plasma and serum. There are currently two FDA-approved serum HER2/*neu* immunoassays. Studies have indicated that serum HER2/*neu* concentrations show strong direct correlation with tumor mass and a worse prognosis. In addition, on tumor removal, serum HER2/*neu* concentrations may be the only realistic way to determine HER2/*neu* status. Monitoring serum HER2/*neu* concentrations may aid in assessing prognosis, response to therapy, and earlier detection of disease progression.[9]

Breast cancer, like most other cancers, is a genetically heterogeneous disease. The intrinsic differences in the types of breast cancer dictate their responsiveness to a given therapy. Elucidating the genetic profile of a given tumor could potentially be useful in designing tailored treatment regimens that avoid unnecessary toxic therapy. Recently, the ability to examine the expression of many genes simultaneously has allowed for the rapid analysis of multiple markers that ultimately may lead to the identification of new tumor markers. Microarray analyses of certain cancers including breast, brain, lung, and prostate cancers and leukemias and lymphomas are beginning to establish a specific "signature" for a given tumor type. In the future detailed genetic analysis of a patient's tumor may provide better prognostic and therapeutic information.[4]

References

1. *CANCER Principles & Practice of Oncology*, 7th ed., V. T. DEVITA, JR., S. HELLMAN, AND S. A. ROSENBERG, eds., Lippincott, Williams & Wilkins, Philadelphia, 2005.

2. TIERNEY, L. M., MCPHEE, S. J., AND PAPADAKIS, M. A., eds.: *2005 Current Medical Diagnosis & Treatment*, 44th ed., Lange Medical Books/McGraw-Hill Medical Publishing Division, New York, 2005.

3. ELMORE, J. G., ARMSTRONG, K., LEHMAN, C. D., AND FLETCHER, S. W.: Screening for breast cancer. *JAMA* 293:1245–56, 2005.

4. ROBISON, J. E., PERREARD, L., AND BERNARD P. S., State of the science: Molecular classifications of breast cancer for clinical diagnostics. *Clin. Biochem.* 37:572–8, 2004.

5. SEREGNI, E., COLI, A., AND MAZZUCCA, N.: Circulating tumour markers in breast cancer. *Eur. J. Nucl. Med. Mol. Imagi.* 1:S15–22, 2004.

6. JANSSENS, J. P., VERLINDEN, I., GUNGOR, N., RAUS, J., AND MICHIELS, L.: Protein biomarkers for breast cancer prevention. *Eur. J. Cancer Prevent.* 13:307–17, 2004.

7. ASCO Special Article:2000 Update of recommendations for the use of tumor markers in breast and colorectal cancer: Clinical practice guidelines of the American Society of Clinical Oncology. *J. Clin. Oncol.* 19:1865–78, 2001.

8. Professional Guide to Diagnostic Tests. Lippincott, Williams & Wilkins, Philadelphia, 2005.

9. CARNEY, W. P., NEUMANN, R., LIPTON, A., LEITZEL, K., ALI, S., AND PRICE, C. P.: Potential clinical utility of serum HER2/*neu* oncoprotein concentrations in patients with breast cancer. *Clin. Chem.* 49:1579–98, 2003.

Case 48

Increasing Abdominal Girth

Nicholas P. Taylor and Randall K. Gibb

A 59-year-old woman, gravida 2 para 1 presented to her primary care physician with a 2-month history of abdominal bloating, early satiety, and increasing abdominal girth. She has a medical history significant only for essential hypertension and depression that have been responding well to medications. She has been postmenopausal for 7 years and has not been on hormone replacement therapy. Prior to menopause she used the copper-T intrauterine device (IUD) for contraception. She denied any vomiting, diarrhea, constipation, or urinary frequency. Screening colonoscopy performed at age 50, routine annual mammography, and annual cytologic screening of the uterine cervix have all been within normal limits. Her only prior operation was a cesarean section. A family history revealed maternal breast cancer, diagnosed at age 62. She does not smoke, drinks occasionally, and does not use any illicit drugs or over-the-counter medications.

On physical exam, she was in no apparent distress. Her cardiac and pulmonary exams were normal. Notable findings included a distended, nontympanitic abdomen with a fluid wave. On pelvic exam, she had normal external genitalia and an atrophic-appearing vagina, and no visible lesions were identified on the cervix. Bimanual exam was difficult because of abdominal distension; however, there was a palpable, mobile mass on the patient's right. The rectovaginal septum was smooth, and stool guaiac test was negative.

An abdominal–transvaginal ultrasound was ordered, as well as serum carcinoembryonic antigen (CEA) and cancer antigen 125 (CA-125) concentrations. The CEA concentration was reported as <0.4 ng/mL (range 0–2.5 ng/mL), and the CA-125 concentration was 1467 U/mL (range 0–35 U/mL). Transvaginal ultrasound revealed a complex right adnexal mass measuring 8 × 6 cm with large amounts of free fluid within the abdominal cavity. The uterus was normal in size and had a regular, thin (3.5-mm) endometrium.

On the basis of these results, a diagnosis of ovarian cancer was presumed, a computed tomography (CT) scan was obtained of the abdomen and pelvis, and the patient was referred to a gynecologic oncologist for further management. The CT scan showed diffuse omental caking, a large complex right adnexal mass, a normal-appearing uterus, ascites, and no pelvic or periaortic lymphadenopathy. The lung bases appeared clear, and there were no bony lesions appreciated.

Three weeks after her initial presentation to her primary care physician, she underwent a total abdominal hysterectomy, bilateral salpingoophorectomy, infracolic

Tietz's Applied Laboratory Medicine, Second Edition. Edited by Mitchell G. Scott, Ann M. Gronowski, and Charles S. Eby

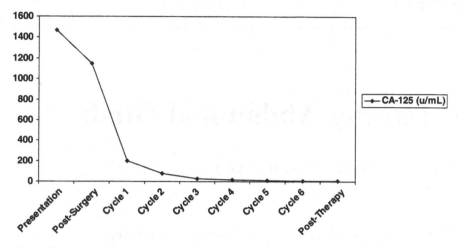

Figure 48.1   CA-125 concentrations in response to therapy. After surgery there is typically a 20–30% decline in CA-125. In chemoresponsive tumors, the CA-125 is expected to return to normal (<35 U/mL) after the third cycle of adjuvant chemotherapy.

omentectomy, and peritoneal tumor debulking to a residual of <1 cm. Intraoperatively, a thickened omentum was noted as well as a large complex right ovarian mass with surface excrescences. Large (>2-cm) tumor plaques were found in the paracolic gutters bilaterally as well as on the small bowel mesentery and sigmoid colon. The final histology was grade 3 papillary serous carcinoma of the right ovary, and her stage, according to the International Federation of Gynecologic Oncologists (FIGO), was IIIC. Figure 48.1 illustrates the decline in the patient's serum CA 125 concentration after her initial surgery followed by six cycles of adjuvant carboplatinum and paclitaxel chemotherapy. Her posttreatment CA-125 was 3 U/mL.

Definition of Disease

Ovarian carcinoma is the leading cause of death from gynecologic cancer in the United States, and is responsible for 5% of all cancer deaths. The median age at diagnosis is 60 years. The lifetime risk of ovarian cancer is approximately 1%. Risk factors for epithelial ovarian cancer include nulliparity and family history of ovarian cancer. A family history of ovarian, breast, endometrial, or colon cancer may indicate a familial cancer susceptibility syndrome. The most common inherited ovarian cancer susceptibility syndrome involves mutations in BRCA1 and BRCA2. Carriers of BRCA1 mutations have a cumulative lifetime risk of ovarian cancer that approaches 44%. Patients are at risk for hereditary ovarian and breast cancer if they have one of the following: (1) premenopausal breast or ovarian cancer, (2) breast cancer diagnosed before age 50 with a first- or second-degree relative with breast or ovarian cancer diagnosed before age 50, (3) breast cancer at any age with two or more family members diagnosed with breast cancer and one or more family members diagnosed with ovarian cancer, (4) family history of a known mutation in BRCA1 or BRCA2, (5) Ashkenazi Jewish heritage with breast cancer diagnosed before age 40, or (6) synchronous breast and ovarian cancers. Similarly, inherited mutations in DNA mismatch repair genes, such as in Lynch syndrome II, increase the lifetime risk of ovarian cancer to approximately 12%. Lynch syndrome II is not a common cause of inherited ovarian cancer, but should be considered in patients who meet any one of the following Bethesda clinical criteria for diagnosis: (1) colorectal cancer diagnosed before age 50, (2) a history of synchronous or metachronous malignancies, (3) one or more first-degree relatives with an Lynch syndrome–related tumor diagnosed before age 50, or (4) two or more relatives with Lynch syndrome–related tumors diagnosed at any age. Protective factors include breastfeeding and use of oral contraceptives.

Epithelial ovarian cancer results from a malignant transformation of ovarian epithelial cells. These cells are histologically indistinguishable from peritoneal epithelium and are thought to transform as the result of an aberrant repair process of the epithelium following ovulation. The most common histologic subtype of epithelial ovarian cancer is serous, accounting for approximately 46% of all ovarian tumors followed by mucinous (36%) and endometrioid (8%). Clear cell, Brenner, and squamous tumors are rare by comparison. Because these tumors arise from the ovarian surface epithelium, malignant cells may shed into the peritoneal cavity and circulate with peritoneal fluid. Surface tumor deposits are frequently identified along the right paracolic gutter, right hemidiaphragm, small and large bowel, and omentum. Tumor spread may also occur via pelvic and aortic lymph nodes.

Epithelial ovarian cancer is usually diagnosed at a late stage. Presenting symptoms are vague, and the differential diagnosis includes a variety of gastrointestinal diseases. Diffuse abdominal pain, bloating, early satiety, dyspepsia, nausea, and increasing abdominal girth secondary to abdominal ascites are common symptoms. Because of the nonspecific symptomatology, approximately 75% of patients have advanced-stage tumor outside of the pelvis at the time of diagnosis.

Differential Diagnosis

The differential diagnosis of ovarian cancer is the same as for an adnexal mass. In a premenopausal patient, pelvic inflammatory disease, tuboovarian abscess, appendiceal abscess, hydrosalpinx, physiologic ovarian cysts, mature cystic teratomas, endometriomas, leiomyomas, benign ovarian masses, and malignant ovarian tumors should be considered. In a postmenopausal patient, there is a greater chance of malignancy. Additional diagnoses in a postmenopausal patient include diverticular abscesses and vascular aneurysms.

The workup of a patient with an adnexal mass generally includes a complete history and physical, transabdominal and transvaginal ultrasonography, and determination of serum CA-125. Results of these tests should be interpreted relative to the patient's reproductive status. In premenopausal women, the sensitivity of CA-125 concentrations is low, so this test should be interpreted with caution. In this population, imaging, along with a complete history and physical, will yield the majority of diagnoses. Premenopausal patients with an asymptomatic adnexal mass that is smaller than 10 cm can be followed. Approximately 70% of these masses will resolve without surgical intervention. A postmenopausal patient with an adnexal mass that is >5 cm, has a complex appearance on ultrasound, or with an elevated CA-125 has a high probability of malignancy. In this group of patients, it is advisable to confirm that routine health maintenance tests such as mammography, cervical cytology, and colonoscopy are within normal limits.

CA-125 is currently the most useful serum marker in epithelial ovarian cancer. CA-125 is a cell surface glycoprotein that is expressed in fetal coelomic epithelium. It is therefore expressed in adults in all tissues derived from coelomic and mullerian epithelium. Normal ovarian epithelial cells, however, do not express CA-125. There are two major antigenic determinants of CA-125: the domain binding murine monoclonal antibody, OC-125; and the domain binding monoclonal antibody M11. Immunoassays to quantify CA-125 concentrations use both monoclonal antibodies, OC-125 and M11 (CA-125 II test). CA-125 is frequently used in the preoperative determination of benign versus malignant adnexal masses. A CA-125 >35 U/mL is considered positive but should not be the sole criterion used for diagnosis. Although CA-125 is elevated in approximately 80% of serous ovarian tumors and has a diagnostic sensitivity of 78%, a specificity of 77% and a NPV approaching 80%, false-positive values are frequent. False-positive CA-125 concentrations can be seen in a variety of benign conditions, including endometriosis, uterine leiomyomas, and pelvic inflammatory disease. Furthermore, in patients younger than 50 years of age, an elevated CA-125 concentration is associated with a malignant mass in less than 25% of patients. In postmenopausal women with a CA-125 >65 U/mL, the sensitivity for a malignancy is 97% with a specificity of 78%.

Retrospective studies have demonstrated that absolute concentrations of CA-125 are not predictive of survival. Changes in CA-125 concentrations are used primarily to follow response to surgery and chemotherapy. As stated previously, the low prevalence of ovarian cancer and the false-positive rate of a single CA-125 makes CA-125 a poor choice for ovarian cancer screening.

Carcinoembryonic antigen (CEA) concentrations are used primarily in gastrointestinal malignancies, particularly colorectal carcinomas. CEA is an antigen present in the fetal colon as well as in cancers. CEA, like CA-125, is a heterogeneic cell surface glycoprotein that is a member of the immunoglobulin superfamily. The function of CEA has not yet been identified. With an upper limit concentration of 2.5 μg/L, the sensitivity for identifying early-stage (Dukes A and B) colorectal cancer is 36% with a specificity of 87%. In advanced-stage disease, the sensitivity improves to approximately 80%. False positives can be found in patients with liver disease, smokers, and patients with small bowel obstruction. CEA is useful (if elevated at diagnosis) in detecting recurrence and liver metastasis. It is not a useful screening test because of poor sensitivity and low prevalence. CEA may be elevated in mucinous epithelial ovarian cancers. If CEA is elevated prior to therapy, it may be a useful marker to follow treatment.

Treatment

One of the most important predictors of survival in patients with ovarian cancer is the amount of residual tumor after initial surgical resection. Therefore, the mainstay of therapy is primary surgical removal of as much tumor as possible (radical optimal tumor debulking). A typical staging operation for ovarian cancer will include total abdominal hysterectomy, bilateral salpingoophorectomy, pelvic and periaortic lymph node dissections, infracololic omentectomy, and multiple peritoneal biopsies. Residual disease of <1 cm is considered optimal. Debulking to microscopic disease is preferable. Given the widespread peritoneal distribution of ovarian cancer, approximately 70% of patients are able to be optimally debulked. Other important prognostic factors include age, tumor stage, histologic grade, and tumor chemoresponsiveness. In early-stage disease, 5-year survival approaches 90% without the use of adjuvant chemotherapy. In advanced-stage disease, 5-year survival without treatment is approximately 10–30%. With adjuvant platinum and taxane-based chemotherapy, 5-year survival increases to approximately 55%. Only 20% of patients will be "cured" of advanced-stage ovarian cancer. However, more than 50% of patients with advanced-stage disease who receive adjuvant platinum and taxane-based chemotherapy will have a complete clinical response. Serial CT scans and CA-125 concentrations are used to monitor for recurrence.

Additional Reading

CANNISTRA, S. A.: Cancer of the ovary. *N. Engl. J. Med. 351*:2519–29, 2004.

DRAKE, J: Diagnosis and management of the adnexal mass. *Am. Fam. Phys. 57*:2471–85, 1998.

DUFFY, M. J.: Carcinoembryonic antigen as a marker for colorectal cancer: Is it clinically useful? *Clin. Chem. 47*:624–30, 2001.

FISHMAN, D. A., COHEN, L., BLANK, S. V. ET AL: The role of ultrasound evaluation in the detection of early-stage epithelial ovarian cancer. *Am. J. Obstet. Gynecol. 192*:1214–22, 2005.

JACOBS, I. J. AND MENON, U.: Progress and challenges in screening for early detection of ovarian cancer. *Mol. Cell. Proteomics 3*:355–66, 2004.

JACOBS, I. J., SKATES, S. J., MACDONALD, N. ET AL.: Screening for ovarian cancer: A pilot randomized control trial. *Lancet 353*:1207–10, 1999.

MUNSTEDT, K., KRISCH, M., SACHSSE, S., AND VAHRSON, H.: Serum CA 125 levels and survival in advanced ovarian cancer. *Arch. Gynecol. Obstet. 259*:117–23, 1997.

OZOLS, R. F., RUBIN, S. C. ET AL.: Epithelial ovarian cancer. In *Principles and Practice of Gynecologic Oncology*, 3rd ed., W. J. HOSKINS ET AL., eds., Lippincott Williams and Wilkins, 2000.

Case 49

To Screen or Not to Screen?

Da-elene van der Merwe and Eleftherios P. Diamandis

A 65-year-old male presented to his family physician reporting elevated blood pressure detected at his local pharmacy. The patient had no significant medical or family history and saw no point in visiting his physician when not ill. On specific questioning, he admitted to getting up about 3–4 times most nights to urinate. He said "I have a cuppa tea before bedtime, doc, so it's OK." He denied disuria, frequencuria, polyuria, and polydipsia. There was no history of weight loss or bone pain, and he denied any sexual dysfunction.

His blood pressure was 170/100. His point of maximum impulse was detected in the 4th–5th intercostal space. Fundoscopy was normal, and no carotid bruit was detected. The rest of his general physical examination appears to be normal.

The physician decided to discuss the issue of screening for prostate disease with him before proceeding with any further testing. After providing information about the outcomes, including the possible benefit and risks of screening and therapy for prostate cancer, the patient decided to proceed with further testing. A digital rectal examination at the time revealed a prostate >0.5 mL in volume. A urine dipstix, a urea–electrolyte profile, and a serum total PSA (s-tPSA) were ordered. Laboratory results were as follows:

Analyte	Value, Conventional Units	Reference Interval, Conventional Units	Value, SI Units	Reference Interval, SI Units
Sodium	146 mmol/L	135–148 mmol/L	Same	
Potassium	4.5 mmol/L	3.5–5.0 mmol/L	Same	
Cl	103 mmol/L	95–107 mmol/L	Same	
tCO_2	22 mmol/L	21–31 mmol/L	Same	
Urea	9 mg/dL	7–18 mg/dL	3.2 mmol/L	2.5–6.4 mmol/L
Creatinine	0.9 mg/dL	0.7–1.3 mg/dL	80 μmol/L	62–115 μmol/L
s-tPSA	7 ng/mL	<4 ng/mL	7 μg/L	<4 μg/L

The patient returned after one week to discuss his results and to repeat his blood pressure measurements. He agreed to a prostate biopsy, realizing that he might be harboring an unknown cancer in his body. Biopsy revealed prostate cancer, and a combined Gleason score of 5 was given (maximum score is 10; higher score means less differentiated cancer). A bone scan did not reveal any metastasis to bone.

Tietz's Applied Laboratory Medicine, Second Edition. Edited by Mitchell G. Scott, Ann M. Gronowski, and Charles S. Eby
Copyright © 2007 John Wiley & Sons, Inc.

The patient was offered the treatment options of either watchful waiting or aggressive therapy, including radical prostatectomy, external beam radiation, or brachytherapy. He chose to have radical prostatectomy after thorough discussion of the possible side effects postprostatectomy.

A s-tPSA 6 weeks after surgery was undetectable. The patient was "delighted" that his cancer was detected in time. However, since his surgery, he is now unable to have an erection.

Definition of the Disease

Adenocarcinoma of the prostate (PCA) is the most common noncutaneous malignancy in men and the second leading cause of cancer-related deaths in the United States. In 2005 it was estimated that more than 200,000 new cases of PCA would be diagnosed and >30,000 men would die of the disease by the end of that year.[1] PCA is unique in several respects. Despite a 30–40% incidence of microscopic PCA in men above the age of 50, only 9–11% of men clinically manifest disease and only 2.6–4.3% die of the disease. Therefore, the majority of histologically evident microscopic cancers do not impact the lifespan of the individual. Most men with prostate cancer are asymptomatic. In contrast to these indolent cancers that are typically found in 8–9 decades, the more aggressive cancers with metastatic potential develop during 5–7 decades. Early diagnosis is vital, and efforts should be made to identify those who will benefit from curative treatment. The following symptoms do not appear until the disease has spread beyond the prostate capsule or has metastasized to lymph nodes or bones: intermittent flow of urine, dribbling of urine before and after urinating, a frequent or urgent need to pass urine, a need to get up several times during the night to urinate, a feeling that the bladder is not completely empty, rarely, blood in the urine, and lower back or bone pain.

Pathophysiology

Prostate cancer develops when the rates of cell division and cell death are no longer equal, leading to uncontrolled tumor growth. Mutations of a multitude of genes, including the genes for p53 and retinoblastoma, can lead to tumor progression and metastasis. In approximately 10% of cases, the development of prostate cancer has been linked to prostate cancer susceptibility genes. The results of a genomewide scan of 91 high-risk prostate cancer families from the United States and Sweden suggested the presence of a major prostate cancer susceptibility locus at chromosome 1q24, designated *HPC1*.

Most (95%) prostate cancers are adenocarcinomas; 70% of prostate cancer cases arise in the peripheral zone, 15–20% in the central zone, and 10–15% in the transitional zone. Most cancers are multifocal, with synchronous involvement of multiple zones of the prostate, which may be due to clonal and nonclonal tumors. Transitional zone cancers spread to the bladder neck, while the peripheral zone tumors extend into the ejaculatory ducts and seminal vesicles. Prostate capsule penetration is a relatively late event. Cancer spreads to bone early; however, the mechanism for distant metastasis is poorly understood. Two theories have been proposed: (1) the "mechanical theory," involving direct spread through the lymphatics and venous spaces into the lower lumbar spine and (2) the "seed and soil" theory, suggesting that tissue factors must be present that allow for preferential growth in certain tissues, such as bone. The doubling time in early-stage disease is as slow as 2–4 years but changes as the tumor grows and becomes more aggressive. The 2002 tumor–node–metastasis (TNM) system is used for the clinical staging of prostate cancer. The Gleason grading system is the most widely accepted system for classifying histological characteristics of prostate cancer. The predominant staining pattern and the second most common pattern are given grades from 1–5; these are then combined to obtain a single score:

- A score of 2–4 is low-grade or well differentiated
- A score of 5–7 is moderate grade or moderately differentiated
- A score of 8–10 is high-grade or poorly differentiated

Differential Diagnosis

The following should be considered in the differential diagnosis of PCA:

    Benign prostatic hypertrophy (BPH)
    Renal calculi
    Prostatic cysts
    Prostatic tuberculosis
    Prostatitis

Diagnosis

Total PSA

Prostate-specific antigen (PSA) is encoded by the human kallikrein gene 3 (KLK3) on chromosome 19q13.4.[2] It is the most abundant protein in seminal fluid and has chymotrypsinlike serine protease activity. A common concern for the measurement of serum PSA for early detection of PCA is that clinically insignificant cancers may be diagnosed and treated. Furthermore, common disorders including BPH and prostatitis elevate PSA in serum to concentrations that overlap significantly with concentrations seen in PCA. Various other factors (exercise, prostate biopsy, etc.) can also increase PSA concentration. Attempts to improve the value of serum PSA measurement in the diagnosis of PCA include PSA velocity, serum concentration of free (unbound) PSA relative to total, PSA density, and age-specific PSA ranges. Currently, total PSA concentrations are interpreted according to three ranges: 0–4 ng/mL, 4–10 ng/mL, and >10 ng/mL. Concentrations <4 ng/mL are considered at low risk for PCA. However, up to 22% of men with s-tPSA <4 ng/mL harbor significant disease. Evidence is mounting to decrease cutoffs to below 4 ng/mL. Proposals include a cutoff of 2.5 ng/mL for younger men. Currently, PSA between 4 and 10 ng/mL is the diagnostic "gray zone" that warrants further workup, such as biopsy. Biopsy-based results showed a positive predictive value of PSA between 12 and 32%. Concerns include cost as well as morbidity of biopsy, since approximately three out of four biopsied men have nonmalignant disease. PSA concentrations >10 ng/mL have a likelihood of 40–50% of PCA; therefore biopsy is highly recommended in these men.

Free PSA

Studies have revealed that 5–45% of serum PSA is free (uncomplexed). The rest is bound to proteinase inhibitors, mainly α_1-antichymotripsin. Measurement of serum free PSA, on its own, does not contribute any enhanced disease-specific information. Measurement of free PSA is used to generate the ratio of free to total PSA (%fPSA). A higher %fPSA has been shown in patients without evidence of PCA, and studies suggest that this significantly enhances the early detection of PCA, particularly in the diagnostic gray zone of s-tPSA (4–10 ng/mL).[3] Furthermore, %fPSA can be useful for predicting prognosis. Because %fPSA is affected by multiple factors (e.g., prostate volume) as well as problems with preanalytical and analytical standardization and equimolarity of PSA assays, it is difficult to define a reference interval. Recommended cutoffs range from 14% to 25%. In conclusion, %fPSA improves specificity while maintaining a high sensitivity for PCA in men with a s-tPSA of 2.6–10 ng/mL. The diagnostic utility of %fPSA decreases in patients with a suspicious DRE or if s-tPSA is >10 ng/mL.

Complexed PSA

PSA forms stable complexes with α1-antichymotrypsin (PSA-ACT), protein C inhibitor (PSA-PCI), α2-macroglobulin (PSA-AMG), and α1-protease inhibitor (API-PSA). PSA-ACT is the major form and is most strongly influenced by PCA. A recently developed assay to measure complexed PSA (cPSA) has shown promising results. Overall, the reports to date have shown that cPSA enhances diagnostic performance (specificity) over s-tPSA in the detection of PCA.[3]

Subfractions of Free PSA

proPSA, BPSA, and iPSA are subfractions of free PSA.[4] Measurement of serum free PSA subfractions for the early detection of PCA looks promising. However, further evaluation is necessary, including precise characterization of each subfraction, as well as refinements in detection techniques.

Human Glandular Kallikrein 2 (hK2)

hK2 and PSA are both serine proteases and gene products of the human kallikrein gene family.[2] They share ~80% sequence homology. Similar to PSA, hK2 forms complexes with inhibitors. hK2 mRNA is expressed in prostatic tissue at concentrations of about 20–50% of PSA mRNA. It has been suggested that there are significant differences in the expression of these two proteins in benign versus malignant prostatic tissue. However, diagnostic enhancements contributed by hK2 measurments, in addition to testing for total and free PSA, is moderate.[5]

Prostatic Acid Phosphatase (PAP)

Acid phosphatases are a group of enzymes capable of hydrolyzing esters of orthophosphoric acid in an acid medium. These enzymes have attracted considerable interest over the past few decades, but experts now agree that PAP analysis has no role in the diagnosis and monitoring of PCA, and PSA is clearly the superior marker. PAP may, however, be helpful in the rare patients who do not produce PSA or in preoperative staging of clinically localized disease.

Insulinlike Growth Factors (IGFs) and Their Binding Proteins (BPs)

Some studies have shown differences between mean concentrations of serum IGF1 and IGFBP3 in controls versus patients with PCA. Until more convincing data are published, it is not recommended to measure either IGF1 or IGFBP3 for screening, diagnosis, prognosis, or risk assessment in PCA.

Screening

Despite international efforts, early detection and treatment of PCA and screening are still controversial issues.[6,7] The National Cancer Institute's prostate, lung, colorectal, and ovarian (PLCO) screening trial and the European Randomized Study of Screening for Prostate Cancer (ERSPC) are major prospective randomized trials to investigate whether PSA screening can reduce mortality from PCA. The American Cancer Society and the American Urological Association recommend annual screening for early detection of PCA for average-risk men beginning at age 50. Men at high risk, including men of African descent and men with a first-degree relative diagnosed before at a relatively young age (i.e., younger than 65 years) should begin testing at age 45. Men with more than one first-degree relative diagnosed with prostate cancer before age 65 could begin testing at age 40. If PSA is <1.0 ng/mL, no additional testing is needed until age 45. If PSA is >1.0 ng/mL but <2.5 ng/mL, annual testing is recommended. If PSA is ≥2.5 ng/mL, further evaluation with biopsy should be considered. However, for PCA screening and treatment, the decision to be aggressive is positively reinforced regardless of outcome. For example, consider the case of a man who decided to undergo PSA screening and is diagnosed with cancer that is localized, as are about 70% of prostate cancers. He chooses radical prostatectomy, as do about 52,000 men annually, but he is impotent after surgery, similar to 60% of men after radical prostatectomy. Even the adverse effects may be associated with positive reinforcements; the patient is happy to be a cancer survivor.[7] Physicians, patients, and policymakers need to understand the power of such thinking. Overenthusiasm without proper outcome data may lead to more harm than good. To curb this possible overenthusiasm, shared decisionmaking will work only if the patient is truly well informed about the pros and cons of screening.[7]

Treatment

The three primary treatment strategies are

- Radical prostatectomy
- Definitive radiation therapy
- Watchful waiting

Several different hormonal approaches can benefit men in various stages of PCA: bilateral orchiectomy, estrogen therapy, LHRH agonists and antagonists, antiandrogens, ketoconazole, and aminoglutethimide. A significant risk exists with all of these therapies. Postsurgery, ~30% suffer from urinary incontinence and ~60% have impotence. Radiation therapy can result in acute cystitis, proctitis, and enteritis.

References

1. JEMAL, A., MURRAY, T., WARD, E. ET AL.: Cancer statistics. *C.A. Cancer J. Clin.* 55:10–30, 2005.
2. BORGONO, C. A. AND DIAMANDIS, E. P.: The emerging roles of human tissue kallikreins in cancer. *Nat. Rev. Cancer* 4:876–90, 2004.
3. RODDAM, A. W., DUFFY, M. J., HAMDY, F. C. ET AL.: Use of prostate-specific antigen (PSA) isoforms for the detection of prostate cancer in men with a PSA level of 2–10 ng/mL: systematic review and meta-analysis. *Eur. Urol.* 48:386–99, 2005.

4. GRETZER, M. B. AND PARTIN, A. W.: PSA markers in prostate cancer detection. *Urol. Clin. North Am.* *30*:677–86, 2003.

5. RITTENHOUSE, H. G., FINLAY, J. A., MIKOLAJCZYK, S. D. ET AL.: Human kallikrein 2 (hK2) and prostate-specific antigen (PSA): Two closely related, but distinct, kallikreins in the prostate. *Crit. Rev. Clin. Lab. Sci. 35*:275–368, 1998.

6. SCHRODER, F. H.: Detection of prostate cancer: The impact of the European Randomized Study of Screening for Prostate Cancer (ERSPC). *Can. J. Urol. 12*:2–6, 2005.

7. RANSOHOFF, D. F., COLLINGS, M. M., AND FOWLER, J. F., JR.: Why is prostate cancer screening so common when the evidence is so uncertain? A system without negative feedback. *Am. J. Med. 113*:663–7, 2002.

Case 50

A Male with Confusing hCG Results

Kingshuk Das

The laboratory was called to explain an apparent inconsistency in the test results for a 40-year-old male with new-onset ascites. He had no history of liver disease, and liver function tests were within normal limits. Exploratory laparotomy revealed a poorly differentiated carcinoma. Values were as follows:

Analyte/Test	Value, Conventional Units	Reference Interval, Conventional Units[a]	Value, SI Units	Reference Interval, SI Units
Quantitative β-hCG (in-house)	552 mIU/mL	<5	552 IU/L	<5
Quantitative β-hCG (outside hospital)	235 mIU/mL	<5	235 IU/L	<5
Qualitative hCG	Negative	Negative	Same	Same

[a]Reference intervals for males and nonpregnant females.

In discussion with the patient's physician, it was revealed that a high quantitative β-hCG concentration was expected because the patient had a germ cell tumor. The qualitative assay was ordered by accident, but the physicians were confused by the results. The two main questions for the laboratory to answer are

1. Why is there a discrepancy between the quantitative and qualitative measurements?
2. Why do the two quantitative test results differ?

Definition of the Disease

Primary germ cell tumors constitute 95% of testicular tumors, most frequently occurring between the ages of 20 and 40. Rarely these neoplasms can arise in extragonadal sites such as the mediastinum and retroperitoneum, and very infrequently in the pineal gland. Germ

Tietz's Applied Laboratory Medicine, Second Edition. Edited by Mitchell G. Scott, Ann M. Gronowski, and Charles S. Eby

cell tumors have some of the highest cure rates of all adult cancers at greater than 90% overall, including 70–80% of those with metastatic disease. These impressive statistics are based on therapies targeted specifically to tumor type and stage; therefore diagnostic accuracy is of utmost importance. Germ cell tumors are categorized into seminomas and nonseminomas, with nonseminomas further subdivided into embryonal carcinomas, teratomas, choriocarcinomas, and yolk sac tumors. Tumor type is primarily diagnosed histologically, but can be aided by measurement of serum hCG and AFP (α-fetoprotein) since the various subsets of germ cell tumors differ in their ability to secrete these markers. In addition to supporting the histological diagnosis, concentrations of serum hCG can be of prognostic value, and can reflect tumor burden and response to therapy of "marker-positive" tumors. Serum hCG concentration is found to be elevated ("marker-positive") in 20–40% of seminomas and 40–50% of nonseminomas, with the following characteristic patterns:[2]

Tumor Type	Serum hCG Elevated	Serum AFP Elevated
Seminoma	Yes (30% β-hCG subunits only)	No
Nonseminoma		
Teratoma	No	No
Embryonal carcinoma	Yes (hCG $\pm$ free β-hCG subunits)	Yes
Choriocarcinoma	Yes (hypergylcosylated hCG $\pm$ free β-hCG subunits)	Yes
Yolk sac tumor	No	Yes

Of note, choriocarcinomas secrete the hyperglycosylated form of hCG (the importance of which will be discussed in later sections). Approximately 30% of marker-positive seminomas secrete only the β subunit of hCG, without detectable intact hCG $\alpha\beta$ dimer, whereas all other marker-positive germ cell tumors secrete intact hCG $\pm$ free β-hCG subunits.[2] Therefore, when measuring hCG as a germ cell tumor marker, it is important to employ testing capable of detecting both intact hCG and free β subunits. Recent studies have also uncovered a small subset of patients with tumors secreting only the α subunit of hCG; and not β subunit or intact hCG; however, the clinical significance of this finding is yet to be determined.[2]

Staging of germ cell tumors is as follows. Stage I disease is limited to testis, epididymis, or spermatic cord; stage II disease is limited to retroperitoneal lymph nodes; and stage III disease extends outside the retroperitoneum to involve supradiaphragmatic lymph nodes or viscera. Higher-grade tumors are more frequently marker-positive, with 87–100% of stage III tumors, 52–82% of stage II tumors, and up to 18% of stage I tumors showing elevated serum hCG.[2] Also, serum hCG concentrations do correlate with marker-positive tumor burden; however, it should be noted that nonseminomas secrete much more hCG than do seminomas, resulting in serum hCG concentrations as high as 3,000,000 IU/L, whereas pure seminomas seldom result in concentrations above 1000 IU/L.[2] Serum hCG concentrations can also be used to monitor marker-positive tumor response to therapy. The half-life of hCG in serum is 24–36 hours, so samples drawn several days apart can be informative. Stage I and II germ cell tumors are treated surgically with orchiectomy, with addition of radiation therapy of the retroperitoneum for seminomas, and resection of retroperitoneal lymph nodes for nonseminomas. For stage III tumors, and stage II disease with extensive lymph node involvement, chemotherapy is used in conjunction with surgery. It is common to assess baseline serum hCG twice before orchiectomy, and then 2–3 times the first week after surgery, or once a week during chemotherapy, to monitor marker-positive tumor response to therapy.

Serum hCG concentrations can also be measured during remission as a marker for recurrent disease. There may be a short-lived increase in serum hCG coinciding with chemotherapy due to release of marker from tumor lysis; however, persistent elevation indicates residual and/or recurrent disease.[2] Unfortunately, a drop in serum hCG to undetectable levels does not necessarily rule out residual or recurrent disease since 20% of marker-positive patients with mixed tumor types (as evidenced by histology) can have a transition during therapy or remission to a marker-negative tumor type such as a teratoma.[2] Serum hCG concentrations can also be of prognostic value in the therapy of stage III disease, or stage II disease with extensive lymph node involvement. Among the "good" prognostic factors are low serum hCG concentrations, low serum AFP concentrations, low tumor burden, and metastases limited to retroperitoneum and lung, which predict cure rates as high as 90%. Among the "poor" prognostic factors are high serum hCG concentrations, primary mediastinal nonseminomas, or nonpulmonary visceral metastases, which predict cure rates of only 35–50%.[2]

Human Chorionic Gonadotropin (hCG)

Human Chorionic Gonadotropin (hCG) is a heavily glycosylated protein composed of two subunits, an α and a β subunit. The α subunit is common to several hormones other than hCG: luteinizing hormone (LH), follicle-stimulating hormone (FSH), and thyroid-stimulating hormone (TSH). However the β subunit is unique to hCG and allows its specific detection.

There are several different forms and degradation products of hCG, as well as different sources of hCG, and this heterogeneity is important to the understanding and interpretation of hCG testing. In contrast to the case scenario presented above, hCG is most often discussed with respect to pregnancy. During pregnancy hCG is initially produced by the developing blastocyst as it implants into the uterine wall. The poorly differentiated cytotrophoblastic cells of implantation and early pregnancy produce the "hyperglycosylated" form of hCG, whereas "regular" hCG is produced later on by the differentiated syncytiotrophoblasts of the placenta.[3,4] It is important to note that hCG is also produced in disease states, such as gestational trophoblastic disease, germ cell tumors, and rarely in liver and epidermal lung tumors.[5]

As far as the different forms of hCG, the predominant form produced during weeks 6–40 of gestation is termed "regular" hCG, and is produced by the placenta. The principal form of hCG secreted by cytotrophoblastic tissue during weeks 3–5 of gestation, as well as that commonly secreted by choriocarcinomas, is hyperglycosylated hCG.[3] The regular and hyperglycosylated forms of hCG can both give rise to a nicked hCG product, which is found in low concentrations during gestation, but is the major hCG variant after delivery or termination of pregnancy.[3] There is also an hCG variant missing a C-terminal peptide from the β subunit that can be detected in gestational trophoblastic disease or carcinoma.[3]

The hCG molecule can also dissociate into its free α and β subunits. As discussed above, certain tumors may produce only free β subunit, which is possible since its locus (*19q13.32*) is distinct from that of the α subunit (*6q12-q21*), and may be differentially regulated during or as a result of oncogenesis.[5,6] Free β subunit generally becomes nicked in serum (nicked β subunit), but a percentage remains unmodified and is found at low levels during pregnancy.[3] The other dissociation product, free α subunit, can be detected as well, however as mentioned earlier it is a nonspecific marker of hCG as it is a common constituent of three other hormones. Hyperglycosylated hCG dissociates into free α subunit and a hyperglycosylated free β subunit.[3] Predictably, this product is prominent when hyperglycosylated hCG predominates, such as early in pregnancy (weeks 3–5) and with choriocarcinomas.[3] Furthermore, both hyperglycosylated and regular hCG can both give rise to nicked hCG, which itself can dissociate into free α subunit and nicked free β subunit.[3,5] The final major metabolite of hCG is the β-core fragment, which is a result of degradation of the nicked free β subunit. This fragment is filtered at the glomerulus, so it is rapidly cleared from the serum, and is the predominant urinary β-hCG species found during weeks 7–40 of gestation.[3,5] Note that in contrast to the rapid renal clearance of the β-core fragment, the other seven metabolic forms of hCG (regular, hyperglycosylated, nicked, hCG minus C-term peptide, nicked free β subunit, free β subunit, and hyperglycosylated free β subunit), as well as the free α-subunit, are all detected in both serum and urine.

hCG Assays

There are many different assays available to detect hCG, including quantitative serum assays, qualitative urine, and qualitative/semiquantitative serum assays. The unifying theme for these assays is that they are all two-site, "sandwich" immunoassays. Quantitative serum hCG testing uses two different antibodies. The first is a capture antibody directed against one site on hCG, with the antibody immobilized by linkage to either a vessel surface or beads. The second antibody is a detection antibody specific for another site on hCG, which is coupled to a tracer (typically an enzyme or radioisotope). The two antibodies are either directed against two different sites on the β molecule (β-hCG assays), or one antibody directed against the α chain and the other against the β chain (intact hCG assays). Patient serum is added to the system and the capture antibody is used to "pull down" the hCG from the serum, creating an immobilized complex of hCG + capture antibody. Then the detection antibody binds to the hCG molecules, creating an immobilized complex or "sandwich" of detection antibody + hCG + capture antibody. After a wash step, the amount of immobilized tracer is assayed by the appropriate method (e.g., adding substrate if the tracer is an enzyme), and the signal generated is directly proportional to the amount of hCG in the patient sample. These quantitative assays can either be a one-step or two-step assay. Two-step assays first incubate the sample with the capture antibody to immobilize the hCG, followed by a wash step, and then the immobilized analyte is incubated with the detection antibody followed by a second wash step. One-step assays do not provide a wash step after the addition of patient sample. One-step assays are more common because of faster assay times and less involved protocols; however, the two-step assays have the advantage of minimizing problems arising from the "hook effect" (which will be discussed shortly).

Qualitative hCG testing is based on the same principles as quantitative hCG testing. Sample is added to the sample well at one end of a test cassette. At this end of the cassette the membrane contains a detection antibody consisting of anti-hCG antibody directed against one chain of the hCG molecule conjugated to a tracer (typically a latex bead). The sample migrates through the matrix via lateral diffusion. Distal to the sample well is a "test" line in the membrane impregnated with immobilized capture antibody (specific for the other chain of hCG). When the antibody + hCG-bead complex reaches this "test" line, migration of the hCG is stopped if intact hCG is present. This results in visualization of the latex particles and a colored line indicating a positive test result. To ensure proper functioning of the assay, there is a control line, located distal to the test line. The control line is impregnated with one of a number of possible substances, but usually with immobilized antibead antibody or immobilized antibodies that recognize the detection antibodies. The ideal control line would contain hCG. Excess free anti-hCG-bead conjugate migrates past the "test" line, and reaches the control line, creating another colored line, indicating that the cassette is working properly. Note that if hCG is coated on the control line, the positive control also indicates that the detection antibody is effective. However, if antidetection antibody is used as the control, a positive control simply indicates that enough sample volume was present to migrate past the test line. These qualitative hCG tests usually use one antibody against α-hCG, and one against the β-subunit, therefore the assays target intact hCG molecules.

Laboratory Investigation

Now that the framework for qualitative and quantitative hCG assays has been described, it is possible to investigate the apparent discrepancies in this case. Consideration should be given to the following:

1. Why is there a discrepancy between the quantitative and qualitative measurements?
   a. Specimen mixup
   b. False negative on the qualitative device
      i. Defective testing device
      ii. Hook effect
      iii. Dilute urine
   c. False positive on the quantitative devices
      i. Heterophile antibodies
   d. Presence of free β (not intact)-hCG

2. Why do the two quantitative test results differ?
   a. Heterophile antibody interference
   b. Improper instrument sampling
   c. Standardization differences

1. Why is there a discrepancy between the quantitative and qualitative measurements?
   a. Specimen mixup should be considered in any situation in which results are inconsistent. Validation of urine is difficult, but blood can by typed to confirm it is from the correct patient. In this case, repeat blood and urine samples were obtained that resulted in the same test values.
   b. False negative on the qualitative device:
      i. Defective qualitative testing devices are always a concern. If it is a random event, it is nearly impossible to confirm. If the problem is seen repeatedly with a given brand or lot number, the problem can be investigated. In this case, because no other false negatives have been reported, and the control line appeared normal, we have to assume the device was working properly.

    ii. The "hook effect" refers to a false-negative result for a one-step assay due to a high concentration of antigen present in the sample. Note that qualitative cassette assays are "one-step" because there is no wash step following addition of patient sample. This occurs because at very high concentrations of analyte, the analyte can occupy virtually all binding sites on both capture and detection antibodies simultaneously. This prevents formation of the "sandwich" complex, resulting in a false negative. In a two-step assay, the hook effect is avoided because the excess analyte is removed after incubation with the capture antibody by a wash, before addition of detection antibody. If a hook effect is suspected, such as when the patient shows clear evidence of pregnancy by ultrasound or clinical presentation but the quantitative or qualitative one-step hCG test is negative or inappropriately low, the patient sample can be diluted 10- or 100-fold and the assay repeated. If a hook effect is present, the diluted sample will appear more concentrated than the undiluted. In this case, dilutions were performed and the sample remained negative.

    iii. Dilute urine can be the cause of false-negative results. Urine is limited because its concentration varies with fluid status. In assays where results are not normalized for creatinine or specific gravity, false negatives are a possibility. In this case, because a duplicate urine sample was obtained, a false negative due to dilute urine was unlikely.

  c. False positive on the quantitative devices:

    i. Heterophile antibodies are antibodies produced by a patient that recognize the antibodies used in a sandwich assay. These antibodies cause interferences in assays by binding simultaneously to the capture and detection antibodies, thereby linking the capture and detection antibodies without the need for antigen. This situation yields a false-positive result. Because antibodies are not filtered through normal glomeruli, these interferences occur only when serum is utilized as a specimen as opposed to urine. Several clues can suggest such an interference: (1) the heterophile antibodies seldom are present in urine, so the combination of positive serum results and negative results in a parallel urine sample would be supportive; (2) if different serum assays are found to yield significantly different hCG results, one might suspect a heterophile antibody specific for the antibodies in one assay, but not another. False positives due to heterophile antibodies can be remedied by pretreating the serum sample with a purified immunoglobulin or commercially available heterophile antibody blocking reagent.[1] In this case, the addition of heterophile blocking reagent demonstrated that the quantitative results were not due to heterophile antibody interference.

  d. Presence of free β (not intact) hCG. Note that the method for the qualitative hCG utilizes a mouse monoclonal antibody against α-hCG and a goat polyclonal against β-hCG. The quantitative assay performed in house utilizes two mouse monoclonal antibodies against β-hCG. The quantitative assay performed at the outside hospital utilizes one monoclonal antibody against β-hCG, and a goat polyclonal against a second site on β-hCG. Since the qualitative assay uses one antibody against the α subunit and one antibody against the β subunit, and the quantitative assays use antibodies directed only toward the β subunit, the qualitative assay recognizes only intact hCG whereas the quantitative assay recognizes both intact hCG and free β-hCG. As discussed earlier, certain hCG-producing tumors produce only β fragment. In this case, the presence of free β-hCG was the cause of the apparent negative qualitative assay.

2. Why do the two quantitative test results differ?

   a. Heterophile antibody interference. As discussed above, heterophile antibodies can cause false-positive results and inconsistent results. In this case, the addition of heterophile blocking reagent demonstrated that the quantitative results were not due to heterophile antibody interference.

   b. Improper instrument sampling is always a concern in automated assays with unusual results. Samples should be examined carefully for bubbles, low sample volume, and clots. Repeat testing should be performed to confirm results. In this case repeat testing was performed on a separate sample gave similar results making improper instrument sampling unlikely.

   c. Standardization differences. As discussed above, there is considerable heterogeneity among hCG species; 10 different antibody preparations have been raised against 10 different β-subunit regions and another preparation, that recognizes the junction of the α and β subunits.[3] Each of these 11 formulations has a unique profile of affinities for the 8 major forms of hCG, with the junctional preparation also recognizing free α subunits. There is also a separate antibody preparation directed against free α subunits. Therefore, the ability of a given assay to detect various hCG forms and degradation products is determined by the combination of capture and detection antibodies employed by that assay.

All hCG tests are standardized using material from the World Health Organization (WHO). This standardization material is produced by extracting hCG from pregnancy urine, and can be further purified to remove the small percentage of nicked hCG present. The problem is that the quantity of these WHO standards are limited and not enough is available for use in calibrating qualitative hCG assays.[3] Therefore, manufacturers have to use limited amounts of WHO standard to calibrate alternative standards obtained from other sources (usually more crude preparations of hCG from pregnancy urine) and then use these alternative standards as calibrators or quality controls. These alternative standards are generally not evaluated as stringently, and may contain varying amounts of the other forms of hCG, including nicked hCG and free β subunits. Therefore, hCG assays may vary in performance from one another according to the particular composition of the standards against which they are calibrated. In the most extreme situation, the same patient sample might give a positive test result with one qualitative assay, and a negative result in another such assay, purely because of differences in calibration materials used in the development of the assays.

In this case, the most likely explanation is that the two quantitative assays are employing different capture/detection antibody combinations, and therefore exhibit different affinities for the hCG variants in the patient's sample.

References

1. BRAUNWALD, E., FAUCI, A., KASPER, D., HAUSER, S., LONGO, D., AND JAMESON, L., eds.: *Harrison's Principles of Internal Medicine*, 15th, McGraw-Hill, New York, 2001.

2. MANN, K., SALLER, B., AND HOERMANN, R.: Clinical use of hCG and hCGβ determinations. *Scand. J. Clin. Lab. Invest. Suppl. 216*:97–104, 1993.

3. GRONOWSKI, A., ed.: *Current Clinical Pathology: Handbook of Clinical Laboratory Testing during Pregnancy*, Humana Press, Totowa, NJ, 2004.

4. BARSS, V. AND BARBIERI, R., eds.: *UpToDate: Obstetrics, Gynecology, and Women's Health*, Up To Date, Waltham, MA, 2005.

5. HARTZ, P., AND MCKUSICK, V., eds.: *Online Mendelian Inheritance in Man* (ID#118860), Johns Hopkins University and National Center for Biotechnology Information, 2004.

6. HAMOSH, A., AND MCKUSICK, V., eds.: *Online Mendelian Inheritance in Man* (ID#118850), Johns Hopkins University and National Center for Biotechnology Information, 2005.

Case 51

Size Greater than Dates

Randall K. Gibb and Nicholas P. Taylor

A 19-year-old gravida 1 para 0 female presented to her physician with vaginal bleeding characterized as moderate in intensity, thin in consistency, and associated with some minimal abdominal cramping. Her pregnancy test was positive approximately 4 weeks ago and per her report, she should be about 9 weeks into her pregnancy. Up until the bleeding, the pregnancy had been uneventful.

On physical examination her vital signs were stable with a normal blood pressure and pulse rate. Her uterine fundal height measured about 16 weeks in size. Attempts at listening for fetal heart tones were unsuccessful. Vaginal examination revealed some bright red serous drainage and blood in the vault with a closed cervix. Bimanual examination confirmed a boggy enlarged uterus with the finding of bilaterally enlarged ovarian cysts measuring about 8 cm each.

An office ultrasound demonstrated absence of an identifiable fetal pole. The uterine cavity on ultrasound was consistent with a "snowstorm" pattern demonstrating diffusely swollen uterine contents. Bilaterally enlarged multicystic ovaries measuring 8 and 7 cm, respectively, were noted with some minimal free fluid in the cul-de-sac.

Laboratory data included the following:

Analyte	Value, Conventional Units	Reference Interval, Conventional Units	Value, SI Units	Reference Interval, SI Units
Urine hCG serum	Positive	Negative	>25 IU/L	<25
Quantitative β-hCG	420,000 mIU/ml	11,500–289,000	420,000 IU/L	11,500–289,000

The patient underwent a chest x-ray that was negative. A complete blood count, and comprehensive metabolic profile, as well as clotting studies were all normal. The patient underwent a suction dilatation and curettage combined with an oxytocin infusion. A large amount of vesicular placental tissue and blood was removed. The patient was monitored postoperatively for any further vaginal bleeding and recovered without incident. The bilateral ovarian cysts were followed by ultrasound and resolved spontaneously after 8 weeks.

Tietz's Applied Laboratory Medicine, Second Edition. Edited by Mitchell G. Scott, Ann M. Gronowski, and Charles S. Eby
Copyright © 2007 John Wiley & Sons, Inc.

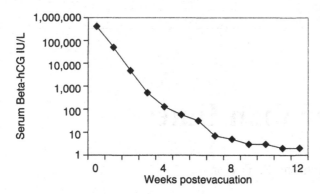

Figure 51.1   Plot of β-hCG concentrations versus time.

The final pathology on the uterine contents revealed absence of any identifiable fetal or embryonic tissues, and a large amount of chorionic villi that exhibited generalized hydatidiform swelling with diffuse trophoblastic hyperplasia. The cytological diagnosis was complete hydatidiform mole. The patient was also instructed to use effective contraception to prevent pregnancy again during the follow-up period. After molar evacuation, the patient was followed by weekly determinations of serum quantitative β-hCG and graphed accordingly (Fig. 51.1). The patient was followed for a total of 6 months with monthly serum quantitative β-hCGs that remained <5 IU/L. After the usual follow-up time the patient was able to discontinue her contraception and attempt pregnancy in the usual fashion.

Definition of the Disease

Gestational trophoblastic disease is actually a spectrum of diseases encompassing complete and partial hydatidiform moles, gestational choriocarcinoma, and placental site trophoblastic tumor (Table 51.1). The incidence of the various forms of gestational trophoblastic disease varies. In the United States, hydatidiform moles are observed in 1

Table 51.1   Gestational Trophoblastic Disease

Hydatidiform Moles		
Complete mole	46XX or 46XY	Evacuation or hysterectomy
	Extensive trophoblastic hyperplasia	
	Fetal tissue absent	
Partial mole	69XXY or 69XXX	Evacuation or hysterectomy
	Focal trophoblastic hyperplasia	
	Fetal tissue present	
Gestational choriocarcinoma	Follows a normal gestation	Surgical excision if possible
	Represents one-fourth of all choriocarcinomas	Multiagent chemotherapy
Placental site trophoblastic tumor	Normally follows a term pregnancy (can be sequela to molar pregnancy or abortion)	Resistant to drug therapy Hysterectomy

in 1500 pregnancies, and in 1 in 600 therapeutic abortions. Gestational choriocarcinoma occurs in 1 in 20,000–40,000 pregnancies; 50% follow after a normal pregnancy, 25% after molar pregnancies, and the remainder after other gestational events. Placental site trophoblastic tumors are even rarer and can develop after any pregnancy related event.

Complete and partial hydatidiform moles are distinct diseases with characteristic histologic, cytogenetic, and clinical features. Despite these differences they are managed in the same fashion. Complete moles have an absence of fetal or embryonic tissue, are associated with diffuse trophoblastic edema and proliferation, and have a 46,XX or 46,XY on karyotype. The amount of trophoblastic proliferation exceeds that observed in partial hydatidiform moles, with the usual symptoms of abnormal bleeding during the first trimester, uterine size greater than dates, absent fetal heart tones, theca lutein cysts on the ovaries, and an abnormally high β-hCG concentration compared to gestational age. Pregnancy-induced hypertension, hyperemesis gravidarum, and thyroid storm are rare clinical entities that can accompany complete hydatidiform moles due to excessive hCG concentrations. Malignant sequela may develop in up to 20% of the patients treated for complete hydatidiform moles.

Partial hydatidiform moles are characterized by the presence of a fetus with only variable to focal trophoblastic proliferation and edema. Cytogenetic analysis demonstrates a triploid karyotype, most commonly 69,XXX or 69,XXY. The most common symptom is first-trimester vaginal bleeding and an elevated β-hCG concentration compared to normal. The other clinical findings seen with complete hydatidiform moles are less likely. Malignant sequela develops in less than 5% of the treated patients with partial hydatidiform moles.

Gestational choriocarcinoma is a malignancy involving both neoplastic synctiotrophoblasts and cytotrophoblasts without identifiable chorionic villi. This condition is also associated with markedly elevated concentrations of β-hCG. This entity tends to develop early systemic metastasis to the vagina, lung, liver, and brain, and chemotherapy is always indicated.

Placental site trophoblastic tumors are rare and are composed of intermediate trophoblast cells. Given the reduced amount of syncytiotrophoblasts the concentration of β-hCG is decreased relative to the other entities. Generally, placental site trophoblastic tumors are not sensitive to chemotherapy and surgical excision or hysterectomy is the mainstay of treatment.

Differential Diagnosis

The most common clinical entity mistaken for an elevated serum quantitative β-hCG that could represent gestational trophoblastic disease is a normal intrauterine pregnancy that is incorrectly dated. An office ultrasound is an easy tool that confirms the finding of pregnancy and can accurately date the pregnancy if necessary.

Another clinical entity that is extremely rare is primary choriocarcinoma of the ovary. In this situation a germ cell cancer develops on one of the ovaries and secretes β-hCG as a tumor marker that can mistakenly be identified as a pregnancy. Again, ultrasonography can identify the features of a solid ovarian tumor that is often unilateral with an empty uterus, indicating that this is a primary ovarian neoplasm.

Rarely, women have persistently elevated β-hCG concentrations as a result of a false-positive assay result. This has been coined "phantom hCG" or "factitious hCG." Most patients with this entity have low-concentration hCG elevations (<100 IU/L), but values higher than 300 IU/L have been reported. This results from interference with the hCG assay most often caused by heterophilic antibodies present in the patient's serum. Heterophilic antibodies are not excreted in the urine, whereas β-hCG from a gestational source would be excreted. A urine pregnancy test would be negative under this situation and is helpful in distinguishing "phantom hCG" from gestational trophoblastic disease. False-positive hCG assays are seldom affected by serial dilution of the patient's sera and will also demonstrate marked variability in the results between assays, with most reflecting undetectable hCG concentrations. False-positive test results should be suspected if hCG concentrations plateau at relatively low concentrations and do not respond to therapeutic maneuvers.

Pathogenesis

Gestational trophoblastic diseases develop from the fetal chorion during pregnancy. Molar pregnancies may be considered to have low malignancy potential as a result of aggressive local proliferation, myometrial invasion, and systemic metastasis. Choriocarcinomas and placental site trophoblastic tumors are true neoplasms, however.

Trophoblastic cells are derived from the outer cell mass of the preimplantation embryo and carry several unique properties. They affect the physical implantation of the embryo, produce sufficient amounts of hCG to maintain early pregnancy, evade maternal immunologic rejection, and invade into the maternal sinuses of the endometrium to nourish and supply the embryo during pregnancy.

Detailed histolopathologic studies coupled with cyogenetic techniques have established two separate molar syndromes. A complete hydatidiform mole is consistently associated with a totally paternally derived diploid genotype known as *diandric diploidy*. The egg is usually fertilized by a single sperm and loses the maternal haploid 23,X component by an unknown mechanism. The paternal haploid set of 23,X is reduplicated, and the normal component of 46 chromosomes is reestablished. A partial hydatidiform mole is associated with complete triploidy as a result of an extra haploid paternal set of chromosomes known as *diandric triploidy*. Partial hydatidiform moles result from dispermic fertilization of an egg with retention of the maternal haploid set, resulting in triploidy. As a result, the partial hydatidiform mole is composed of both maternal and paternal chromosomes, while the complete hydatidiform mole is entirely paternal.

Gestational choriocarcinoma is a malignant transformation of molar tissue or a de novo lesion that arises spontaneously from the placenta of any antecedent pregnancy. Placental site trophoblastic tumor's pathogenesis is poorly understood.

Many studies have documented an increase risk for women to develop gestational trophoblastic disease at each end of the range of reproductive life, namely, the very young and the very old who become pregnant. These age-related differences may reflect defective gametogenesis at the extremes of reproductive life, which predispose to the androgenic conceptus, giving rise to molar pregnancies. It is, however, well recognized that the greatest risk is a prior history of hydatidiform mole in which the risk may increase 10-fold.

Treatment

Hydatidiform moles are initially managed by dilatation and suction curettage. As long as β-hCG concentrations continue to decrease after evacuation, there is no need for chemotherapy. Serial quantitative β-hCG determinations should be performed every $1-2$ weeks while elevated until normal (<5 IU/L), and then at monthly intervals for an additional 6 months. However, if β-hCG concentrations increase or plateau over the course of several weeks, reevaluation for possible malignant postmolar gestational trophoblastic disease is indicated. A variety of hCG criteria have been used to diagnose postmolar gestational trophoblastic disease. The following are readily accepted criteria:

1. An hCG concentration plateau for four values $\pm 10\%$ recorded over a 3-week duration

2. An hCG concentration increase of $>10\%$ of three values recorded over a 2-week duration

3. Persistence of detectable hCG for more than 6 months after molar evacuation.

A new intrauterine pregnancy needs to be ruled out on the basis of hCG concentrations and ultrasonography when an increase in hCG concentration is detected. Once the diagnosis of malignant gestational trophoblastic disease is established, immediate evaluation for metastasis and risk factors is mandatory. A repeat physical exam is performed as well as a chest x-ray and/or computerized tomography (CT) scan of the chest, abdomen, and pelvis with contrast to detect potential metastatic sites. If lung lesions are identified on the chest x-ray, an abdominal pelvic CT is mandatory to rule out liver or other solid organ involvement that may go undetected by physical exam. Baseline serum quantitative β-hCG is also needed as a new pretherapy concentration. A complete blood count, liver, and renal function tests are also obtained in anticipation for the need for chemotherapy.

Patients with malignant gestational trophoblastic disease are classified as having nonmetastatic gestational trophoblastic disease or metatstatic gestational trophoblastic disease. Metastatic gestational trophoblastic disease is further subdivided into good prognosis and poor prognosis disease based on risk factors. Risk factors associated with good prognosis disease are duration of disease <4 months, pretreatment hCG concentration <40000 IU/L, no brain or liver metastases, no antecedent term pregnancy, and no prior chemotherapy. High-risk disease is essentially the reverse of these risk factors.

Patients with nonmetastatic and good prognosis metastatic gestational trophoblastic disease can be successfully treated with initial single-agent regimens. The two most commonly used drugs are methotrexate and dactinomycin. Chemotherapy is given until normalization of the serum quantitative β-hCG (<5 IU/L) and extended for $1-2$ cycles after the first normal β-hCG. Essentially all of these patients will achieve complete remission. Recurrence rates are less than 5% among successfully treated patients.

Patients with poor prognosis metastatic gestational disease and choriocarcinoma require multiagent chemotherapy. The standard chemotherapy regimen is EMA-CO, or etoposide, methotrexate, dactinomycin, cyclophosphamide, and vincristine. Localized or persistent lesions not responding to chemotherapy can be addressed with surgical resection or irradiation. Survival rates as high as 84% have been reported. Despite this aggressive chemotherapy regimen, up to 13% of patients with poor prognosis disease will develop recurrence after achieving a clinical remission.

The mainstay for the treatment of placental site trophoblastic tumors is hysterectomy and surgical resection of any metatstases. Given the low response rate to chemotherapy, early intervention with aggressive surgical resection is paramount.

Additional Reading

SOPER, J. T., MUTCH, D. G., AND SCHINK, J. C.: Diagnosis and treatment of gestational trophoblastic disease: ACOG Practice Bulletin No. 53. *Gynecol. Oncol. 93*:575–85, 2004.

SOPER, J. T., LEWIS, J. L., AND HAMMOND, C. B.: Gestational trophoblastic disease. In *Principles and Practice of Gynecologic Oncology*, 2nd ed., W. J. HOSKINS, C. A. PEREZ, AND R. C. YOUNG, eds., Lippincott-Raven, Philadelphia, 1997, pp. 1039–77.

COLE, L. A.: PHANTOM hCG and phantom choriocarcinoma. *Gynecol. Oncol. 71*:325–9, 1998.

HAMMOND, C. B., BORCHET, L. G., TYREY, L., CREASEMAN, W. T., AND PARKER, R. T.: Treatment of metastatic trophoblastic disease: Good and poor prognosis. *Am. J. Obstet. Gynecol. 115*:451–7, 1973.

Part Thirteen

Hematologic Malignancies

Cases of chronic lymphocytic leukemia (CLL) concomitant with autoimmune hemolytic anemia (AHA), acute promyelocytic leukemia (APL) concomitant with disseminated intravascular coagulation (DIC), peripheral T-cell leukemia–lymphoma, chronic myelogenous leukemia, and polycythemia vera are reported and discussed in Cases 52, 53, 54, 55, and 56, respectively (all edited by CSE).

Tietz's Applied Laboratory Medicine, Second Edition. Edited by Mitchell G. Scott, Ann M. Gronowski, and Charles S. Eby
Copyright © 2007 John Wiley & Sons, Inc.

Case 52

A Man with Anemia and Lymphocytosis

Sylva Bem, Robert E. Hutchison, and Naif Z. Abraham, Jr.

A 58-year-old Caucasian man presented to the emergency room with the chief complaint of fatigue and weakness for the previous 3–4 days. He described dyspnea on exertion without chest pain, cough, sore throat, dizziness, myalgias, arthralgias, fever, or sweats. Past medical history was unremarkable, and he was not taking any prescribed medications. Physical examination was notable for normal vital signs, pallor, and mild scleral icterus. Oral pharynx was benign, lung sounds were vesicular, and cardiac exam was normal. A liver edge was not palpable, but the spleen was mildly enlarged. A careful exam for peripheral adenopathy was negative. The results of laboratory studies performed on admission were as follows:

Analyte	Value, Conventional Units	Reference Interval, Conventional Units	Value, SI Units	Reference Interval, SI Units
WBC	$28.7 \times 10^3/\mu L$	4–10	$28.7 \times 10^9/L$	4–10
Neutrophil count	$7.0 \times 10^3/\mu L$	1.8–7.0	$7.0 \times 10^9/L$	1.8–7.0
Lymphocyte count	$21.1 \times 10^3/\mu L$	1.2–4.0	$21.1 \times 10^9/L$	1.2–4.0
Monocyte count	$0.6 \times 10^3/\mu L$	0–0.6	$0.6 \times 10^9/L$	0–0.6
Hemoglobin	5.6 g/dL	13.5–18	56 g/L	135–180
Hematocrit	16%	41–53	0.16 volume	0.41–0.53
Platelets	$76 \times 10^3/\mu L$	150–400	$76 \times 10^9/L$	150–400
BUN	24 mg/μL	9–20	8.57 mmol/L	3.21–7.14
Creatinine	1.2 mg/μL	0.8–1.5	105.96 mmol/L	70.64–132.45
Bilirubin, total	2.1 mg/μL	0.2–1.3	31.5 mmol/L	3–19.5
LDH	350 U/L	110–210 U/L	5.9 μkat/L	1.9–3.6
Haptoglobin	<6 mg/μL	30–180	<60 mg/L	300–1800
Direct Coombs test	Positive	Negative	Same	

The patient was admitted by the medicine team for an acute presentation of anemia, which most likely was autoimmune-mediated hemolytic type (given the increased LDH, the low haptoglobin, and a positive direct Coombs test). To evaluate the patient's lymphocytosis, a blood sample was submitted for flow cytometry analysis. Results showed a monoclonal

Tietz's Applied Laboratory Medicine, Second Edition. Edited by Mitchell G. Scott, Ann M. Gronowski, and Charles S. Eby
Copyright © 2007 John Wiley & Sons, Inc.

B-cell population with expression of CD19, CD20, CD22, CD23, and CD38 and with coexpression of CD5, consistent with chronic lymphocytic leukemia (CLL). Interphase nuclei evaluated by fluorescence in situ hybridization (FISH) cytogenetic assay for the presence of abnormalities associated with CLL showed all the cells to have a deletion of the short arm of chromosome 17 at the p53 locus.

He was started on prednisone to treat the hemolytic anemia and rituximab (monoclonal anti-CD20) for treatment of CLL. He also received folic acid as a supplementation to compensate for excess hemolysis.

Diagnosis

Chronic lymphocytic leukemia/small lymphocytic lymphoma (CLL/SLL) is an indolent monoclonal proliferation of mature lymphocytes, generally of B-cell lineage. It is a systemic disease and usually involves blood, lymph nodes, and bone marrow. The lymphocyte count is typically greater than $10 \times 10^3/\mu L$; however, diagnosis is possible even with counts less than that if the morphology and immunophenotype are typical of CLL (see Fig. 52.1 and Table 52.1). When there is predominant blood involvement, it is called *chronic lymphocytic leukemia*; when there is predominant lymph node involvement, the term *small lymphocytic lymphoma* is usually used; however, they are considered a single entity. Most cases present as CLL, and a majority occur in people over the age of 60 with men affected twice as frequently as women. It is a rare disease in people under 40. The onset is usually insidious and frequently is discovered by accident. Anemia may develop, most often later in the course of disease as a result of impaired production due to bone marrow replacement by leukemic cells. The platelet count can be reduced for the same reasons. Autoimmune hemolytic anemia develops in about 10% of patients.

Examination of a peripheral blood smear shows an increase in mature lymphocytes with coarsely condensed nuclear chromatin arranged in "blocks" sharply separated by parachromatin. Cytoplasm is typically slight to moderate and size variation is minimal, with overall monotonous appearance. In typical cases of CLL, there are fewer than 10% prolymphocytes (larger mature lymphocytes with prominent nucleoli and moderately abundant cytoplasm). The presence of more than 55% prolymphocytes with a high white count suggests prolymphocytic leukemia (PLL), which is a more aggressive disease. Some cases of CLL show increased prolymphocytes (10–55%) and the term "CLL/PLL" is used. This may, on occasion, herald a "prolymphocytoid" transformation of CLL. Lymph node involvement in CLL appears as a diffuse infiltrate of small mature lymphocytes with clumped nuclear chromatin and small amounts of cytoplasm, scattered prolymphocytes, and the presence of proliferation centers. These are small collections of lymphocytes with increased cytoplasm, prolymphocytes, and paraimmunoblasts (the latter of which are slightly larger and with more prominent nucleoli than prolymphocytes). Mitotic figures are minimal. Bone marrow involvement is frequently seen and can be nodular, interstitial, or diffuse. Nodular and interstital patterns are usually present in early stages of CLL; advanced disease is usually associated with a diffuse pattern.

By immunohistochemistry or by flow cytometry, CLL/SLL shows a characteristic phenotype. Lymphocytes expresses B-cell markers CD20, CD19, CD79a, CD23, often dim CD22, and dim surface immunoglobulin (Ig) of IgM or IgD subtype with either κ (60%) or λ (40%) monoclonal light-chain expression. The coexpression of CD5 (normally

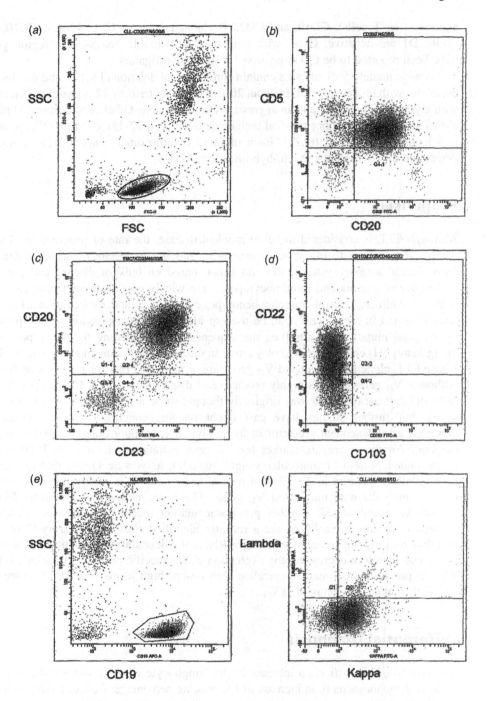

Figure 52.1 Typical CLL immunophenotype (*a*). Small lymphocytes are circled: low forwardscatter (*x* axis) indicates small cell size and low side-scatter (*y* axis) indicates minimal cytoplasm and nuclear complexity. (*b–d*) Binding intensity of fluorescent-labeled antibodies that recognize different epitopes on the surface of lymphocytes highlighted in (*a*). (*b*) Coexpression of CD5 and CD20. (*c*) Coexpression of CD20 and CD23. (*d*) Expression of CD22 but not CD103 (specific for hairy cell leukemia; see Table 52.1). (*e*) A population of small, CD19-positive B lymphocytes have been selected for gating. (*f*) The B lymphocytes express only one type of light chain; kappa, confirming that it is a malignant, clonal population.

expressed on T cells), CD19, and CD23 is characteristic for CLL. FMC7, CD10, and cyclin D1 are negative. Cases with unmutated Ig variable heavy-chain region genes have been reported to be CD38-positive by some investigators.

Approximately 50% of cases contain chromosomal deletion (13q14), and this finding correlates with longer survival. In about 20% of the cases trisomy 12 is present, correlating with atypical morphology and an aggressive clinical course. Other chromosomal abnormalities associated with poor survival include deletion (11q 22-23), deletion (17p13) at the p53 locus, and deletion (6q21). Each of these chromosomal abnormalities is usually detectable by fluorescence in situ hybridization (FISH).

Prognosis

Although CLL is considered to be an indolent disease, the rate of progression, disease complications, time to initiation of treatment, and life expectancy vary considerably. Two clinical staging systems, Rai and Binet, based on bulk of disease and presence or absence of anemia and thrombocytopenia, are widely used to predict patients' prognosis. In addition, several immunophenotype, cytogenetic, and molecular markers that have emerged in recent years can be used to identify high risk asymptomatic patients. Ig V_H gene mutational status [i.e., the sequence of DNA coding for the V portion of the Ig heavy (H) chain] seems to play a role in disease progression and outcome. Patients whose CLL clone has unmutated V_H genes are at increased risk for progressive disease. Although V_H gene status is highly predictive of disease outcome in CLL, it is a technically difficult assay. CD38 was originally thought to be a reliable marker for V_H gene status, but further studies have cast doubt on this conclusion. Its expression is, however, an independent predictor of aggressive disease, poor outcome, and shortened survival. Another surrogate marker for V_H gene mutational status is ZAP-70 protein (ζ-associated protein of molecular weight 70 kDa), a tyrosine kinase that appears to be normally expressed in T cells and natural-killer cells. It is highly overexpressed in CLL tumor cells with unmutated V_H genes. However, methods of assessing ZAP-70 are not yet standardized. Another prognostic marker recently reported is microRNA expression profile. MicroRNAs are a recently identified class of regulatory RNAs that function by targeting specific messenger RNAs for degradation or inhibition of translation and therefore decreasing the expression of the specific proteins. A specific microRNA expression was found to correlate with low or high levels of ZAP-70 expression and with mutational status of IgV_H.

Differential Diagnosis

Absolute lymphocytosis is an increase in the lymphocyte count in the peripheral blood. *Relative lymphocytosis* is an increase of lymphocyte percentage. Absolute lymphocytosis can be divided into two main categories: secondary (reactive) and primary (clonal).

Secondary lymphocytosis is frequently accompanied by neutropenia and is usually associated with viral infections, including Epstein–Barr virus (EBV), acute infectious lymphocytosis, hepatitis, and numerous others. Lymphocytosis in children and young adults is usually of viral origin, while chronic lymphocytosis in middle-aged and older adults is often due to CLL or other lymphoproliferative disorders.

Infectious mononucleosis due to EBV infection is frequent in adolescents and young adults, but can also be observed in older adults. It usually presents with sore throat, malaise, lymphadenopathy and hepatosplenomegaly. Typical peripheral blood findings include increased WBC, ranging within $12-25 \times 10^3/\mu L$, and absolute lymphocytosis with numerous large, transformed lymphocytes with immature nuclear chromatin and increase in the amount of basophilic cytoplasm or "monocytoid" lymphocytes. These changes are not pathognomonic for EBV, and can be seen in other infections, such as cytomegalovirus, toxoplasmosis, and infectious hepatitis. EBV virus attaches to C3d complement receptor (CD21) on B lymphocytes and stimulates proliferation and production of polyclonal immunoglobulin. The cellular immune response consists of activation and proliferation of T lymphocytes, usually during the second week of illness, and occurs as a reaction to B-cell activation. These actually represent the atypical lymphocytes present in the blood. Diagnosis is based on detection of a specific humoral immune response (increase in titer of IgG and IgM viral capsid antibodies), or of heterophil antibodies that bind to the red cells of other species, such as horse or sheep. Cytomegalovirus infection is a syndrome similar to infectious mononucleosis. There is no rise in heterophil antibody, and diagnosis is made by CMV culture or serology. Persistent polyclonal B-cell lymphocytosis is a rare condition in adults, predominantly female smokers, and in the postsplenectomy state. It is a benign polyclonal B-cell proliferation of clefted or lobated lymphocytes with increased polyclonal serum IgM.

Pertussis (whooping cough) previously was the frequent cause of lymphocytosis in children but has now been reduced by routine immunization. The lymphocytes are small mature T cells. It can occur in adults whose immunity has waned since childhood immunization, and also in unimmunized children. There is a significant lymphocytosis with WBC usually $>30 \times 10^3/\mu L$ accompanied by characteristic clinical symptoms (paroxysm of coughing with thick sputum production). The lymphocyte count is highest during the first 3 weeks of illness and then decreases. Human T-lymphotropic virus type 1 (HTLV-1) can present as transient T-cell lymphocytosis with 10–40% of the lymphocytes consisting of atypical and immature forms. Some HTLV-1 carriers can eventually develop adult T-cell leukemia/lymphoma.

Primary lymphocytosis is typically due to mature B-cell neoplasms. Numerous lymphoproliferative disorders other than CLL can present as lymphocytosis, with or without lymph node, bone marrow, or splenic involvement. The differential diagnosis includes, in addition to chronic lymphocytic leukemia, B-cell prolymphocytic leukemia, lymphoplasmacytic lymphoma/Waldenström's macroglobulinemia, hairy cell leukemia, splenic marginal zone lymphoma, and plasma cell myeloma. In general, disseminated B-cell neoplasms are relatively indolent. Rarely, a leukemic phase of mantle cell lymphoma or follicular lymphoma can occur. Distinction is made on the basis of morphology, immunophenotype, and molecular characteristics (Table 52.1).

B-Cell prolymphocytic leukemia (mentioned previously) is a malignancy of B prolymphocytes (medium-sized round lymphoid cells with prominent nucleoli). Prolymphocytes must exceed 55% of lymphoid cells in the blood. They strongly express surface IgM/IgD as well as CD19, CD20, CD22, and FMC7. CD5 is present in one-third of cases, and CD23 is typically absent.

Lymphoplasmacytic lymphoma/Waldenström's macroglobulinemia is a neoplasm of small B lymphocytes, plasmacytoid lymphocytes, and plasma cells, usually lacking CD5, and secreting a serum monoclonal protein (IgM) that may cause symptomatic

Table 52.1 Immunophenotype of Mature B-Cell Neoplasms: Surface Immunoglobin (SIg)

Neoplasm	SIg	CD5	CD23	CD103	Cyclin D1	CD10
B-CLL/SLL	dim+	+	+	−	−	−
B-Prolymphocytic leukemia	++	−/+	−	−	−	−
Lymphoplasmacytic lymphoma	++	−	−	−	−	−
Splenic marginal zone B-cell lymphoma	+	−	−	−	−	−
Hairy cell leukemia	+	−	−	++	+/−	−
Plasma cell myeloma	−	−	−	−	−/+	−/+
Mantle cell lymphoma	++	+	−	−	+	−
Follicular lymphoma	+	−	−	−	−	+

hyperviscosity or cryoglobulinemia. Translocation t(9;14)(p13;q32) and rearrangement of the PAX-5 gene is reported in up to 50% of cases.

Splenic marginal zone lymphoma is a B-cell malignancy consisting of small lymphocytes of the marginal zone in the splenic germinal centers of white pulp. Lymphoma cells can be found in the peripheral blood as villous lymphocytes (presence of short polar villi). Tumor cells are positive for CD20 and CD79a; they are negative for CD23, CD5, CD10, CD43, and CD103. Allelic loss of chromosome 7q21-32 is present in up to 40% of the cases. Dysregulation of CDK6 gene located at 7q21 has also been reported.

Hairy cell leukemia is a tumor of small B-lymphoid cells with oval nuclei and abundant cytoplasm with "hairy" projections, strongly expressing CD103, CD22, and CD11c. CD5, CD10, and CD23 are negative. Most patients present with splenomegaly and peripheral cytopenias.

Plasma cell neoplasms are disorders of terminally differentiated B cells. They usually involve bone marrow or extramedullary masses (plasmacytomas); significant peripheral involvement is rare (2%). Plasma cell leukemia is defined as greater than 20% or $>2 \times 10^3/\mu L$ plasma cells in blood. The prognosis is considerably worse when multiple myeloma presents with plasma cell leukemia.

Mantle cell lymphoma is a neoplasm composed of monomorphous small to medium-sized lymphocytes with slightly irregular nuclei. Proliferation centers are absent. They are monoclonal B cells with moderate to strong surface IgM expression, and are typically CD5-positive, FMC7-positive and CD23- and CD10-negative. All cases are bcl-2 protein–positive, and almost all cases express cyclin D1. Bcl-2 is a member of a large family of proteins involved in regulation of apoptosis (programmed cell death). Expression of bcl-2 protects lymphocytes from apoptosis and leads to reduced cell death and steady accumulation. Cyclin D1 belongs to group of proteins involved in regulating the cell cycle. Dysregulation of the activity of cyclins favors cell proliferation Seventy to seventy-five percent of cases demonstrate t(11;14)(q13;q32) translocation.

Follicular lymphoma is a nodal lymphoma composed of follicle center B cells (centrocytes—small cleaved cells, and centroblasts—large noncleaved cells), which has a predominantly follicular pattern. It can also involve blood, spleen, bone marrow, and extranodal sites. The tumor cells are surface Ig–positive, CD10-positive, and CD5-negative and express B-cell-associated antigens (CD19, CD20, CD22). Tight meshworks of CD21 and CD23 follicular dendritic cells are present in follicular areas. Of all cases reported, 70–90% have t(14;18), involving rearrangement of the bcl-2 gene.

Therapy

Therapeutic options for CLL include a "watch and wait" approach until the course of the disease is declared. Patients requiring treatment may be treated with a variety of chemotherapy regimens, including chlorambucil, cyclophosphamide, purine analogs like fludarabine, CHOP (cyclophosphamide, doxorubicin, vincristine, prednisone), CVP (cyclophosphamide, vincristine, prednisone), FND (fludarabine mitoxantrone, dexamethasone), and FC (fludarabine and cyclophosphamide). Typical response rates with these treatments range from 80–90% in treatment-naive patients to 30–40% in those with relapsed or refractory disease. Currently, two monoclonal antibodies are approved for use in the United States. Rituximab (Rituxan), an anti-CD20 antibody, is approved for relapsed or refractory low-grade non-Hodgkin, CD20-positive lymphoma, including CLL/SLL. Its use in CLL sometimes results in loss of CD20 expression due to blockade of the antigen or emergence of a CD20-negative clone. Campath-1H (Alemtuzumab), which targets CD52-positive lymphocytes, is indicated for treatment of B-cell CLL in patients who have been treated with alkylating agents and who have failed fludarabine therapy.

Additional Reading

CALIN, G. A., FERRACIN, M., CIMMINO, A., ET AL.: A MicroRNA signature associated with prognosis and progression in chronic lymphocytic leukemia. *N. Engl. J. Med. 353*:1793–801, 2005.

CRESPO, M., BOSCH, F., VILLAMOR, N. ET AL.: ZAP-70 expression as a surrogate for Immunoglobulin-variable-region mutations in chronic lymphocytic leukemia. *N. Engl. J. Med. 348*:1764–75, 2003.

HARRIS, N. L., JAFFE, E. S., STEIN, H. ET AL.: A revised European-American classification of lymphoid neoplasms: A proposal from the International Lymphoma Study Group. *Blood 84*:1361–92, 1994.

HUTCHISON, R. E. AND ABRAHAM, N. Z. JR.: Leukocyte disorders. In *Henry's Clinical Diagnosis and Management by Laboratory Methods*, 21st ed., R. A. MCPHERSON AND M. R. PINCUS, eds., London, Elsevier, 2005.

VENUGOPAL, P., BYRD, J. C., ENGERT, A. ET AL.: Changing the outcome of chronic lymphocytic leukemia: Prognostic tools and novel therapeutic modalities. *Clin. Adv. Hematol. Oncol. 3*:2–15, 2005.

World Health Organization Classification of Tumours: *Pathology and Genetics of Tumours of Haematopoietic and Lymphoid Tissues*, E. S. JAFFE, N. L. HARRIS, H. STEIN, AND J. W. VARDIMAN, eds., Lyon, IARC Press, 2001.

A Teenager with Pneumonia, Leukopenia, and Ecchymoses

Anna Halldórsdóttir

The patient, a 15-year-old white male, presented to the emergency department of the university hospital because of weakness and a fever of 102°F (38.9°C). There was no prior history of illness. At the time of admission, the patient appeared pale and had tenderness over the sternum. There were ecchymoses over the anterior abdominal wall and right buttock. Blood pressure was 110/65 mm Hg, pulse 105/bpm and regular. Examination of the chest showed dullness over the right posterior lung fields. Breath sounds were bronchial in this area with rales. The liver was palpable at the costal margin, but the spleen was not palpated. A chest x-ray was normal except for linear streaks in the region of the right lower lobe.

The following laboratory values were reported on admission:

Analyte	Value, Conventional Units	Reference Interval, Conventional Units	Value, SI Units	Reference Interval, SI Units
WBC	$3.4 \times 10^3/\mu L$	3.8–9.8	$3.4 \times 10^9/L$	3.8–9.8
Platelet count	$31 \times 10^3/\mu L$	150–450	$31 \times 10^9/L$	150–450
Hemoglobin	10.4 g/dL	12.3–16.6	104 g/L	123–166
MCV	98.7 fL	83–97	Same	
Neutrophil	$0.9 \times 10^3/\mu L$	1.8–6.6	$0.9 \times 10^9/L$	1.8–6.6
Lymphocytes	$1.7 \times 10^3/\mu L$	1.2–3.3	$1.7 \times 10^9/L$	1.2–3.3
Monocytes	$0.8 \times 10^3/\mu L$	0.2–1.2	$0.8 \times 10^9/L$	0.2–1.2
Sodium	141 mmol/L	138–145	Same	
Potassium	4.5 mmol/L	4.0–5.3	Same	
Chloride	105 mmol/L	98–108	Same	
CO_2, total	21 mmol/L	22–29	Same	
Urea nitrogen	15 mg/dL	7–18	5.4 mmol urea/L	2.5–6.4
Creatinine	0.8 mg/dL	0.2–1.0	71 μmol/L	18–88
Glucose	100 mg/dL	70–115	5.6 mmol/L	3.9–6.4
Protein, total	6.0 g/dL	6.0–8.0	60 g/L	60–80
Albumin	3.6 g/dL	3.5–5.5	36 g/L	35–55
Urate	8.8 mg/dL	2.0–6.0	523 μmol/L	119–357

Tietz's Applied Laboratory Medicine, Second Edition. Edited by Mitchell G. Scott, Ann M. Gronowski, and Charles S. Eby
Copyright © 2007 John Wiley & Sons, Inc.

Analyte	Value, Conventional Units	Reference Interval, Conventional Units	Value, SI Units	Reference Interval, SI Units
Bilirubin, total	0.7 mg/dL	0.2–1.0	12 μmol/L	3–17
AST	55 U/L	15–35	0.92 μkat/L	0.25–0.58
ALT	35 U/L	10–30	0.58 μkat/L	0.17–0.50
LDH	320 U/L	150–250	5.33 μkat/L	2.50–4.17
PT	16.5 s	10.2–13.5	Same	
aPTT	45 s	28–35	Same	
Fibrinogen	110 mg/dL	210–400	1.1 g/L	2.1–4.0
Fibrin-split products	1 : 80	<1 : 20	Same	
D-dimer test	2000 mg/mL FEU*	<500		

*FEU = Fibrinogen equivalent units

A review of a peripheral blood smear was notable for a left shift with 8% band forms, 2% myelocytes, and 3% promyelocytes. No blasts were detected. Platelets were normal in morphology but decreased. Red cell morphology was notable for moderate variation in size (anisocytosis) and shape (poikilocytosis), but there was no dominant morphologic abnormality.

Diagnosis

Thrombocytopenia, abnormal PT and PTT, decreased fibrinogen, and increased fibrin-split products and D-dimer, in conjunction with peripheral ecchymoses, suggested a diagnosis of disseminated intravascular coagulation (DIC). Because of the presence of pancytopenia, a bone marrow biopsy and aspirate were obtained from the posterior iliac crest. The aspirate was scanty and obtained with difficulty. The bone marrow biopsy core was white rather than pink in gross appearance. The bone marrow aspirate specimen was dilute and contained fat but no spicules. No megakaryocytes were seen. Fifty-eight percent of cells were mononuclear and contained azurophilic granules. The cells varied considerably in size and shape; many nuclei were either kidney-shaped or bilobated. The biopsy specimen was markedly hypercellular and contained few fat globules. There were few megakaryocytes and erythroid precursors. The cells had a uniform, monotonous appearance; many contained nucleoli, and most contained azurophilic granules.

Portions of the aspirate were sent for cytogenetic studies and immunological marker determination. Flow cytometry showed that many cells were positive for CD13, CD15, CD32, and CD33; T-cell and B-cell markers were nonreactive. Cytogenetic analysis revealed occasional aneuploidy, and many cells showed a t(15 : 17) translocation; no Philadelphia (Ph[1]) chromosome was seen. The findings supported a diagnosis of acute promyelocytic leukemia complicated by disseminated intravascular coagulation.

The patient presented with pancytopenia and pneumonia with sternal tenderness. The sternal tenderness suggested that the pancytopenia was caused by a hypercellular marrow rather than an aplastic marrow. The physical evidence of pneumonia predominated over the radiological findings because marked neutropenia precluded granulocytic infiltration. The ecchymoses were explained by the laboratory studies showing evidence of DIC.

The combination of pancytopenia and hyperplastic bone marrow containing a predominance of immature cells was compatible with a diagnosis of acute leukemia. The peripheral blood findings were not diagnostic because the patient was leukopenic without blasts in the peripheral smear. However, the bone marrow was hyperplastic, and most of the cells were promyelocytes. The presence of DIC in a patient with a hyperplastic bone marrow and cells that contain azurophilic granules strongly suggests that the patient has acute promyelocytic leukemia (APL). Results of cell surface marker studies were typical of those found in granulocytic cell lines and were compatible with a myeloid leukemia. The finding of t(15 : 17) chromosomal translocation was characteristic of APL.

Acute Leukemia

Most patients presenting with acute leukemia have pancytopenia and circulating blasts. WBC can be increased, normal, or decreased, although counts between 5000 and 30,000 are most common. Peripheral blood smear is usually diagnostic and shows the presence of immature forms (blasts) with a high nuclear : cytoplasmic ratio and fine chromatin. About 10% of patients, however, do not have circulating blasts. In these cases a bone marrow biopsy and aspirate are necessary to establish the diagnosis. The classic bone marrow findings are hypercellularity and decreased megakaryocytes with clusters or sheets of blasts, which may almost completely replace normal hematopoietic elements. The French–American–British (FAB) classification states that at least 30% of nucleated cells have to be blasts for a diagnosis of acute leukemia, whereas the more recent WHO classification decreased that percentage to 20%.[5,6]

The two main forms of acute leukemias are acute lymphoblastic (ALL) and acute myeloid leukemias (AML). ALL is more common in children, whereas AML is more common in adults. The two types have an equal incidence in teenagers. Although certain morphological features are characteristic of each type, there is a considerable morphological overlap. Cytochemcal stains such as myeloperoxidase (MPX) and nonspecific esterase (NSE) are often helpful in distinguishing AML from ALL. MPX stain is positive in myeloid cells, whereas NSE is positive in monocytic cells but lymphoid cells are mostly negative. Flow cytometry can also be helpful as it is able to detect a variety of cell surface markers characteristic of different cell types.

The FAB classification divides AMLs into eight categories (M0–M7) according to morphological, cytochemical, and immunophenotypical features. These include the undifferentiated leukemia (M0), granulocytic leukemias (M1–M3), myelomonocytic (M4), monocytic leukemia (M5), erythroleukemia (M6), and acute megakaryocytic leukemia (M7). The natural course of AML can range from a disease of progressive cytopenias to one of acute virulence; the subacute form is more commonplace in the elderly. M3, also known as *acute promyelocytic leukemia* (APL), is usually acute in onset. The diagnostic features of APL are as follows: (1) bone marrow findings of ≥20% blasts and abnormal promyelocytes combined, (2) intense MPX reactivity, (3) multiple Auer rods in blasts and promyelocytes, and (4) translocation 15 : 17 (q22 : q22).[6]

Acute Promyelocytic Leukemia

APL or M3 accounts for approximately 10–15% of all AML cases. It is relatively more common in younger patients and Hispanics. There are actually two variants of M3: the hypergranular and hypogranular (M3v) types. The hypergranular form is more common (75%) and usually presents with a low WBC count, often <5000. The promyelocytes contain an abundance of eosinophilic primary granules, often in aggregates called *Auer rods*. The hypogranular form is less common and has a worse prognosis, presenting with a very high WBC count, frequently >50,000. The immature cells in this variant contain few granules visible by light microscopy. However, cytochemistry reveals strong MPX reactivity in APL cells and immunophenotypic studies by flow cytometry show positivity for CD33 and CD13, but little or no expression of CD34 and HLA DR.

The most impressive clinical features of APL compared to other AMLs are the severe coagulopathy frequently present at diagnosis (discussed in a subsection below) and the therapeutic response to retinoic acid. The empiric observation that ATRA (all-trans retinoic acid) induces remission in patients with APL led to a dramatic change in both the understanding and management of this disorder. Most APL patients harbor a specific balanced reciprocal translocation involving the RARα (retinoic acid receptor α) gene on chromosomes 17 and the PML (promyelocytic leukemia) gene on chromosome 15, which gives rise to a PML-RARα fusion protein. Four other translocations, all involving the RARα gene, have been reported in rare cases of APL.[16] PML-RARα is a dominant negative inhibitor of retinoid-induced transactivation resulting in a block in differentiation at the promyelocytic stage of development. This fusion protein aberrantly recruits the nuclear corepressor complex, causing decreased RARα activity and repression of target gene transcription. ATRA binds to PML-RARα and reverses the repression of target genes required for normal hematopoietic development.

In addition to interfering with normal RARα function, the PML-RARα fusion protein also interferes with the function of the native PML protein. PML is a component of a nuclear structure called *nuclear bodies* (NBs) and is essential for multiple stress/DNA damage-activated apoptotic pathways.[10] In APL cells the integrity of the NB is disrupted and a microspeckled distribution of PML-RARα is observed. Treatment of APL cells with ATRA causes the NBs to regenerate, with proper relocalization of PML.

Diagnosis of APL requires the confirmation of the translocation t(15 : 17) either by conventional cytogenetics, fluorescence in situ hybridization (FISH) or reverse transcriptase polymerase chain reaction (RT-PCR).[4] Classic cytogenetics involves staining and karyotyping of cultured cells in metaphase. This requires viable cells from bone marrow aspirate or peripheral blood and can take up to 2 weeks. The FISH technique does not require viable cells as the nuclei are stained in interphase and takes only 24–72 hours. However, FISH requires probes against specific genes and does not give information about other possible genetic lesions. RT-PCR testing for the presence of the PML-RARα fusion product in blood or bone marrow is rapid, is sensitive, and defines targets for detection of minimal residual disease (MRD). However, technical problems with RT-PCR include poor RNA yield at diagnosis, contamination, and artifacts. Finally, detection of microspeckled nuclear distribution of the PML protein by immunofluorescence or immunohistochemistry has been described. This technique is rapid, simple, and specific, but gives no information on the type of PML-RARα fusion and is subject to artifacts due to cellular degradation. Because molecular remission has been recently established as a therapeutic objective in APL, RT-PCR should be performed at presentation to precisely characterize the target for amplification, even in patients with confirmed t(15 : 17) by other methods. However, this assay should be performed only by reference laboratories, to avoid technical pitfalls such as false positives.[13]

Treatment of APL is curative in most patients since the introduction of ATRA. Prognostic factors such as WBC and platelet counts help guide the choice of treatment. Induction chemotherapy with anthracyclines and ATRA is now standard of care and leads to complete remission in >90% of patients. Early laboratory evaluation of MRD (minimal residual disease) after ATRA-based induction is not recommended except as a part of investigational studies as several large clinical trials have failed to find any correlation between the postinduction PCR status and subsequent patient outcome. Consolidation therapy with 2–3 cycles of intensive chemotherapy leads to molecular remission in 90–99% of patients.[12] RT-PCR is regarded mandatory after completion of consolidation therapy to determine the relapse risk in individual patients, preferably using a bone marrow specimen. Maintenance therapy with ATRA, after ATRA-based induction and subsequent consolidation chemotherapy, has been shown to improve prognosis so that 5-year survival now exceeds 70%.[14]

Arsenic trioxide (ATO), the notorious poison, has been shown to have a dramatic effect in the treatment of APL, and is not associated with severe toxicity in this context. The mechanism of arsenic cytotoxicity is thought to involve posttranslational modification followed by degradation of the PML-RARα fusion protein, targeting of PML to nuclear bodies with restoration of its physiologic functions, and production of reactive oxygen species (ROS) by NADPH oxidase in leukemic cells. The role of ATO in APL treatment is still under investigation. The combination of ATRA and ATO in patients with newly diagnosed APL has yielded more durable remission than monotherapy and ATO may be superior to ATRA in relapsed APL.[1]

The most important complication of ATRA-based therapy is the retinoic acid syndrome (RAS), a cardiorespiratory syndrome manifested by dyspnea, pulmonary infiltrates, pleural or pericardial effusions, episodic hypotension, and occasionally acute renal failure. Initial studies in which ATRA was administered as a single agent for induction reported an incidence of approximately 25%. With earlier recognition, the mortality rate of the patients with this syndrome has declined from approximately 30% to 5–10%. Diagnosis can be difficult as the symptoms are nonspecific. The pathogenesis of the syndrome is not completely understood, but tissue infiltration is always observed in RAS. Myeloid precursors and mature granulocytes, presumably the differentiating ATRA-treated APL cells, infiltrate into several organs, due to changes in their adhesive capacity and cytokine production. The best treatment approach is early recognition and initiation of dexamethasone.[7]

The patient described above was simultaneously administered platelets and fresh-frozen plasma to correct the coagulopathy. Allopurinol was administered to prevent tumor lysis syndrome, a potential complication for chemotherapy for malignancies with a high proliferation index. The preferred treatment options at the time of chemotherapy were either cytosine arabinoside and daunomycin or ATRA. ATRA was chosen, and after four weeks of therapy, the patient entered complete remission without developing severe pancytopenia.

Disseminated Intravascular Coagulation (DIC) and APL

Dissseminated intravascular coagulation is not a disease or a symptom but a syndrome, which is always secondary to an underlying disorder. The syndrome is characterized by a systemic activation of the blood coagulation system, which results in the generation and deposition of fibrin, leading to microvascular thrombi in various organs and the development of multiorgan failure. Consumption and subsequent exhaustion of coagulation proteins and platelets because of the ongoing activation of the coagulation system may induce severe bleeding complications. Hence, a patient with DIC can present with a simultaneously occurring thrombotic and bleeding problem.

Many disease states may lead to the development of DIC. The most common diseases in patients with DIC are leukemia, infections, solid cancers, obstetric complications, and aortic aneurysm.[15] In general there are two major pathways that may cause DIC: (1) a systemic inflammatory response, leading to activation of the cytokine network and subsequent activation of coagulation (such as in sepsis or major trauma) and/or (2) release or exposure of procoagulant material (in)to the bloodstream (such as in malignancies or in obstetrical cases). Procoagulant molecules include tissue factor (TF) and a cancer procoagulant, a cysteine protease with factor X–activating properties.[8]

Several simultaneously occurring mechanisms play a role in the pathogenesis of DIC: (1) increased thrombin generation due to activation of the tissue factor/FVIIa pathway; (2) dysfunctional anticoagulant pathways, including reduction in antithrombin and depression of the protein C system; and (3) impaired fibrinolysis, caused mainly by a sustained increase in plasma levels of PAI-1 (plasminogen activator inhibitor 1).

No single routinely available laboratory test is sufficiently sensitive or specific to enable a diagnosis of DIC. However, in clinical practice a diagnosis of DIC can often be made by a combination of platelet count, measurement of global clotting times [activated partial thromboplastin time (aPTT) and PT], measurement of one or two clotting factors and inhibitors (such as antithrombin), and a test for FDPs (fibrin degradation products). Serial coagulation tests are usually more helpful than single laboratory results in establishing the diagnosis of DIC. FDPs may be detected by specific enzyme-linked immunosorbent assays (ELISAs) or by latex agglutination assays. The main problem with these assays is low specificity since many other conditions such as inflammation or recent surgery are associated with elevated FDPs. More recently developed tests such as D-dimer, which are specifically aimed at the detection of neoantigens on degraded crosslinked fibrin, also suffer from low specificity.

To aid in diagnosis, a scoring system has been proposed by the ISTH (International Society of Thrombosis and Hemostasis). In the presence of an underlying disorder known to be associated with DIC, global coagulation tests are ordered (platelet count, PT, fibrinogen, FDPs). Using the results of these tests, a score is calculated that separates cases into overt DIC and nonovert DIC. The scoring system is a strong independent predictor of fatal outcome in intensive care patients. Some studies suggest that these traditional coagulation markers are not sensitive enough to diagnose nonovert DIC (or pre-DIC), which responds better to treatment than does overt DIC. Investigational hemostatic molecular markers include thrombin–antithrombin complex (TAT), prothrombin activation fragment F1 + 2, plasmin–plasmin inhibitor complex (PPIC), and aPTT biphasic waveforms, but these are not widely available and their clinical usefulness has not been proved.

The key of DIC treatment is the specific and forceful management of the underlying disorder. This may not always be sufficient, though, as DIC may proceed after proper treatment has been initiated, especially in patients with sepsis. Unfortunately, there are few scientifically validated treatment modalities for DIC. Supportive treatment is important, and plasma or platelet substitution therapy is indicated in patients with active bleeding and in those requiring an invasive procedure. Heparin has been used in the past, but a benefit has never been demonstrated in controlled clinical trials. Therefore, therapeutic doses of heparin are recommended only in patients with clinically overt thromboembolism or extensive fibrin deposition. One novel therapeutic agent, recombinant-human-activated protein C, has been shown to reduce mortality in patients with sepsis (with or without DIC) and is recommended in sepsis patients at high risk of death. Heparin should be withheld during administration of this drug.[3]

A life-threatening hemorrhagic diathesis consistent with DIC is present in 80–90% of APL patients at presentation and may be exacerbated by chemotherapy. It tends to be particularly severe in the microgranular variant of APL. Laboratory manifestations typical of DIC are typically present: low platelets, increased PT and aPTT, elevated fibrinogen degradation products (FDP), and decreased fibrinogen. Similar to other DIC conditions, there is laboratory evidence of both activation of the coagulation system and increase in fibrinolysis. One feature that distinguishes the coagulopathy of APL from typical DIC is the maintenance of relatively normal levels of the coagulation inhibitors antithrombin and protein C. The DIC is attributed to the spontaneous or chemotherapy associated release of a tissue factor with procoagulant activity present in the granules of the leukemic promyelocytes. In addition there is proteolysis due to release from the leukemic cells of lysosomal neutrophilic enzymes, including leukocyte elastase, which are able to cleave fibrinogen. APL cells also express high levels of annexin II, which is a fibrinolytic protein that increases the efficiency of plasmin formation. However, the role of primary fibrinolysis in the pathogenesis of DIC in APL is uncertain.[2]

Prior to the introduction of ATRA for the management of APL patients, fatal hemorrhage was a major cause of morbidity and mortality, thus contributing to failure of remission induction. In one large retrospective study the rate of early hemorrhagic deaths was about 10% and this was not affected by treatment with either heparin or antifibrinolytic drugs.[9] ATRA rapidly reverses the coagulopathy in most patients with APL, so ATRA therapy should be started as soon as possible. Some have suggested that ATRA should be given as soon as APL is suspected, instead of waiting for genetic confirmation of diagnosis, because a fraction of patients develop fatal hemorrhages during the diagnostic evaluation before beginning antileukemic therapy or during the first days of induction. In a 2001 multicenter study of patients receiving ATRA for induction therapy, mortality due to early hemorrhage was about 5%.[11] Therefore, rapid institution of supportive measures to reverse the coagulopathy may lower the risk of life-threatening hemorrhages in these patients. Treatment should be based on liberal transfusion of fresh-frozen plasma, fibrinogen, or both, as well as on aggressive platelet support to maintain the fibrinogen level above 150 mg/L and the platelet counts above $30-50 \times 10^9$/L until clinical signs of coagulopathy have disappeared.[13]

References

1. CHOU, W. C. AND DANG, C. V: Acute promyelocytic leukemia: Recent advances in therapy and molecular basis of response to arsenic therapies. *Curr. Opin. Hematol. 12*:1–6, 2005.

2. FALANGA, A. AND RICKLES, F. R.: Pathogenesis and management of the bleeding diathesis in acute promyelocytic leukemia. *Best Pract. Res. Clin. Haematol. 16*:463–82, 2003.

3. FOURRIER, F.: Recombinant human activated protein C in the treatment of severe sepsis: An evidence-based review. *Crit. Care Med. 32*:S534–41, 2004.

4. GRIMWADE, D. AND LO COCO, F.: Acute promyelocytic leukemia: A model for the role of molecular diagnosis and residual disease monitoring in directing treatment approach in acute myeloid leukemia. *Leukemia 16*:1959–73, 2002.

5. HOFFMAN, R. ET AL.: *Hematology, Basic Principles and Practice*, Elsevier, Churchill Livingstone, 2005.

6. JAFFE, E. S. ET AL.: *Pathology and Genetics of Tumours of the Haematopoietic and Lymphoid Tissues. World Health Organization Classification of Tumours*, P. KLEIHUES AND L. H. SOBIN, eds., IARC Press, Lyon, France, 2001.

7. LARSON, R. S. AND TALLMAN, M. S.: Retinoic acid syndrome: Manifestations, pathogenesis, and treatment. *Best Pract. Res. Clin. Haematol. 16*:453–61, 2003.

8. LEVI, M.: Current understanding of disseminated intravascular coagulation. *Br. J. Hematol. 124*:567–76, 2004.

9. RODEGHIERO, F. ET AL.: Early deaths and antihemorrhagic treatments in acute promyelocytic leukemia. A GIMEMA retrospective study in 268 consecutive patients. *Blood 75*:2112–7, 1990.

10. SALOMONI, P. AND PANDOLFI, P. P.: The role of PML in tumor suppression. *Cell 108*:165–70, 2002.

11. SANZ, M. A. ET AL.: Risk-adapted treatment of acute promyelocytic leukemia with all-trans-retinoic acid and anthracycline monochemotherapy: A multicenter study by the PETHEMA group. *Blood 103*:1237–43, 2004.

12. SANZ, M. A., MARTIN, G., AND LO COCO, F.: Choice of chemotherapy in induction, consolidation and maintenance in acute promyelocytic leukemia. *Best Pract. Res. Clin. Haematol. 16*:433–51, 2003.

13. SANZ, M. A., TALLMAN, M. S., AND LO-COCO, F.: Tricks of the trade for the appropriate management of newly diagnosed acute promyelocytic leukemia. *Blood 105*:3019–25, 2005.

14. TALLMAN, M. S. ET AL.: All-trans retinoic acid in acute promyelocytic leukemia: long-term outcome and prognostic factor analysis from the North American Intergroup protocol. *Blood 100*:4298–302, 2002.

15. WADA, H.: Review: Disseminated intravascular coagulation. *Clin. Chim. Acta 344*:13–21, 2004.

16. ZELENT, A. ET AL.: Translocations of the RARalpha gene in acute promyelocytic leukemia. *Oncogene 20*:7186–203, 2001.

Case 54

A Middle-Aged Man with Chronic Foot Ulcer

Brian Watson

A 60-year-old man presented to the emergency room with complaints of malaise, fatigue, and a nonhealing foot ulcer. Three weeks earlier, he had been diagnosed with pyoderma and prescribed prednisone 80 mg/day and cyclosporine 500 mg/day. His past medical history was significant for pyoderma gangrenosa, a severe form of pyoderma associated with chronic disease that occurs on the trunk, diagnosed 3 years prior to presentation. He also had a history of steroid-induced hypertension and diabetes.

The patient was mildly tachycardic, afebrile, and normotensive. His physical exam was notable for a large, erythematous ulcer involving the dorsum and plantar surfaces of his right foot, and two separate (3 cm in maximum dimension) raised, erythematous lesions on his left scapula and midback. No lymphadenopathy was identified.

The following laboratory results were obtained:

Analyte	Value, Conventional Units	Reference Interval, Conventional Units	Value, SI Units	Reference Interval, SI Units
WBC	$26.9 \times 10^3/\mu L$	3.8–9.8	$26.9 \times 10^9/L$	3.8–9.8
Neutrophils, absolute	$22.2 \times 10^3/\mu L$	1.8–6.6	$22.2 \times 10^9/L$	1.8–6.6
Lymphocytes, absolute	$2.9 \times 10^3/\mu L$	1.2–3.3	$2.9 \times 10^9/L$	1.2–3.3
Monocytes, absolute	$1.6 \times 10^3/\mu L$	0.2–1.2	$1.6 \times 10^9/L$	0.2–1.2
Eosinophils, absolute	$0.2 \times 10^3/\mu L$	0.0–0.5	$0.2 \times 10^9/L$	0.0–0.5
Basophils, absolute	$0.1 \times 10^3/\mu L$	0.0–0.2	$0.1 \times 10^9/L$	0.0–0.2
Hemoglobin	14.6 g/dL	13.8–17.2	146 g/L	138–172
Hematocrit	43%	41–51	0.43 volume	0.41–0.51
Platelets	$753 \times 10^3/\mu L$	140–440	$753 \times 10^9/L$	140–440
ESR	90 mm/h	0–20	Same	

Initial management focused on local wound care and oral antibiotics to treat a possible cellulitis. Over the next month, the patient underwent multiple skin biopsies to determine the etiology of his chronic foot ulcer. While some of the biopsies showed a nonspecific

Tietz's Applied Laboratory Medicine, Second Edition. Edited by Mitchell G. Scott, Ann M. Gronowski, and Charles S. Eby
Copyright © 2007 John Wiley & Sons, Inc.

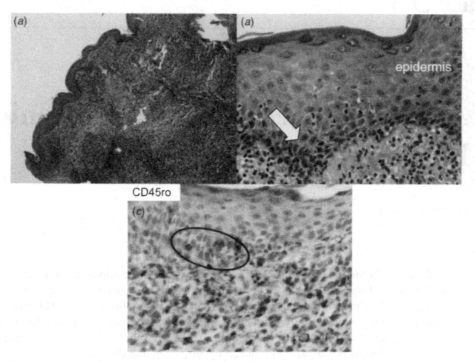

Figure 54.1 Medium (a) and high power (b) photomicrographs of tissue from the right arm show a lymphohistocytic dermal infiltrate with epidermotropic component (arrow). The lymphocytes are small and round, lacking the classic features of a cutaneous T-cell lymphoma. A CD45ro stain (c) highlights T cells constituting about half of the dermal infiltrate with some expression seen in lymphocytes in the epidermis (circle).

atypical, mixed inflammatory infiltrate; others showed atypical lymphocytic infiltrates with lymphocytes extending into the epidermis (epidermaltropic component; Fig. 54.1). Immunohistochemical studies to determine if these processes represented a hematopoietic malignancy were inconclusive. While review of multiple specimens by multiple pathologists favored a reactive process, the possibility of a primary cutaneous T-cell lymphoma could not be excluded.

Differential Diagnosis

Clinically, lesions suspicious for a T-cell lymphoma overlap with a wide variety of other malignant and benign lesions. Presenting first usually as plaques or patches, more advanced disease can present as tumor nodules. The plaque stage has wide overlap with infectious lesions and inflammatory processes such as atopic dermatitis, contact dermatitis, fungal infection, psoriasis, and parapsoriasis. While the presence of tumors is more associated with malignancy, other benign conditions such as pseudolymphoma and lymphomatoid papulosis are also in the differential. Histologically, there is a great overlap between reactive lymphoid infiltrates and malignant cutaneous lymphomas as both benign and malignant lesions can demonstrate dense lymphocytic infiltrates with cytologic atypia that spread from the dermis to involve the epidermis. To determine the presence of a clonal process, the two most suspicious specimens were evaluated for T-cell receptor

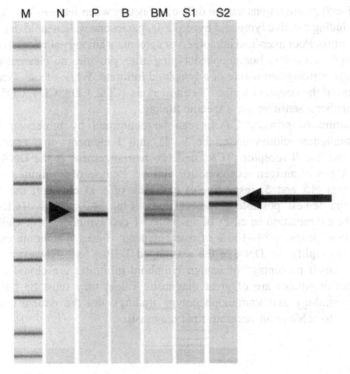

M   N   P   B   BM   S1   S2

Figure 54.2   A representative computer generated gel of TCR-γ rearrangements of the patient's skin (S1—right calf; S2—left scapula) and bone marrow (BM). The large arrow indicates clonal rearrangement of both TCR-γ genes in a lymphocyte clone detected in the patient's skin samples and an oligoclonal background in a bone marrow sample. The arrowhead indicates a monoclonal product in the positive control (P). Polyclonal products are seen in the negative control lane (N). The marker lane shows the sizing ladder (M). The amplification control lane shows no products (B).

gamma (TCR-γ) rearrangement status, and both samples showed the same clonal rearrangement (Fig. 54.2), leading to the diagnosis of a cutaneous T-cell lymphoma (CTCL).

Incidence and General Characteristics

Following the gastrointestinal tract, the skin is the second most common site of extranodal non-Hodgkin lymphomas (NHLs). Overall, the incidence of primary cutaneous NHLs is 1 : 100,000. Mycosis fungodies, the most common type of primary cutaneous NHL, accounts for approximately 0.5% of hematopoietic neoplasms. While T-cell lymphomas represent the majority of primary cutaneous lymphomas, the diagnosis is often difficult, requiring multiple biopsies and complex immunophenotypic and molecular diagnostic tests. Further complicating the diagnosis is the heterogeneity of entities that fall into the CTCL category. While mycosis fungoides is the most common type, anaplastic large cell lymphoma and CD30-negative peripheral T-cell lymphomas are also included in this category. The microscopic features of CTCLs are varied. Mycosis fungoides consists of small epidermal collections of lymphocytes with folded, "cleaved" nuclei, and Pautrier microabscesses. Anaplastic large T-cell lymphoma presents with large pleomorphic cells with effacement of the dermal and epidermal architecture. When the histology is classic, a diagnosis of CTCL is easier.

However, clonal T-cell proliferations can be difficult to detect when features overlap with benign entities, including reactive lymphoid hyperplasia, parapsorasis, lichenoid dermatitis, and spongotic dermatitis. Poor inter- and intraobserver agreement among pathologists further complicates diagnostic accuracy. Immunophenotyping often provides no clearcut answer regarding the benign or malignant nature of a lymphoid infiltrate. While clonal T-cell disorders may lose one of the common surface T-cell markers (CD2, CD3, CD4, CD5, CD7, and CD8), this is neither a sensitive nor a specific finding.

The clonal nature of primary CTCLs can be confirmed by molecular testing methods. When malignant clones arise, the V, D, and J elements that encode the peptide chains of the T-cell receptor (TCR) undergo rearrangement at the DNA level. T Cells have two types of antigen receptors: $\alpha\beta$ and $\gamma\delta$. Beause of its limited number of V and J elements (15 and 5, respectively) and lack of a D element, the TCR-γ family produces the fewest possible recombinations (Fig. 54.3). Thus, TCR-γ has become a target for examination in cases of suspected T-cell lymphomas. T-Cell clonality can be identified in about 79–100% of true cutaneous T-cell lymphoma cases by primers designed to amplify the DNA of the rearranged TCR-γ loci. However, studies have shown that a small percentage of benign lymphoid infiltrates are clonal as well. Thus, while molecular studies are of great diagnostic value, they must be combined with skin biopsy histology and immunophenotype findings and the patient's clinical features and history to achieve an accurate final diagnosis.

Treatment

The treatment of CTCLs is governed by the stage of the disease. Early stages of mycosis fungoides, with limited involvement of the skin (patch–plaque stage), are treated with psoralens

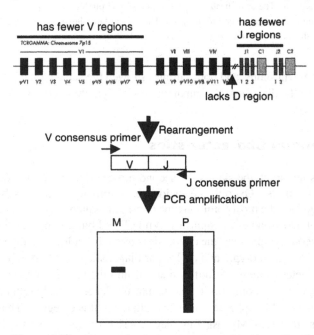

Figure 54.3   Since TCR-γ lacks a D region and has fewer V and J regions than other members of the TCR family, it is an ideal target for PCR amplification due to the production of fewer products with V and J region consensus primers. Monoclonal processes will produce a single dominant product (M), where as polyclonal process usually produces multiple products (P).

and ultraviolet light A (PUVA therapy), and topical agents: steroids, nitrogen mustard, BCNU, and spot electron-beam radiation. Systemic therapy is indicated for bulky skin tumors and erythroderma due to diffuse skin involvement, with or without circulating Sezary cells (leukemic malignant T cells). Treatment options include immunomodulatory regimens such as interferons, interleukin 12, and cytotoxic fusion antibodies, total skin electron beam therapy, single-agent chemotherapy with purine analogs such as fludarabine or methotrexate, and retinoids such as bexarotene. When the leukemic phase of mycosis fungoides occurs (Sezary syndrome), extracorporal photopheresis is another immunomodulatory treatment option. Patients undergo leukopheresis to temporarily isolate circulating leukocytes. Following exposure to psoralen and UVA radiation to produce DNA damage, the leukocytes are reinfused. In advanced disease, lymph node and visceral involvement by malignant lymphocytes is observed and treatment includes skin directed therapies with the addition of combination cytoxic chemotherapy. The other less common CTCLs are usually treated with multiagent chemotherapy similar to those used in treating advanced stages of mycosis fungoides/Sezary syndrome, including doxorubicin. Survival decreases as the disease becomes more advanced. Patients with limited skin disease have a life expectancy that is similar to age-, gender-, and race-matched controls. Ten-year survivals for more advanced stages of mycosis fungoides range within ∼20–40%.

Additional Reading

ABD-EL-BAKI, J., STEFANATO, C. M., KOH, H. K., DEMIERRE, M. F., AND FOSS, F. M.: Early detection of cutaneous lymphoma. *Oncology* (Williston Park) *12*:1521–30, 1998.

BRADY, S. P., MAGRO, C. M., DIAZ-CANO, S. J., AND WOLFE, H. J.: Analysis of clonality of atypical cutaneous lymphoid infiltrates associated with drug therapy by PCR/DGGE. *Hum. Pathol.* *30*:130–6, 1999.

BURG, G., ZWINGERS, T., STAEGEMEIR, E., AND SANTUCCI, M.: Interrater and intrarater variabilities in the evaluation of cutaneous lymphoproliferative T-cell infiltrates. EORTC-Cutaneous Lymphoma Project Group. *Dermatol. Clin.* *12*:311–4, 1994.

FOSS, F.: Lymphoma and experimental therapies. *Curr. Opin. Oncol.* *16*:421–8, 2004.

GUTZMER, R., MOMMERT, S., KIEHL, P., WITTMANN, M., KAPP, A., AND WERFEL, T.: Detection of clonal T-cell receptor gamma gene rearrangements in cutaneous T-cell lymphoma by LightCycler-polymerase chain reaction. *J. Invest. Dermatol.* *116*:926–32, 2001.

HODGES, E., KRISHNA, M. T., PICKARD, C., AND SMITH, J. L.: Diagnostic role of tests for T-cell receptor (TCR) genes. *J. Clin. Pathol.* *56*:1–11, 2003.

HOLM, N., FLAIG, M. J., YAZDI, A. S., AND SANDER, C. A.: The value of molecular analysis by PCR in the diagnosis of cutaneous lymphocytic infiltrates. *J. Cutan. Pathol.* *29*:447–52, 2002.

MURPHY, M., FULLEN, D., AND CARLSON, J. A.: Low CD7 expression in benign and malignant cutaneous lymphocytic infiltrates: Experience with an antibody reactive with paraffin-embedded tissue. *Am. J. Dermatopathol.* *24*:6–16, 2002.

ORMSBY, A., BERGFELD, W. F., TUBBS, R. R., AND HIS, E. D.: Evaluation of a new paraffin-reactive CD7 T-cell deletion marker and a polymerase chain reaction-based T-cell receptor gene rearrangement assay: implications for diagnosis of mycosis fungoides in community clinical practice. *J. Am. Acad. Dermatol.* *45*:405–13, 2001.

SANTUCCI, M., BURG, G., AND FELLER, A. C.: Interrater and intrarater reliability of histologic criteria in early cutaneous T-cell lymphoma. An EORTC Cutaneous Lymphoma Project Group study. *Dermatol. Clin.* *12*:323–7, 1994.

SIGNORETTI, S., MURPHY, M., CANGI, M. G., PUDDU, P., KADIN, M. E., AND LODA, M.: Detection of clonal T-cell receptor gamma gene rearrangements in paraffin-embedded tissue by polymerase chain reaction and nonradioactive single-strand conformational polymorphism analysis. *Am. J. Pathol.*, *154*:67–75, 1999.

WILLEMZE, R., JAFFE, E. S., BURG, G., LORENZO, C. ET AL.: WHO-EORTC classification for subcutaneous lymphomas. *Blood 105*:3768–85, 2005.

YAZDI, A. S., MEDEIROS, L. J., PUCHTA, U., THALLER, E., FLAIG, M. J., AND SANDER, C. A.: Improved detection of clonality in cutaneous T-cell lymphomas using laser capture microdissection. *J. Cutan. Pathol.* *30*:486–91, 2003.

Case 55

A Man with Progressive Effort Intolerance and Splenomegaly

Mrinal M. Patnaik and Ayalew Tefferi

A 56-year-old male presented to the clinic with complaints of progressive effort intolerance, which he noted over the last 6 months, associated with early satiety and sensation of fullness in the left upper quadrant of his abdomen.

A clinical exam revealed the presence of pallor, sternal tenderness, and massive splenomegaly. The spleen was firm and was felt 8 cm below the left costal margin. The liver span was increased up to 16 cm and the liver was felt 2 cm below the right costal margin. He did not have any petechiae, purpura, or ecchymosis.

Laboratory values obtained from him were as follows:

Analyte	Value, Conventional Units	Reference Interval, Conventional Units	Value, SI Units	Reference Interval, SI Units
Hemoglobin	9.5 g/dL	13.1–17.2	95 g/L	131–172
Hematocrit	30%	40–50	0.30 volume	0.40–0.50
WBC	$170 \times 10^3/\mu L$	4.5–11.0	$170 \times 10^9/L$	4.5–11.0
Platelet count	$850 \times 10^3/\mu L$	150–400	$850 \times 10^9/L$	150–400
Reticulocyte %	1.5%	0.5–2.0%	0.015 fraction	0.005–0.020
Differential count				
Blast cells	$1.7 \times 10^3/\mu L$	0	$1.7 \times 10^9/L$	0
Promyelocytes	$8.5 \times 10^3/\mu L$	0	$8.5 \times 10^9/L$	0
Neutrophil myelocytes	$35.7 \times 10^3/\mu L$	0	$35.7 \times 10^9/L$	0
Metamyeocytes	$153 \times 10^3/\mu L$	0	$153 \times 10^9/L$	0
Neutrophils	$85 \times 10^3/\mu L$	1.5–6.7	$85 \times 10^9/L$	1.5–6.7
Eosinophils	$6.8 \times 10^3/\mu L$	0–$0.7 \times 10^3/\mu L$	$6.8 \times 10^9/L$	0–0.7
Basophils	$10.2 \times 10^3/\mu L$	0–0.2	$10.2 \times 10^9/L$	0–0.2
Monocytes	$3.4 \times 10^3/\mu L$	0.2–0.9	$3.4 \times 10^9/L$	0.2–0.9
Lymphocytes	$3.4 \times 10^3/\mu L$	1.5–4.0	$3.4 \times 10^9/L$	1.5–4.0

Tietz's Applied Laboratory Medicine, Second Edition. Edited by Mitchell G. Scott, Ann M. Gronowski, and Charles S. Eby
Copyright © 2007 John Wiley & Sons, Inc.

Differential Diagnosis

From the investigations discussed above, it is seen that the patient has an anomaly involving proliferation of at least two cell lines, the myeloid cells and the platelets. This is most likely to be due to a myeloproliferative disorder (Table 55.1). It is imperative to first rule out a leukemoid reaction, which is a white cell response to various infectious, stressors, and inflammatory states. In a leukemoid reaction there is generally an identifiable

Table 55.1   Myeloid Malignant Disorders

Acute—acute myeloid leukemia
Chronic—chronic myeloid disorders
   Philadelphia chromosome–positive—CML
   Philadelphia chromosome–negative
Myeloproliferative disorders
   Classical
      Polycythemia rubra vera
      Essential thrombocytosis
      Agnogenic myeloid metaplasia with myelofibrosis
   Atypical
      Chronic myelomonocytic leukemia
      Juvenile myelomonocytic leukemia
      Chronic neutrophilic leukemia
      Chronic eosinophilic leukemia
      Hypereosinophilic syndrome
      Chronic basophilic leukemia
      Systemic mastocytosis
      Unclassified myeloproliferative disorders
Myelodysplastic disorders

Table 55.2   Causes of Thrombocytosis

Reactive
   Acute blood loss, acute infections, and acute inflammatory states
   Iron deficiency anemia
   Hemolytic anemia
   Asplenia, and after splenectomy
   Cancers
   Chronic inflammatory states: connective tissue disorders, temporal arteritis,
      inflammatory bowel disease, tuberculosis
   Drugs: vincristine, ATRA (all-trans retinoic acid), cytokines, and growth
      factors
Clonal
   Polycythemia rubra vera
   CML
   Essential thrombocytosis
   Agnogenic myeloid metaplasia with myelofibrosis
   Atypical myeloproliferative disorders

Table 55.3   Massive Splenomegaly with Anemia

Infections
   Chronic malaria
   Kala azar
   Infectious mononucleosis
Portal hypertension
Infiltrative disorders
   Gaucher's disease
   Niemann–Pick disease
Hematological causes
   Myeloproliferative disease
   Amyloidosis
   Hodgkin's disease
   Hairy cell leukemia
   Waldentrom's macroglobulinemia

precipitating factor, which can be temporally associated with a rise in the white count. The white cells are predominantly segmented and band neutrophils, and the total count rarely exceeds $50,000 \times 10^3/\mu L$. There are no blasts seen on the peripheral smear, although immature forms such as promyelocytes and metamyleocytes may be seen in small numbers. The peripheral smear is also useful in identifying toxic granules and leukocyte Dohle bodies, which represent the leukocytes' response to inflammation. Since most of these cells in the leukemoid reaction are mature, the leukocyte alkaline phosphatase enzyme activity, determined by scoring enzymatic activity after applying substrate on a peripheral blood smear, within 0–4+, will be elevated. The elevated platelet count may be reactive or a marker of a clonal myeloproliferative disorder (Table 55.1).

It is also important to consider the differential diagnosis of the elevated platelet count in the context of the case (Table 55.2).

This 56-year-old male presented with features of progressive anemia, along with massive splenomegaly. The differential diagnosis of massive splenomegaly with anemia is shown in Table 55.3.

The patient did not have a history of travel or exposure to endemic regions to acquire malaria. On a clinical exam there were no stigma of chronic liver disease like spider nevi, frontal balding, gynecomastia, caput medusa, or loss of axillary and pubic hair to support advanced liver disease. The infiltrative disorders listed above are rare, and are more commonly seen in pediatric populations. This patient was thought to have symptoms and signs that were hematological in origin.

Disease

In order to confirm the diagnosis of chronic myeloid leukemia, the following tests were done and the results were as follows.

Test	Result	Interpretation
Bone marrow aspiration and biopsy	Increased cellularity involving all three cell lines—the granulocytes, megakaryocytes, and erythrocytes; morphologically the cells had a normal maturation	The bone marrow points to a clonal proliferation involving all three cell lines, typical of a myeloproliferative disorder

Test	Result	Interpretation
Cytogenic analysis	26/26 karyotypes showed a shortened chromosome 22, due to a t(9 : 22) translocation	This is the Philadelphia chromosome, a very specific cytogenic anomaly for the diagnosis of CML
Leukocyte Alkaline Phosphatase (LAP)	6 (normal range 40–130)	Helps differentiate a leukemoid reaction and polycythemia rubra vera (PRV) from CML
Cyanocobalamin	1100 pg/mL (normal range 100–700)	Marked elevations are seen in PRV and CML
Uric acid	10 mg/dL (normal range 4.5–8.2)	Notable prior to therapy as urate is an important component of the tumor lysis syndrome

Chronic Myelogenous Leukemia

CML is a clonal myeloproliferative disorder characterized by the presence of anemia, splenomegaly, and a typical left shift granulocytosis. CML was probably the first form of leukemia to be recognized as a distinct clinical entity. In 1960 Nowell and Hungerford detected a consistent chromosomal abnormality in patients with CML, later named *Philadelphia* (Ph) *chromosome*, due to a reciprocal translocation between chromosomes 9 and 22 designated as t(9;22) (q34;q11). The Ph chromosome translocation produces a fusion protein, BCR-ABL, which is responsible for much of the clinical and pathological features of CML. CML evolves through three phases, the chronic phase (average 4–6 years), accelerated phase, and blast crisis. The duration of the chronic phase is variable and influenced by timing and type of treatment and additional cytogenetic abnormalities. The blast phase disease resembles acute leukemia. Its phenotype is myeloblastic in 70–80% of patients and lymphoblastic in 20–30%.

Cytogenetics of CML

The cytogenetic hallmark of CML is the Philadelphia chromosome, and when it is acquired by a pleuripotent, hematopoetic stem cell, expression of the BCR-ABL fusion gene/ protein confers a proliferative advantage. The mechanism behind the survival advantage is not well defined but is believed to be a combination of a constitutive expression of growth factors like G-CSF and IL-3 by the leukemia progenitor cells along with a defective apoptotic response to stimuli, that should have led to physiological cell death. The Ph-positive clone proliferates and displaces normal hematopoesis and is susceptible to additional genetic aberrations, which is responsible for the diseases evolving from chronic phase to accelerated phase and blast crisis. The advent of genetic microarray techniques that permit comparisons of gene expression profiles should help identify the genes involved in blastic transformation. The BCR-ABL fusion gene translates into a 210-kDa oncoprotein referred to as $p210^{BCR-ABL}$. Other variant breakpoints and fusions can give rise to full-length, functionally oncogenic proteins $p190^{BCR-ABL}$ and $p230^{BCR-ABL}$.

The fusion protein results in unregulated activity of BCR tyrosine kinase by the ABL gene. This tyrosine kinase then acts by deregulating cellular proliferation, decreasing the adherence of leukemic cells to the bone marrow stroma, and decreasing apoptosis. The ABL protein is found normally in both the nucleus and the cytoplasm, and nuclear ABL is a proapoptotic protein. However, BCR-ABL is unable to enter the nucleus, probably because of its constitutively activated tyrosine kinase.

Genetic Diagnosis of CML

Conventional cytogenetics involves the light microscopic examination of chromosomes in order to identify either numerical or structural abnormalities. Cells are induced to divide and arrested at the metaphase stage of mitosis. Giemsa staining (also termed "G banding") creates bright and dark bands of varying length and brightness to permit identification of chromosome pairs and large deletions, translocations, and partial or complete chromosome duplications.

In CML, standard cytogenetics reveals a balanced reciprocal translocation between chromosomes 9 and 22 that results in a shortened chromosome 22 (Ph chromosome). Standard cytogenetics in CML is usually performed on bone marrow samples. Test results are routinely available in 2–3 weeks, but preliminary results can be requested and may be available in 3 days.

Fluorescence in situ hybridization (FISH) uses fluorochrome-labeled DNA probes that are hybridized to unstained interphase or metaphase nuclei on a microscopic glass slide. Hybridization is accomplished by first denaturing genomic DNA (i.e., converting it from a double- to single-strand conformation) and then incubating it with the specific FISH probes. The FISH signals are detected by fluorescence microscopy. FISH probes are prepared to be complementary to repetitive DNA sequences usually situated at the centromere or specific loci to detect structural chromosomal lesions, including translocations (e.g., the *Bcr/Abl* fusion sequence in CML), deletions (e.g., 5q in acute leukemia and other myeloid disorders), and gene amplification (e.g., *HER2* oncogene in breast cancer). FISH may be applied to a standard cytogenetic chromosome preparation as well as unstained glass slides of fresh or fixed specimens from blood, bone marrow, or other tissue, and sensitivity ranges within 0.1–1%. In CML, interphase FISH is performed with a green probe for *bcr* and a red probe for *abl*. A yellow signal denotes *Bcr/Abl* fusion.

Reverse transcriptase polymerase chain reaction (RT-PCR) is currently the most sensitive technique for detecting a CML clone. In RT-PCR, disease-specific mRNA is first converted to cDNA and subsequently subjected to a standard PCR reaction. RT-PCR can either be qualitative or quantitative. In qualitative RT-PCR the amplified product is assessed by gel electrophoresis after the entire PCR reaction (30 cycles) is completed. Assay specificity as well as sensitivity in RT-PCR is further enhanced by the use of nested primers (nested RT-PCR). In nested RT-PCR, two pairs of PCR primers are used for the same target molecule. The first pair of primers amplifies the target in the standard manner, and then the second pair of primers (nested primers) binds within the amplified PCR product to produce a second PCR product that will be shorter than the first one. Quantitative real-time RT-PCR is based on measurement of fluorescence emission during the PCR reaction. Turnaround time for real-time RT-PCR is measured in hours, and test sensitivity is estimated at 0.001% ($1 : 10^5$).

Standard cytogenetic studies of the bone marrow disclose the Ph chromosome, t(9;22)(q34;q11), in approximately 95% of CML patients at diagnosis. In the remaining 5%, the Ph chromosome might be either masked (submicroscopic *Bcr/Abl* fusion) or part of a complex/variant chromosomal translocation (the involvements of other chromosome breakpoints in addition to 9q34 and 22q11). These latter "Ph-negative" as well as the Ph-positive cases are readily identified by either FISH or RT-PCR, thus giving the molecular methods superior sensitivity. However, neither overall survival nor treatment response appears to be influenced by variant versus typical Ph chromosome translocations.

The molecular assays used to detect the Ph translocation do not require the presence of dividing cells and can be performed on both the peripheral blood and bone marrow specimens with equivalent results. However, only standard cytogenetics enables the detection of additional cytogenetic abnormalities (e.g., trisomy 8, isochromosome 17q), which, when found at the time of diagnosis, might predict a shorter duration of chronic-phase disease. Furthermore, baseline karyotype information is important in interpreting subsequent clonal evolution, and cytogenetic monitoring of treatment effect. Therefore, standard cytogenetic studies should be considered at the time of CML diagnosis in all patients.

Detection of the Ph chromosome, or its molecular equivalent, within the context of a chronic myeloid disorder is diagnostic of CML regardless of the presentation phenotype, which can sometimes mimic either essential thrombocytosis or myelofibrosis with myeloid metaplasia. On the other hand, the absence of the Ph chromosome does not exclude CML, and if the clinical scenario dictates, FISH or PCR for *Bcr/Abl* should be performed.

Prognosis

Various staging systems have been developed in order to prognosticate CML. Two commonly used indices in CML are the Sokal index and the Euro score. Clinical variables are age, platelet count, spleen size, and percentage of blood blasts, basophils, and eosinophils. The Sokal index was derived from data for patients treated with busulfan and hydroxyurea, and the Euro score, from patients treated with interferon-α, respectively. It is important to note that these scores are limited in their ability to predict survival in any particular patient.

Therapy for CML

Allogeneic stem cell transplantation is the only curative therapy available for CML, and is the standard treatment for patients less than 40 years of age who have an HLA identical sibling. In general, transplant outcome is best in chronic-phase ($\approx$60% long-term remissions) disease as opposed to either accelerated ($\approx$30%) or blast-phase disease ($\approx$14%). In a long-term study of 373 patients with CML who were transplanted with chronic phase disease, the 8-year leukemia-free survival was 47% (69 cases). Approximately 50% of the patients experienced both acute and chronic graft-versus-host disease (GVHD). Transplant-related mortality was 41%. Furthermore, quality of life is generally compromised in long-term survivors of AHSCT (allogeneic hematopoetic stem cell transplantation), and there is a constant risk of relapse even after the first decade of transplant. Several factors modify transplant outcome in AHSCT. In general, younger age, timing of transplant in the first year of diagnosis, the use of unmanipulated stem cells (i.e., non-T-cell-depleted), and the use of matched sibling donors (as opposed to unrelated donors) significantly improves AHSCT outcome. The use of nonmyeloablative stem cell transplants has increased the response rates in this age group of patients based on a two-pronged approach to eradication of the leukemic clone: milder cytotoxic conditioning regimine preceding stem cell infusion followed by graft-versus-leukemia effect.

Before the advent of the oral drug imatinib, patients with CML, who were not transplant candidates or were awaiting transplant, were treated with hydroxyurea or interferon-α (INF-α) to control chronic phase myeloid proliferation. Hydroxyurea is an oral ribonucleotide reductase inhibitor and is well tolerated. INF-α requires subcutaneous administration, causes substantial side effects, but produces major and complete cytogenic response in chronic phase patients of 25% and 10%, respectively, and extends survival 1–2 years compared to hydroxyurea. CML in blast phase is resistant to both hydroxyurea and INF-α. Multiagent chemotherapy induces responses in only about 20% of patients with myeloblastic transformation and 50% of those with lymphoblastic transformation, but responders relapse quickly and die of progressive disease.

In 1996, clinical trials were started with imatinib; an oral tyrosine kinase inhibitor, for treatment of CML refractory to INF-α. Imatinib induced complete hematological response in more than 95% and major cytogenetic responses in 40–50% of patients. As a result, imatinib (brand name Gleevec) has become a mainstay in treatment for patients diagnosed with CML who are not candidates for allogeneic stem cell transplantation. Imatinib responses are superior in chronic-phase versus advanced-phase disease as well as in low-risk versus high-risk chronic-phase patients. One approach to management of a patient with newly diagnosed CML would be a trial of imatinib for 6–9 months, and in those who do not achieve a near-complete or complete cytogenic response, allogeneic stem cell transplantation should be offered, provided the estimated transplantation related mortality is low.

Regardless of the impressive results outlined above for imatinib, it is unlikely to be curative, considering increasing reports of resistance. Most relapses are due to reactivation of the BCR/ABL tyrosine kinase as a result of point mutations scattered throughout the ABL kinase gene or amplification of BCR/ABL at the genomic or transcript level. After the discovery of imatinib for the treatment of CML, other candidate molecules for targeted therapy in CML have been rapidly emerging. These include (1) SRC tyrosine-kinase inhibitors, (2) adaphostin—ABL tryphostin, (3) geldanamycin—inhibitor of BCR/ABL chaperone protein, (4) farnesyltransferase inhibitors, and (5) leptomycin B—blocks the nuclear export of BCR/ABL once it is able to enter the nucleus, and is used in conjunction with imatinib.

Additional Reading

BARRETT, A. J.: Allogeneic stem cell transplantation for chronic myeloid leukemia. *Semin. Hematol.* 40:59–71, 2003.

COX, M. C., MAFFEI, L., BUFFOLINO, S. ET AL.: A comparative analysis of FISH, RT-PCR, and cytogenetics for the diagnosis of bcr-abl-positive leukemias. *Am. J. Clin. Pathol.* 109:24–31, 1998.

DRUKER, B. J., TALPAZ, M., RESTA, D. J. ET AL.: Efficacy and safety of a specific inhibitor of the BCR-ABL tyrosine kinase in chronic myeloid leukemia. *N. Engl. J. Med.* 344:1031–37, 2001.

GEARY, C. G.: The story of chronic myeloid leukemia. *Br. J. Haematol.* 110:2–11, 2000.

GUILHOT, F., CHASTANG, C., MICHALLET, M. ET AL.: Interferon alfa-2b combined with cytarabine versus interferon alone in chronic myelogenous leukemia. *N. Engl. J. Med.* 337:223–9, 1997.

KISS, T. L., ABDOLELL, M., JAMAL, N., MINDEN, M. D., LIPTON, J. H., AND MESSNER, H. A.: Long-term medical outcomes and quality-of-life assessment of patients with chronic myeloid leukemia followed at least 10 years after allogeneic bone marrow transplantation. *J. Clin. Oncol.* 20:2334–43, 2002.

SCHAEFER, A. J.: Thrombocytosis. *N. Engl. J. Med.* 350: 1211–19, 2004.

SPURBECK, J. L., ADAMS, S. A., STUPCA, P. J., AND DEWALD, G. W.: Primer on medical Genomics. Part XI: Visualizing human chromosomes. *Mayo Clin. Proc.* 79:58–75, 2004.

TEFFERI, A., WIEBEN, E. D., DEWALD, G. W., WHITEMAN, D. A., BERNARD, M. E., AND SPELSBERG, T. C.: Primer on medical genomics part II: Background principles and methods in molecular genetics. *Mayo Clin. Proc.* 77:785–808, 2002.

Case 56

A Man with Splenic Vein Thrombosis and Polycythemia

Karen Austin

A 55-year-old man presented to the emergency room with a 2–day history of frequent black, tarry stools. He also complained of persistent facial flushing and pruritis and occasional epistaxis during the previous 4 months. Past medical history was negative for hypertension, smoking, diabetes, and previous venous or arterial thrombosis. He also noted that he was a frequent blood donor, giving blood approximately 3–4 times per year for the last 30 years. Physical findings were notable for normal vital signs, plethora, a palpable spleen 5 cm below the left costal margin, and a strongly positive fecal occult blood test. An upper endoscopy revealed large gastric varices as the source of the bleeding. An abdominal CT scan demonstrated splenomegaly and possible splenic vein thrombosis. In addition to routine laboratory analytes, testing for inherited and acquired hypercoagulable risk factors was performed:

Analyte	Value, Conventional Units	Reference Interval, Conventional Units	Value, SI Units	Reference Interval, SI Units
WBC	$9.8 \times 10^3/\mu L$	$3.8–9.8 \times 10^3/\mu L$	$9.8 \times 10^9/L$	3.8–9.8
Hemoglobin	18.2 g/dL	13.8–17.2 g/dL	182 g/L	138–172
Hematocrit	57%	41–50%	0.57 volume	0.41–0.50
MCV	82.0 fL	80–90.6	Same	
Platelet count	$1200 \times 10^3/\mu L$	$140–440 \times 10^3/L$	$1200 \times 10^9/L$	$140–440 \times 10^9/L$
Antithrombin activity	99%	80–140	0.99 IU	0.80–1.40
Protein C activity	115%	60–132	1.15 IU	0.60–1.32
Protein S free antigen	72%	58–169	0.72 IU	0.58–1.69
Lupus anticoagulant	Negative	Negative	Same	

Tietz's Applied Laboratory Medicine, Second Edition. Edited by Mitchell G. Scott, Ann M. Gronowski, and Charles S. Eby
Copyright © 2007 John Wiley & Sons, Inc.

The patient was taken to the operating room for an open splenectomy. He was found to have splenomegaly with very large dilated gastric varices and short gastric vessels. Pathologic examination of the spleen revealed a fresh blood clot in the splenic hilum as well as congestive splenomegaly with marked expansion of the red pulp and dilated sinuses. He had an uncomplicated recovery and was referred to a hematologist for further evaluation of erythrocytosis and thrombocytosis.

Clinical Case Follow-up

Therapeutic phlebotomy was started and the target hematocrit of 45% was obtained. However, the platelet count remained $>1000 \times 10^3/L$. Hydroxyurea was begun with lowering of this platelet count to $<500 \times 10^3/L$. Pruritis resolved, and the patient has not experienced any thrombotic complications.

Differential Diagnosis of Erythrocytosis and Thrombocytosis

Causes of erythrocytosis and thrombocytosis are reviewed in Tables 56.1 and 56.2. Congenital erythrocytosis is extremely rare. Various mutations that disable the negative regulatory domain of the erythropoietin (EPO) receptor have been identified in autosomal dominantly inherited familial erythrocytosis. Congenital erythrocytosis may also result

Table 56.1   Classification of Erythrocytosis

Primary
  Congenital
    EPO receptor hypersensitivity
    Hypoxia sensor hypersensitivity
  Acquired
    Polycythemia vera
Secondary
  Appropriate (chronic tissue hypoxia)
    High altitude
    Pulmonary diseases
    Hypoventilation
    Cyanotic heart disease
    Smoking
    Hemoglobinopathies:
      High oxygen affinity
      Congenital methemoglobinemia
  Inappropriate
    Malignant tumors (renal, brain, liver, adrenal)
    Benign tumors (uterine fibroids, renal cysts)
    Androgen therapy
    Blood doping
Relative (normal red cell volume, decrease in plasma volume)
  Gaisbock syndrome

Table 56.2   Classification of Thrombocytosis

Primary
    Myeloproliferative disorders
        Chronic myeloid leukemia
        Essential thrombocytosis
        Polycythemia vera
        Myelofibrosis with myeloid metaplasia
Secondary
    Acute anemia (hemorrhage, hemolysis)
    Infections
    Inflammatory states
    Iron deficiency
    Postsplenectomy
    Malignancy

from gene mutations that alter cellular sensitivity to hypoxia leading to inappropriate secretion of erythropoietin (EPO).

Polycythemia vera (PV) is the only acquired, clonal, primary cause of erythrocytosis. However, before diagnosing PV, it is essential to rule out other causes for erythrocytosis, which includes both secondary and apparent increases in erythrocyte volume. Apparent polycythemia may result from acute situations in which the plasma volume is greatly depleted (i.e., involving severe dehydration, diarrhea, vomiting, aggressive diuresis, severe burns) and the hematocrit becomes elevated. In addition, some otherwise healthy people will have hematocrits that are slightly above the upper limit of the reference interval, due to decreased plasma volume rather than increased red cell volume (apparent erythrocytosis). This condition is poorly understood, but is associated with obesity, hypertension, and smoking, and does not warrant an evaluation for PV in the absence of other diagnostic features of the disease as discussed below.

Secondary polycythemia represents a true increase in erythrocyte volume. Causes include chronic exposure to carbon monoxide as is seen in long-term smokers, chronic hypoxia due to cardiopulmonary diseases, obstructive sleep apnea or living at high altitudes, erythropoietin (EPO)-producing tumors, and congenital high-oxygen-affinity hemoglobins, to name only a few.

Congenital thrombocytosis is also extremely rare. Typically, acquired thrombocytosis is a reaction to an underlying process (Table 56.2), even when the platelet count exceeds $1000 \times 10^3/\mu L$. If secondary causes are not identified, a diagnosis of a myeloproliferative disorder requires further evaluation to differentiate primary thrombocytosis from chronic myeloid leukemia, primary myelofibrosis with myeloid metaplasia, and polycythemia vera since the prognoses and treatments are different.

In the case presented above, there were no apparent secondary explanations for either the thrombocytosis or erythrocytosis, and the preliminary diagnosis was polycythemia vera. First, poycythemia was confirmed by performing red cell and plasma volume determinations in the nuclear medicine department. Venous blood was sterilely collected, and known quantities of ^{51}Cr, to label red cells, and ^{125}I-labeled albumin were added. Following reinfusion of the labeled whole blood, a second sample was collected and isotope concentration measured. Based on the degree of isotope dilution, red cell volume and plasma volume were calculated. The patient's red blood cell volume was 38.9 mL/kg (reference interval 18.9–31.6 mL/kg), and plasma volume was 36.6 mL/kg (reference interval 27.7–46.2 mL/kg), confirming an absolute erythrocyctosis. Findings from a bone marrow biopsy were typical for polycythemia vera: a hypercellular marrow, with expansion of myeloid, erythroid, and megakaryocytic lineages with abnormal clusters of megakaryocytes; no evidence of myelodysplasia; and no stainable iron. Finally, DNA testing revealed that the patient was positive for the JAK2-V617F mutation. This further supported the diagnosis of polycythemia vera in this patient.

Definition of Disease

Polycythemia vera (PV) is one of the chronic myeloproliferative disorders (MPD), a group that also includes essential thrombocytosis (ET), myelofibrosis with myeloid metaplasia (MMM), and chronic myelogenous leukemia (CML; see Case 55). The myeloproliferative disorders are characterized by various degrees of bone marrow hypercellularity and atypical megakaryocytic hyperplasia and clustering, and may or may not display splenomegaly, increased myeloid cells of any or all lineages in the peripheral blood, and clonal cytogenetic changes. The distinction between these disorders rests in the demonstration of clonal erythrocytosis in PV, significant bone marrow fibrosis in MMM, isolated thrombocytosis in ET, and bcr/abl translocation in CML. PV has an incidence of approximately 2.3 in 100,000 cases per year with a slight male predominance. The median age at diagnosis is approximately 60 years.

Most patients present with symptoms related to expanded blood volume and increased blood viscosity, the most serious of which are myocardial infarction, stroke, and venous thromboses, often involving the hepatic (Budd–Chiari syndrome), portal, or splenic veins. Some reports have indicated that thrombosis is the presenting symptom for PV in 10–50% of patients, as it was in this case, occurring in ≤40% of patients during the course of their disease, and is the leading cause of death. Almost counterintuitively, patients with PV may be at risk for hemorrhagic complications, most often occurring when platelet counts exceed 1,000,000/μL. This is thought to be due to multiple factors, including poor platelet aggregation in response to platelet agonists, such as ADP, epinephrine, and thrombin; low intraplatelet levels of serotonin; and acquired von Willebrand disease. Acquired von Willebrand disease is due to a decrease in large von Willebrand factor multimers secondary to adsorption onto the surface of the increased platelet mass and subsequent enhanced proteolysis.

Aside from thrombosis and bleeding, some patients with PV present with vague, nonspecific complaints including headache, dizziness, fatigue, blurry vision, and tinnitus. The majority of patients have splenomegaly, although it may or may not be palpable on physical exam. Other symptoms include erythromelalgia, which is a throbbing and burning sensation of the hands and feet, and severe generalized pruritis, often occurring after a warm bath or shower, which is related to histamine release from the increased number of circulating basophils.

Diagnosis

PV should be considered in any patient suspected of having an increased red cell mass when the hematocrit is >54% for men and >51% for women. In addition, white blood cell counts and platelet counts are often increased. The Polycythemia Vera Study Group (PVSG) developed diagnostic criteria for PV in the 1970s by combining clinical

Table 56.3   Proposed Diagnostic Criteria for Polycythemia Vera

Criterion[a]
A1. Increased red cell mass (>25% above predicted) or hematocrit >60% in males and >56% in females
A2. Absence of secondary causes of erythrocytosis (normal arterial oxygen saturation and no elevation of serum EPO)
A3. Palpable splenomegaly
A4. JAK2 V617F mutation or other cytogenetic abnormality (excluding BCR-ABL)
B1. Thrombocytosis
B2. Neutrophilia
B3. Splenomegaly based on imaging

[a]A1, A2, and either another A or two B criteria are required for a diagnosis of polycythemia vera.
Source: Adapted from *Hematology* 2005, pp. 201–208.

and laboratory findings. The essential components of a PVSG diagnosis of PV included an elevated red blood cell mass (RCM), normal oxygen saturation, and splenomegaly. In the absence of splenomegaly, patients must have two of the following: leukocytosis >12,000/μL, thrombocytosis >400,000/μL, serum B_{12} >900 pg/mL or unbound B_{12} binding capacity >2200 pg/mL, and leukocyte alkaline phosphatase score (LAP) >100. Serum B_{12} is elevated because of the secretion of transcobalamin protein from granulocytes in myeloproliferative disorders. LAP enzymatic activity is diminished (<100), in neutrophils derived from chronic myelogenous leukemia clones, but normal in PV clones.

While some physicians continue to use the PVSG criteria to diagnosis PV, recent debate among hematologists has focused on the sensitivity and specificity of some of the tests as well as the utility of alternative diagnostic algorithms. Most experts agree that PV should be a clinical diagnosis, with laboratory data used to confirm suspicions. However, there is a dispute over the utility of determining RCM, and some experts assert that the measurement may be affected by comorbid conditions such as iron deficiency or chronic hypoxia that can decrease the sensitivity and specificity of the test. Other experts argue that the secondary criteria—leukocytosis, thrombocytosis, LAP, and B_{12} measurements—lack sensitivity and specificity and should not be relied on to make a diagnosis of PV. Proponents for changing the diagnostic criteria advocate using EPO levels (low or normal in PV, despite increased red blood cells) and bone marrow biopsy as part of the investigation. While certain bone marrow histopathologic abnormalities, including hypercellularity of all three cell lines, clustered megakaryocytes, loss of fat spaces, and very low iron stores, are commonly found in PV, they are not specific for the disorder. With the discovery of the JAK2-V617F, the diagnostic algorithm for PV may be altered to include this mutation (Table 56.3).

Pathogenesis

PV is a clonal stem cell disorder that leads to increased production of all three myeloid cell lines, most prominently the red blood cells. Its specific etiology remains elusive, as the clonal molecular lesion has not been established. Karyotypic changes are found in less than 20% of people with PV, and are often nonspecific for the disorder. Researchers have examined erythropoietin (EPO) and its relationship to PV, and it has been shown that erythroid precursors in PV may not require exogenous EPO for growth, unlike normal controls and patients with erythrocytosis due to another etiology. However, whether the clonal erythroid growth in PV is independent of EPO stimulation or is simply hypersensitive to EPO remains unclear. Other areas of investigation in PV include molecular analyses of the EPO receptor, levels of circulating thrombopoietin (TPO) and the relationship to platelet production, and the pathogenetic properties of the polycythemia rubra vera 1 (PRV-1) gene product that has been isolated from granulocytes of patients with PV but not in normal controls or those with a secondary erythrocytosis.

Recently, researchers have discovered an association between PV and a somatic point mutation in the Janus kinase 2 (JAK2) gene, which is located on chromosome 9p. The mutation predicts replacement of a valine with phenylalanine at position 617 of the JAK2 protein (JAK2-V617F) and leads to a constitutively active tyrosine kinase. JAK2 binds to the cytoplasmic region of the EPO receptor and is activated when EPO binds to the extracellular EPO receptor domain. Following activation, JAK2 activates signaling pathways that promote erythroid survival, proliferation, and differentiation. When expressed in mice, JAK2-V617F produces erythrocytosis. While it is clear that the JAK2 kinase plays a central role in the development of non-CML myeloproliferative disorders, additional research is under way to identify the complex molecular biology. The mutation is found in non-CML forms of MPD with frequencies of 74–97% in PV, 35–50% in MMM, and 33–57% in ET. Importantly, this mutation is not found in people with secondary polycythemia or normal control subjects.

One of the hallmarks of the myeloproliferative diseases is an exaggerated response to growth factors. The discovery of the JAK2 mutation may help explain some of the hypersensitivity to growth factors, including EPO, interleukins, and TPO, which has been demonstrated in patients with PV. Studies have shown that kinase inhibitors can block the in vitro proliferation of EPO-independent erythroid progenitors in PV, suggesting that the underlying cause of their propagation is due to the constituent activation of the tyrosine kinase itself; due to mutations in the kinase domain of the JAK2 gene. Also, much like the story of Gleevec for CML (see Case 55), the identification of a specific tyrosine kinase that is abnormal in PV may lead to molecular treatments targeting this gene to provide more effective management of the disease.

Treatment

Thrombosis accounts for the majority of morbidity and mortality in PV, and preventing such events dictates much of the treatment for the disorder. The mainstay of treatment is phlebotomy, with the goal of maintaining the hematocrit below 45%. Although repeated phlebotomy worsens iron deficiency, patients should be instructed not to take supplemental iron, as the resultant iron deficiency decreases production of red blood cells, and reduces the need for subsequent phlebotomy. Some patients need myelosuppressive therapy, and alkylating agents such as busulfan were used in the past. However, they produced an unacceptable increased risk for leukemic conversion, and are not the standard of care today. Now, hydroxyurea is the most commonly used therapy. It is usually dosed at 500–1500 mg/day, adjusted to maintain platelet counts less than 500,000/µL without reducing the neutrophil count to less than 2000/µL. Interferon-α (IFN-α) has shown promise in reducing erythrocytosis and also some of the pruritis associated with PV. Anagrelide specifically lowers platelet counts, although the exact mechanism is not known, and is used to decrease the risk of hemorrhage and reduce some of the symptoms of PV, including erythromelalgia, headache, dizziness, and blurry vision, which are thought to be due to microvascular occlusion secondary to thrombocytosis. Low-dose aspirin is recommended, unless contraindicated or if platelet count is $>1500 \times 10^3/L$, based on evidence from a randomized trial in PV patients showing that aspirin reduced the combined endpoint of death, myocardial infarction, stroke, and venous thrombosis, but not death. Finally, symptomatic treatment of pruritis can be accomplished with antihistamines and selective serotonin reuptake inhibitors.

Prognosis

PV is an indolent but incurable disease with a median survival of over 10 years if treated appropriately. The most common cause of death is arterial thrombosis. In addition, PV may progress to myelofibrosis, CML, or a highly aggressive form of acute leukemia that is usually refractory to chemotherapy.

Additional Reading

SPIVAK, J. L.: Polycythemia vera: Myths, mechanisms and management. *Blood 100*:4272–90, 2002.

STUART, B. J. AND VIERA, A. J.: Polycythemia vera. *Am. Fam. Phys. 69*:2139–44, 2004.

TEFFERI, A.: Polycythemia vera: A comprehensive review and clinical recommendations. *Mayo Clin. Proc. 78*:174–94, 2003.

TEFFERI, A. AND SPIVAK, J. L.: Polycythemia vera: Scientific advances and current practice. *Semin. Hematol. 42*:206–20, 2005.

VAINCHENKER, W. AND CONSTANTINESCU.: A unique activating mutation in JAK2 (V617F) is at the origin of polycythemia vera and allows a new classification myeloproliferative diseases. *Hematology* 195–200, 2005.

Part Fourteen

Benign Hematologic Disorders

Cases of sickle cell disease, anemia due to renal failure, pernicious anemia, heparin-induced thrombocytopenia, hemophilia, qualitative platelet disorder, von Willebrand disease, thrombotic thrombocytopenic purpura, cold agglutinin disease, and jaundice are presented and discussed in Cases 57, 58, 59, 60, 61, 64, 65, 66, 67, and 69, respectively (all edited by CSE); Cases 62 and 63 (both edited by CSE) discuss cases of inherited and acquired venous thromboembolism, respectively; and Rh hemolytic disease of the newborn is the topic of Case 68 (edited by AMG).

Tietz's Applied Laboratory Medicine, Second Edition. Edited by Mitchell G. Scott, Ann M. Gronowski, and Charles S. Eby
Copyright © 2007 John Wiley & Sons, Inc.

Case 57

A Child with Pneumonia

John A. Koepke

A 12-year-old African-American male child was admitted to the hospital through the emergency room because of severe illness marked by high fever [103°F (39.6°C)] and rapid, shallow breathing. Physical examination indicated consolidation of the left lower lung fields where no breath sounds could be auscultated. Examination of the abdomen revealed that the liver was enlarged, but the spleen could not be palpated. The patient had several healed scars and open sores on his ankles. Portable x-ray examination of the chest showed consolidation of the left lower lobe of the lung. Pulse oximetry on room air was 87%, improving to 95% while receiving supplemental oxygen (3-L nasal prong).

A blood sample drawn in the emergency room provided the following results:

Analyte	Value, Conventional Units	Reference Interval, Conventional Units	Value, SI Units	Reference Interval, SI Units
WBC	$28 \times 10^3/\mu L$	3.2–9.8	$3.2–9.8 \times 10^9/L$	3.2–9.8
RBC	$3.88 \times 10^6/\mu L$	4.50–5.70	$3.88 \times 10^{12} L$	4.50–5.70
Hemoglobin	10.0 g/dL	13.6–17.2	110 g/L	136–172
MCV	82 fL	80–110	Same	
RDW	23	11–14.5	Same	
Reticulocyte %	8%	0.5–1.5	0.08 fraction	0.005–0.015
Platelet count	$658 \times 10^6/\mu L$	140–440	$658 \times 10^9/L$	140–440
Bilirubin, total	2.0 mg/dL	0.3–1.1	34.2 μmol/L	5.1–18.8
LDH	334 U/L	100–250	5.7 μkat/L	1.7–4.3
Haptoglobin	10 mg/dL	27–220	100 mg/L	270–2200

Review of the peripheral blood film showed poikilocytosis with crescent-shaped erythrocytes (Fig. 57.1). There was a granulocytosis with a marked left shift, that is, with many immature granulocytes in the circulation. Many granulocytes contained toxic granulations and had Döhle bodies. Chemical urinalysis showed proteinuria, but screening tests for urinary tract infection (i.e., nitrite and leukocyte esterase) were negative. Examination of stained sputum showed many Gram-positive cocci in pairs and short chains, sometimes within granulocytes. Sputum culture grew *Streptococcus pneumoniae*,

Tietz's Applied Laboratory Medicine, Second Edition. Edited by Mitchell G. Scott, Ann M. Gronowski, and Charles S. Eby
Copyright © 2007 John Wiley & Sons, Inc.

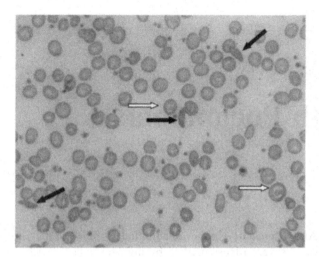

Figure 57.1   Peripheral smear showing sickle cells (black arrows) and target cells (white arrows).

which was consistent with the initial Gram stain of the sputum. The diagnosis of acute pneumonia was made based on the laboratory and radiological findings, and the patient was treated with antibiotics for bacterial (pneumococcal) pneumonia. Additional tests were performed to evaluate his anemia. He did well and was discharged from the hospital in 5 days.

Differential Diagnosis

The combination of anemia and pneumococcal pneumonia in an African-American child directs attention to consideration of another underlying disorder possibly involving a hemoglobinopathy. The findings of proteinuria and mild hepatomegaly without apparent splenomegaly or lymphadenopathy also provide the clinician with leads that can be pursued with appropriate laboratory examination.

Laboratory investigation of anemia begins with an automated complete blood count (CBC) that differentiates anemias into normocytic (MCV, 80–100 fL), microcytic (MCV, <80 fL), or macrocytic (MCV, >100 fL) types. Normocytic anemia, such as this case showed, mandates examination of the peripheral blood smear for unusual or abnormal erythrocytes that demonstrate microcytosis, hypochromia, spherocytosis, aniso-cytosis, poikilocytosis, or presence of target or sickle cells. Howell–Jolly bodies in some erythrocytes indicate a nonfunctioning spleen that can result from sickle cell disease. Multiple episodes of crisis cause splenic ischemia and infarction, finally culminating in splenic fibrosis and atrophy (i.e., autosplenectomy).

A reticulocyte count is very useful in differentiating hemolytic anemias with increased erythropoiesis from nonhemolytic anemias in which erythrocyte production is diminished. The reticulocyte count is elevated in most hemolytic anemias [in this case, the absolute reticulocyte count (RBC × reticulocyte %) was $310 \times 10^3/\mu L$ (reference range 24–84)], although a normal or low reticulocyte count may occur in aplastic crises.

The diagnosis of hemolytic anemia was made on the basis of a moderate anemia coupled with an elevated reticulocyte count. Because the patient was African-American, sickle cell disease (with a prevalence of 1 in 600 African-Americans) was at the top of the list of possible diagnoses. In this patient, the sickle cell solubility test was positive. This test checks for the decreased solubility of reduced sickle hemoglobin (HbS) in a specially constituted buffer solution causing increased turbidity that can be distinguished by visual inspection when compared to control hemoglobin incubated under similar conditions.

Glucose-6-phosphate dehydrogenase (G6PD) deficiency should also be considered in the differential diagnosis. The gene for G6PD is carried on the X chromosome, and consequently G6PD deficiency is a sex-linked disorder. Its incidence in African-American males is roughly 1 in 8. Erythrocytes of these individuals contain levels of G6PD that, although low, usually maintain an adequate reserve of reduced glutathione to prevent oxidation of hemoglobin. However, exposure to oxidizing substances (e.g., primaquine for prophylaxis of malaria, nitrofurantoin for urinary tract infection, or fava beans) or an acute febrile illness may overwhelm the fragile system operating with marginal levels of G6PD and lead to phagocytosis of red cells containing denatured hemoglobin (Heinz bodies). In interim periods, the erythrocytes of patients deficient in G6PD survive normally. G6PD deficiency is detected with a screening procedure followed by quantitative assay for specific enzymatic activity. The G6PD screening test was negative in this patient, indicating normal G6PD activity.

African-American patients may be afflicted with thalassemia or thalassemia–sickle cell disease, and therefore the possibility of these conditions must not be ignored. Hemoglobin electrophoresis plus measurement of the concentrations of fetal hemoglobin and hemoglobin A_2 are necessary to make these diagnoses. The exact delineation of the various kinds of thalassemia can at times be quite difficult, and family studies as well as more sophisticated laboratory studies (e.g., isoelectric focusing method of separating hemoglobin types, direct amino acid sequencing, α- and β-hemoglobin chain synthetic ratios, α-globin gene deletion and β-globin coding and noncoding mutations by DNA analysis) may be required in certain cases.[1,2] Prenatal diagnosis of a hemoglobinopathy is best done by DNA analysis of fetal cells obtained by sampling the chorionic villi.

Additional studies such as assays for total and conjugated bilirubin, urine urobilinogen, haptoglobin, and LDH are usually abnormal in cases of accelerated hemolysis, regardless of cause. These determinations may be useful for following the severity and progression of a hemolytic process, but they do not add more to establishing a specific diagnosis.

On the basis of the positive sickle cell solubility test, hemoglobin electrophoresis was performed to confirm the diagnosis (Fig. 57.2), because false-positive (paraproteins) or false-negative (severe anemia, elevated haemoglobin F) results may be obtained with the hemoglobin solubility screening test. Hemoglobin electrophoresis uses cellulose acetate or agarose gels at pH 8.6 for convenient resolution of hemoglobins A, F, C, and S. A second supplemental electrophoretic procedure is performed at acid pH (6.0) to separate abnormal hemoglobins, such as hemoglobins D and G, which migrate with hemoglobin S at pH 8.6.

In the electrophoretic procedure, the relative proportions of normal as well as abnormal hemoglobins can be quantitated. In this case, the proportion of hemoglobin S (HbS) was 82%, fetal hemoglobin (HbF) 14%, and hemoglobin A_2 (HbA$_2$) 4%. Many laboratories use high-performance liquid chromatography (HPLC) instruments for hemoglobin analysis. The advantages of HPLC compared to electrophoresis include accurate quantification of hemoglobins F and A_2, and labor-saving automation (Fig. 57.3).

The patient had not received any erythrocyte transfusions in the previous several weeks, and therefore there was no contamination of the specimen with normal adult hemoglobin A (HbA) from transfused blood. A mistaken diagnosis of sickle cell *trait* could be

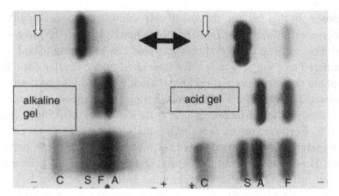

Figure 57.2   Cellulose acetate (pH 8.6, on left) and acid (pH 6.2 on right) electrophoresis gels; free hemoglobin is applied in wells cut into gel (white arrows) and gel is placed in buffer oriented with positive (+) and negative (−) electrodes. At the conclusion of electrophoresis, hemoglobin is stained and scanned in a densitometer to semiquantitate hemoglobin species. Top lane, ◄► contains patient's hemoglobin (F, 14%; S, 84%; A₂, not visible). Middle lane contains hemoglobins A and F from another patient. Bottom lane contains control hemoglobins.

made in a patient with sickle cell disease who had recently been transfused with red cells containing normal HbA. Whereas diagnostic electrophoresis should be restricted to a time long after transfusion, effectiveness of a transfusion can be monitored by hemoglobin electrophoresis. By measuring HbA and HbS periodically, the proportion of HbS can be monitored and new transfusions invoked and thus avert complications of sickle cell disease in selected patients at high risk for ischemic cerebral events, acute chest syndrome, complications during pregnancy, or prior to elective major surgery.

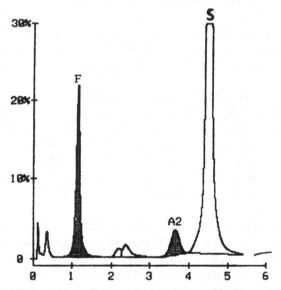

Figure 57.3   HPLC analysis of patient with sickle cell disease. Following lysis of red cells, free hemoglobin solution is applied to a cation exchange column. The column is perfused with a solution of increasing cation concentration causing different hemoglobin species to elute at specific times. Hemoglobin A would elute between peak F (HbF) and A₂ (HbA₂), but is absent on this graph because the patient was homozygous for hemoglobin S.

Inherited conditions involving HbS in African Americans include sickle cell trait (HbS plus normal HbA; prevalence 1 in 12), sickle cell disease (homozygous HbS; Prevalence in 1:600) or combined with other hemoglobinopathies or thalassemias: SC hemoglobinopathy (HbS plus HbC; prevalence 1 in 800), SD hemoglobinopathy (HbS plus HbD, rare), and S-β-thalassemia (prevalence 1 in 600). Sickle cell trait is an asymptomatic condition except under extreme hypoxic conditions. The other conditions are usually less severe clinically than sickle cell disease (HbSS).

Pathophysiology

Substitution of valine for glutamic acid at amino acid position 6 of the β-globin chain increases the affinity of deoxygenated hemoglobin S tetramers for each other, producing spontaneous polymerization, and crescent-shaped red cells. The rigid sickle cells have shortened lifespans and cause microvascular occlusions leading to ischemic injury in multiple tissues. A mild to moderate leukocytosis is common in sickle cell patients, and is associated with increased morbidity and mortality, consistent with a role of inflammatory mediators in vascular complications. The spleen and bone marrow are common sites of vasoocclusive crises and tissue infarctions.

Treatment

Pain crises due to vasoocclusive events are the most frequent complaint of patients with sickle cell disease. Bone pain, particularly in the legs and ribs, is the most common symptom, as well as joint pain, headache, and abdominal pain. The standard approach to management of pain crises is to evaluate and treat possible precipitating causes such as infection, provide oral and intravenous hydration and supplemental oxygen, and to relieve pain, typically with parenteral narcotics administered via a patient-controlled analgesic pump. Red cell transfusions are not usually indicated for uncomplicated pain crises. However, some patients with sickle cell disease do require intermittent transfusions for severe anemia, complicated crises, prior to surgical procedures, or stroke prophylaxis.[3]

The many transfusions that these patients receive increase the risk of developing various antibodies to donor erythrocytes. About one-quarter of sickle cell patients will develop antibodies, and procuring compatible blood becomes more difficult. The use of designated, related donors whose erythrocyte antigen phenotypes match those of the recipient lessens the rate of immunization and also improves the chances of finding compatible blood.[4]

Another problem associated with chronic transfusions is transfusion hemosiderosis, the buildup of stored iron in the patient's body. Each unit of transfused erythrocytes contains 150–250 mg of elemental iron. When the transfused cells finally are cleared, the iron from their hemoglobin is stored in the reticuloendothelial cells. In addition, intestinal absorption of dietary iron increases in patients with chronic hemolytic anemia. Both of these mechanisms can cause massive storage of iron, which can lead to parenchymal organ (liver, heart) and endocrine gland (especially pancreas) dysfunction.

Iron overload is a major concern for children at high risk for stroke based on transcranial Doppler studies showing high blood flow rates in the middle cerebral or internal carotid arteries. Chronic transfusions reduce strokes, but when stopped, the stroke risk returns.[5] The risk of iron overload may be lessened by use of partial red cell exchange transfusions and iron chelation. Until recently, iron chelation therapy required daily prolonged subcutaneous infusion of deferoxamine. A long-awaited oral iron chelator, deferasirox (Exjade), was approved by the FDA in 2005, and offers the potential for reduction of iron overload complications in patients with chronic hemolytic anemia, especially those with sickle cell disease and severe forms of thalassemia.[6]

The complications of vasoocclusive crises involve many organs including lung, liver, brain (cerebrovascular accidents), penis (priapism), bone (aseptic necrosis), retina, kidney, spleen, and skin (leg ulcers).[7] Erythrocyte exchange transfusion can lead to healing of skin ulcers such as this patient displayed, and primary and secondary prevention of strokes, as well as reduction of morbidity from acute cerebral ischemia, priapism, and acute chest syndrome. Congestive heart failure, chronic pulmonary hypertension, renal insufficiency, and joint damage are common long-term complications. In children, the necrosis and periosteitis of metacarpal and metatarsal bones causes a painful deformation termed the "hand–foot syndrome." Aplastic crisis (acute failure to produce erythrocytes) may result from infection with human parvovirus B19 that selectively affects erythroid precursors in bone marrow. A further complication of any hereditary hemolytic disorder is formation of bilirubin gallstones to a degree that may require cholecystectomy.

Infection is the major cause of death in children with sickle cell disease because, after loss of splenic function, susceptibility increases for infections with encapsulated organisms, such as *Streptococcus pneumoniae* and *Haemophilus influenzae*. Osteomyelitis with *Salmonella* is also common in patients with sickle cell disease. General preventive measures include immunization with a polyvalent pneumococcal vaccine and chemoprophylaxis with antibiotics. Folate supplementation should also be administered to prevent depletion in the presence of lifelong brisk hematopoiesis.

A number of innovative therapeutic initiatives are currently under active investigation; they include trials of drugs that reduce hemoglobin S polymerization, bone marrow transplantation, and gene therapy. Currently, the chemotherapeutic agent, hydroxyurea, which increases synthesis of HbF, is the only medication that can alter the clinical severity of sickle cell disease.[8] Increased concentration of intracellular HbF increases the minimum gelling concentration of deoxygenated HbS solutions and reduces the likelihood of sickling. Other affects of hydroxyurea that are associated with clinical improvement in patients with sickle cell disease include reduction in neutrophil count and reduces red cell adhesion to endothelial cells. Some medical centers are now performing bone marrow transplant for hemoglobinopathies, primarily for treatment of thalassemia, but there exists a potential for application to sickle cell disease for children at high risk of stroke.

References

1. STEINBERG, M. H.: The interactions of α-thalassemia with hemoglobinopathies. *Hematol. Oncol. Clin. North Am.* 5:453–73, 1991.

2. KAUFMAN, R. E.: Analysis of abnormal hemoglobins. In *Practical Laboratory Hematology*, J. A. KOEPKE, ed., Churchill Livingstone, New York, 1991.

3. DANIELSON, C. F. M.: The role of red blood cell exchange transfusion in the treatment and prevention of complications of sickle cell disease. *Ther. Apheresis* 6:24–31, 2001.

4. KANTER, M. H. AND HODGE, S. E.: The probability of obtaining compatible blood from related directedd donors. *Arch. Pathol. Lab. Med.* 114:1013–16, 1990.

5. STOP2 Trial Investigators: Discontinuing prophylactic transfusions used to prevent stroke in sickle cell disease. *N. Engl. J. Med.* 353:2769–78, 2005.

6. CAPPELLINI, M. D.: Iron-chelating therapy with the new oral agent ICL679 (Exjade®). *Best Pract. & Res. Clin. Haematol.* 18:289–98, 2005.

7. CLASTER, S. AND VICHINSKY, E. P.: Managing sickle cell disease. *Br. Med. J.* 327:1151–55, 2003.

8. HALSEY, C. AND ROBERTS, I. A. G.: The role of hydroxyurea in sickle cell disease. *Br. J. Haematol.* 120:177–86, 2003.

Additional Reading

SAFKO, R.: Anemias of abnormal globin development-hemoglobinopathies. In *Clinical Hematology—Principles, Procedures, Correlations*, 2nd ed., E. A. STIENE-MARTIN, C. A. LOTSPEICH-STEININGER, AND J. A. KOEPKE, eds., Lippincott, Philadelphia, 1992, pp. 192–216.

Case 58

A Man with a Tender Toe and Anemia

John A. Koepke

A 50-year-old African-American man came to the emergency room complaining of several weeks of left great toe pain. During the past month, he had not felt well. Food tasted different, his appetite was decreased, and he had lost 20 lb. His skin was itchy, and he noted occasional leg and hand cramping. At times he felt mentally slow and forgetful.

He was employed and smoked one pack of cigarettes and drank one pint of liquor each day. Preexisting medical problems included hypertension, hypercholesterolemia, and type 2 diabetes, but he did not consistently see a physician or take prescribed medications. Laboratory data from 3 years earlier were notable for: hemoglobin 13.9 g/dL and creatinine 1.3 mg/dL.

Physical examination showed a chronically ill-appearing man with an inflamed tophaceous area on the medial aspect of his left great toe. BP was 144/80, pulse 92, and temperature 36°C. Lung, heart, and abdominal exams were unremarkable. There was +2 pedal edema.

The following laboratory test results were obtained:

Analyte	Value, Conventional Units	Reference Interval, Conventional Units	Value, SI Units	Reference Interval, SI Units
Sodium	144 mmol/L	135–145	Same	
Potassium	3.9 mmol/L	3.3–4.9	Same	
Chloride	108 mmol/L	97–110	Same	
CO_2, total	22 mmol/L	22–32	Same	
Glucose	113 mg/dL	54–99	6.3 mmol/L	3.0–5.5
Urea nitrogen	114 mg/dL	9–25	40.7 mmol/L	3.2–8.9
Creatinine	13.9 mg/dL	0.7–1.3	1229 μmol/L	62–115
Hemoglobin	9.6 g/dL	13.8–17.2	96 g/L	138–172
MCV	91.3 fL	80–97.6	Same	
RDW	14.0%	11–14.5	0.14 fraction	0.11–0.45

Tietz's Applied Laboratory Medicine, Second Edition. Edited by Mitchell G. Scott, Ann M. Gronowski, and Charles S. Eby
Copyright © 2007 John Wiley & Sons, Inc.

Analyte	Value, Conventional Units	Reference Interval, Conventional Units	Value, SI Units	Reference Interval, SI Units
Reticulocyte %	1.2%	0.5–1.5	0.012 fraction	0.005–0.015
Erythropoietin	1.0 mU/mL	4.0–21	Same	
Iron	32 μg/dL	45–160	5.7 μmol/L	8.1–28.6
Iron binding capacity	189 μg/dL	220–420	33.8 μmol/L	39.8–75.2
Transferin saturation	17%	20–50	0.17 fraction	0.2–0.5
Ferritin	1436 ng/ml	20–323	1436 μg/L	20–323
Soluble transferrin receptor	2.80 mg/L	0.85–3.05	Same	
Vitamin B$_{12}$	814 pg/mL	223–1132	600 pmol/L	165–835
Folic acid	15.5 μg/L	>5.4	35 nmol/L	>12.2
Joint aspirate				
Microscopic	Crystals (negative birefringent)	No crystals		
Urinalysis				
Protein	+3	Negative		
pH	6.0	4.5–8.0		
Microscopic				
WBC	25/hpf	0–5		
RBC	50/hpf	0–3		
Urine culture	No growth	No growth		

Abdominal ultrasound showed a liver that was normal in size and echogenicity and bilateral small kidneys with increased echotexture consistent with renal parenchymal disease. A renal biopsy showed arterial thickening and diffuse glomerulosclerosis, consistent with chronic hypertension.

The gout was treated with an intraarticular steroid injection, hemodialysis was initiated, and hypertension, diabetes, and alcohol and smoking cessation were managed medically. Recombinant human erythropoietin (Epogen) injections were begun for treatment of anemia. He did not require red blood cell transfusion.

Differential Diagnosis

The initial diagnosis, based on the history and initial laboratory data, was anemia of chronic disease (ACD). This is a large group of conditions second only to iron deficiency as a cause of anemia. This class of anemias can be due to chronic infectious or inflammatory conditions, carcinoma, autoimmunity, or chronic renal disease.[1] Patients with ACD typically have a mild, normocytic anemia and inappropriately low reticulocyte response. Cytokines, including interleukin-1 (IL-1), interferon gamma (IF-γ), and tumor necrosis factor α (TNF-α), produced in response to chronic inflammatory states, such as gout, cause anemia through multiple mechanisms, including direct suppression of erythropoiesis, blunted renal production of erythropoietin (EPO) in response to anemia, and increased uptake and sequestration of iron within macrophages. A key effecter of iron sequestration is hepcidin, a peptide synthesized by hepatocytes in response to IL-6 and liposaccharide. Hepcidin blocks release of iron from duodenal enterocytes and macrophages, causing hypoferremia and anemia.

Indirect measurements of iron stores can be confusing in ACD. Serum iron and transferrin saturation are typically low, but unlike simple iron deficiency, transferrin concentration is not elevated. Intracellular iron is bound to ferritin, and serum ferritin concentration accurately reflects iron stores in most individuals. However, serum ferritin concentrations can be elevated in ACD states, reflecting increased hepatic synthesis of apoferritin (non-iron-containing ferritin), reducing the sensitivity and negative predictive value of a normal or elevated ferritin concentration for excluding iron deficiency. An alternative to performing a bone marrow biopsy to assess iron stores in patients with ACD and possible coexisting iron deficiency is to measure serum soluble transferrin receptor (sTfR).[2] In iron deficiency, both transferrin receptor expression on the surface of erythroid progenitors and soluble shed TfR are increased. Optimal detection of iron deficiency in patients with ACD is achieved by determining the ratio of sTfR to the logarithm of serum ferritin.[3] A sTfR/log ferritin ratio >2 is consistent with ACD and iron deficiency, while a ratio <1 is predictive of ACD alone. While evelated sTfR is a sensitive indicator of iron deficiency, it is nonspecific, and will be elevated in patients with chronic hemolytic anemias such as sickle cell disease, thalassemias, and hereditary spherocytosis. Currently, sTfR assays are not available on most automated chemistry instruments, and demand for the test is low. In this case presentation, a sTFs/log transferrin ratio of 0.9 is consistent with ACD with adequate iron stores despite the low serum iron and transferrin saturation. While chronic inflammation due to untreated gout may contribute to the patient's anemia, the markedly low serum erythropoietin concentration, blood chemistries, and loss of renal parenchyma point to renal disease as the primary cause of his anemia.

Treatment

The only therapy for chronic renal failure, other than renal transplantation is renal dialysis. The usual treatment consists of several sessions of either intravenous or peritoneal dialysis 2 or 3 times each week. Also periodic red cell transfusions may be required to maintain even a low normal blood hemoglobin concentration. Since the discovery, synthesis, and widespread use of the erythrogenic hormone, erythropoietin (Epogen, Procrit), the administration of this product has significantly changed the quality of life for patients on long-term dialysis.

In this patient, hemodialysis 3 times a week was initiated. Recombinant human erythropoietin (Epogen) injections (50 U/kg IV with each dialysis) were begun for the treatment of the anemia in addition to iron injections, which are recommended for patients with chronic renal failure since iron deficiency occurs in 25–37% of these patients when the patient's marrow becomes erythropoietic following the treatment with EPO.[4] Causes of iron deficiency include frequent phlebotomies, blood loss in dialysis tubing, and chronic gastrointestinal blood loss. Dialysis patients require 400–500 mg of supplemental iron (equivalent to the iron in two units of blood) every 3 months to compensate for ongoing losses. Recognizing that transferrin saturation <20% and ferritin <100 pg/mL lack ideal sensitivity and specificity, the National Kidney Foundation guidelines for management of anemia of chronic kidney disease nevertheless recommend these cutoffs for diagnosing function iron deficiency.[4] Since oral iron therapy has seldom been successful, intravenous iron therapy is usually added to the treatment regimen.

By the second month of therapy the patient's hemoglobin reached the recommended target level of 11–12 g/dL. Table 58.1 documents this improvement. It was sought to

Table 58.1   National Kidney Foundation Outcome Quality Initiative Guidelines[a]

	Outpatient hemodialysis, (months)				
	1	2	3	4	5
Hemoglobin (g/dL)	9.6	11.9	14.3	13.1	11.9
Serum iron (μg/dL)	67	58	165	129	98
Transferrin (μg/dL)	224	229	291	269	249
Saturation	23%	20%	57%	48%	39%
Ferritin (ng/mL)	1598	563	—	—	750
EPO dose (units IV)*	↑ 25%	n/c	↓ 25%	↓ 15%	↑ 10%
IV Ferrlicit	125 mg/week × 4	125 mg/week × 4			

[a]These guidelines were used during outpatient dialysis.
*Arrows indicate percent increase or decrease of erythropoietin dose based on hemoglobin.

maintain this target level of hemoglobin and the dose of EPO was lowered in order to accomplish this. It was also decided to treat the patient with parenteral ferrous gluconate therapy (Ferrlecit®), during the first 2 months based on transferrin saturations.

In addition to using hemoglobin, transferrin saturation, and ferritin results to adjust EPO doses and guide iron supplementation, automated reticulocyte analysis can provide additional guidance. Automated hematology analyzers are able to accurately and precisely count reticulocytes, including the performance of differential reticulocyte counts based on measuring intracellular mRNA. Immature reticulocytes, termed the *immature reticulocyte fraction* (IRF), contain increased amounts of mRNA, are released from the bone marrow within a couple of days after stimulation by EPO, and thus allow for an early determination if EPO is indeed effective treatment for the patient.[5] This is also important to note since EPO is an expensive hormone and if EPO is not effective in some patients, significant savings can be found if the hormone is discontinued. On the other hand, since the effective dosage is quite variable among patients, the IRF can be useful as the dosage is titrated during the early weeks of treatment. Circulating hypochromic reticulocytes are the earliest indicators of iron-restricted erythropoiesis. Some automated hematology analyzers report reticulocyte hemoglobin concentration. Prospective studies in renal dialysis patients comparing traditional transferrin saturation and ferritin cutoffs to a hypochromic mean reticulocyte hemoglobin concentration threshold for I.V. iron supplementation concluded that the reticulocyte parameter was a more accurate predictor of response to parenteral iron.[6]

In patients with ACD due to conditions other than renal failure, anemia is usually considered to be a secondary problem, and mild to moderate anemia is tolerated while treatment is focused on the underlying disease process. However, the possibility that anemia is an independent risk factor for important functional morbidities and morality in patients with ACD as well as in elderly people without evidence of renal disease, iron deficiency, or ACD is now being considered.[7] If prospective studies confirm important benefits to correction of anemia in these populations with current (EPO) or novel therapeutics, diagnostic tests to differentiate the causes of anemia and to monitor therapy will expand as well.

References

1. WEISS, G. AND GOODNOUGH, L. T.: The anemia of chronic disease. *N. Engl. J. Med. 352*:1011–23. 2005.

2. LEWIS, J. P. AND MEYERS, F. J.: The anemia of renal insufficiency. In *Laboratory Hematology*, J. A. Koepke, ed., Churchill Livingstone, New York, 1984, pp. 43–57.

3. PUNNOENEN, I., IRJALA, K., AND RAJAMAKI, A.: Serum transferrin receptor and its ratio to serum ferritin in the diagnosis of iron deficiency. *Blood 89*:1052–7, 1997.

4. National Kidney Foundation: K/DOQI Clinical practice guidelines for anemia of chronic disease, 2000. *J. Kidney Dis. 37*(Suppl 1):S182–238, 2001.

5. KOEPKE, J. A.: Update on reticulocyte counting. *Lab. Med. 30*:339–43, 1999.

6. FISHBANE, S., GALGANO, C., LANGLEY, JR., F. C., CANFIELD, W., AND MAESKA, J. K.: Reticulocyte hemoglobin content in the evaluation of iron status of hemodialysis patients. *Kidney International 52*:217–22, 1997.

7. GURANLNIK, J. M., EISENSTAEDT, R. S., FERRUCCI, L., KLEIN, H. G., AND WOODMAN, R. C.: Prevalence of anemia in persons 65 years and older in the United States: Evidence for a high rate of unexplained anemia. *Blood 104*:2263–8, 1997.

Case 59

A Woman with Fatigue and Pallor

Naif Z. Abraham, Jr. and Robert E. Hutchison

A 59-year-old secretary was feeling increasing fatigue and weakness that had developed insidiously over a few months. Recently she had become very pale and exhibited irritability, forgetfulness, personality change, and mood swings. She did report changes in taste. Her well-being had deteriorated so greatly that she sought medical attention. In addition, she described the recent onset of tingling and prickling sensations (paresthesias) localized symmetrically in her feet. Although the patient admitted to having episodes of weakness and lightheadedness, she denied hallucinations or other disturbances of mentation. On physical examination, she appeared very pale with slightly icteric skin and sclerae. Her pulse was rapid, and auscultation revealed a systolic flow murmur. Her tongue was not sore, but it appeared smooth and beefy red (atrophic glossitis) on inspection. In addition, diminished vibration and position sense as well as impaired cutaneous touch and pain sensation was present in the lower extremities.

Initial laboratory results were as follows:

Analyte	Value, Conventional Units	Reference Interval, Conventional Units	Value, SI Units	Reference Interval, SI Units
WBC	$3.8 \times 10^3/\mu L$	4.5–11.0	$3.8 \times 10^9/L$	4.5–11.0
Hemoglobin	6.1 g/dL	11.7–16.0	61 g/L	117–160
Hematocrit	18%	35–47	0.18 volume	0.35–0.47
MCV	131 fL	81–101	Same	
MCH	44.9 pg	27–34	Same	
MCHC	34.3 g Hb/dL	31–36	Same	
Reticulocyte %	0.2%	0.5–1.5	0.002 fraction	0.005–0.015
Platelet count	$83 \times 10^3/\mu L$	150–450	$83 \times 10^9/L$	150–450
LDH	1535 U/L	140–280	25.59 μkat/L	2.33–4.67
Bilirubin	2.1 mg/dL	0.2–1.0	36 μmol/L	3–17

Review of peripheral blood smear yielded the following:

Erythrocyte morphology—marked anisocytosis (cell size variation); moderate poikilocytosis (cell shape variation); mild polychromasia; moderate macrocytosis,

Tietz's Applied Laboratory Medicine, Second Edition. Edited by Mitchell G. Scott, Ann M. Gronowski, and Charles S. Eby
Copyright © 2007 John Wiley & Sons, Inc.

including oval macrocytes, schistocytes or helmet cells, and broken erythrocyte fragments

Leukocyte morphology—occasional hypersegmented (i.e., 6 or more nuclear lobes) neutrophils present; nucleated erythrocytes present (3 per 100 leukocytes counted)

Results from the patient's complete blood count indicated a macrocytic (MCV > 101; normal ranges vary slightly with laboratory and population) anemia. The differential diagnosis of macrocytic anemia includes megaloblastic anemia, aplastic anemia, alcohol abuse, liver disease, autoimmune hemolytic anemia, and the myelodysplastic syndromes. The elevated RDW and decreased reticulocyte count with the peripheral blood findings of numerous oval macrocytes and hypersegmented neutrophils favored the diagnosis of megaloblastic anemia. In addition, the elevated LDH and total bilirubin are consistent with ineffective erythropoiesis, and the neurological findings could be due to cobalamin (vitamin B_{12}) deficiency.

Additional laboratory tests were performed:

Analyte	Value, Conventional Units	Reference Interval, Conventional Units	Value, SI Units	Reference Interval, SI Units
Folate	3.1 ng/mL	3–16	7.2 nmol/L	7–36
Folate (red cell)	155 ng/mL	130–628	352 nmol/L	294–1422
Methylmalonic acid	6.5 μg/dL	0.85–4.35	552 nmol/L	72–370
Homocysteine	19.5 μmol/L	5.1–13.9	19.5 μmol/L	5.1–13.9
Cobalamin	114 μg/mL	200–900	84 μmol/L	148–664

The low serum cobalamin (cbl), normal serum and red cell folate, and elevated serum levels of methylmalonic acid (MMA) and homocysteine supported a diagnosis of cbl deficiency as the cause of the macrocytic anemia. In the United States, cbl deficiency is due mainly to malabsorption, and thus a Schilling test (results presented below) was performed in order to distinguish lack of gastric production of intrinsic factor (IF), which binds to free cbl in the upper small intestine, from disease of the terminal ileum (the site for IF–cbl complex absorption). Although the Schilling test does not directly diagnose cbl deficiency, it can help elucidate the mechanism of cbl deficiency.

Schilling Test of Cobalamin Absorption

Stage I. The fasting patient is given an oral dose of radiolabeled (tracer) cobalamin and also receives, at the same time, a large, parenteral dose of unlabeled cobalamin in order to saturate the cbl binding sites; saturation allows the orally absorbed labeled cobalamin to be excreted in the urine. Radioactivity is then measured in the urine collected over the next 24 hours. Normal levels of radioactivity in the urine indicate normal absorption of cobalamin, which suggests either dietary deficiency or food-bound cobalamin malabsorption. An abnormally low level of radioactivity in the urine indicates poor absorption of cobalamin and necessitates further testing.

Stage II. If stage I is abnormal, the test is repeated, and this time the oral dose of labeled cobalamin is given together with intrinsic factor. Normal radioactivity in the 24-hour urine specimen indicates that a lack of intrinsic factor in the patient is the cause of cobalamin deficiency, whereas abnormally low radioactivity in the stage II sample strongly suggests intestinal malabsorption. Complete collection of urine for 24 hours for both stage I and stage II is required for correct interpretation of this test. Additional tests can be run (if both stage I and II are abnormal) with either prior treatment with antibiotics or with pancreatic extract to rule out, respectively, bacterial overgrowth or pancreatic insufficiency as potential causes of abnormal cobalamin absorption.

The results indicated that the patient had impaired absorption of cobalamin (stage I) that was corrected in the presence of exogenously administered intrinsic factor (stage II). In the absence of evidence of gastric disease or history of gastric surgery, the Schilling test provided strong evidence for the diagnosis of pernicious anemia.

Results of Schilling test in this patient were as follows:

Analyte	Value, Conventional Units	Reference Interval, Conventional Units	Value, SI Units	Reference Interval, SI Units
Stage I	3%	>9%	0.03	>0.09
Stage II	15%	>9%	0.15	>0.09

The patient was initially treated with administration of hydroxocobalamin (1000 μg/day, intramuscularly, for 2 weeks). She began to feel better within the first few days after therapy was begun. Laboratory results were obtained after 2 weeks of therapy:

Analyte	Value, Conventional Units	Reference Interval, Conventional Units	Value, SI Units	Reference Interval, SI Units
WBC	$15.5 \times 10^3/\mu L$	4.5–11.0	$15.5 \times 10^9/L$	4.5–11.0
Hemoglobin	11.3 g/dL	11.7–16.0	113 g/L	117–160
Hematocrit	34%	35–47	0.34 volume	0.35–0.47
MCV	104.7 fL	81–101	Same	
MCH	34.5 pg	27–34	Same	
MCHC	32.9 g Hb/dL	31–36	Same	
Platelet count	$460 \times 10^3/\mu L$	150–450	$460 \times 10^9/L$	150–450
Reticulocyte count	5.0%	0.5–1.5	0.05 fraction	0.005–0.015
Cobalamin	1037 pg/mL	200–900	765 pmol/L	148–664

Despite marked improvement in her hematologic status, the patient's neurological manifestations were not entirely reversed. She showed a persistent deficit in vibration sense, and her paresthesias showed minimal change. However, the prognosis for eventual neurological improvement was good, because of the relatively short duration of symptoms before treatment. The longer the duration of neurological symptoms before diagnosis and treatment, the more likely that they will not be totally reversed by therapy and that some neurological deficit will remain.

Pernicious Anemia (PA)

Pernicious anemia is a type of megaloblastic anemia caused by cyanocobalamin, or vitamin B_{12}, deficiency, and much of the time is attributable to an autoimmune chronic gastritis. The autoimmune gastritis causes atrophy and destruction of the gastric mucosal oxyntic (parietal) cells, which secrete hydrochloric acid and intrinsic factor (IF— a glycoprotein with a high affinity for cbl) into the gastric fluid. IF is required for normal absorption of cbl in the ileum, and the loss of IF secretion causes cbl malabsorption and PA. The deficiency becomes apparent only after 4 or 5 years because the stores of the vitamin in normal liver tissue are sufficient for that length of time.

Cbl is a generic term for analogs of cyanocobalamin or vitamin B_{12}, and refers to the entire molecule excluding the cyano (—CN) group attached to the β position of the cobalt atom. Different ligands attached to this position produce different forms of cbl. Although multiple forms of cbl exist in the human body, only two are biologically active (methylcobalamin and adenosylcobalamin); each functions as a coenzyme in different metabolic reactions. In our discussion, we shall use the term "cobalamin" (cbl) as a general term for this family of cobalt coordination compounds, unless otherwise stated.

Cobalamins are required for normal metabolic functioning of the body; however, these compounds are synthesized by bacteria and cannot be synthesized by humans. Meat, liver, fish, and dairy products are the main food sources of cbl; cbl is not found in plants. The acidic gastric environment, along with proteases, releases cbl bound to food proteins, which makes free cbl accessible for absorption by the body. R protein (RP), produced in salivary glands, can now bind with free cbl and then transport the RP–cbl complex to the duodenum. In the presence of a more neutral pH and pancreatic proteases, cbl is released from RP and can now bind with IF. The IF–cbl complex is then transported to the ileum, where the complex binds to cubilin (the intestinal IF receptor) and absorption (i.e., receptor-mediated endocytosis) of cbl occurs, most likely with the interaction of the general transport membrane receptor, megalin. The bulk of normal cbl absorption occurs via receptor-mediated endocytosis; at times, however, if free cbl concentration is great enough, some cbl absorption can occur by simple diffusion across the cell membrane (mass action). Once inside the ileal enterocyte, the complex dissociates, and cbl can now be transported into the portal blood bound with another cbl transport protein called *transcobalamin II*.

In addition to the normal uptake of ingested cbl, an enterohepatic circulation of cbl exists, where intestinal absorption of cbl secreted into bile takes place. Absorption is IF-dependent and will not take place in the absence of IF. Excretion of cbl occurs predominantly in the feces.

If gastritis abolishes the secretion of IF, however, the IF–cbl complex is not formed and malabsorption of cobalamin will usually occur, which, over time, leads to cobalamin deficiency. Chronic gastritis is histopathologically defined by increased plasma cells and lymphocytes within the gastric mucosa, and at least three types of chronic gastritis (defined by location and/or etiology) are recognized: multifocal chronic atrophic gastritis (with focal atrophy and inflammation throughout the stomach), autoimmune chronic atrophic gastritis (inflammation and atrophy spare the antrum), and diffuse antral, or *Helicobacter pylori*–associated, chronic gastritis (antral predominant inflammation). Consequently, in some types of gastritis, serum gastrin levels may be elevated (hypergastrinemia), due to significant destruction of the oxyntic glands and loss of feedback inhibition by hydrochloric acid on neuroendocrine cells that produce gastrin. Similarly, serum pepsinogen I levels may be significantly reduced on destruction of chief cells. Prolonged chronic inflammation and epithelial cell destruction may also produce a secondary change in gastric mucosa, intestinal metaplasia within the stomach. Either change can ultimately lead to either neuroendocrine carcinoma or adenocarcinoma of the stomach in some patients. In addition, chronic lymphoid hyperplasia in the stomach may, over time, give rise to lymphoma.

An autoimmune process (and possibly genetic susceptibility) causes loss of the parietal cell mucosa in PA. Patients affected by PA frequently develop other autoimmune diseases such as Graves disease, Hashimoto's thyroiditis, and vitiligo. Three types of autoantibodies have been identified in many (but not all) patients with PA: blocking antibodies that bind IF and prevent its binding with cbl, binding antibodies that react with IF–cobalamin complexes, and parietal cell antibodies directed against the H+/K + -adenosine triphosphatase (ATPase) of the gastric parietal cell. The ATPase is the proton pump responsible for acid secretion in the stomach. It is thought, however, that parietal cell injury and cell death occur by cell-mediated direct T-lymphocyte cytotoxicity.

Although IF antibodies are highly specific, they are positive in only about 50–75% of patients with PA. Conversely, antiparietal cell antibodies are present in a higher proportion of patients with disease, but specificity of this test is low since the test can be positive in normal individuals as well as individuals with other types of autoimmune disease.

The loss of specific cells from the gastric mucosa and consequent changes in serum levels may be utilized to biochemically diagnose gastritis and PA. Thus, the serum gastrin and serum pepsinogen I assays are ancillary tests that may be useful in assessing the significance of a low serum cbl level. Other tests, including tests for *H. pylori* infection and serum antibody tests for anti-parietal-cell and anti-intrinsic-factor antibodies may also be useful in the diagnosis of pernicious anemia. While a definitive diagnosis of PA in a patient is obtained with a Schilling test, which assesses *the actual absorption of cobalamin with and without IF*, the importance of this test is controversial given its complexity and availability of alternative serum analytes.

Pathophysiology

Either cbl deficiency or folate deficiency can impair DNA synthesis throughout the body by interfering with the utilization of tetrahydrofolate (THF) and its derivatives and can produce megaloblastic anemia. A form of THF is required for both purine and pyrimidine synthesis, which also serves as a rate-limiting step in DNA synthesis. A form of THF is also required for methionine synthesis, the only reaction requiring both cbl and folate. Homocysteine is converted to methionine utilizing methylcobalamin as a required coenzyme (Fig. 59.1). Consequently, tissues in which rapid cell division occurs are the most seriously affected by either cbl or folate deficiency, including the bone marrow and the lining of the gastrointestinal tract. In the bone marrow, impaired DNA synthesis leads

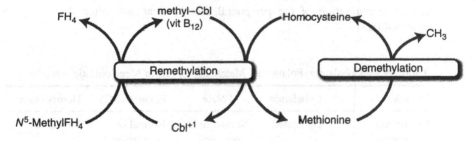

Figure 59.1 *Reaction 1*: homocysteine metabolism—methionine undergoes demethylation to form homocysteine. During periods of increased demand for methionine, homocysteine undergoes remethylation, a multienzymatic step that requires both folic acid and vitamin B_{12} as cofactors to provide methyl groups. A deficiency of either vitamin B_{12} or folic acid produces an increase in plasma homocysteine concentration. N^5-MethylFH$_4$ = N^5 methyltetrahydrofolate, reduced form of folic acid, FH$_4$ = tetrahydrofolate.

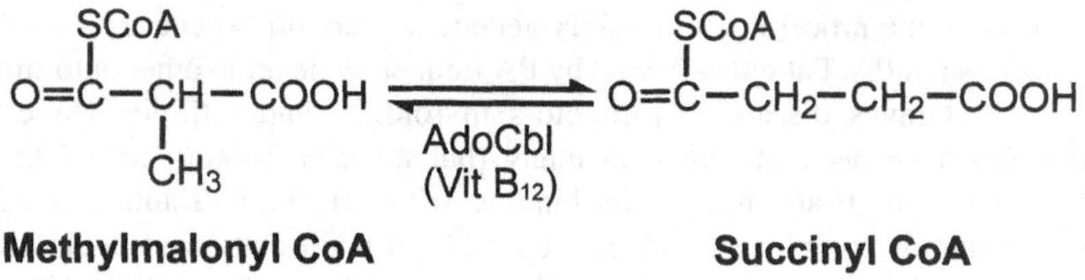

$$O{=}\overset{\overset{\displaystyle SCoA}{|}}{C}{-}\underset{\underset{\displaystyle CH_3}{|}}{CH}{-}COOH \rightleftharpoons O{=}\overset{\overset{\displaystyle SCoA}{|}}{C}{-}CH_2{-}CH_2{-}COOH$$

$$\underset{\displaystyle (Vit\ B_{12})}{AdoCbl}$$

Methylmalonyl CoA   **Succinyl CoA**

Figure 59.2   *Reaction 2*: conversion of methylmalonyl CoA to succinyl CoA requires vitamin B_{12}. A deficiency of vitamin B_{12} produces an increase in serum methylmalonic acid.

to characteristic megaloblastic hematopoiesis. Nuclear maturation is retarded compared with cytoplasmic maturation; specifically, nuclear–cytoplasmic asynchrony occurs. The result is larger cell size with immature-appearing nuclei. These changes occur in erythroid, granulocytic and megakaryocytic cell lineages. In addition, reaction 1 (Fig. 59.1) is important in regulating serum homocysteine levels (i.e., can produce hyperhomocysteinemia), while inhibition of reaction 2 (Fig. 59.2) can produce increases in methylmalonic acid.

Folate deficiency can produce a hematologic picture of megaloblastic anemia identical to that of cbl deficiency. However, the two deficiencies must be distinguished since cbl deficiency causes potentially irreversible neurological change, which is seldom seen with deficiency of only folic acid. Folate deficiency can be identified primarily by low serum and erythrocyte folate levels, elevation of homocysteine with normal levels of MMA, and correction of anemia in response to physiological (not pharmacological) doses of folate (see Table 59.1).

Subacute combined degeneration (SCD) of the spinal cord, or "neuroanemic syndrome," due to cbl deficiency may not be directly related to the block in DNA synthesis responsible for megaloblastic anemia. Pathologic changes affect primarily the white matter, and may affect the brain and peripheral nervous system as well as the spinal cord. Histopathologic features of SCD include myelin sheath swelling, degeneration, and spongy vacuolation, and, with progression, axonal degeneration and astrocytic gliosis. Recent experimental evidence suggests that SCD may be due to interference of a regulatory role of cbl in the mammalian central nervous system (CNS) involving homeostasis of myelin production and lysis via CNS cytokines and growth factors. This delicate balance becomes "upset" with cbl deficiency, and SCD can result. Neurologic disease can occur in the setting of a normal CBC and MCV in 40–50% of patients with PA. However, careful examination of the peripheral blood smear will often detect hypersegmented neutrophils.

Table 59.1   Cobalamin, Folate, and Metabolite Levels in Megaloblastic Anemia

Disorder	Cobalamin	Folate	Folate (RBC)	Homocyseine	MMA
Cobalamin deficiency	Decreased	Normal or increased	Normal or decreased	Increased	Increased
Folate deficiency	Normal	Decreased or normal	Decreased	Increased	Normal
Cobalamin and folate deficiency	Decreased	Decreased	Decreased	Increased	Increased

Clinical Features

PA is insidious in its onset. Classically, as in the case presented above, the patient presents with nonspecific signs and symptoms of anemia and with characteristic neurological abnormalities. In some patients, however, involvement may be selective, affecting either bone marrow or nervous system and having little or no effect on other organ systems. PA usually occurs after age 40 and is seen particularly in persons of northern European origin.

Weakness, fatigue, syncope, angina, lightheadedness, palpitations, pallor, dyspnea, and cardiac flow murmurs are due to the anemia per se. A minimal fever may occur; slight jaundice and scleral icterus may develop as a result of increased heme metabolism due to accelerated apoptosis of red cell precursors in the bone marrow. Purpura due to severe thrombocytopenia occurs rarely. Gastrointestinal signs and symptoms include a smooth, beefy red tongue (atrophic glossitis) with or without pain, anorexia, weight loss, and constipation or diarrhea.

Classic neurological signs and symptoms include (1) symmetric tingling and numbness in the lower extremities, progressing to diminished fine touch, vibratory, and position sense (*posterior* column degeneration) and (2) weakness, spasticity, and hyperactive deep reflexes (*lateral* column degeneration). Disease of the upper extremities is similar, but usually less severe. Irritability, forgetfulness, visual impairment, or other disturbances in mentation (confusion, depression, dementia), are less common neurological symptoms. It is important to remember that neurological sequelae of cbl deficiency may occur in the absence of anemia. Thus, neurological complaints may be the initial, presenting symptoms in patients with deficiency.

Diagnosis

Patients with PA usually have an anemia with significant macrocytosis. The peripheral blood film shows poikilocytosis and anisocytosis as well as large, fully hemoglobinized, oval macrocytes. The red blood cell distribution width (RDW) is typically increased, and reticulocyte production is usually decreased. If megaloblastic anemia develops in an individual with iron deficiency or with thalassemia minor (disorders that are characterized by microcytosis), the MCV may be in the normal range. Mild thrombocytopenia is common, as is mild leukopenia. The presence of large neutrophils with hypersegmented nuclei (>5 lobes per nucleus) is a distinctive feature of megaloblastic anemia.

Bone marrow examination characteristically shows megaloblastic hematopoiesis: marked erythroid hyperplasia with megaloblasts, giant band neutrophils, giant metamyelocytes with immature chromatin, and large megakaryocytes with nuclear separation and nuclear fragments. Iron stores are increased. However, bone marrow examination is not necessary when peripheral blood films show morphological changes consistent with megaloblastic anemia and noninvasive tests yield clear results. Bone marrow examination is indicated in a patient with macrocytic anemia that has not resolved despite therapy with folate and cobalamin.

Serum lactate dehydrogenase (LDH) is markedly elevated because of the increased intramedullary destruction of cells. *Serum iron* may be increased because of decreased erythropoiesis and iron utilization. A mild increase in *serum unconjugated bilirubin* results from ineffective erythropoiesis and hemolysis of abnormal erythrocytes.

Once megaloblastic anemia is suspected or identified, serum cbl, homocysteine, MMA, and erythrocyte and serum folate assays should be performed. Although the erythrocyte folate level may be decreased in cbl deficiency, the serum folate level is usually normal or high (see Table 59.1). This is in contrast to folate deficiency, in which serum and erythrocyte folate levels are both decreased. Clinical signs generally appear when serum cbl levels fall below 150 pg/mL, although elevations of serum homocysteine and MMA are more sensitive indicators of intracellular cbl depletion. Increases of MMA and/or homocysteine may have causes other than cbl deficiency. Observing an increased reticulocyte percent 5–7 days after administering vitamin B_{12} can differentiate cbl deficiency from folate deficiency or other causes of macrocytic anemia.

The Schilling test allows differentiation of cbl deficiency due to a small intestinal malabsorption defect due to lack of IF (PA) from other causes of deficiency. The result of stage I testing indicates ability or inability to absorb cbl in the small intestine. If inability is demonstrated, the result of stage II testing usually indicates whether malabsorption is due to lack of IF from the gastric mucosa or to an absorption defect in the small intestine. Normal absorption of labeled cbl provided with exogenous IF in the stage II test is strong evidence for a diagnosis of PA (provided that the patient has not had a gastrectomy).

A significant proportion of older people have elevated homocysteine and MMA concentrations with normal or "low–normal" serum cbl levels and an absence of classic features of PA or megaloblastic anemia. Potentially irreversible neurological diseases, including neuropsychiatric disorders, do occur in patients who are functionally cbl-deficient, suggesting that some patients may have potentially reversible disease due to unrecognized cbl deficiency. At present, patients with neurological symptoms and low–normal cbl levels should be tested for functional evidence of cbl deficiency (elevated serum homocysteine and MMA) and, if appropriate, treated and followed for signs of improvement. It is, however, unclear whether treatment of all patients (i.e., in the absence of signs or symptoms) with "low–normal" serum cbl concentrations should be undertaken.

Treatment

The mainstay of treatment of PA is replacement therapy with cbl by either oral or intramuscular injection of pharmacologic doses of synthetic cbl (cyanocobalamin or hydroxocobalamin). While parenteral cbl bypasses ileal absorption, a small amount of oral cbl is absorbed across mucosal surfaces independent of intrinsic-factor-mediated uptake. Therefore, a daily 1.0 mg oral dose of cbl compensates for the daily 1–5 μg physiologic loss. Maintenance therapy must be continued for the rest of the patient's life. Because patients with PA have an increased incidence of gastric cancer, long-term follow-up should include prompt evaluation of abnormal gastrointestinal signs and symptoms and routine periodic examinations for occult blood in stool, but routine upper endoscopy has not been shown to be cost-effective.

During the early treatment of patients with severe PA, hypokalemia may suddenly develop as a result of potassium requirements of hematopoietic cells. To prevent the possibility of cardiac arrhythmia and sudden death secondary to hypokalemia, oral potassium supplements can be started at the same time as the cbl therapy and continued during the first 10 days of treatment. Cbl deficiency should never be treated with folic acid alone. Although the hematologic abnormalities may respond partially to folic acid therapy, the neurological lesions do not respond and may progress and become irreversible.

Response to replacement therapy occurs within 1–2 days as patients experience an improved sense of well-being. Megaloblastic features of the marrow revert to normal within 2–3 days, and reticulocytosis peaks within 10 days. Normal hemoglobin levels are usually achieved within 1–2 months. Marked improvement occurs in neurological symptoms of recent onset; however, a lesser degree of improvement can be expected for longstanding neurological symptoms.

Additional Reading

BRIDDON, A.: Homocysteine in the context of cobalamin metabolism and deficiency states. *Amino Acids 24*:1–12, 2003.

CARMEL, R.: Current concepts in cobalamin deficiency. *Ann. Rev. Med. 51*:357–75, 2000.

CARMEL, R., GREEN, R., ROSENBLATT, D. S., AND WATKINS, D.: Update on cobalamin, folate and homocysteine. *Hematology* 62–81, 2003.

CHRISTENSEN, E. I. AND BIRN, H.: Megalin and cubilin: Multifunctional endocytic receptors. *Nat. Rev. Mol. Cell Biol. 3*:258–68, 2002.

DIXON, M. F., GENTA, R. M., YARDLEY, J. H. ET AL.: Classification and grading of gastritis: The updated Sydney system. *Am. J. Surg. Pathol. 20*:1161–81, 1996.

KYRLAGKITSIS, I. AND KARAMANOLIS, D. G.: Premalignant lesions and conditions for gastric adenocarcinoma: Diagnosis, management, and surveillance guidelines. *Hepato-Gastroenterology 50*:592–600, 2003.

SCALABRINO, G.: Cobalamin (vitamin B_{12}) in subacute combined degeneration and beyond: Traditional interpretations and novel theories. *Exp. Neurol. 192*:463–79, 2005.

TEFFERI, A.: Anemia in adults: A contemporary approach to diagnosis. *Mayo Clin. Proc. 78*:1274–80, 2003.

TOH, B-H., ALDERUCCIO, F.: Pernicious anemia. *Autoimmunity, 37*:357–361, 2004.

WARD, P.C.J.: Modern approaches to the investigation of vitamin B12 deficiency. *Clin. Lab Med., 22*:435–445, 2002.

WEIR, D.G. AND SCOTT, J.M.: The biochemical basis of the neuropathy in cobalamin deficiency. *Bailliere's Clin Haematol., 8*:479–97, 1995.

WHITTINGHAM, S. AND MACKAY, I.R.: Autoimmune gastritis: Historical antecedents, outstanding discoveries, and unresolved problems. *Int Rev Immunol., 24*:1–29, 2005.

Case 60

Pulseless Leg 9 Days after a Myocardial Infarction

Majed Refaai

A 32-year-old woman developed preeclampsia during her first pregnancy. Premature labor progressed to delivery of a viable infant at 31 weeks' gestation. The mother remained hypertensive, and one week postpartum awoke with severe chest pain. Emergency room evaluation was notable for systolic blood pressure 50 mm Hg, heart rate 75 bpm, and chest auscultation revealed bilateral rales. Chest radiograph interpretation was cardiomegaly with pulmonary edema. Electrocardiogram showed sinus rhythm and ST elevations in leads I, AVL, and V2, consistent with an acute anteriolateral myocardial infarction.

On admission, laboratory values were as follows:

Analyte	Value, Conventional Units	Reference Interval, Conventional Units	Value, SI Units	Reference Interval, SI Units
WBC	$15.8 \times 10^3/\mu L$	4.8–10.8	$15.8 \times 10^9/L$	4.8–10.8
Hemoglobin	12.1 g/dL	12.0–16.0	121 g/L	120–180
Hematocrit	36%	37–47	0.36 volume	0.37–0.47
MCV	101 fL	81–99	Same	
Platelet count	$406 \times 10^3/\mu L$	130–400	$406 \times 10^9/L$	130–400
aPTT	21.4 s	18–35	Same	
PT	9.0 s	9.8–11.0	Same	
LDH	269 U/L	100–190	4.6 μkat/L	1.7–3.2
Creatine kinase	9000 U/L	10–80	153 μkat/L	0.17–1.36

Cardiac catheterization identified a left main coronary artery dissection with occlusion of the left anterior descending artery. The patient underwent urgent four-vessel coronary artery bypass surgery with insertion of an intraaortic balloon pump through the right femoral artery and a left ventricular assist device (LVAD), in order to wean her from cardiopulmonary bypass. Continuous heparin infusion was begun to prevent formation of clots within the LVAD tubing and hypokinetic left ventricle. Postoperative bleeding

Tietz's Applied Laboratory Medicine, Second Edition. Edited by Mitchell G. Scott, Ann M. Gronowski, and Charles S. Eby
Copyright © 2007 John Wiley & Sons, Inc.

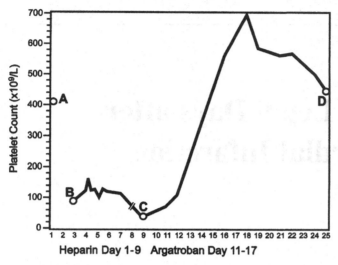

Figure 60.1   Time course of platelet count: (A) admission with acute MI, (B) after coronary artery bypass surgery; (C) pulseless right leg; (D) at discharge.

required multiple blood product transfusions and reexploration of the mediastinum to control bleeding.

The patient's cardiac function gradually improved, and on day 4 the left ventricular assist device and intraaortic balloon were removed and she was extubated. During days 4–7 platelet counts fluctuated between 163×10^9/L and 99×10^9/L while heparin infusion continued (Fig. 60.1). A platelet count was not obtained on day 8. On day 9, the patient's right leg became cold and pulseless, and her platelet count was 34×10^9/L. Heparin-induced thrombocytopenia with thrombosis (HITT) was suspected, heparin administration was stopped, and a right femoral artery thrombectomy was performed. A clinical diagnosis of HITT was supported by detection of heparin-induced thrombocytopenia (HIT) antibodies in the patient's day 9 serum, based on a positive serotonin release assay.

Analyte	Value, Conventional Units	Reference Interval, Conventional Units	Value, SI Units	Reference Interval, SI Units
Seratonin release assay				
No heparin	5%	<20%	0.05 fraction	<0.20
1.0 U/mL heparin	87%	<20%	0.87 fraction	<0.20
100 U/mL heparin	11%	<20%	0.11 fraction	<0.20

In order to prevent additional arterial or venous thromboembolic events, anticoagulation was resumed with a continuous infusion of argatroban. Infusion rate was titrated to obtain an aPTT corresponding to 1.5–3.0 × laboratory's mean normal aPTT, and warfarin was begun 3 days later. Over the next 6 days, argatroban infusion rate and warfarin dose were adjusted to obtain an INR of 2–3. The patient's platelet count rapidly recovered, and she experienced no bleeding complications or new thromboembolic events. Platelet count at discharge was 445×10^9/L (Fig. 60.1). Indefinite anticoagulation with warfarin was recommended due to severe left ventricular hypokinesis and the risk of intraventricular thrombus formation.

Differential Diagnosis

A significant decline of platelet count following 5–14 days of heparin exposure is consistent with the development of heparin-induced thrombocytopenia (HIT). However, thrombocytopenia can occur in many clinical conditions (Table 60.1), and a careful review of clinical and laboratory data is required before accepting a diagnosis of HIT. First, a low platelet count from an automated hematology analyzer must be confirmed by reviewing the peripheral blood smear to rule out pseudothrombocytopenia. Ex vivo platelet clumping may be caused by autoantibodies that only bind platelets when calcium ions are chelated by the anticoagulant in the collection tube (EDTA), or in the presence of the drug abciximab, a monoclonal antibody that blocks platelet aggregation. A rarer cause of inaccurate automated platelet counts occurs in patients with congenital macrothrombocytopenia (May–Hegglin anomaly). If the peripheral smear exam confirms thrombocytopenia, then the possible etiologies listed in Table 60.1 should be considered.

Table 60.1 Causes of Acquired Thrombocytopenia

Decreased production
  Primary bone marrow disease
  Leukemia
  Aplastic anemia
  Ionizing radiation
  Chemotherapy
  Idiosyncratic drug reactions
Increased consumption
  Immunity-mediated
    Autoantibody-mediated
      Immune thrombocytopenia purpura (ITP)
      Posttransfusion purpura (PTP)
      Thrombotic thrombocytopenia purpura (TTP)
    Drug-induced
      Heparin-induced thrombocytopenia (HIT)
      Quinine, antibiotics (vancomycin, rifampin), nonsteroidal antiinflammatory drugs, platelet
        glycoprotein IIb/IIa inhibitors: abciximab, tirofiban, eptifibatide
  Non-immunity-mediated
    Disseminated intravascular coagulation (DIC) due to sepsis, trauma, cancer
    Obstetric complications (preeclampsia, amniotic fluid embolism)
    Extracorporal circulation (heart–lung bypass)
Sequstration
  Hypersplenism due to portal hypertension
  Arteriovenous malformations
Dilution
  Acute blood loss replacement with only fluids and red blood cells

Definition

HIT is defined as an otherwise unexplained decline in platelet count, during or shortly after heparin exposure, accompanied by formation of heparin-dependent autoantibodies. Because of its relatively high frequency and association with venous and arterial thromboses, HIT is considered to be the most serious form of drug-induced thrombocytopenia.

The typical presentation of HIT is a decline in platelet count starting during days 5–10 of heparin exposure. Usually, the platelet count falls more than 50% below the pre-heparin exposure baseline platelet count, and the nadir is less than $100 \times 10^9/L$ but rarely less than $20 \times 10^9/L$. However, patients who develop HIT may have a normal platelet count ($>150 \times 10^9/L$) if their baseline platelet counts were elevated. Despite thrombocytopenia, bruising and bleeding are not features of HIT. Instead, thrombotic complications occur in 30–50% of HIT patients, either concurrent with the onset of thrombocytopenia, or up to 30 days later. Venous thromboses are more common than arterial events, except in patients with underlying chronic or acute arterial damage such as the femoral artery trauma associated with intraaortic balloon pump placement as in this patient. Skin necrosis at injection sites with or without thrombocytopenia can occur in patients who develop HIT while receiving subcutaneous injections of UFH. Rarely, HIT can present with disseminated intravascular coagulation, transient global amnesia, and adrenal cortical necrosis.

Following discontinuation of heparin exposure, the platelet count typically begins to recover within several days. Subsequent reexposure to heparin may lead to rapid (<24 hours) thrombocytopenia in a patient with persistence of HIT antibodies. Fortunately, HIT antibodies usually are undetectable 2–3 months after heparin discontinuation, and brief reexposure can be done successfully in special circumstances when alternative anticoagulants are not practical. For example, cardiothoracic surgery using heparin during cardiopulmonary bypass has been successfully performed in patients with a history of HIT more than 100 days before surgery in whom HIT antibodies were no longer detectable.

The incidence of HIT varies among patient populations. Frequencies of $\leq 1\%$ have been reported in patients receiving UFH for initial treatment of venous thrombosis, atrial fibrillation, and acute coronary syndrome. Higher frequencies were noted in patients undergoing different medical or surgical procedures that required UFH such as hemodialysis (3.9%), cardiothoracic surgery (2.3%), and orthopedic surgery (5%). HIT also occurs in patients who receive prophylactic or therapeutic doses of low-molecular-weight heparin (LMWH), but the incidence is much lower compared to UFH. HIT has been linked to minimal exposure to UFH from arterial and venous line flushes and heparin-coated catheters as well, although these appear to be rare events.

Pathophysiology

HIT is an acquired, autoantibody-mediated, prothrombotic state resulting in platelet activation, aggregation, and consumption (Fig. 60.2). Heparin binds to circulating platelet factor 4 (PF4), a member of the C–X–C subfamily of chemokines, which is stored in platelet α granules. Heparin–PF4 complexes expose neoepitopes on PF4 that trigger the formation of PF4 autoantibodies (predominantly IgG isotype), in a minority of patients. Binding of heparin–PF4–IgG immune complexes to immunoglobin heavy-chain (Fc) receptors on the platelet surfaces initiates platelet activation in a subset of at-risk patients. Activated platelets release more PF4 and perpetuate the platelet activation cycle. Activation also leads to platelet aggregation and the production of platelet

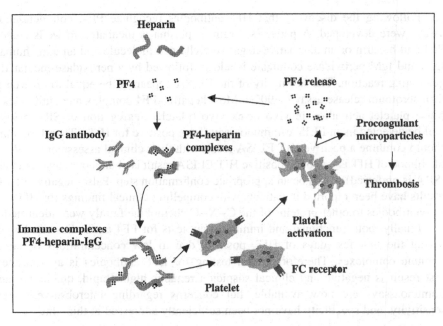

Figure 60.2   Pathophysiology of HIT. (Adapted from Aster, R. H.: *N. Engl. J. Med. 332*:1374–6, 1995.)

microparticles, leading to platelet consumption and thrombin generation, respectively. In addition, heparin sulfate, a heparin-like molecule expressed on the surface of endothelial cells, may contribute to the HIT procoagulant state. Heparan sulfate–PF4–IgG immune complexes can induce endothelial cell expression of tissue factor. This may partially explain the occurrence of delayed thrombotic complications in HIT patients following removal of heparin exposure.

Laboratory Detection of HIT Antibodies

Since HIT is a clinical–pathologic diagnosis, laboratory tests that detect HIT antibodies can be useful when combined with the patient's clinical picture. HIT antibodies can be detected with functional assays that monitor activation of fresh, control platelets when exposed to a patient's serum in the presence of heparin, and immunoassays that detect antibodies that bind to PF4. Platelet aggregation is a popular method because of the availability of aggregometer instruments, despite its low sensitivity (50–81%), and specificity of almost 100%. Aggregation of control platelets in the presence of a patient's serum and therapeutic concentration of UFH will essentially confirm the diagnosis of HIT, but a negative result cannot exclude it.

The platelet serotonin release assay (SRA) is more sensitive than the platelet aggregation assay, however, it is offered by only a handful of reference laboratories. Patient serum is incubated with control platelets containing ^{14}C-labeled serotonin and a range of heparin concentrations. In the presence of serum containing HIT antibodies and a therapeutic UFH concentration, the control platelets are activated and release radiolabeled serotonin. Specificity is improved by requiring minimal activation in the absence, or at supratherapeutic concentrations, of UFH. The sensitivity of this test ranges within 85–94%, with a specificity approaching 100%.

Following the discovery that HIT antibodies recognize PF4, commercial ELISA assays were developed. A patient's serum or plasma is incubated in wells coated with PF4 and heparin or an alternative negatively charged molecule and an anti–human IgG, IgA, and IgM-peroxidase conjugate is added, followed by a peroxidase-mediated color-generating reaction. The sensitivity of the ELISA appears to be equal to or even greater than serotonin release assay (>90%). Most heparin–PF4 complex autoantibodies do not cause platelet activation in vivo or ex vivo (platelet aggregation or SRA assays), yet will be detected in an ELISA immunoassay (false positive for HIT). Therefore, clinicians should combine a positive HIT ELISA result with their clinical assessment. If the pretest likelihood of HIT is low but a positive HIT ELISA result is obtained, a functional HIT test (SRA is preferred) would be an appropriate confirmation step. False-negative PF4 ELISA results have been reported in patients with compelling clinical findings for HIT in whom autoantibodies to other proteins of the C–X–C chemokine family were identified.

Finally, both functional and immunoassay tests for PF4 antibodies can be negative during the first few days of HIT, possibly due to low concentrations of circulating immune complexes. Therefore, serial testing for HIT antibodies is appropriate if the first result is negative and clinical suspicion remains high. Rapid, qualitative anti-PF4 immunoassays are now available, but concerns regarding interobserver agreement, sensitivity, and specificity have not been sufficiently addressed at this time.

Management

In order to diminish the consequences of concurrent thromboses, and prevent subsequent ones, all forms of heparin exposure must be discontinued immediately when HIT is suspected, and a different anticoagulant should be started. Heparin is replaced by saline in pressure monitoring lines and intravenous flush solutions, and heparin-bonded catheters are removed. Since HIT patients rarely bleed, platelet transfusions, which theoretically might contribute to platelet activation and thrombosis, are not routinely indicated.

Starting warfarin in a thrombocytopenic HIT patient may increase the risk for dermal and subcutaneous venous thromboses and venous limb gangrene since warfarin introduces an additional prothrombotic risk factor by decreasing protein C before adequate suppression of prothrombin activity. Low-molecular-weight heparin preparations are also unacceptable substitutions since HIT antibodies can cross-react with LMWHs, prolonging thrombocytopenia and the risk of thrombotic complications. Fortunately, three parenteral drugs that directly inhibit the catalytic site of thrombin and do not cross-react with HIT antibodies have been available since the late 1990s. Lepirudin is a recombinant form of hirudin, a direct thrombin inhibitor (DTI) found in the saliva of the medicinal leech. Bivalirudin is another recombinant direct thrombin inhibitor derived from hirudin. They both bind irreversibly to thrombin and are excreted renally. Some patients may form antibodies to lepirudin that prolong the drug's half-life. Argatroban is a synthetic, reversible, direct thrombin inhibitor that undergoes hepatic metabolism. Similar to UFH, DTIs are administered as continuous infusions with immediate anticoagulant activity, require therapeutic monitoring using the aPTT, and have short half-lives (0.5–1.5 hours). Unlike UFH, which can be rapidly neutralized by protamine, there are no reversal agents for DTIs. This is particularly important for HIT patients undergoing cardiopulmonary bypass surgery in which anticoagulation with a DTI increases the risk of severe postoperative bleeding due to prolonged anticoagulation. HIT patients who require prolonged anticoagulation may be started on warfarin once thrombocytopenia is resolved, continuing a DTI until a therapeutic INR is obtained. Clinical trials of oral DTIs are under way and may soon be an alternative anticoagulant for HIT patients.

Danaparoid (Orgaran) and fondaparinux (Arixtra) are anticoagulants that may be used in HIT patients under certain circumstances. Danaparoid is prepared from porcine tissue and contains heparinlike molecules that predominantly accelerate antithrombin inhibition of factor Xa, while Arixtra is a synthetic molecule that specifically accelerates antithrombin inhibition of factor Xa. They are given subcutaneously, have long half-lives (25 and 17 hours, respectively), and both show either absent (Arixtra) or negligible (danaparoid) in vitro cross-reactivity with HIT antibodies.

Summary

Close monitoring of platelet counts is indicated for all patients receiving heparin to assure prompt recognition of HIT. Clinical assessment combined with laboratory tests to detect heparin–PF4 autoantibody complexes are helpful in establishing the diagnosis of this acquired hypercoaguable state. Alternative anticoagulantion options are effective in reducing serious morbidity and mortality from thromboembolic complications.

Additional Reading

AREPALLY, G., REYNOLDS, C., TOMASKI, A. ET AL.: Comparison of PF4/Heparin ELISA assay with the ^{14}C-serotonin release assay in the diagnosis of heparin-induced thrombocytopenia. *Am. J. Clin. Pathol.* *104*:648–54, 1995.

AREPALLY, G. M., ORTEL, T. L., Heparin-induced thrombocytopenia. *N. Engl. J. Med.* *355*:809–17, 2006.

ASTER, R. H.: Immune thrombocytopenias casued by glycoprotein IIb/IIIa inhibitors. *Chest 127*(suppl 2):53S–59S, 2005.

BERKMAN, N., MICHAELI, Y., Or, R., AND ELDOR, A.: EDTA-dependent pseudothrombocytopenia: A clinical study of 18 patients and review of the literature. *Am. J. Hematol. 36*:195–201, 1991.

CHONG, B. H., BURGERSS, J., AND ISMAIL, F.: The clinical usefulness of platelet aggregation test for the diagnosis of heparin-induced thrombocytopenia. *Thromb. Haemost. 69*:344–50, 1995.

CINES, D. B., TOMASKI, A., AND TANNENBAUM, S.: Immune endothelial-cell injury in heparin-associated thrombocytopenia. *N. Engl. J. Med. 316*:581–9, 1987.

DAVOREN, A. AND ASTER, R. H.: Heparin-induced thrombocytopenia and thrombosis. *Am. J. Hematol. 81*:36–44, 2006.

HIRSH, J., HEDDLE, N., AND KELTON, J. G.: Treatment of heparin-induced thrombocytopenia. *Arch. Intern. Med. 64*:361–9, 2004.

SHERIDAN, D., CARTER, C., AND KELTON, J. G.: A diagnostic test for heparin-induced thrombocytopenia. *Blood 67*:27–30, 1986.

WARKENTIN, T. E. AND GREINACHER, A.: Heparin-induced thrombocytopenia: Recognition, treatment, and prevention. *Chest 126*:311S–337S, 2004.

WARKENTIN, T. E. AND KELTON, J. G.: A 14-year study of heparin-induced thrombocytopenia. *Am. J. Med. 101*:502–7, 1996.

WARKENTIN, T. E., LEVINE, M. N., HIRSH, J. ET AL.: Heparin-induced thrombocytopenia in patients treated with low-molecular weight heparin or unfractionated heparin. *N. Engl. J. Med. 332*:1330–5, 1995.

Case 61

Young Girl with a Bloody Knee Effusion

Danielle Stueber

A 2-year-old girl was seen at a university hospital for a swollen left knee. The knee was tender, and the child was tearful and had refused to walk over the last 48 hours. x-Ray studies revealed an opaque effusion. The knee was aspirated and frank blood returned. The child had an extensive history of unexplained bruising and prolonged excessive bleeding with mouth trauma.

The following laboratory results were reported:

Analyte	Value, Conventional Units	Reference Interval, Conventional Units	Value, SI Units	Reference Interval, SI Units
Platelet count	$348 \times 10^3/\mu L$	140–400	$348 \times 10^9/L$	140–400
PT	12.7 s	11–15 s	Same	
aPTT	80 s	23–35	Same	
aPTT 50 : 50 mix	35 s	23–35	Same	
Factor XI activity	78%	50–150	0.78 IU	0.05–1.50
Factor IX activity	109%	50–150	1.09 IU	0.05–1.50
Factor VIII activity	4%	50–200	0.04 IU	0.50–200
Von Willebrand factor antigen	94%	50–200	0.94 IU	0.05–2.00
Von Willebrand factor activity	88%	50–200	0.88 IU	0.50–2.00

Based on a factor VIII activity of 4% and a normal von Willebrand factor (vWF) activity, a diagnosis of moderate hemophilia A was made. She was treated with whole-blood replacement therapy from private donors and recovered. At age 4, she experienced a severe bleed into the right ankle joint and was treated with a commercial factor VIII concentrate prior to the era of mandatory testing of plasma for pathogens and viral inactivation treatment of concentrates. Approximately one month later, she presented with lethargy, nausea, vomiting, and icteric sclerae. A diagnosis of non-A, non-B viral hepatitis was made and she was given a guarded prognosis for recovery. Over the course of the

Tietz's Applied Laboratory Medicine, Second Edition. Edited by Mitchell G. Scott, Ann M. Gronowski, and Charles S. Eby
Copyright © 2007 John Wiley & Sons, Inc.

443

following year, she gradually regained strength and seemed to recover completely, although no follow-up viral studies were done at that time.

She continued to do well with sporadic hemarthroses after minimal trauma. She was treated conservatively at home with bed rest, ace wraps, and ice for these infrequent episodes, and was rarely treated with antihemophilic factor. Although susceptible to mucous membrane hemorrhage, she did not experience disabling menorrhagia. A trial of DDAVP did not appreciably increase circulating factor VIII activity.

Family history was negative for other males or females with clinical or laboratory evidence of factor VIII deficiency, including one sister and three brothers.

As an adult, the patient and her parents underwent genetic testing for factor VIII mutations. She was heterozygous for an intron 22 inversion that was not detected in either parent. Routine laboratory studies at the time revealed immunity to hepatitis C with undetectable viral load by polymerase chain reaction. Liver enzymes were also in the normal range.

Pregnancy was planned, and the following year she gave birth to a healthy, term daughter. The mother was maintained on prophylactic antihemophilic factor from the onset of labor until day 10 postpartum and experienced no hemorrhage or soft tissue hematoma. Four years later, she gave birth to a healthy, term son. Cord blood samples taken at delivery showed a PTT of 73 s and undetectable factor VIII activity, consistent with severe hemophilia A. The infant underwent routine CT scan of the brain to detect any bleeding, which was normal. Prophylactic recombinant factor VIII was infused immediately prior to circumcision and every 12 hours for three subsequent days to prevent hemorrhage from the site.

Clinical Aspects of the Disease

Hemophilia is a sex-linked bleeding disorder that affects 1 in 5000 males and 1 in 5 million females worldwide. Hemophilic persons are deficient in either factor VIII (FVIII) or factor IX (FIX) coagulation proteins. Historically, these two forms are known as *hemophilia A*, or "classic hemophilia," and *hemophilia B*, or "Christmas disease," respectively. Other proteins or factors can also be deficient, leading to a bleeding tendency or a frank bleeding disorder. A brief summary of hereditary bleeding disorders follows at the end of this case. All bleeding disorders require a thorough workup in order to properly administer therapy, which is specific to each disorder.

Factor VIII deficiency is 6 times more common than factor IX deficiency, but the two are clinically indistinguishable. Because of the diversity in genetic mutations, there is a wide range of clinical severity in both types of hemophilia. Persons with FVIII or FIX activities <40% are considered hemophilic. They are classified according to the percent of circulating active FVIII or FIX in venous blood samples, which corresponds to three clinical phenotypes: mild (6–40%), moderate (1–5%), or severe (<1% or undetectable). The bleeding diathesis is lifelong, and the type and frequency of bleeding complications are consistent within each class. The phenotypic expression of hemophilia is constant throughout the life of an individual and is similar in all affected members of a given family. Characteristic for all forms of hemophilia is the lack of excessive bleeding from superficial cuts, due to normal primary hemostasis achieved by platelets and vWF.

The differences among the clinical pictures of severe and mild hemophilia are remarkable (see Table 61.1). A severely affected hemophilic patient, like the infant described above, shows hemorrhagic diathesis during the neonatal period. In about 50% of unanticipated patients, the first bleeding episode occurs at the time of circumcision. Later in life,

Table 61.1 Clinical Forms of Hemophilia

Severity (% of normal)	aPTT (sec)	Clinical manifestations
Severe (<1%)	>65	Severe bleeding into skin, joints, muscles, often with a delayed onset, may occur even after unrecognized trauma; the disorder is usually evident in the first year of life; prophylactic therapy is recommended to prevent and arrest hemorrhage
Moderate (1–5%)	50–65	Extensive bleeding occurs after trauma, but spontaneous bleeding and hemarthrosis are less common; the need for replacement varies from sporadic to relatively frequent
Mild (6–40%)	35–45	Absence of spontaneous bleeding; excessive bleeding occurs only after major trauma or surgery; the patient may remain undiagnosed for several years

untreated severe hemophilic patients experience around 15 bleeding episodes per year into joints and muscles, which leads to debilitating arthropathy. In contrast, a mildly affected patient may remain free of serious bleeding for a long period of time and is seldom diagnosed before adolescence or early adulthood. This woman expresses a phenotype that falls in between the extremes. She was diagnosed in childhood, experiences hemarthrosis and intramuscular bleeding at irregular intervals, usually after an identifiable trauma, and does not suffer from spontaneous hemorrhage. In addition, she is also susceptible to intraabdominal bleeding from ovulation.

Genetics

Hemophilia A and B are transmitted by different genes on the long arm of the X chromosome and so manifest a complex, sex-linked inheritance pattern. The sons of a hemophilic man do not inherit hemophilia because they receive a paternal Y, not X, chromosome; their maternal X chromosome bears normal genes. All daughters of a hemophilic father receive his X chromosome and are therefore obligatory carriers of hemophilia. Since their second, maternal, chromosome presumably is normal, they will transmit hemophilia with a 50% probability to their sons. Similarly, the probability is 50% for their daughters to be carriers. Very rarely, a hemophilic father and asymptomatic carrier mother will produce a hemophilic daughter.

Unequal partitioning of genetic material on the XY pair is responsible for X-linked recessive diseases, and recessive mutations on the X chromosome are expressed in males (resulting in hemophilia or colorblindness) and usually silent in females. The Lyon hypothesis of X inactivation in somatic cells predicts that carriers should have FVIII activities of approximately 50% when half of the maternal X and half of the paternal X genes are randomly inactivated. What is seen clinically and molecularly in female patients resembles a Gaussian distribution of X inactivation rather than an ideal 50/50 phenotypic mosaic. In other words, a woman with one normal and one hemophilic gene could have FVIII activity ranging from 1% to 100%, averaging around 50%. Therefore, some women with one hemophilic gene will experience hemorrhagic symptoms. As a child, this patient sought medical attention for multiple mucosal membrane hemorrhages and extensive bruising of the skin and soft tissues. However, the diagnosis of hemophilia A was not made until she presented with hemarthrosis. Bleeding into the joints is uncommon except in patients with bleeding disorders. While hemophilia in women is rare, bleeding disorders in women are not rare and any abnormal bleeding deserves careful hematologic investigation.

About 30% of A and B hemophiliacs have "sporadic" hemophilia; that is, there is no family history of the disorder. Typically, a de novo mutation occurs during spermatogenesis in the maternal grandfather, and the affected boy's mother is an asymptomatic carrier. Thousands of different mutations have been identified in hemophiliacs, ranging from large deletions, inversions, and non-sense mutations that severely limit or prevent production of factor VIII or IX, to minor deletions, insertions, or missense mutations that produce more subtle quantitative or qualitative protein modifications. Approximately 50% of patients with severe hemophilia A inherit an X chromosome on which the factor VIII gene has undergone an inversion and homologous recombination between intron 22(45%) or 1(5%) and a nearby region outside of the gene, disrupting transcription of a complete FVIII mRNA. The first step in genetic testing of patients and female carriers of severe hemophilia A is to apply molecular diagnostic methods that detect FVIII inversions as was performed in this case.

Complications of Hemophilia

Until the advent of AIDS, the major causes of mortality and morbidity were hemorrhage and severe arthropathies. Acute hemarthroses are exquisitely painful. Recurrent joint bleeds cause synovial hypertrophy, which is even more vulnerable to spontaneous bleeding and local inflammatory responses that damage cartilage and subchondral bone. Inadequately treated joint bleeds in knees, elbows, and ankles eventually lead to severe contractions, reduced mobility, muscle wasting, and consideration of joint replacement surgery.

The wide availability of commercial factor VIII and IX concentrates in the 1970s reduced the severity and frequency of bleeding complications, but came at the cost of hepatitis C and HIV infections. There have been no new cases of HIV infection linked to plasma-derived factor concentrates since 1986, due to effective screening of plasma donors and viral inactivation procedures during the manufacturing process. Similar success has been achieved in prevention of hepatitis C transmission. However, there are many hemophilics still coping with HIV infection and progressive liver disease due to chronic hepatitis C infection.

Up to one-third of patients with severe hemophilia A and 3–5% of patients with severe hemophilia B who have been treated with blood products develop neutralizing alloantibodies to factor VIII or factor IX, respectively, due to mutations that prevent synthesis of complete FVIII or FIX proteins. Antibodies to infused FVIII and FIX rarely occur in patients with moderately severe or mild hemophilia who have diminished amounts of full-length FVIII or FIX protein circulating. Although presence of an antibody, also called an "inhibitor," does not increase the frequency of hemorrhage, it will complicate management of bleeding episodes if the inhibitor is potent (high-titer), and/or inducible. A persistent, high-titer inhibitor will neutralize an initial infusion of clotting factor. A low-titer but inducible inhibitor minimally neutralizes infused factor at first, but within a few days, the antibody titer rises rapidly (amnestic response). When replacement therapy is withheld, the inhibitor activity gradually decreases or even disappears but will reappear with the next infusion. Regimens of immune tolerance have been developed to eliminate inhibitors, but these therapies are costly and often require intensive treatment over a year or more.

Laboratory Diagnosis

Both factor IX and factor VIII participate in the process of blood coagulation as an enzyme–cofactor complex (FIXa–FVIIIa) essential for the activation of factor X (Fig. 61.1). Selective deficiency of either factor IX or factor VIII contributes to a more or less extensive prolongation of the aPTT while other screening clotting assays (prothrombin time, thrombin time) remain normal. Coagulation factor activities are performed by combining patient plasma with plasma completely deficient in the specific factor of interest, and then performing an aPTT for intrinsic factors or a PT for extrinsic and common pathway factors (Fig. 61.1). The degree of correction of the factor-deficient plasma's prolonged aPTT or PT following mixing with patient plasma is compared to the correction obtained with dilutions of normal pooled plasma (NPP), and expressed as percent activity. Reference intervals for coagulation factor activities typically range within 50–150%.

For detection of an inhibitor, a simple screening test can be used. If an inhibitor is present, incubation of a 50 : 50 mixture of patient plasma and NPP will lengthen the aPTT of normal plasma to a pronounced degree. Once a positive mixing study is obtained, the strength of the inhibitor is quantitated by performing mixing studies with NPP and

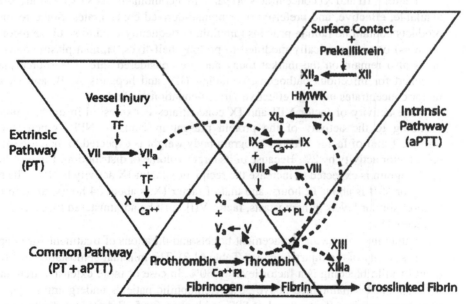

Figure 61.1 Coagulation cascade. Coagulation is initiated by exposure of blood to tissue factor (TF), which combines with factor VII/VIIa to activate factors X and IX. Factor Xa converts prothrombin to thrombin, which activates cofactors V and VIII and factor XI to produce a rapid and sustained generation of thrombin. Thrombin converts fibrinogen to fibrin, which spontaneously polymerizes with other fibrin molecules to form a weak gel. It is at this point that coagulation instruments detect clot formation. Covalent crosslinking of fibin molecules by factor XIIIa (another substrate of thrombin) produces a durable fibrin clot.

serial dilutions of the patient's plasma, then measuring the residual factor FVIII or FIX activity after incubation for 2 hours at 37°C. The *Bethesda titer* is defined as the reciprocal of the dilution of patient plasma that neutralizes 50% of factor VIII or factor IX activity present in NPP.

When a decreased factor VIII activity is detected, as seen in the young woman in this case, further testing of von Willebrand factor is necessary in order to distinguish hemophilia A from von Willebrand disease (see Case 64). The von Willebrand factor is a multimeric plasma protein with two important functions in hemostasis: (1) it mediates platelet adhesion to the vessel wall at the site of injury and (2) it transports and stabilizes factor VIII in the circulation. Consequently, an apparent deficiency of factor VIII may be secondary to deficiency of von Willebrand factor. In the case presented, the concentration of von Willebrand factor was normal.

Treatment

Replacement therapy in hemophilia is geared to prevent debilitating arthropathies from day-to-day living as well as to prevent excessive bleeding from accidental traumas and invasive procedures. Patients with severe disease are recommended to start prophylactic, regular infusions every other day to maintain circulating factor VIII or factor IX levels above 1%. Prophylactic infusions begin in infancy between the first and second years of life or after the first joint bleed. Patients with moderate or mild hemophilia are treated with factor replacement as needed for trauma and before surgery or dental work.

Factor VIII and XI concentrates prepared in recombinant DNA expression systems are available, effective, and preferred over human-derived concentrates. Some recombinant products contain no human proteins (albumin is frequently used to stabilize recombinant proteins) or are genetically modified to prolong half-lives. Human-plasma-derived products also remain on the market today and are considered safe. The source plasma is screened for infectious pathogens, including HIV and hepatitis A, B, and C, and the factor concentrates undergo effective viral attenuation methods.

The activity of factor VIII and IX concentrates is expressed in units, 1 unit corresponding to the activity of the protein present in 1 mL of NPP. When calculating dosage, 1 unit of factor VIII per kilogram body weight is expected to increase the recipient's factor activity by 2%. Because of its larger volume of distribution, 1 unit of factor IX per kilogram is expected to increase the recipient's factor IX activity by 1%. The half-life of factor VIII is about 12 hours, and that of factor IX is about 24 hours; thus, in order to support similar levels of hemostasis, factor VIII must be administered twice as frequently as factor IX.

Guidelines for factor replacement targets and durations of treatment vary depending on the severity of the injury (e.g., see Table 61.2). The minimal hemostatic level for treatment of mild bleeding is a factor level of 30%. In case of more extensive trauma, factor level should be maintained above 50%. Hemophilic patients undergoing major surgical operations require a factor level of 80%, or higher, for 5–7 days in order to remain free of hemorrhage.

Hemophiliacs with clinically significant inhibitors (Bethesda titers >5–10) cannot achieve reliable hemostasis by simply increasing the amount of infused factor VIII or IX. In 1998, recombinant factor VIIa was approved for treatment of hemophiliacs with

Table 61.2   Clinical Indications for Coagulation Factor Concentrates

Derived from human plasma	
Intermediate-purity FVIII	Von Willebrand factor replacement
Prothrombin complex concentrate	Factors FX and FII deficiencies
Highly purified using monocloncal antibodies	
Monoclonal FVIII	Hemophilia A
Monoclonal IX	Hemophilia B
Recombinant factor concentrates	
Complete factor VIII molecule	Hemophilia A
B-Domain-deleted factor VIII	Hemophilia A
Complete factor IX molecule	Hemophilia B
Factor VIIa	Hemophilics with inhibitors; FVII deficient

inhibitors. In pharmacologic doses, rFVIIa activates factor X, which generates adequate thrombin at sites of vessel injury to produce a hemostatic fibrin plug. To prevent bleeding complications from major surgery or trauma, rFVIIa must be infused every 2–3 hours because of its short half-life. Thrombotic complications are extremely rare in hemophiliacs with inhibitors who receive rFVIIa, However, off-label use of rFVIIa in nonhemophiliacs with various hemorrhagic emergencies has been associated with an increased risk of arterial thromboembolic events.

1-Desamino-8-D-arginine vasopressin (DDAVP), an analog of the hormone vasopressin, is helpful for treatment of some patients with mild and moderate hemophilia A during dental and other minor surgical procedures. DDAVP stimulates release of factor VIII and von Willebrand factor from endothelial stores into the circulation. Antifibrinolytic agents such as ε-aminocaproic acid and tranexamic acid inhibit clot lysis by blocking the binding of plasmin to its substrate, fibrin. These drugs are useful adjuvants to factor infusions or DDAVP treatment.

Other treatment modalities are currently under development and include new methods of modifying the gene to increase protein half-life, to upregulate expression in transgenic models and gene transfer through viral vectors, among others. The factor VIII gene is one of the best characterized in the genome and the clinical, and laboratory features of the disease make it a good model for gene therapy trials since there are both small and large hemophilia animal models, the protein can be manufactured in more than one tissue bed in vivo, and there is a broad therapeutic range (1–100%). In addition, clinical aspects of the disease are closely linked to discrete protein activities and can be measured by a blood test. Gene therapy trials in humans to date have demonstrated safety and variable efficacy.

Other Bleeding Disorders

With the exception of factor XII, prekallikrein, and high-molecular-weight kininogen (HWMK), deficiency of any component of the coagulation cascade can lead to clinically significant bleeding (Table 61.3). In addition, inherited disorders of collagen (Ehlers–Danlos syndrome) and platelet function (Glanzman's thrombasthenia, Bernard–Soulier syndrome; see Case 64) also manifest bleeding symptoms ranging from mild bruising to life-threatening hemorrhage.

Table 61.3   Common and Uncommon Heritable Bleeding Disorders

Coagulation protein deficiency	Inheritence pattern	Prevalence	Symptoms
Factor V (labile factor)	Autosomal recessive	1 per 1 million births	Can have profuse bleeding
Factor VII	Autosomal recessive	1 per 500,000 births	Variable severity, including mucosal bleeding (epistaxis, menorrhagia, dental extractions), hemarthrosis, intramuscular hemorrhage, postsurgical, and trauma hemorrhage
Factor VIII (antihemophilic factor)	X-linked recessive	1 per 5000 male births, 1 per 5 million female births	Mucosal bleeding (epistaxis, dental extractions), hemarthrosis, intramuscular hemorrhage, postsurgical, and trauma hemorrhage
von Willebrand disease, type 1 and 2 variants	Usually autosomal dominant	~0.1% prevalence	Considered a risk factor for postsurgical hemorrhage, mucosal bleeding (epistaxis, menorrhagia, dental extractions), hemarthrosis rare except in type 3 variant, postsurgical, and trauma hemorrhage
Type 3 variant	Autosomal recessive	1 per 1 million births	
Factor IX (Christmas factor)	X-linked recessive	1 per 30,000 male births	Mucosal bleeding (epistaxis, dental extractions), hemarthrosis, intramuscular hemorrhage, postsurgical, and trauma hemorrhage
Factor X (Stuart–Prower factor)	Autosomal recessive	1 per 500,000 births	Mucosal bleeding (epistaxis, dental extractions), hemarthrosis, intramuscular hemorrhage, postsurgical, and trauma hemorrhage
Factor XI (hemophilia C)	Autosomal dominant; severe type is autosomal recessive	~4% Ashkenazi Jews; 1 per 1 million general population	Less severe than other deficiencies; increased risk for postsurgical hemorrhage of mucosal membranes (prostate, tonsillectomy, dental extractions)
Factor XIII	Autosomal recessive	1 per 3 million births	Cranial bleeding with mild trauma, easy bruisability, poor wound healing, scar dehiscence, hemarthroses

Additional Reading

BERNTORP, E. AND MICHIELS, J. J.: A healthy hemophilic patient without arthropathy: From concept to clinical reality. *Semin. Thromb. Hemostatsis 29*:5–10, 2003.

BOLTON-MAGGS, P. AND PASI, J. K.: Haemophilias A and B. *Lancet 361*:1801–9, 2003.

HIGH, K. A.: Gene transfer as an approach to treating hemophilia. *Semin. Thromb. Hemostatsis 29*:107–19, 2003.

LETHAGEN, S.: Desmopressin in mild hemophilia A: Indications, limitations, efficacy, and safety. *Semin. Thromb. Hemostatsis 29*:101–6, 2003.

PEYVANDI, F., ASSELTA, R., AND MANNUCCI, P. M.: Autosomal recessive deficiencies of coagulation factors. *Rev. Clin. Exp. Hematol. 5*:369–88, 2001.

PRUTHI, R. K.: Hemophilia: A practical approach to genetic testing. *Mayo Clin. Proc. 80*:1485–99, 2005.

SHAPIRO, A. D.: Recombinant factor VIIa in the treatment of bleeding in hemophilic children with inhibitors. *Semin. Thromb. Hemostatsis 26*:413–41, 2000.

SRIVASTAVA, A.: Dose and response in haemophilia—optimization of factor replacement therapy. *Br. J. Haematol. 227*:12–25, 2004.

Case 62

A Young Man with Chest Pain Following a Knee Injury

Ganesh C. Kudva

A previously healthy 32-year-old Caucasian man suffered a ligament injury to his left knee while playing soccer. His leg was immobilized in a long leg splint. A few days later he was admitted to the hospital with left-sided chest pain and dyspnea. Physical examination revealed no swelling in either lower extremity. Ventilation–perfusion scan demonstrated a left lower lobe pulmonary embolism (PE). Ultrasonography of his lower extremities failed to show evidence of deep venous thrombosis (DVT). He was anticoagulated initially with intravenous unfractionated heparin and subsequently with warfarin. Family history revealed that his maternal grandmother had a DVT in her 40s. Routine laboratory tests included a normal CBC and basic and complete metabolic panel.

Laboratory results for thrombophilia risk factors were as follows:

Analyte	Value, Conventional Units	Reference Interval, Conventional Units	Value, SI Units	Reference Interval, SI Units
aPTT	29 s	25–36	Same	
PT	13.1 s	12.1–14.4	Same	
Activated protein C resistance ratio	1.2	>1.6	Same	
Factor V Leiden mutation	Heterozygous	Not detected	Same	
Prothrombin G20210A mutation	Heterozygous	Not detected	Same	
Antithrombin activity	129%	85–130	1.29 IU	0.85–1.30
Fasting homocysteine	20.9 μmol/L	4.0–12	Same	
Fibrinogen	299 mg/dL	170–400	2.99 g/L	1.70–4.00
Factor VIII activity	117%	45–225	1.17 IU	0.45–2.25
Factor IX activity	150%	70–180	1.50 IU	0.7–1.80
Anticardiolipin antibodies	Negative	Negative	Same	
Lupus anticoagulant	Negative	Negative	Same	

Tietz's Applied Laboratory Medicine, Second Edition. Edited by Mitchell G. Scott, Ann M. Gronowski, and Charles S. Eby
Copyright © 2007 John Wiley & Sons, Inc.

Table 62.1   Transient VTE Risk Factors

Venous catheters
Heart failure
Immobilization
Trauma
Surgery
Heparin-induced thrombocytopenia (HIT; see Case 60)
Pregnancy and postpartum
Estrogen therapy (birth control pills and hormone replacement therapy)
Prolonged travel (especially air travel)

He remained on warfarin (target INR 2-3) with no further recurrences for $3\frac{1}{2}$ years when anticoagulation was stopped because the venous thromboembolism was provoked by knee injury and subsequent immobilization of the leg. He continues to take Foltx (vitamins B_6, folic acid, and B_{12}) for hyperhomocysteinemia.

Definition

Deep venous thrombosis (DVT) of the lower extremities and consequent pulmonary embolism (PE) is a major cause of morbidity and mortality with an estimated incidence of over 600,000 cases and 60,000 deaths annually in the United States. The incidence of venous thromboembolism (VTE) rises with age, becoming increasingly common over the age of 60.

Risk factors for VTE can be divided into those that are transient (Table 62.1), which are present in about 50–60% of patients, and persistent; the latter is referred to as *thrombophilia* (Table 62.2). In about 50% of cases without transient risk factors (unprovoked) clinical and/or laboratory risk factors are not identified (idiopathic). Estimates of the frequency of inherited thrombophilia risk factors in unprovoked VTE cases are listed in Table 62.2.

Diagnosis of Venous Thromboembolism

VTE should be suspected in any patient at risk for this condition who present with signs and symptoms of pulmonary embolism (dyspnea, chest pain, hemoptysis, syncope, hypotension, hypoxia) or deep vein thrombosis of the extremities (swelling, pain, discoloration). Occasionally, VTE may be silent and discovered incidentally during imaging for other reasons such as staging cancer.

Diagnosis of deep venous thrombosis is usually confirmed by ultrasonography, a simple, noninvasive, and totally safe imaging modality, although insensitive for detection of pelvic and distal calf venous thromboses. Computerized tomography (CT) and magnetic resonance imaging (MRI) are more sensitive methods for detecting DVT throughout the entire lower limb. Contrast venography is the historical gold standard method for diagnosing DVT, but it is invasive and rarely available in most hospitals.

Pulmonary embolism is usually diagnosed by CT scanning, MRI, or radionuclide ventilation–perfusion scanning, although pulmonary angiography remains the gold standard. With the introduction of multidetector–row spiral CT, visualization of small peripheral pulmonary arteries and detection of small peripheral emboli has been considerably improved. Frequently, as in this case, pulmonary embolism is diagnosed without evidence

Table 62.2 Persistent VTE Risk Factors

Hereditary thrombophilia
    Antithrombin deficiency (2%)
    Protein C deficiency (2%)
    Protein S deficiency (2%)
    Factor V Leiden mutation (30%)
    Prothrombin gene mutation G20210A (10%)
    Dysfibrinogenemia (<1%)
Acquired thrombophilia
    Polycythemia
    Essential thrombocythemia
    Paroxysmal nocturnal hemoglobinuria (PNH)
    Cancer
    Obesity
    Antiphospholipid syndrome
Thrombophilias involving genetic and environment interactions
    Hyperhomocysteinemia
    Elevated fibrinogen
    Elevated factor VIII
    Elevated factor IX
    Elevated factor XI

of deep venous thrombosis. This is usually because ultrasonography fails to identify a pelvic or calf DVT, or the entire thrombus may have embolized.

Multiple prospective, randomized studies have confirmed that when a phyisican determines a low pretest probability for a DVT or PE, and a sensitive, quantitative D-dimer test result is not elevated, then lower extremity or pulmonary imaging studies can be deferred and the patient does not require anticoagulation. D-Dimer is a degradation product of crosslinked fibrin whose levels are typically elevated in patients with acute VTE. D-Dimer levels may also be increased by a variety of other disorders, including recent surgery, hemorrhage, trauma, pregnancy, cancer, or acute arterial thrombosis and may occasionally be elevated in apparently normal persons for unclear reasons. Thus, D-dimer assay is a sensitive but nonspecific test that does not help "rule in" VTE when positive but is useful to "rule out" the diagnosis when negative.

Testing for Thrombophilia

Testing for thrombophilia is indicated in patients who are young (<55 years) and develop unprovoked VTE. Patients who have a family history of VTE and those who develop recurrent, unprovoked VTE may also be considered for laboratory evaluation. Testing, other than molecular methods (factor V Leiden, prothrombin gene mutation G20210A), should be deferred until several weeks after the event because acute thrombosis can cause a temporary lowering of the natural anticoagulants: antithrombin and proteins C and S. Testing should also be done when patients are not anticoagulated because warfarin lowers protein C and S activities and falsely low antithrombin activity may be obtained during treatment with heparin. Testing, when appropriately done, besides identifying risk factors, helps estimate risk of recurrence and thus enables determination of the duration of anticoagulation therapy.

Hereditary Thrombophilia

Ever since the discovery of antithrombin in 1965, progress in uncovering hereditary risk factors for thrombophilia has been slow. Proteins C and S were discovered in the 1980s. These are naturally occurring anticoagulants whose partial deficiency confers an increased risk for venous thrombosis. Each one accounts for a small proportion of cases of hereditary thrombophilia. In 1993, Dahlbeck described activated protein C resistance (APCR) followed by the discovery in 1994 by Bertina of the factor V Leiden mutation, which accounts for this phenomenon, the most common type of hereditary thrombophilia. In 1996 the prothrombin gene mutation G20210A was discovered and soon found to be the second most common hereditary thrombophilic risk factor.

Activated Protein C Resistance and Factor V Leiden

Protein C is activated by a thrombin–thrombomodulin complex on the surface of endothelial cells. In the presence of its cofactor, protein S, activated protein C (aPC) degrades activated coagulation factors V and VIII (Va and VIIIa) in a feedback loop, thereby damping down the coagulation cascade. The factor V Leiden mutation substitutes glutamine for arginine at position 506 of factor V, eliminating an aPC cleavage site. This mutation, which is present almost exclusively in Caucasians, is found in about 5–7% of the population and in about 30% of patients with idiopathic VTE. It is the most common cause of inherited thrombophilia and heterozygotes have a 7-fold increase in the risk of VTE compared with the normal population. Homzygotes, in contrast, have an 80-fold risk.

Prothrombin Gene Mutation G20210A

A single nucleotide substitution of adenine for guanine at the 20210 position in the 3' untranslated region of the prothrombin gene (G20210A) results in increased prothrombin activity and a 2–3 times increase in the risk of VTE. Like factor V Leiden mutation, the prothrombin gene mutation is also found almost exclusively in the Caucasian population with a frequency of about 2%. Approximately 10% of patients with an idiopathic VTE are heterozygous for the prothrombin mutation.

Hyperhomocysteinemia

An association has been demonstrated between fasting hyperhomocysteinemia and deep venous thrombosis through case control studies. Homocysteine is produced by demethylation of methionine, and is either converted to cysteine and excreted in the urine, or remethylated to regenerate methionine. Hyperhomocysteinemia may occur as a result of acquired or genetic causes. Mutations C677T and A1298C of the methyl tetrahydrofolate reductase (MTHFR) enzyme render it thermolabile and reduce its activity. As a result, patients with these mutations, which are very common, are at increased risk for elevated fasting homocysteine concentrations. There is, however, no association between the MTHFR mutations and VTE. Acquired causes of fasting hyperhomocysteinemia include hypothyroidism and renal failure and deficiencies of vitamins B_6, folic acid (B_9), and B_{12}. It is unclear whether the hyperhomocysteinemia is a cause or consequence of the VTE. Homocysteine levels can be effectively reduced with folic acid supplementation alone or with combinations of vitamins B_6, B_9, and B_{12}. However, preliminary results from a randomized control trial showed that reducing homocysteine concentrations did not decrease the rate of VTE recurrence. Thus, even if primary causation is not disproved, correction of the abnormality does not appear to reduce the risk of recurrent VTE.

Treatment of VTE

The treatment of venous thromboembolism consists of anticoagulation initially with intravenous unfractionated heparin or subcutaneous low-molecular-weight heparin to prevent extension of the thrombosis and subsequently oral warfarin, an inhibitor of the hepatic synthesis of vitamin K–dependent coagulation factors X, IX, VII, and II (prothrombin), and natural anticoagulants protein C and S, for an extended period to prevent recurrence.

In those individuals where a transient risk factor such as surgery, temporary immobilization, birth control pill, or venous catheter precipitates the venous thrombosis, anticoagulation for 3–6 months is adequate provided the risk factor is no longer present. For those who have a persistent risk factor such as permanent immobility or decompensated heart failure and in those who have unprovoked venous thromboembolism, extended anticoagulation may be considered after only one or two events. At present there is evidence to support that extended anticoagulation for up to 2 years is beneficial in preventing recurrences in idiopathic or unprovoked VTE after a single event. For those who have three events (two recurrences) indefinite anticoagulation is the accepted norm.

Indefinite anticoagulation is also considered beneficial in individuals with idiopathic VTE due to the antiphospholipid syndrome, antithrombin deficiency, protein C deficiency, protein S deficiency, homozygous factor V Leiden, or combined heterozygous factor V Leiden and prothrombin gene 20210 mutation. Individuals with only one risk factor such as heterozygous factor V Leiden or prothrombin gene mutation G20210A do not benefit from extended anticoagulation. Persistence of residual thrombosis and persistently elevated D-dimer have recently been identified as independent risk factors for recurrent VTE and thus may also need to be considered in determining the duration of anticoagulation. Elimination of risk factors such as estrogen therapy, obesity, heart failure, and cancer may also contribute significantly to reducing the recurrence rate.

Additional Reading

BAUER, K. A.: Hypercoagulable states. In *Hematology, Basic Principles and Practice*. R. HOFFMAN ET AL., eds., Churchill Livingstone, Philadelphia, 2000, pp. 2009–39.

BLANN, A. D. AND LIP, G. Y. H.: Venous thromboembolism. *Br. Med. J. 332*:215–9, 2006.

BOS, G. J. M. ET AL.: Homocysteine lowering by B vitamins and the secondary prevention of deep vein thrombosis and pulmonary embolism: A first randomized placebo-controlled double blind trial. *Blood* (Suppl.; Abstract 489) 2004.

DE STEFANO, V., MARTINELLI, I., MANNUCCI, P. M. ET AL.: The risk of recurrent deep venous thrombosis among heterozygous carriers of both factor V Leiden and the G20210A prothrombin mutation. *N. Engl. J. Med. 341*:801–6, 1999.

PALARETI, G. AND COSMI, B.: Predicting the risk of recurrence of venous thromboembolism. *Curr. Opin. Hematol. 11*:192–7, 2004.

SCHOEPF, U. J., GOLDHABER, S. Z., AND COSTELLO, P.: Spiral computed tomography for acute pulmonary embolism. *Circulation 109*:2160–7, 2004.

WELLS, P. S., OWEN, C., DOUCETTE, S., FERGUSSON, D., AND TRAN, H.: Does this patient have deep vein thrombosis? *JAMA 295*:199–207.

Case 63

A Young Woman with Postpartum Cerebral Venous Thrombosis and Abnormal Coagulation Tests

Hans-Joachim Reimers

An 18-year-old young woman was transferred from an outside hospital to the neurology service for evaluation of headaches, seizures, and a parietooccipital infarct on a computed tomography scan. She had undergone an emergency caesarean section in the 34th week of her second pregnancy 4 weeks earlier. The baby did not survive. After the delivery, she started having severe, continuous, throbbing temporooccipital headaches. One week prior to admission, she had four episodes of generalized, tonic–clonic seizures. Apart from the headaches, she had no other symptoms, and the physical examination was normal. However, a magnetic resonance venogram and arteriogram showed a left transverse venous sinus thrombosis and a left temporal lobe infarct. Review of her past medical history revealed that she had one prior miscarriage at gestational age month 2. The family history was noticeable for a cousin with possible cerebrovascular accident in her 20s.

The following laboratory tests were performed:

Analyte	Value, Conventional Units	Reference Interval, Conventional Units	Value, SI Units	Reference Interval, SI Units
WBC	$5.5 \times 10^3/\mu L$	4.0–10.0	$5.5 \times 10^9/L$	4.0–10.0
Hemoglobin	12.6 g/dL	12.0–15.0	126 g/L	120–150
Platelet count	$140 \times 10^3/\mu L$	140–400	$140 \times 10^9/L$	140–400
Activated partial thromboplastin time (aPTT)	79.8 s	24–36	Same	
aPTT 50 : 50 mix	76.5 s	24–36	Same	
Factor VIII activity	38% (83%)	60–160	0.38 IU	0.60–1.60
Factor XI activity	21% (67%)	60–160	0.21 IU	0.60–1.60
Factor IX activity	21% (39%)	60–160	0.21 IU	0.60–1.60

Tietz's Applied Laboratory Medicine, Second Edition. Edited by Mitchell G. Scott, Ann M. Gronowski, and Charles S. Eby
Copyright © 2007 John Wiley & Sons, Inc.

Analyte	Value, Conventional Units	Reference Interval, Conventional Units	Value, SI Units	Reference Interval, SI Units
Factor XII activity	20% (39%)	60–160	0.20 IU	0.60–1.60
Lupus anticoagulant testing:				
Staclot-LA Δ	47.8 s	<9.0	Same	
Dilute Russell viper venom time	Positive	Negative	Same	
Dilute prothrombin time index	1.85	<1.31	Same	
Anticardiolipin antibodies				
IgG	23 GPL	<12	Same	
IgM	55 MPL	<12	Same	
Antinuclear antibody (ANA)	Negative	Negative	Same	

Laboratory evaluation revealed a prolonged activated partial thromboplastin time (aPTT), but a normal prothrombin time (PT) and thrombin time. There was incomplete correction of the prolonged aPTT in the 50:50 mix consistent with an aPTT inhibitor. The intrinsic pathway factor activites (XII, XI, IX, and VIII) were diminished when measured by an aPTT-based method on a 1:10 dilution of plasma. However, when performed on 1:40 dilutions of the patient plasma, factor activities increased (see values in parentheses in laboratory results tabulation), consistent with dilution of an nonspecific inhibitor in her plasma. There was evidence of an IgM anticardiolipin antibody of moderate strength as measured by a β_2 glycoprotein I–dependent ELISA test. The possibility of an antiphospholipid antibody was tested further in three assays in which the phospholipid dependence of the prolonged clotting time is examined in either the intrinsic pathway (Staclot-LA), the extrinsic pathway (dilute prothrombin time), or the common pathway (dilute Russell viper venom time). All three tests were positive, and thus supported the presence of an antiphospholipid antibody. Additional tests for inherited thrombophilia risk factors (protein C, protein S, antithrombin activities, factor V Leiden, and prothrombin G20210A mutations) were normal or negative, and fasting plasma homocysteine concentration was normal.

The patient was started on a therapeutic dose of low-molecular-weight heparin (LMWH) and warfarin and discharged. When her outpatient PT-INR prolonged to the therapeutic target range of 2–3, LMWH was stopped. Repeat MRI was scheduled in 3 months.

However, 10 weeks later, the patient presented with pleuritic chest pain. A spiral computed tomography scan and a ventilation–perfusion scan were indicative of pulmonary embolism. Admission laboratory studies showed that the PT-INR was not therapeutic (1.4), the aPTT remained prolonged, and the Staclot-LA test remained abnormal with a Δ value of 20.6 s (normal less than 9 s) indicative of the persistence of a lupus anticoagulant.

Treatment with LMWH and warfarin was reinstituted with the same target INR of 2–3 but with more frequent monitoring. One year later, the patient became pregnant again. Her anticoagulation with warfarin was changed to adjusted dose LMWH (enoxaparin 1 mg/kg body weight every 12 hours) during the pregnancy. She delivered a healthy baby, resumed warfarin oral anticoagulation postpartum, and has remained free from thrombotic and hemorrhagic complications for the last 2 years.

Table 63.1   Clinical Criteria for the Diagnosis of Antiphospholipid Antibody Syndrome

Vascular thrombosis
   One or more episodes of arterial, venous, or small vessel thrombosis, affecting any tissue or organ
Pregnancy-related morbidity
   Unexplained death of a morphologically normal fetus at or after week 10 of gestation
   Premature birth of morphologically normal neonate at or before week 34 of gestation because of
      severe eclampsia or preeclampsia, or severe placental insufficiency
   Three or more unexplained consecutive spontaneous abortions before week 10 of gestation

Adapted from *J Haemastasis and Thrombosis* 4:295–306, 2006.

The Antiphospholipid Syndrome

The *antiphospholipid syndrome* (APS) is a noninflammatory autoimmune disease defined by the presence of antiphospholipid antibodies APA in the plasma of patients with venous or arterial thrombosis, or complications of pregnancy (Table 63.1). APS occurs predominantly in young women and is characterized by recurrence and high morbidity.

Primary antiphospholipid syndrome refers to patients with the syndrome who do not have any other rheumatological or autoimmune conditions such as lupus erythematosus. Associated (but not defining) conditions include thrombocytopenia, vasculitic rashes, arthralgias, dermal necrosis of digits, livedo reticularis, and pulmonary hypertension. A thrombotic cause of these additional manifestations is unlikely since anticoagulant treatment does not result in a remission of these complaints.

The presence of APL antibodies can be detected by either a phospholipid-dependent prolongation of a coagulation test [lupus anticoagulant (LAC)] or as anticardiolipin antibodies (ACA) in a β_2-glycoprotein I (β_2-GPI)-dependent enzyme-linked immunosorbent assay (ELISA). LAC activity and ACA are closely related but not identical. Patients should be tested with both types of assays (immunologic and clot-based) to rule out the diagnosis of antiphospholipid syndrome in a patient with a clinical presentation consistent with this disorder.

Diagnosis of Antiphospholipid Syndrome

Criteria for the definite diagnosis of APS were agreed on at an international workshop in 1999 and recently updated in 2005. These "Sapporo criteria" require at least one clinical criterium (vascular thrombosis or pregnancy-related morbidity (see Table 63.1) and one laboratory criterion (anticardiolipin antibodies isotype IgG or IgM at moderate or high levels, i.e., greater than 20 GPL or MPL units or a lupus anticoagulant (see Table 63.2).

ACA are antibodies against β_2-GPI that have been detected in an ELISA containing cardiolipin as the phospholipid that binds β_2-GPI (which is present in the assay). LAC is defined as an antibody against a phospholipid binding protein such as prothrombin or β_2-GPI that induces prolongation of a phospholipid-dependent clotting assay. Thus, antiphospholipid antibodies (APA), or more accurately antiphospholipid–protein antibodies, can be described as LA or as ACA. Antibodies that recognize purified β_2-GPI not associated with phospholipid are currently not included in the diagnostic laboratory criteria for APL syndrome. However, many investigators consider the presence of these antibodies to be more specific for the syndrome. The ACA or LA must be demonstrated on two or more

Table 63.2   Laboratory Criteria for Diagnosis of Antiphospholipid Antibody Syndrome

Anticardiolipin IgG or IgM antibodies present at moderate to high levels (>20 GPL or MPL units) on two or more occasions separated by at least 12 weeks
Lupus anticoagulant detected in the blood on two or more occasions separated by at least 6 weeks
International Society of Thrombosis and Haemostasis criteria for lupus anticoagulant include
Prolongation of a phospholipid dependent screening assay (e.g., aPTT, dilute prothrombin time, dilute Russell viper venon time)
Evidence of inhibitory activity in mixing studies
Evidence that the inhibitory activity is phospholipid-dependent
Exclusion of other coagulopathies or specific factor inhibitors

GPL and MPL unit-cardiolipin binding activity of a purified IgG or IgM respectively at 1 μs/mL from a reference standard.
Adapted from *J Haemastasis and Thrombosis* 4:295–306, 2006.

occasions at least 12 weeks apart since transient presence of these antibodies can be observed during acute illness such as an infection, and does not qualify for the diagnosis of APL syndrome. (However, there is no evidence that transient APAs are less important than persistent antibodies.)

Association of Antiphospholipid Antibodies and Thrombosis

The prevalence of LAC has been reported to be as high as 8% in healthy blood donors, and IgG-ACA and IgM-ACA were identified in 6.5% and 9.4% of healthy subjects, respectively. However, it is unusual to find healthy subjects who are persistently positive for APA. In a general obstetric population the prevalence of LAC was 0.3% and the prevalence of ACA was 2.2–9.1%, similar to a nonpregnant population. In contrast, the prevalence of APA in patients with thrombosis has been reported to be 4–21%, suggesting an increased risk of thrombosis in patients with APA.

The Framingham Heart Study found an increased risk of transient ischemic attacks and strokes associated with ACA in women (HR 2.6; absolute risk 3.2%) but not in men. A retrospective review of more than 13,000 women found a prevalence of APA of 20% among women with recurrent fetal loss compared with 5% in healthy women. The association between APA and thrombosis is stronger with LAC than with ACA. In a metaanalysis of 25 studies involving more than 7000 patients, the odds ratio for thrombosis was 1.6 for ACA and 11.0 for LAC.

Pathophysiology of Antiphospholipid Syndrome

As pointed out above, it has become apparent that the so-called APA are not directed against anionic phospholipids but against plasma proteins with affinity for anionic phospholipids. Thus, the term APA is a misnomer but remains well established. Besides prothrombin and β_2-glycoprotein I (a protein of unknown function that avidly binds to negatively charged phospholipids), more than 20 other possible target proteins for APA have been described, including protein C, protein S, and tissue plasminogen activator. Recently, some attention has been given to the possible role of annexin V in pregnancy-related antiphospholipid syndrome or APS. Annexin V is a protein synthesized by placental trophoblasts and present on villous surfaces. Annexin V is thought to shield phospholipids on the villi from contact with the flowing blood and thereby prevent thrombosis. Binding of the antiphospholipid antibody to phospholipid–protein complexes may displace the annexin V on the placental surfaces, thus disrupting the antithrombotic shield and allowing exposed anionic phospholipids to serve as surfaces for promoting pro-coagulant activity. However, at the present time, only β_2-GPI antibodies and prothrombin antibodies are accepted as relevant for APS.

It has remained difficult to understand why antibodies to these proteins prolong the clot-ting times in vitro but are prothrombotic in vivo. One possible explanation is that the protein antibody complex (e.g., β_2-GPI–β_2-GPI antibody) binds more avidly to a phospholipid surface in vitro as compared to β_2-GPI alone, and thereby interferes with rapid assembly of the tenase (enzyme factor IXa, cofactor VIIIa, and substrate factor X) and prothrombinase (enzyme factor Xa, cofactor Va, and substrate prothrombin) complexes on the lipid surface and thus delays formation of a fibrin clot. In contrast, in vivo, APL antibody–protein com-plexes may bind to receptors (such as the LDL-R family) on platelets, monocytes, and endo-thelial cells, causing their activation (e.g., expression of tissue factor) and thus a prothrombotic state. While APAs are probably too weak to fully activate these cells, these antibody–protein complexes may increase the responsiveness to their other agonists (e.g., collagen stimulation of platelets). This would explain why, although antibodies are persistently circulating, the patient does not suffer continuously from thrombotic compli-cations. Laboratory evidence also supports APA inhibition of proteins C and S, as well as interference in fibrinolytic, inflammatory, and apoptosis pathways. Given the hetero-geneous clinical and biological behavior of APAs, it is likely that a combination of these interactions contributes to the pathology of these autoantibodies. Presently, insights into mechanisms that link APA with pregnancy complications are even more incomplete.

Clinical Presentation of Antiphospholipid Syndrome

The most common thrombotic events are deep vein thrombosis with or without pulmonary embolism. However, venous thromboses in unusual locations including intrabdominal, cerebral, and upper extremities should alert clinicians to test for APAs. Neurologic com-plications of the antiphospholipid syndrome include single or recurrent cerebral infarcts, transient ischemic attacks, severe vascular headaches, and visual disturbances. In a pro-spective study, 18% of young adults (age 15–44 years) who had sustained an ischemic stroke or TIA tested positive for ACA. Whether ACA is also a risk factor for older patients is still debated. Thus, current data suggest that testing for ACA and LAC is warranted at least for younger patients who present with ischemic stroke or TIA. Strokes due to embo-lization of sterile vegetations on mitral or aortic valves (marantic endocarditis) have been reported, but myocardial infarctions are rarely associated with the presence of APA.

Rarely, patients present with catastrophic antiphospholipid syndrome: mulitorgan failure due to diffuse microvascular thromboses, no evidence of an underlying cause of disseminated intravascular coagulopathy, and laboratory confirmation of APAs. Despite anticoagulation, immune suppression, plasmapheresis, and aggressive supportive therapy, the prognosis for these patients is very poor.

Defining and recognizing the role of antiphospholipid syndrome in pregnancy-related complications has remained difficult. First-trimester spontaneous pregnancy loss is rela-tively common, and definitive exclusion of anatomic, genetic, or hormonal causes of early pregnancy losses is seldom possible. While withholding a label of APS until a woman has had three or more consecutive spontaneous early pregnancy failures may improve the specificity of the diagnosis, in clinical practice, laboratory testing for APA is often performed after one or two losses, and if positive, the cause is likely to be attributed to APS. Nor is it always possible to determine whether APAs were the likely cause of a late fetal death in utero. Gross and histologic evidence of placental insufficiency is neither sensitive nor specific for pregnancy complications that occur in the presence of APAs.

Treatment of Antiphospholipid Antibody Syndrome

Venous thromboembolism is the most common presentation of antiphospholipid syndrome and occurs in about 30% of patients. Initial treatment consists of at least 5 days of unfractionated heparin or LMWH overlapping with warfarin. Moderate-intensity oral anticoagulation (target INR 2-3) reduces the risk of recurrent thrombosis by about 80–90%. High-intensity oral anticoagulation (INR > 3) has not been shown to be more effective in preventing recurrent thrombosis in two prospective trials.

The optimal duration of anticoagulation for prevention of recurrent thrombosis in patients with APL antibodies is unknown. The risk of recurrence appears to peak in the first 6 months after discontinuation of anticoagulation, and is higher for patients with antiphospholipid antibodies compared to patients who are antibody-negative. Retrospective studies report recurrence rates as high as 53–69%. Therefore, the general consensus is to anticoagulate patients with APS and venous thrombosis indefinitely. It is unknown whether anticoagulation can be discontinued in patients whose lupus anticoagulant and/or ACA testing has become negative, or if the only laboratory finding is a persistent low-titer ACA. Therefore, indefinite anticoagulation is recommended.

Arterial events in APL syndrome most commonly involve the cerebral circulation (stroke 13%; TIA 7% initial manifestation). Moderate-intensity warfarin (INR 1.4–2.8) and aspirin (325 mg) are equivalent for the prevention of thromboembolic complications in patients with a first ischemic stroke and antiphospholipid antibodies. The 2-year recurrence rate is about 24%.

The optimal treatment of pregnant women with APL antibodies and a history of fetal losses but no prior thrombosis is unknown. Consensus recommendations suggest that women with antiphospholipid antibodies and a history of three or more early pregnancy losses or one or more late pregnancy losses who have no prior history of thrombosis receive combined treatment of aspirin and unfractionated or LMWH (prophylactic dose) during pregnancy. Aspirin should be started with attempted conception.

Additional Reading

WILSON, W. A., GHARAVI, A. E., KOIKE, T., ET AL.: International consensus statement on preliminary classification criteria for definite antiphospholipid syndrome: Report of an international workshop. *Arthritis Rheum.* *42*:1309–11, 1999.

LEVINE, J. S., BRANCH, D. W. AND RANCH, J.: The antiphospholipid syndrome. *N. Engl. J. Med.* *346*:752–63, 2002.

RAND, J. H.: The antiphospholipid syndrome. *Ann. Rev. Med.* *54*:409–24, 2003.

LIM, W., CROWTHER, M. A., AND EICKELBOOM, J. W.: Management of antiphospholipid antibody syndrome. A systematic review. *JAMA 295*:1050–7, 2006.

ORTEL, T. L.: Thrombosis and the antiphospholipid syndrome. In *Hematology* (Am. Soc. Hematol. Educ. Program), 2005, pp. 4062–68.

ALVING, B. M.: The antiphospholipid syndrome: Clinical presentation, diagnosis and patient management. In *Consultative Hemostasis and Thrombosis*, C. S KITCHENS, B. M. ALVING, AND C. M. KESSLER, eds., Saunders, Philadelphia, 2002, pp. 269–78.

ELDER, A.: Management of thrombophilia and antiphospholipid syndrome during pregnancy. In *Consultative Hemostasis and Thrombosis*, C. S. KITCHENS, B. M. ALVING, AND C. M. KESSLER, eds. Saunders, Philadelphia, 2002, pp. 449–60.

BATES, S. M., GREER, I. A., HIRSH, J., AND GINSBURG, J. S.: Use of antithrombotic agents during pregnancy: The Seventh ACCP Conference on Antithrombotic and Thrombolytic Therapy. *Chest 126*:S627–44, 2004.

DE GROOT, P. G, AND DERKSEN, R. H. W. M.: Pathophysiology of the antiphospholipid syndrome. *J. Thromb. Haemost. 3*:1854–60, 2005.

Case 64

A Baby with Petechiae and Bruises

Lori Luchtman-Jones

A well-appearing, term infant was born by vaginal delivery to a healthy 27-year-old mother with a benign prenatal and postpartum course. Within an hour of birth he developed generalized petechiae and bruising over his trunk and left arm. His CBC was normal for a term newborn: WBC $10 \times 10^3/\mu L$, hemoglobin 18.4 g/dL, and platelets $173 \times 10^3/\mu L$. An extensive evaluation for sepsis was begun, and he was treated empirically with antibiotics and an antiviral agent until cultures of spinal fluid, urine, and blood were negative at 72 hours. A herpes simplex virus PCR was negative on blood and spinal fluid as well. The CSF was described as "bloody," and he bled from the puncture site for over an hour. Prothrombin time (PT) and activated partial thromboplastin time (aPTT) were normal for age. At 6 days of life, he had a generalized seizure. MRI of his head showed a hemorrhagic infarction of the left centrum ovale region. The baby was begun on an anticonvulsant. After discharge to home, his mother noticed intermittent bruising of his arms, leg, and ear. After intramuscular injection of childhood immunizations at 2 months of age, the site bled intermittently for several hours. The baby also had occasional epistaxis. Serial evaluations of platelet count, prothrombin time (PT), and activated partial prothrombin time (aPTT) were normal.

At 6 months of age he was referred for a pediatric hematology evaluation. He was taking no medications except phenobarbital. There was no family history of bleeding problems, and his parents and older brother (full sibling) were in good health. Physical exam revealed a well-developed, well-nourished, developmentally appropriate 6-month-old infant with a band of petechiae around the lower third of the left upper arm, where the phlebotomist's tourniquet had been placed.

Laboratory results at age 6 months were as follows:

Analyte	Value, Conventional Units	Reference Interval, Conventional Units	Value, SI Units	Reference Interval, SI Units
WBC	$10.8 \times 10^3/\mu L$	6–17.5	$10.8 \times 10^9/L$	6–17.5
Hemoglobin	8.5 g/dL	9.5–13.5	85 g/L	95–135

Analyte	Value, Conventional Units	Reference Interval, Conventional Units	Value, SI Units	Reference Interval, SI Units
Hematocrit	26%	29–41	0.26 volume	0.29–0.41
MCV	68 fL	74–108	Same	
Reticulocyte count	2%	0.5–1.5	0.02 fraction	0.005–0.015
Platelet count	$390 \times 10^3/\mu L$	140–400	$390 \times 10^9/L$	140–400
PT	13.8 s	12.2–14	Same	
aPTT	36.2 s	30.5–37	Same	
Fibrinogen	283 mg/dL	218–306	2.83 g/L	2.18–3.06
Factor VIII activity	92%	60–160	0.92 IU	0.6–1.6
Factor IX activity	72%	60–160	0.72 IU	0.6–1.6
Platelet function screen: col/epi	>300 s	70–170	Same	
Platelet function screen: col/ADP	>250 s	50–150	Same	

Given the evidence of a significant bleeding disorder from infancy onward with normal platelet count and coagulation tests, and abnormal platelet function screening results, a congenital qualitative platelet disorder was suspected. Platelet aggregometry was performed on the patient (see Fig. 64.1).

To confirm that the patient's platelets lacked GpIIb/IIIa receptors for fibrinogen binding, peripheral blood was incubated with fluorescent antibodies to CD41 (GpIIb) and 61 (GpIIIa) and analyzed by flow cytometry. Compared to control platelets, the patient's platelets were CD41/CD61-negative, while the parents' platelets stained with approximately 50% of the intensity of control platelets. On the basis of these test results, the infant was diagnosed with Glanzmann thrombasthenia.

After the seizure, he was begun on phenobarbital, which will probably be discontinued in early childhood if no other seizures occur. Iron drops were prescribed for his microcytic, hypochromic anemia, presumed to be iron deficiency anemia secondary to chronic blood loss. Because of his bleeding problems shortly after delivery, he was not circumcised at that time. Given the risk of alloimmunization (see definition of *alloimmunization* later, under Treatment section) and the potential need for a platelet transfusion with elective circumcision, this patient's mother decided against the procedure. She and his physicians will consider circumcision in the future should he require a platelet transfusion for another reason.

This baby received his subsequent childhood immunizations subcutaneously, rather than intramuscularly, in order to prevent intramuscular hematoma. His parents made sure that he had soft toys to play with and padded sharp corners and ledges at home. When his mobility increases over the next few months, he will be fitted with a soft helmet. Soft helmets may prevent or lessen head trauma in toddlers and children, but many families and older patients dislike the stigmatization. Dental hygiene practices are especially important in patients with bleeding tendencies, both because gingivitis is associated with bleeding, and also because tooth extraction is associated with risk of hematoma and bleeding.

Differential Diagnosis of Qualitative Platelet Disorders

Platelets participate in hemostasis by adhering to the subendothelium at the site of vascular disruption, binding agonists to specific surface receptors to promote activation

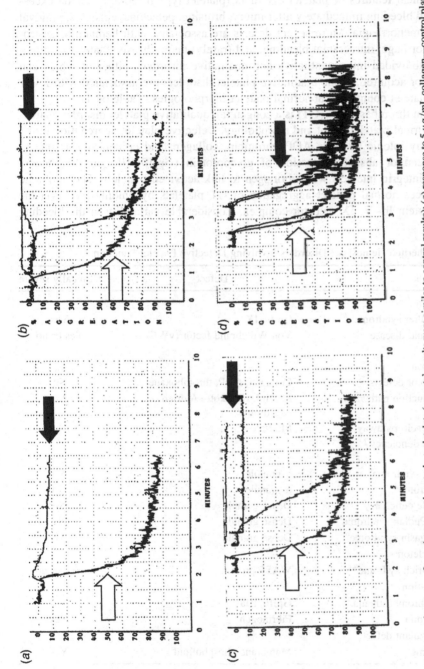

Figure 64.1 Aggregation curves for patient ◀ and control ▷ platelets (parents' results were similar to control results): (*a*) response to 5 μg/mL collagen—control platelets rapidly aggregate, and light transmission through cuvette increases to ~90% while light transmission is <10% with patient's platelets; (*b*) response to 0.25 and 0.50 mg/mL arachadonic acid—control platelets rapidly aggregate while light transmission through patient's platelets remains at baseline indicating no aggregation; (*c*) response to 20 μm ADP and 300 μm epinephrine—control platelets rapidly aggregate, patient's platelets show no aggregation; (*d*) response to 1.2 and 1.5 mg/mL ristocetin—both control and patient's platelets rapidly aggregate and light transmission is >80%.

of downstream signaling pathways that lead to spreading to breach the disruption and secreting granular contents to recruit and activate additional platelets, promoting activation of factor X and prothrombin, forming a platelet aggregate, and initiating clot retraction. Clinical features of platelet disorders (platelet-type bleeding) include excessive, prolonged bleeding immediately after injury, bruising, petechiae, epistaxis, gingival bleeding, and menorrhagia. More severe defects are associated with hematuria, gastrointestinal hemorrhage, intracranial bleeding, and (rarely) hemarthrosis. Platelet dysfunction can be subdivided into quantitative and qualitative disorders, either of which can be congenital or acquired. Some qualitative platelet disorders are associated with lower than normal platelet counts and abnormal platelet morphologies (Table 64.1).

Glanzmann thrombasthenia (GT) is a congenital, qualitative platelet disorder characterized by a normal platelet count and morphology. Defective platelet aggregation in the presence of physiologic agonists ADP, thrombin, collagen, and epinephrine is due to severely reduced or absent expression of glycoprotein (Gp)IIb/IIIa on the platelet surface. This integrin interacts with fibrinogen to link activated platelets. The antibiotic ristocetin induces normal platelet aggregation of GT platelets by binding vWF via the intact glycoprotein Ib–V–IX receptor complex. Considerable variability in the bleeding

Table 64.1   Inherited Hemostasis Disorders Involving Defective Platelet Function

Affected function	Defect	Clinically severe
Platelet adhesion		
Bernard–Soulier syndrome[a,b]	Gp Ib/IX	Yes
Von Willebrand disease (vWD)[a]	Von Willebrand factor (vWF)	Yes or no
Platelet activation		
Platelet receptor defects	Collagen, ADP, thromboxane A_2	No
Signal transduction pathways	Multiple/Wiskott–Aldrich syndrome[a,c]	No
Arachadonic acid pathway	Multiple	No
Platelet granule deficiency/ defects		
Gray platelet syndrome[a]	α granule	No
Quebec syndrome[a]	α granule	No
Dense granule deficiency	Dense granule	No
Hemansky–Pudlak syndrome[d]	Dense granule	No
Chediak–Higashi syndrome[d]	Dense granule	No
Platelet cytoskeleton		
Wiskott–Aldrich sydrome[a,c]	WASP protein	Yes or no
Platelet aggregation		
Glanzmann thrombasthenia	GpIIb/IIIa	Yes
Afibrinogenemia	Fibrinogen	Yes
Platelet procoagulant defect		
Scott syndrome	Membrane phospholipid	Yes

[a]Can be associated with decreased platelet count.

[b]Inherited macrothrombocytopenia.

[c]X-linked inheritance, microthrombocytopenia.

[d]Accompanied by albinism.

symptoms of patients with GT has been reported. Mucocutaneous bleeding and menorrhagia are very common, but hemarthroses are rare. Many patients are identified in infancy; most are diagnosed before 5 years of age. Severe bleeding symptoms are often associated with iron deficiency anemia due to blood loss.

This rare disorder is inherited in an autosomal recessive fashion. In this family, platelet flow cytometry results showed the parents to be in the low–normal range for GpIIb/IIIa, while the patient's platelets were deficient. The parents are likely heterozygotes for GT, and, as is typical, they are asymptomatic and have normal platelet aggregation study results. Each subsequent pregnancy from these parents carries a 1 : 4 risk of disease, a 1 : 2 chance of heterozygous (carrier) status, and a 1 : 4 chance of normal genotype.

Bernard–Soulier–syndrome (BSS) is an even rarer (<1 per 1,000,000) autosomal recessive, qualitative platelet disorder. Mutations in the genes coding for GPIba or GPIX, which constitute parts of the GPIb–V–IX receptor, impair platelet adhesion to the damaged subendothelium via vWF, resulting in a severe bleeding phenotype. BSS is an example of an inherited macrothrombocytopenia. Some platelets are so large that automated cell counters fail to recognize them as platelets, producing erroneous low platelet counts. However, more accurate manual platelet counts frequently confirm a moderate to mild thrombocytopenia. Platelet aggregometry demonstrates defective ristocetin-mediated aggregation and reduced thrombin-induced aggregation since intact GPIb is necessary for maximum activation reponse to thrombin. Normal responses to other physiologic agonists (ADP, collagen, epinephrine, arachadonic acid) are expected; however, thrombocytopenia may prevent adequate concentration of platelets to perform aggregation studies. Flow cytometry using monoclonal antibodies to GPIb and GPIX can be used to make the diagnosis by confirming a lack of one or the other component.

Laboratory Diagnosis of Qualitative Platelet Disorders

Laboratory analysis of patients with apparent bleeding problems utilizes initial testing of the cellular and fluid-phase components of hemostasis, followed by more specialized testing of the suspected problematic aspect (Fig. 64.2). A platelet count will identify patients with a quantitative platelet defect, although one must remember that some qualitative defects are associated with lower platelet counts as well (Table 64.1). The possibility of coagulation factor inhibitors and deficiencies should be assessed using the prothrombin time (PT) and the activated partial thromboplastin time (aPTT). A prolonged aPTT can occur in vWD and should be explored by confirmatory testing of vWF activity, vWF antigen, factor VIII activity, (see Case 65), or hemophilia A (FVIII), B (FIX), or C (FXI) (see Case 61). The bleeding time (BT) and platelet function screen (PFA-100, Dade-Behring, Deerfield, IL, USA) are screening tests of primary hemostasis that include, but are not limited to, evaluation of platelet function. Platelet function screening tests should be performed on patients with adequate ($>100 \times 10^3/\mu L$) platelet counts, and in the absence of drugs known to cause platelet dysfunction. An abnormal result in the absence of a diagnosis of vWD should be pursued with definitive testing by platelet aggregometry. In some cases where clinical suspicion of platelet dysfunction remains high despite normal BT or PFA-100 results, platelet aggregometry should be considered because of its greater sensitivity for detecting some mild qualitative disorders.

The Ivy bleeding time (BT), or a modification of the technique, is used to assess the integrity of the subendothelium–von Willebrand factor (vWF)–platelet–fibrinogen

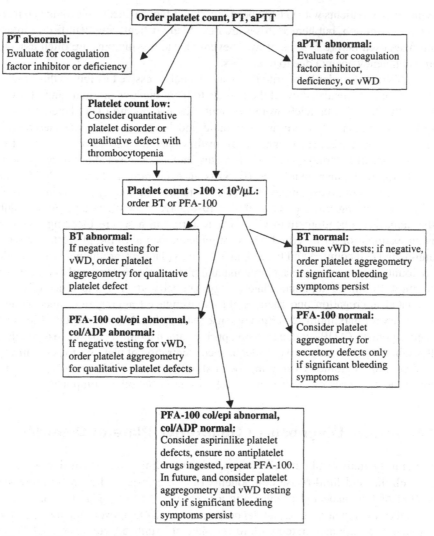

Figure 64.2   Algorithm for evaluation of patient with abnormal bleeding history (PT—prothrombin time; aPTT—activated partial thromboplastin time; vWD—von Willebrand disease; BT—bleeding time; PFA-100—platelet function screen, Dade-Behring, Deerfield, IL, USA; col/epi—collagen/epinephrine cartridge on PFA-100; col/ADP—collagen/ADP cartridge on PFA-100).

system. A specially trained laboratory technician performs this bedside test. A blood pressure cuff placed on the upper arm is inflated to 40 mm Hg as a lancet device is used to deliver a standardized incision on the patient's forearm. A stopwatch tracks the time elapsed before incisional bleeding ceases. This time, in minutes, is compared to the normal range for the person's age. While the BT holds the advantage of in vivo testing of the subendothelial interaction with blood components, the test has fallen out of favor in most modern laboratories. The requirement for a specially trained technician to perform the test on the patient limits its availability and increases laboratory costs. Because it involves laceration of the forearm, associated with bleeding and scarring, repetitive testing is relatively contraindicated. Normal test ranges in healthy adults can be generated and validated with effort, but pediatric normal ranges for this invasive test are usually inferred from published reference ranges. Many technical and patient variables affect the precision and accuracy of the bleeding time. For example, variations in skin thickness with age and nutritional status can affect the depth of the laceration, even when age range-specific lancet devices are used. BT results may be prolonged when platelet counts fall below $100 \times 10^3/\mu L$, so verification of a platelet count of at least $100 \times 10^3/\mu L$ should always precede BT testing. BT normal ranges are usually given for newborn infants to age 6 months, and for all others >6 months of age. The shortened BT result in early infancy is attributed to the preponderance of larger vWf multimers at this age.

An alternative to the BT for evaluation of vWF–platelet–fibrinogen interactions is the PFA-100 two-cartridge test system. Citrated whole blood is added to test cartridges with a collagen-coated membrane and either epinephrine (col/epi) or adenosine diphosphate (col/ADP). The sample is pulled through a capillary tube and the central aperture of the membrane to generate high shear flow as a physical platelet activator, in addition to the physiologic activators collagen, epinephrine, and ADP. Activated platelets adhere to the membrane and to each other until the aperture is occluded. The interval from sample application to occlusion, in seconds, is designated the closure time (CT). CT is dependent on platelet number; intact platelet adhesion, activation, and aggregation; and interactions of platelets with fibrinogen and vWF. Hematocrit and platelet count should be obtained prior to PFA-100 testing, since values for hematocrit of <25 or >50% and platelet count <$100 \times 10^3/\mu L$ may cause inaccurate closure times.

The PFA-100 has been validated to differentiate between the effect of aspirin or other nonsteroidal antiinflammatory drugs (NSAIDs), which should prolong the col/epi cartridge results only, and other congenital or acquired qualitative platelet defects, vWD, and dysfibrinogenemia, which should result in prolonged CTs of both col/epi and col/ADP cartridges. However, the PFA-100 test has not been validated for predicting the risk of bleeding in asymptomatic, unselected patients prior to surgery or invasive procedures. Published CT normal ranges for newborns (cord blood) are shorter than those for toddlers through adulthood, consistent with BT results and the prediction that the high-molecular-weight vWf multimers in babies enhance platelet performance in platelet function screening tests. In pediatric patients with suspected bleeding problems, the sensitivity and specificity of the PFA-100 was superior to the BT in identifying patients with qualitative platelet disorders or vWD. The utility of the PFA-100 to detect patients with qualitative platelet defects has been assessed using platelet aggregometry as the gold standard, with favorable results for vWD and for severe platelet dysfunction syndromes such as Glanzmann thrombasthenia and Bernard–Soulier syndrome. Both the BT and the PFA-100 have been shown to be less effective at identifying patients with congenital defects of platelet secretion. Therefore, a patient with significant platelet-type symptoms and an otherwise negative evaluation should be considered for platelet aggregation studies.

Platelet aggregometry remains the gold standard for evaluation of in vitro platelet function in response to physiologic agonists and also to ristocetin. Citrated whole blood is centrifuged at 900 r/min (revolutions per minute) for 10 minutes to pellet red cells and white cells, but not platelets, to obtain platelet-rich plasma (PRP). Platelet-poor plasma (PPP) is prepared by centrifuging the residual cell pellet at 15,000 r/min for 10 minutes. The PRP is diluted, if necessary, with PPP to obtain a platelet count of 200–250 $\times 10^3/\mu L$. PRP is added to a glass tube containing a magnetic stir bar to maintain platelets in suspension, and the tube of PRP is placed within the light path of the aggregometer instrument. Platelet agonists are added to separate tubes, and as platelets undergo activation and aggregate, more light passes through the tube and reaches the detector (PRP = 0% light transmission = PPP, 100%).

Treatment

Mild bleeding events may be controlled with local measures such as pressure or hemostatic agents such as fibrin glue or topical thrombin. The antifibrinolytic agent ε-aminocaproic acid (Amicar) can stabilize the fibrin clot and delay fibrinolysis by interfering with the binding of plasmin and plasminogen to fibrinogen. Platelet transfusion to override the dysfunctional platelets is the most common intervention for severe bleeding and is also used prophylactically in situations with high risk of serious hemorrhage. Since bleeding times typically normalize at a platelet count of about $100 \times 10^3/\mu L$ in a person with normal platelet function, a substantial number of platelets must be transfused before a patient with Glanzmann thrombasthenia can be expected to approach normal platelet function test results. Single-donor pheresis platelet products have the advantage of minimizing donor exposures while maximizing the increase in platelet count. Unfortunately, in addition to the usual risks of blood transfusion, alloimmunization to a missing glycoprotein or to human leukocyte antigens (HLA) on transfused platelets is a major problem in these patients. Alloimmunized patients may become refractory to further platelet transfusions and have increased risk of graft rejection when undergoing bone marrow transplantation. Attempts are made to reserve platelet transfusion for episodes of severe bleeding.

Case reports of effective primary hemostasis following the use of DDAVP (a vasopressin analog) in patients with qualitative platelet disorders exist. However, neither bleeding time nor platelet function screening tests have been reported to normalize after DDAVP use. More recently, the use of recombinant coagulation factor VIIa (Novo-Seven, Novo Nordisk, Bagsvaerd, Denmark) has been reported from the results of an international survey of patients with GT, many of whom were alloimmunized and most of whom had severe disease. The intention to treat success rate of evaluable episodes for surgical procedures was 85%, and the intention to treat success rate for evaluable episodes of bleeding was 64%. The optimal dose, dose interval, number of doses, and incidence of side effects are unresolved at present.

Allogenic bone marrow transplantation from an HLA-matched sibling offers the only true cure for Glanzmann thrombasthenia, but is associated with significant and life-threatening potential side effects such as graft–host disease, nonengraftment, and infection. The older sibling and the patient in this case could be HLA-tested for compatibility. If bone marrow transplantation from a sibling is a consideration, the patient should not receive blood (platelet) transfusions from first-degree relatives, in order to minimize risks of graft rejection.

In the absence of better treatment options, supportive and preventive care remain the most important aspects of management in patients with moderate to severe qualitative platelet disorders. Patients are advised to wear a bracelet or necklace identifying their platelet dysfunction and bleeding risk. Medications with antiplatelet effects should be avoided.

Additional Reading

BREDDIN, H. K.: Can platelet aggregometry be standardized? *Platelets 16*:151–8, 2005.

CARIAPPA, R., WILHITE, T. R., PARVIN, C. A., AND LUCHTMAN-JONES, L.: Comparison of PFA-100® and bleeding time testing in pediatric patients with suspected hemorrhagic problems. *J. Ped. Hem. Oncol. 25*:474–9, 2003.

FLOOD, V. H., JHINSON, F. L., BOSHKOV, L. K., ET AL.: Sustained engraftment post bone marrow transplant despite antiplatelet antibodies in Glanzmann thrombasthenia. *Pediatr. Blood Cancer 45*:971–5, 2005.

HARRISON, P.: The role of PFA-100® testing in the investigation and management of haemostatic defects in children and adults. *Br. J. Haematol. 130*:3–10, 2005.

MATZDORFF, A.: Platelet function tests and flow cytometry to monitor antiplatelet therapy. *Semin. Thromb. Hemost. 31*:393–9, 2005.

NURDEN, A. T.: Qualitative disorders of platelets and megakaryocytes. *J. Thromb. Haemost. 3*:1773–82, 2005.

Case 65

Evaluation of a Reference Range Outlier

Charles Eby

A 44-year-old woman donated blood for a coagulation test reference range study. Her activated partial thromboplastin time (aPTT) was >2 standard deviations above the reference interval mean, and she was referred to a hematologist by her internist. During a bleeding history interview, she reported that she had always bruised easily, bled severely following surgery to repair a congenital mandible defect during adolescence, and had a hysterectomy in her 30s for menorrhagia. However, her three pregnancies and deliveries had been uneventful. Her family history was positive for a father who bled extensively after tonsillectomy, and recently had repeated gastrointestinal hemorrhages requiring multiple blood transfusions since starting on warfarin following mitral valve replacement. One sister also bled excessively after tonsillectomy. Four other siblings were asymptomatic. Her three teenage daughters also had negative bleeding histories. Vital signs were normal and physical exam was unremarkable, including normal appearance of surgical scars, no increased joint laxity or decreased skin elasticity, and no abnormal bruises or petechiae.

The following laboratory studies were obtained:

Analyte	Value, Conventional Units	Reference Interval, Conventional Units	Value, SI Units	Reference Interval, SI Units
WBC	$6.4 \times 10^3/\mu L$	4.8–10.8	$6.4 \times 10^9/L$	4.8–10.8
Hemoglobin	12.4 g/dL	12.0–16.0	124 g/L	120–160
Platelet count	$298 \times 10^3/\mu L$	140–400	$298 \times 10^9/L$	140–400
aPTT	38 s	23–35	Same	
Prothrombin time	14.1 s	11.5–14.5	Same	
Factor VIII activity	40%	60–160%	0.45 IU	0.60–1.60

Tietz's Applied Laboratory Medicine, Second Edition. Edited by Mitchell G. Scott, Ann M. Gronowski, and Charles S. Eby
Copyright © 2007 John Wiley & Sons, Inc.

Analyte	Value, Conventional Units	Reference Interval, Conventional Units	Value, SI Units	Reference Interval, SI Units
Von Willebrand antigen	48%	60–160%	0.48 IU	0.60–1.60
Ristocetin cofactor Activity	15%	60–160%	0.15 IU	0.60–1.60
PFA-100 closure time				
ADP	180 s	50–150	Same	
Epinephrine	214 s	70–170	Same	

Based on the positive family history, persistently prolonged aPTT, abnormal primary hemostasis screening test, mild reduction in factor VIII activity, and von Willebrand factor (vWF) antigen and marked reduction in vWF activity, a diagnosis of type 2 von Willebrand disease was considered. Two additional tests were performed; von Willebrand multimer analysis (Fig. 65.1), and ristocetin induced platelet agglutination (RIPA, Fig. 65.2). Multimer analysis demonstrated loss of large and intermediate von Willebrand multimers, and RIPA showed a blunted platelet agglutination response to increasing concentrations of the antibiotic ristocetin. On the basis of these findings, a diagnosis of type 2A von Willebrand disease was made. The patient's symptomatic father and sister were evaluated at another medical center, and diagnoses of type 2 A von Willebrand disease were confirmed.

Differential Diagnosis of Hemostasis Disorders

Evaluation of a patient suspected of having a hemostatic defect begins with a detailed personal and family bleeding history. Positive responses to questions such as "Do you bruise easily or bleed freely from minor cuts?" are nonspecific. Most adults have experienced some bleeding challenges, either physiologic (menstruation, labor, and delivery), accidental, or iatrogenic, and quantitative information about such events should be obtained. For example, if a patient states that she bled freely after extraction of wisdom teeth, ask follow-up questions to estimate the volume (teaspoons, tablespoons, cups), onset (immediately afterward, or starting days later), and duration (hours or days) of bleeding, and whether additional medical interventions were required (emergency room visit, sutures, blood component transfusion, or other hemostatic agents). When patients provide vague or incomplete personal or family histories about key events or diagnoses, efforts should be made to obtain primary data (request medical records and laboratory test results, or contact previous healthcare providers). These efforts will improve diagnostic accuracy and may prevent redundant testing.

Hemostasis disorders may be grouped by onset—lifelong (inherited) versus acquired, and defect—primary versus secondary hemostasis. Disorders of primary hemostasis involve platelet or vWF quantitative or qualitative defects. Typical symptoms include excessive bleeding from mucosal surfaces: epistaxis, gingival and gastrointestinal bleeding, and menorrhagia; and multiple, small (1–2-mm) subcutaneous hemorrhages (petechiae) on dependent (lower extremities) or traumatized (blood pressure cuff) skin areas. Onset of bleeding tends to be immediate after trauma, and inheritance patterns may be autosomal recessive or dominant with variable penetrance (see the case reported in

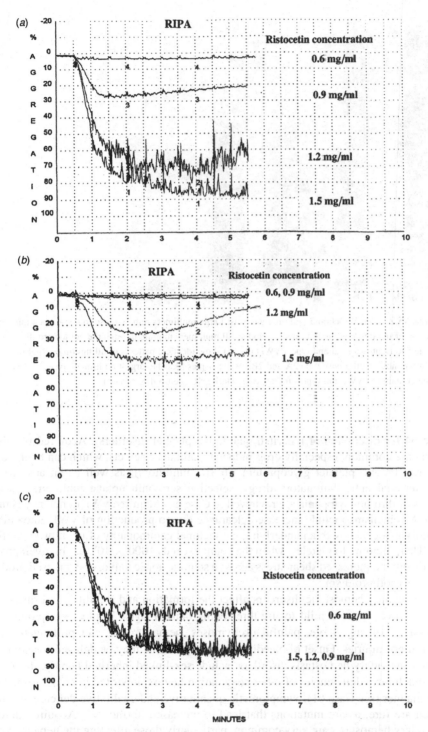

Figure 65.1   Ristocetin-cofactor-induced agglutination (RIPA) results: (*a*) increasing light transmission due to agglutination of normal platelets and vWF when ristocetin is >0.6 mg/mL. (*b*) blunted agglutination in response to ristocetin ≥0.9 mg/mL in platelet-rich plasma from patient described in this case (type 2A vWD); (*c*) exaggerated agglutination response to ristocetin at 0.6 and 0.9 mg/dL in platelet-rich plasma from a patient with type 2B vWD.

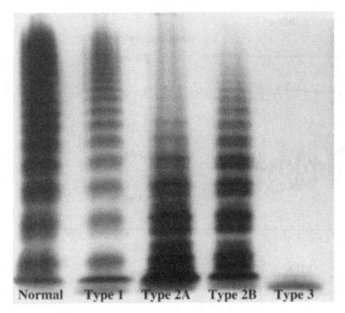

Figure 65.2   von Willebrand multimer analysis: Large multimers remain close to the application point at the top of the figure while intermediate and small multimers migrate through the gel toward the bottom. From left to right—normal and type 1 vWD plasma show identical patterns of all multimers (gel is qualitative, not quantitative); type 2A and 2B vWD plasmas lack the largest multimers; type 3 vWD plasma contains no vWF multimers (courtesy of Marlies R. Liedford-Kraemer.)

Case 64 for discussion of inherited qualitative platelet disorders). Acquired platelet disorders are common, especially drug-induced qualitative defects, which can be therapeutic (aspirin, Plavix, platelet glycoprotein IIb/IIIa inhibitors), as well as an adverse effect (nonsteroidal antiinflammatory drugs, selective serotonin uptake inhibitors). Acquired causes of thrombocytopenia are reviewed in Case 60. Acquired vWF deficiency is uncommon. Mechanisms include increased clearance due to production of vWF autoantibodies [usually associated with an underlying monoclonal gammopathy of unknown significance (MGUS)], binding to platelets when the count exceeds $1000 \times 10^6/\mu L$ in myeloproliferative disorders, increased shear stress across a stenotic aortic valve, or decreased production due to hypothyroidism.

Secondary hemostatic disorders affect the formation and stability of fibrin clots, and vary in severity from mild to life-threatening hemorrhages. Typical symptoms include excessive bruising, large, painful ecchymoses, hemarthroses, and prolonged bleeding from minor injuries. Onset of bleeding following trauma may be delayed for hours. Congenital secondary hemostasis disorders include sex-linked inherited hemophilia A and B, and much rarer deficiencies of other coagulation factors, inherited in an autosomal recessive manner (see Case 61). Symptomatic quantitative and qualitative deficiencies of fibrinogen are rare, as are mutations that lead to increased fibrinolysis. Acquired defects of secondary hemostasis are very common, particularly those affecting the hepatic synthesis of vitamin K–dependent coagulation factors X, IX, VII, and II (prothrombin). Mechanisms include acute or chronic liver diseases, nutritional deficiency of vitamin K, and therapeutic (oral anticoagulation with warfarin) or toxic (poisoning with rodentacides) vitamin K antagonism. Other classes of anticoagulant drugs reduce the rate of fibrin clot formation by directly inhibiting thrombin (hirudin, argatroban, and bivalirudin; see Case 60), or by accelerating inhibition of activated factors X and II (factor Xa and thrombin) by the natural inhibitor antithrombin (unfractionated heparin, low-molecular-weight heparin, and fondaparinux). Rarely, adults may produce inhibiting autoantibodies to coagulation factors, typically against factor VIII, and present with sudden onset of severe bleeding complications. Management strategies include immediate correction of the acquired coagulopathy to control bleeding, and immune suppression to stop production of the inhibitor (see Case 61). Acquired hyperfibrinolysis is an extremely rare event, associated with some malignancies, and bites from poisonous spiders and snakes. However, thrombolytic drugs (recombinant tissue plasminogen activator, urokinase, and streptokinase) are effective interventions to lyse acute coronary and cerebral thrombi as well as hemodynamically significant pulmonary emboli. Increased rates of thrombin generation and fibrinolysis are frequent complications of many illnesses, producing a clinical and laboratory condition called *disseminated intravascular coagulopathy* (DIC, see Case 53).

Unfortunately, the clinical signs and symptoms of primary and secondary disorders of hemostasis are not specific, and screening laboratory testing should be performed initially (platelet count, bleeding time, PFA-100, prothrombin time, and activated partial thromboplastin time), in order to guide subsequent laboratory evaluation of a patient with a significant bleeding history (see Case 64 for an algorithm).

Von Willebrand Factor

Megakaryocytes and endothelial cells are the only sites of von Willebrand factor synthesis. Within the endoplasmic reticulum, two vWF molecules undergo C-terminal linkage to form a dimer, and in the golgi apparatus, N-terminal linkage of dimers produces a range of intermediate and large multimers. vWF is stored in platelet α granules and released on activation. Endothelial cells constitutively secrete vWF and also store vWF in cytoplasmic vesicles (Weibel–Palade bodies) whose contents are released into the blood in response to activation of the endothelial membrane vasopressin V2 receptor. A plasma metaloprotease enzyme, ADAMTS-13, acts on circulating vWF multimers (cleavage between Tyrosine 1605 and Methionine 1606), shortening the very large multimers. Congenital or acquired deficiency of ADAMTS-13 can lead to thrombocytopenia and microangiopathic hemolytic anemia due to agglutination of platelets by unusually large vWF multimers.

Different domains of the vWF molecule are critical for the protein's multiple hemostatic functions. A collagen binding domain supports vWF adhesion to subendothelial collagen. When collagen-bound vWF is exposed to a high shear force, as is produced by damage to arterial vessels, the conformation of the platelet glycoprotein Ib binding region is altered, facilitating platelet adhesion and subsequent exposure to collagen, thrombin, and other platelet activators at the site of vascular injury. However, only the large vWF multimers have a role in platelet adhesion. Subsequent platelet aggregation is dependent on fibrinogen and vWF joining activated platelets by binding to platelet glycoprotein IIb/IIIa receptors. Another region of vWF binds coagulation factor VIII (FVIII), protecting it from rapid clearance and delivering FVIII to the site of vascular injury.

Von Willebrand Disease

Von Willebrand disease (vWD) is the most common inherited hemostatic disorder. The prevalence of vWD is approximately 100 per million worldwide when diagnostic criteria include a history of symptomatic bleeding and appropriate laboratory findings. vWD disease is divided into quantitative and qualitative vWF multimer defects. Type 1 vWD is a partial deficiency of vWF, with autosomal inheritance and incomplete penetrance, accounting for 70–80% of the diagnoses of vWD. Bleeding symptoms are typically mild to moderate. Most individuals with decreased vWF have plasma concentrations of 30–50%, have mild and inconsistent bleeding histories, lack an impressive family bleeding history, and do not have causal mutations in the vWF gene. Labeling these patients with a diagnosis of type I vWD is controversial. A person's blood type is an important, but incomplete explanation, for low vWF antigen concentrations. A typical vWF antigen range for type O blood donors is 36–157% compared to 48–239% for type A, 57–241% for type B, and 64–238% for type AB blood donors. A more complete understanding of the genetic and environmental factors that contribute to the wild variability of vWF levels is needed. One could consider reductions in vWF level to be a weak, continuous risk factor for bleeding complications, reserving the diagnosis of type I vWD for patients with vWF levels <20%, and personal and family bleeding histories consistent with autosomal dominant inheritance with high penetrance. Many, but not all, patients meeting these criteria will have a candidate causal vWF gene mutation.

Type 3 vWD is a rare, severe quantitative deficiency of vWF with an autosomal recessive inheritance pattern. Plasma vWF is usually undetectable, and FVIII activity is markedly reduced (≤5%) in the absence of its protective carrier molecule. Some type 3 vWD patients are homozygous or compound heterozygotes for a variety of vWF mutations, while others inherit normal vWF genes. Bleeding complications are severe, including spontaneous hemarthroses. While parents of type 3 vWD children are obligate carriers, most are asymptomatic.

Type 2 vWD consists of four different inherited qualitative vWF defects, and constitutes approximately 20–30% of vWD diagnoses. The severity of bleeding complications among patients with type 2 forms of vWD vary widely, but are typically intermediate between types 1 and 3 patients. Type 2A vWD (10–15% of vWD diagnoses) results from mutations that either impair secretion of large multimers or increase vWF susceptibility to proteolysis, leading to a reduction in circulating large vWF multimers. In vitro assays of vWF adhesion activity are dependent on the presence of large multimers. As a result, patients with type 2A vWD will typically have a mild reduction in vWF antigen and FVIII, and a moderate to severe reduction in vWF activity. Type 2B vWD (~5% of vWD diagnoses) is due to gain of function mutations in the platelet GPIb binding region of vWF, causing increased spontaneous binding of large and intermediate multimers to circulating platelets, and sometimes a mild thrombocytopenia due to shortened platelet survival. Type 2M vWD (very rare) is caused by mutations in the GPIb binding region that reduce vWF adhesion to platelets, but do not affect multimer patterns. Inheritance of types 2A, 2B, and 2M vWD is autosomal dominant with high penetrance. Finally, type 2N (rare) vWD is due to mutations in the FVIII binding domain that reduce vWF affinity for FVIII, leading to reduced FVIII half-life and decreased plasma FVIII activity, but do not affect vWF concentration, platelet adhesion function, or multimer pattern. Symptomatic patients are either type 2N homozygous, or compound heterozygous for type 1 and type 2N vWD.

Laboratory Diagnosis

Laboratory evaluation of patients suspected of von Willebrand disease relies on a panel of functional and immunologic tests, often performed on more than one occasion. Initial testing should include determination of plasma FVIII activity (method described in Case 61), von Willebrand factor antigen concentration, and platelet adhesion activity. In the absence of a definite family history of vWD, these specific tests may be preceded by performing a platelet count and global screening test of primary hemostasis (bleeding time or PFA-100 (see Case 64 for a discussion of these tests), and secondary hemostasis screening tests (aPTT may be prolonged as a result of FVIII deficiency). While the PFA-100 is considered to be a sensitive screening test for vWD, the bleeding time and aPTT are insensitive, and normal results for the latter two should not deter further testing when clinical suspicion exists for an increased bleeding risk.

There are several comparable methods for quantifying WF antigen, including immunoelectrophoresis, ELISA, and nephelometry. The ristocetin cofactor assay measures vWF platelet adhesion activity. Ristocetin is an antibiotic that binds to vWF multimers and enhances binding to platelet glycoprotein Ib in the absence of an increased shear force. Different concentrations of ristocetin are added to clear glass tubes containing formalin-fixed control platelets, and a patient's platelet poor plasma. The tubes are placed in an aggregometer instrument that measures increased light transmission through the tube as vWF multimers bind to and agglutinate the platelets. The increase in light transmission at different concentrations of ristocetin obtained with a patient's plasma is compared to dilutions of normal pooled plasma (NPP, which is assigned an activity of 100%) to determine ristocetin cofactor activity. A similar assay can be performed on some automated coagulation instruments. Ristocetin cofactor activity is dependent on the presence of larger vWF multimers since they are more effective at binding to platelet GPIb receptors.

Large vWF multimers also bind to collagen more avidly than do intermediate and small multimers. This property can be assessed in a collagen binding assay. Patient plasma is incubated in microtier wells with collagen type III bound to the bottom. After washing, an ELISA assay is performed with antihuman vWF antibodies to measure bound vWF. While this method accurately measures high-molecular-weight vWF multimers and has a lower level of detection compared to ristocetin cofactor assay, the physiologic importance of measuring in vitro binding of vWF to collagen has not been confirmed. In addition, if collagen binding were used instead of ristocetin cofactor assay to assess vWF function, patients with type 2M vWD would be misclassified since their plasma contains a full complement of vWF multimers with normal binding to collagen, but defective adhesion to platelets. Typical results for this test panel in different types of vWD are listed in Table 65.1.

Due to both biological and analytical variability, a different pattern of normal and abnormal results could be obtained when testing of patients with vWD is repeated, especially for type 1 vWD. For example, a patient with a convincing personal bleeding history and a first-degree relative with clinical and laboratory findings consistent with type 1 vWD could have a normal panel of results on one encounter, and some or all abnormal results when retested. Clinicians and laboratory technicians must take this into account when evaluating patients. In addition, oral contraceptives and pregnancy will increase vWF antigen and activity as well as FVIII levels, making it difficult to "rule out" type 1 vWD under these circumstances.

Table 65.1   Typical Laboratory Results in von Willebrand Disease

Type	FVIII:C	vWF:Ag	vWF:RCo	Multimers	RIPA
1	↓	↓	↓	NL	
2A	↓	↓	↓↓	Large, ↓	Blunted
2B	↓	↓	↓↓	Large, ↓	Exaggerated
2M	↓	↓	↓↓	NL	Blunted
2N[a]	↓↓	NL/↓	NL/↓	NL	
3	↓↓↓	↓↓↓	↓↓↓	Absent	

[a]vWF:Ag and vWF:RCo may be decreased in presence of compound heterozygote type 2N/type 1.

Key: FVIII:C, factor VIII activity; vWF:Ag, von Willebrand factor antigen; vWF:RCo, von Willebrand factor ristocetin cofactor activity; RIPA, ristocetin-induced platelet agglutination.

Type 2, B, or M vWD should be suspected when the vWF antigen : activity ratio is <0.7 (0.3 for patient in this case study) and type 2N suspected if the ratio of vWF Ag: FVIII is <0.7. To confirm a loss (type 2A or 2M) or gain (type 2B) of platelet adhesion function, a variation of the ristocetin cofactor assay is performed: ristocetin-induced platelet agglutination (Fig. 65.1). Increasing concentrations of ristocetin are added to platelet-rich plasma prepared from the patient's citrated whole blood, and agglutination is measured in an aggregometer. Patients with types 2A and 2M vWD will exhibit a blunted agglutination response, as did the patient in this case, due to a lack of (type 2A) or dysfunctional (type 2M) large vWF multimers. Patients with type 2B vWD will demonstrate an exaggerated agglutination response due to gain of function mutations that will enhance adhesion of intermediate vWF multimers to platelets in the presence of ristocetin. However, before diagnosing type 2B vWD based on a hyperresponse to ristocetin, an alternative, much rarer disorder must be considered: platelet-type pseudo–von Willebrand disease due to gain of function mutations in platelet GPIb. Repeating the RIPA test on mixtures of (1) patient's platelet-poor plasma and washed, fresh control platelets and (2) patient's washed platelets and normal platelet poor plasma should confirm whether the "gain of function" mutation is due to the patient's vWF or platelets. To confirm a diagnosis of type 2N vWD, a quantitative ELISA vWF: FVIII binding assay is available through some reference laboratories.

vWF multimer analysis is technically difficult, and is performed by selected reference laboratories. Separation of vWF multimers by agarose gel electrophoresis and identification of bands using radiolabled or chemoluminescent vWF antibodies will confirm a normal pattern of multimers in healthy controls and patients with types 1, 2M, and 2N vWD; the loss of large multimers in types 2A and 2B; and an absence of multimers in rare patients with type 3 vWD (Fig. 65.2). The utility of molecular diagnostic techniques to diagnose vWD is currently limited because of the incomplete understanding of the genetics of type 1 vWD. However, most causative mutations of type 2 forms of vWD are localized to exons coding for specific protein domains. While some laboratories perform genetic testing for type 2 vWD, it is rarely necessary to confirm a diagnosis of type 2 vWD that is based on the hemostasis testing described previously.

Management

A few months later the patient was scheduled for elective extraction of a molar. She received an intravenous infusion of desmopressin (DDAVP). A sample of citrated blood was collected one hour postinfusion, and the following results were obtained: FVIII activity, 187%; vWF antigen, 93%; and vWF ristocetin cofactor activity, 66%. On the basis of the excellent responses, the extraction was performed the same day and the patient was instructed to take 1000 mg of Amicar every 6 hours for the next 5 days. She tolerated the extraction without excessive immediate or delayed bleeding.

Treatment options for vWD include pharmacologic and transfusion therapies, depending on the type of vWD, historical response to bleeding challenges, and severity of anticipated intervention. DDAVP, a synthetic analog of vasopressin originally developed for treatment of diabetes insipidus, stimulates the release of stored vWF and factor VIII, producing a 3–5-fold increase in plasma vWF and FVIII levels within ~60 minutes followed by a gradual return to baseline over 8–12 hours. Two to three repeated doses at 12–24-hour intervals may be indicated in some circumstances, but tachyphylaxis (reduced response to a repeated stimulus) is common with multiple doses of DDAVP, and hyponatremia may occur, especially in young children. In general, DDAVP is an excellent hemostatic agent for management of menorrhagia, minor traumas, and surgical procedures in type 1 and some type 2 vWD patients. Most patients with type 1, and some with types 2A and 2M vWD, will respond to DDAVP. However, a response should be confirmed by monitoring vWF and FVIII after a test dose. DDAVP is not administered to type 2B vWD patients because they may develop transient thrombocytopenia after treatment due to release of large vWF multimers that avidly bind platelets. Type 2N patients do respond to DDAVP, but the increase in FVIII is relatively transient, due to the vWF-FVIII binding defect. Type 3 vWD patients do not respond to DDAVP. Antifibrinolytic drugs (ε-aminocaproic acid; Amicar) are useful adjuncts to DDAVP to prevent bleeding from mucous membranes, especially after dental procedures. Amicar binds to plasminogen, preventing attachment to fibrin, and delaying fibrinolysis.

vWF is copurified with factor VIII when FVIII concentrates are prepared from plasma by chromatography methods. These "intermediate-purity" FVIII concentrates are the preferred source of vWF replacement for major trauma or surgery in type 1 vWD patients, and for both mild and severe bleeding challenges in some type 2 and all type 3 vWD patients. However, FVIII concentrates purified from plasma using monoclonal FVIII antibodies and recombinant FVIII concentrates do not contain vWF, and should not be used to treat vWD patients. Cryoprecipitate is enriched in both FVIII and vWF, and would be an appropriate vWF replacement product if an intermediate-purity FVIII concentrate is not readily available. Since vWF antigen and activity results are rarely performed as STAT tests, vWF replacement is typically monitored by following FVIII activity.

Additional Reading

SCHNEPPENHEIM, R. AND BUDDE, U.: Phenotypic and genotypic diagnosis of von Willebrand disease: A 2004 update. *Semin. Hematol.* 42:15–28, 2005.

SADLER, J. E.: New concepts in von Willebrand disease. *Ann. Rev. Med. 56*:173–91, 2005.

MANNUCCI, P. M.: Treatment of von Willebrand's disease. *N. Engl. J. Med. 351*:683–94, 2004.

SADLER, J. E.: von Willebrand disease type 1: A diagnosis in search of a disease. *Blood 101*:2089–93, 2003.

FAVALORO, E. J.: von Willebrand factor collagen-binding (activity) assay in the diagnosis of von Willebrand disease: A 15-year journey. *Semin. Thrombo. Hemost. 28*:191–202, 2002.

Case 66

A Woman with Abdominal Pain and Thrombocytopenia

Ji Lu

A 42-year-old African-American woman developed dull crampy abdominal pain without accompanying nausea, fever, or diarrhea. Pain persisted over the next 4 days, and she noticed blurred vision and two bruises on her legs, although she did not recall ever falling or bumping into anything. When her symptoms did not improve, her sister brought her to the hospital. The patient worked as a nurse's aide, took no prescribed or over-the-counter medications, and did not acknowledge consumption of alcohol or illicit drugs. She was not sexually active.

On physical exam she was normotensive and afebrile; there were several 4–7-cm ecchymoses on the right knee and left tibia; neurological exam was nonfocal; her abdomen was mildly tender without palpable liver, spleen, or mass. The remainder of her exam was normal. Initial laboratory findings were as follows:

Analyte	Value, Conventional Units	Reference Interval, Conventional Units	Value, SI Units	Reference Interval, SI Units
WBC	$17.6 \times 10^3/\mu L$	4–10	$17.6 \times 10^9/L$	4–10
Hemoglobin	5.0 g/dL	12–15	50 g/L	120–150
Hematocrit	19%	36–48%	0.19 volume	0.36–0.48
MCV	61 fL	80–98	Same	
Reticulocyte %	8.2%	0.5–1.5%	0.082 fraction	0.005–0.015
Platelet count	$17 \times 10^3/\mu L$	140–400	$17 \times 10^9/L$	140–400
Prothrombin time	14 s	11–15	Same	
aPTT	26.45	23–36	Same	
Fibrinogen	454 mg/dL	140–400	4.54 g/L	1.4–4.0
Bilirubin, total	3 mg/dL	0.3–1.2	51.3 mmol/L	5.1–20.5
Bilirubin, indirect	2.5 mg/dL	<0.2	42.8 mmol/L	<3.42
Lactate dehydrogenase	4500 U/L	50–150 U/L	76.5 μkat/L	2.50–4.17
Creatinine	1.4 mg/dL	0.6–1.1	124 mmol/L	53–97
Haptoglobin	<7 mg/dL	35–164	<7 mg/L	350–1640

Tietz's Applied Laboratory Medicine, Second Edition. Edited by Mitchell G. Scott, Ann M. Gronowski, and Charles S. Eby

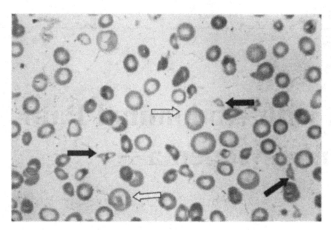

Figure 66.1   100× magnification of peripheral blood smear showing schistocytes (black arrows) and polychromatophilic red cells (white arrows).

A review of the patient's peripheral blood smear confirmed the low platelet count and elevated WBC consisting of neutrophils with immature forms limited to bands and metamyelocytes (left shift). Red cell morphology was notable for severe poikilocytosis (variation in shape) and anisocytosis (variation in size) dominated by many schistocytes (small, irregular, fragmented red cells) and polychromatophilic red cells (larger, blue–gray cells, consistent with increased reticulocyte count) (Fig. 66.1). The history, laboratory studies, and peripheral blood smear findings were consistent with microangiopathic hemolytic anemia due to thrombotic thrombocytopenia purpura (TTP). She was infused with four units of fresh-frozen plasma and two units of red cells while waiting for a central venous catheter to be inserted for plasma exchange.

Daily plasma exchange was initiated and abdominal pain resolved within several days, but platelet count (range 18–62 × 10^3/μL) and LDH did not normalize after 15 days despite addition of prednisone and replacement with cryoprecipitate-poor plasma. The patient tolerated a laproscopic splenectomy on day 16 without serious bleeding complications, and daily plasma exchange was continued, but her platelet count did not improve until rituximab was started. She was discharged on day 25 with a platelet count of 333 × 10^3/μL, and has remained in clinical remission for 38 months.

Differential Diagnosis

Microangiopathic hemolytic anemia (MAHA) refers to red cell fragmentation leading to hemolysis. In contrast to autoimmune hemolytic anemia, hemolysis in MAHA is caused by mechanical disruption of the red cell membrane, usually due to passage through abnormal arterioles. Fragmentation of red cells can be observed in the peripheral smear as schistocytes. Although rare schistocytes may be observed in normal peripheral smears, >1% schistocytes is abnormal. MAHA may be caused by any condition that increases physical stress on red cells. The most common causes are listed in Table 66.1.

TTP—Clinical Presentation

Thrombotic thrombocytopenic purpura (TTP) is a rare life-threatening disorder that has historically been recognized by the pentad of thrombocytopenia, microangiopathic

Table 66.1   Causes of Microangiopathic Hemolytic Anemia (MAHA)

Thrombotic thrombocytopenic purpura
Disseminated intravascular coagulation
Preeclampsia, eclampsia, HELLP syndrome
Disseminated cancer
Malignant hypertension
Vasculitis
Vascular malformations
Native or prosthetic heart valve dysfunction
Intraarterial balloon pump
Drugs (quinine, cyclosporine, ticlopidine, mitomycin C)
Burns

hemolytic anemia (MAHA), neurological symptoms, renal function abnormalities, and fever. Neurological symptoms are present in most patients diagnosed with TTP. The most common symptoms include confusion and severe headaches, but focal neurological symptoms, seizures, and coma can also occur. In patients with TTP, renal impairment is variable, and the urine analysis may be abnormal due to mild proteinuria and microhematuria with or without red cell casts. Fever is noted in about 60% of patients. Abdominal pain, possibly due to gastrointestinal ischemia, and neutrophilia are also sometimes observed.

The presentation of TTP shares many similarities with hemolytic uremic syndrome (HUS). Both can present with thrombocytopenia and MAHA, but TTP tends to have predominantly neurological symptoms while acute renal insufficiency is dominant in HUS. However, patients presenting with sporadic MAHA and predominantly renal dysfunction should still receive plasma exchange unless they have a prodrome of bloody diarrhea. Patients presenting with MAHA immediately preceded by bloody colitis are typically children and have HUS caused by a Shiga toxin released by enterohemorrhagic *Escherichia coli*, usually O157:H7. The associated thrombocytopenia and MAHA are seldom severe, and plasma exchange and antibiotic therapy have not been shown to be effective for those patients who typically recover with supportive care. At one point TTP and HUS were thought to be different presentations of the same disease process. However, more recent findings regarding the pathophysiology of TTP may distinguish it as a separate entity from HUS.

The incidence of TTP in the United States is estimated to be 11 per million. Idiopathic/sporadic TTP is the most common type, with an incidence of 4.5 per million. Very rare, autosomal recessive and dominant familial forms of TTP have been described, characterized by unpredictable TTP episodes typically beginning in childhood. TTP may also be associated with other conditions. Approximately 10–25% of cases of TTP occur during pregnancy or post-partum. A possible risk factor is an increased secretion of unusually large von Willebrand factor (ULVWF) during the third trimester of pregnancy (see TTP—Pathophysiology section below). Pregnancy-associated TTP does not resolve spontaneously following delivery, and plasma exchange is still the treatment of choice. MAHA and thrombocytopenia can also be a complication of systemic autoimmune disorders, cancers, bone marrow transplantation, HIV infections, and certain medications such as quinine, ticlopidine, clopidogrel, mitomycin C, and cyclosporine.

TTP—Pathophysiology

TTP is associated with the deposition of platelet-rich hyaline thrombi within the microcirculation of the brain, kidneys, heart, pancreas, spleen, adrenal glands, and other organ systems. In a majority of patients with TTP, the formation of these thrombi has been attributed to the abnormal accumulation of unusually large (UL) von Willebrand factor (vWF) multimers. vWF is synthesized in endothelial cells and assembled into multimers ranging in size from small dimers to huge unusually large multimers (ULvWF). When released into the plasma, ULvWF multimers are quickly reduced in size by a vWF-specific protease called ADAMTS-13 (*a d*isintegrinlike *a*nd *m*etalloprotease with *t*hrombo*s*pondin type 1 repeats). Very low or absent *ADAMTS13* activity is associated with accumulation of ULvWF multimers, which can then attach to platelets and promote platelet activation and aggregation, leading to the formation of platelet thrombi. Patients with the familial form of TTP have severe deficiencies of *ADAMTS13* activity and mutated *ADAMTS13* genes located on chromosome 9q34.

Most patients with sporadic/idiopathic TTP have very low or undetectable *ADAMTS13* activity at presentation. Inhibitory antibodies against ADAMTS-13 are detected in some, but not all, patients, which may be due to the insensitivity of current assay methods. As is seen in other autoimmune diseases, there is an increased incidence of sporadic/idiopathic TTP, ADAMTS-13 deficiency, and autoantibodies in African- American women. In patients diagnosed clinically with HUS, however, *ADAMTS13* activity is usually normal or only moderately decreased, and autoantibodies are not detected.

Laboratory Testing for Diagnosis and Management of TTP

While the classic pentad of TTP includes thrombocytopenia, microangiopathic hemolytic anemia (MAHA), neurological symptoms, renal dysfunction, and fever, the clinical symptoms are not consistently seen in all patients, and the decision to initiate potentially lifesaving treatment is made based solely on findings of unexplained acute thrombocytopenia and MAHA. Thrombocytopenia may be significant (mean $25 \times 10^3/\mu L$, range $5-120 \times 10^3/\mu L$), but severe bleeding complications are rare. A peripheral blood smear showing red blood cell fragmentation and >1.0% schistocytes is consistent with MAHA. The MCV can also be decreased as a result of red blood cell fragmentation, and hemolysis can cause elevated serum LDH and unconjugated bilirubin and reduced serum haptoglobin as seen in the case presented above.

Until recently, assays for *ADAMTS13* activity and ADAMTS-13 inhibitor titers were complex, labor-intensive, and available only through some reference laboratories. However, the development of synthetic substrates that are cleaved by *ADAMTS13* has facilitated development of simple and rapid commercial fluorescent enzyme assays. Nevertheless, due to a lack of clinical experience, it is premature to diagnose TTP or make management decisions based solely on *ADAMTS13* activity and inhibitor results.

Treatment

Thrombotic thrombocytopenic purpura has a mortality rate as high as 90% if left untreated. Plasma exchange, also known as *plasmapheresis*, reduces the mortality rate to 25% and should be initiated even if the diagnosis is uncertain. Plasma exchange removes ULvWF multimers and acquired *ADAMTS13* antibodies while replacing the ADAMTS-13 protease. Plasma infusion alone is not as effective as plasma exchange, but it can be used temporarily if plasma exchange is not immediately available. Although it would seem reasonable to assume that replacing a patient's plasma with cryoprecipitate-poor plasma, which is depleted of vWF, would be beneficial, small comparison studies have not shown a definite clinical benefit compared to fresh-frozen plasma (FFP). The recommended regiment is to exchange 1–1.5 estimated plasma volumes per treatment or 40–60 mL/kg body mass, performed daily until clinical and laboratory evidence indicates that hemolysis and platelet consumption have stopped. The effect of treatment can be evaluated by observation of end-organ, particularly neurologic, ischemic symptoms, normalization of LDH, and resolution of thrombocytopenia. Neurological symptoms and LDH tend to improve before thrombocytopenia, while schistocytes may persist for days or weeks following clinical remission. Recovery of renal function is not a reliable endpoint since chronic renal failure can occur in up to 25% of patients. Once clinical remission is achieved, plasma exchange can be tapered over 1–2 weeks and then stopped.

Complications of plasma exchange occur in 30–60% of patients treated. Complications can be major or minor and are usually due to immune reactions to transfused FFP or related to central venous catheter placement. Patients with a previous anaphylactoid reaction to plasma can be pretreated with prednisone, and diphenhydramine. Platelet transfusions are contraindicated and should be done only if absolutely necessary as they may exacerbate neurological symptoms or renal insufficiency.

Of patients receiving plasma exchange therapy for TTP, 10–20% do not respond after 5–7 days of treatment. For resistant disease, therapeutic options include increasing the frequency of plasma exchange to twice daily, which more efficiently exchanges plasma than increasing the volume of daily exchange; immunosuppressive agents such as prednisone; replacement with cryoprecipitate-poor plasma; vincristine; cytoxan; and intravenous immune globulin (IVIG). Splenectomy may benefit some patients by elimination of anti-ADAMTS-13-antibody-producing B cells and removing the sequestration site of platelets and red blood cells. Several recent case studies suggest that rituximab, a monoclonal antibody against CD20 antigen on B lymphocytes, may be able to reduce ADAMTS-13 inhibitor titers and increase enzymatic activity, and clinical remissions have been reported following rituximab therapy despite failure of other treatment modalities. Unfortunately, no prospective, controlled studies have been performed for any of these salvage therapies to determine the best approach to managing refractory TTP patients. Patients who recover from TTP may have relapses and require monitoring for recurrence of ischemia symptoms along with periodic CBC and LDH measurements. Patients who achieve a clinical remission but have persistent ULvWF multimers and low *ADAMTS13* activity appear to be at higher risk for relapse. The 10-year relapse rate is 36%, but mortality and morbidity of relapses are lower than the initial episode because of a predictable response to plasma exchange and early diagnosis.

Additional Reading

BOYCE, T. G., SWERDLOW, D. L., AND GRIFFIN, P. M.: *Escherichia coli* O157:H7 AND the hemolytic-uremic syndrome. *N. Engl. J. Med. 333*:364–8, 1995.

BURNS, E. R., LOU, Y., AND PATHAK, A: Morphologic diagnosis of thrombotic thrombocytopenic purpura. *Am. J. Hematol. 75*:18–21, 2004.

COPPO, P., BENGOUFA, D., VEYRADIER, A. ET AL.: Severe ADAMTS13 deficiency in adult idiopathic thrombotic microangiopathies defines a subset of patients characterized by various autoimmune manifestations, lower platelet count, and mild renal involvement. *Medicine* (Baltimore) *83*:233–44, 2004.

FURLAN, M., ROBLES, R., GALBUSERA, M. ET AL.: Von Willebrand factor-cleaving protease in thrombotic thrombocytopenic purpura and the hemolytic-uremic syndrome. *N. Engl. J. Med. 339*:1578–84, 1998.

MOAKE, J. L.: Thrombotic microangiopathies. *N. Engl. J. Med. 347*:589–600, 2002.

RIZVI, M. A., VESELY, S. K., GEORGE, J. N. ET AL.: Complications of plasma exchange in 71 consecutive patients treated for clinically suspected thrombotic thrombocytopenic purpura-hemolytic uremic syndrome. *Transfusion 40*:896–901, 2000.

ROCK, G. A.: Management of thrombotic thrombocytopenic purpura. *Br. J. Haematol. 109*:496–507, 2000.

RUGGENENTI, P., NORIS, M., AND REMUZZI, G.: Thrombotic microangiopathy, hemolytic uremic syndrome, and thrombotic thrombocytopenic purpura. *Kidney Int. 60*:831–46, 2001.

SHUMAK, K. H., ROCK, G. A., NAIR, R. C., and the Canadian Apheresis group: Late relapses in patients successfully treated for thrombotic thrombocytopenic purpura. *Ann. Intern. Med. 122*:569–72, 1995.

VEYRADIER, A., OBERT, B., HOULLIER, A., MEYER, D., AND GIRMA, J. P.: Specific von Willebrand factor-cleaving protease in thrombotic microangiopathies: A study of 111 cases. *Blood 98*:1765–72, 2001.

VON BAEYER, H.: Plasmapheresis in thrombotic microangiopathy-associated syndromes: Review of outcome data derived from clinical trials and open studies. *Ther. Apher. 6*:320–8, 2002.

WONG, C. S., JELACIC, S., HABEEB, R. L., WATKINS, S. L., AND TARR, P. I.: The risk of the hemolytic-uremic syndrome after antibiotic treatment of *Escherichia coli* 0157 : H7 infections. *N. Engl. J. Med. 342*:1930–6, 2000.

Case 67

Sudden Jaundice and Painful Fingers

Arnel Urbiztondo

The patient is a 60-year-old Caucasian male who went to see his physician with complaints of progressive fatigue and shortness of breath with exertion over the past month. He also noted intermittent painful, purple fingers when he worked outdoors in the cold, which resolved when he went indoors. Four years ago he was diagnosed with chronic lymphocytic leukemia (CLL), based on an incidental finding of a clonal lymphocytosis, and had not required treatment. Physical examination was notable for pale conjunctiva and mild scleral icteris. No peripheral adenopathy was detected, and his liver and spleen were not enlarged.

The following laboratory tests were ordered, and the results are shown:

Analyte	Value, Conventional Units	Reference Interval, Conventional Units	Value, SI Units	Reference Interval, SI Units
WBC	$43 \times 10^3/\mu L$	4.0–10.0	$43 \times 10^9/L$	4.0–10.0
Neutrophil count	1.5	1.8–7.7	$1.5 \times 10^9/L$	1.8–7.7
Lymphocyte count	41.5	1.0–4.8	$41.5 \times 10^9/L$	1.0–4.8
Hemoglobin	7.7 g/dL	14–17	77 g/L	140–170
RBC	$2.70 \times 10^3/\mu L$	4.50–5.70	$2.70 \times 10^{12}/L$	4.50–7.50
Hematocrit	23%	40–50	0.23 volume	0.40–0.50
Platelets	$160 \times 10^3/\mu L$	140–400	$160 \times 10^9/L$	140–400
MCV	85.4 fL	80–98	Same	
Reticulocyte %	11%	0.5–1.5%	0.11 fraction	0.005–0.015
Reticulocyte count	$295 \times 10^3/\mu L$	20–90	295 $10^9/L$	20–90
Bilirubin total	3.2 mg/dL	0.2–1.3	54.7 μmol/L	3.4–22.2
Bilirubin indirect	2.0 mg/dL	<0.3	34.2 μmol/L	<5.1
LDH	394 U/L	110–210	6.7 μkat/L	1.9–3.6
Haptoglobin	<7 mg/dL	27–220	<70 mg/L	270–2200

Examination of a peripheral blood smear showed an increased number of mature lymphocytes and scattered clumps of agglutinated red cells, rare spherocytes, and increased polychromasia (red cells recently released from the bone marrow contain residual RNA that stains purple on Wright–Giemsa staining).

Tietz's Applied Laboratory Medicine, Second Edition. Edited by Mitchell G. Scott, Ann M. Gronowski, and Charles S. Eby
Copyright © 2007 John Wiley & Sons, Inc.

A blood sample was sent to the blood bank for blood typing. The patient was A positive. A screen for red cell antibodies in his serum was positive, leading to testing his serum against a panel of commercial red cells of known phenotype. The patient's serum caused +2 agglutination of each red cell in the panel, as well as his own red cells, when examined at room temperature. However, when commercial red cells and patient serum were preincubated at 37°C before mixing, no agglutination occurred either spontaneously, or after the addition of Coombs antiserum (anti–human IgG and complement). Incubating the patient's red cells with Coombs antiserum at room temperature [direct antibody test (DAT)], caused +2 agglutination. When repeated with specific antiserum, the DAT was negative with anti-IgG and +2 with anticomplement. Finally, serial dilutions of the patient's serum were combined with test red cells at 4°C and agglutination was observed up to a dilution of 1 : 1024. The clinical, laboratory, and blood bank serology findings supported a diagnosis of cold agglutinin disease complicating chronic lymphocytic leukemia.

Definition

Cold autoantibodies are IgM antibodies that bind to the patient's own red cells at low temperatures (0–4°C). Most healthy people have low-titer ($\leq 1 : 32$) polyclonal cold autoantibodies in their sera, and they are considered benign and harmless because they have low thermal amplitudes, rarely agglutinating red cells in vitro above 25°C. Sometimes cold agglutinins will produce spurious erythrocyte results (increased MCV, decreased red cell number, inaccurate calculated hematocrit) due to agglutination at ambient temperature.

However, if the thermal amplitude of cold autoantibodies reaches temperatures close to acral body temperature (≥ 30°C), they may be harmful and cause hemolytic anemia. When hemolysis occurs, this is referred to as *cold agglutinin disease* (CAD), or *cold autoimmune hemolytic anemia*. Cold autoimmune hemolytic anemia accounts for 16–32% of immune mediated hemolytic anemias (see Case 92 for a discussion of warm autoimmune hemolytic anemia). CAD may be subdivided into two groups: chronic and transient.

Chronic cold agglutinin disease is characterized by a stable, mild to moderate anemia, occasional episodes of acute exacerbations of hemolysis and jaundice, or a combination of these presentations. Some patients will also report symptoms of peripheral vasoocclusion (cyanosis, numbness, pain) due to red cell agglutination by IgM within the arterioles of the fingers, toes, nose, and earlobes precipitated by exposure to cold temperatures. A mixture of intravascular and extravascular hemolysis occurs as a result of IgM-mediated complement activation on the red cell membrane. Patients with chronic CAD usually present in their fifth to eighth decades, sometimes in association with lymphoma, Waldenström macroglobulinemia, or chronic lymphocytic leukemia, as occurred in this case. While most cases are idiopathic, the IgM autoantibodies are produced by a monoclonal B cell population, and the disorder may eventually evolve into a malignant proliferative disease.

Transient cold agglutinin disease is a postinfectious disorder, in which the polyclonal IgM cold autoantibodies appear while the patient is recuperating from *Mycoplasma pneumonia* and less often infectious mononucleosis. Transient CAD has rarely been associated with cytomegalovirus, influenza, and human immunodeficiency virus (HIV) infections. Compared to the chronic form, transient CAD affects younger ages, is self-limited, and is usually asymptomatic, although rarely hemolysis can be severe.

Typically, the antigenic target of cold agglutinins is the Ii blood group system. This is a carbohydrate blood group similar to the ABO blood group. Newborn red cells express i antigen, and adult red cells predominantly express I antigen. Rare adults are homozygous ii. Chronic CAD IgM antibodies with I antigen specificity express unique heavy-chain variable regions and predominantly κ light chains, while transient polyclonal cold agglutinins associated with *Mycoplasma pneumoniae* are also specific for I antigen. Infectious mononucleosis-associated cold agglutinin IgM antibodies are polyclonal, and recognize the i antigen.

Differential Diagnosis

Signs and symptoms of cold-associated distal vasooclusion are neither specific (other causes include cryoglobulinemia and Raynaud phenomenon) nor sensitive for chronic cold agglutinin disease. The presence of spherocytes on peripheral smear could be due to a congenital red cell cytoskeleton defect (hereditary spherocytosis), or warm auto-immune hemolytic anemia.

However, distinguishing immune-mediated hemolytic anemias from inherited and acquired causes of nonimmune hemolytic anemia can be reliably achieved by obtaining a positive direct antibody test (DAT). The test is performed by incubating (at 37°C) a patient's rinsed red cells with a polyspecific antiserum that recognizes both human IgG and complement proteins. If red cells are coated with IgG and/or complement 3d, cross-linking of red cells by the antiserum will cause visible agglutination (scored +1 to +4). Subsequent testing with specific antisera to IgG and complement will complete the characterization of the autoimmune process. A diagnosis of chronic cold agglutinin disease is confirmed by additional serologic testing demonstrating only complement bound to red cells, a markedly elevated cold agglutinin titer, and none or minimal agglutination of cord blood red cells due to lack of expression of I antigen. Some drug-induced hemolytic anemias will have complement-only-positive DAT, without elevated cold agglutinin titers. Rarely, patients will have a mixed warm–cold autoimmune hemolytic anemia with IgG-positive DAT and high-titer cold agglutinin.

The presence of a high-titer cold agglutinin with high thermal amplitude can cause false-positive agglutination in other red cell serologic tests performed at room temperature such as ABO, Rh typing, and antibody screens. This interference can be removed by pre-warming cells and reagents or absorbing the cold agglutinin prior to testing, in order to correctly type the patient and identify possible underlying alloantibodies.

Pathophysiology

Agglutination and activation of the classical complement pathway occurs when cold agglutinins bind to red cells in the colder climate of the tips of the fingers, toes, nose, and earlobes. As red cells reenter the warmer visceral circulation, complement activation can go to completion and causing intravascular hemolysis if the IgM cold autoantibody has a very high thermal amplitude, delaying dissociation from the warming red cell. If complement activation is arrested at the C3b stage as a result of early dissociation of IgM cold agglutinins with lower thermal amplitudes, red cells are sequestered and partially or completely phagocytized predominantly in the liver by hepatic macrophages, which have a greater affinity for C3b than do splenic macrophages. Extravascular hemolysis, therefore, occurs primarily in the liver. Phagocytosis is dependent on the amount of C3b attached to the red cell membrane. Red cells with insufficient C3b density escape destruction and are released back into the circulation, where the C3b inactivator system further degrades C3b into C3d, C3dg, or both. These red cells not only escape the initial hepatic phagocytosis but also become resistant to further sequestration and destruction despite heavy coating with C3b degradation products for two reasons: (1) hepatic macrophages do not recognize C3b degradation products, and (2) red cells coated with C3d and C3dg are protected from further deposition of complement when exposed to IgM cold agglutinins in the distal circulation.

Treatment of Chronic Cold Agglutinin Disease

For the majority of cases, supportive therapy is all that is needed for chronic and transient cold agglutinin disease. In cases with mild anemia, keeping the patient's extremities warm, even moving to a warmer climate, is generally effective. Steroids are, by and large, not effective. However, certain subgroups of patients whose cold autoantibodies operate with high thermal amplitude have been reported to respond favorably with prednisone. α-Interferon has been effective as have oral chemotherapy drugs, including chlorambucil and cyclophosphamide. A prospective study using rituximab, to target mature B cells for destruction, in patients experiencing significant hemolysis and anemia showed the CD20 monoclonal antibody to be effective and well tolerated. Plasma exchange can be used in acute situations to lower the titer of IgM autoantibodies. Because the main organ of sequestration in chronic cold agglutinin disease is the liver, splenectomy is usually ineffective. Red cell transfusions should be reserved for exceptionally severe anemia since a considerable percentage of donor cells will be promptly agglutinated and undergo complement-mediated intra- or extravascular hemolysis.

In this case presentation, the patient's underlying CLL was responsible for his symptomatic CAD with evidence of both intravascular and extravascular hemolysis. He responded to four weekly infusions of rituximab, anti-CD20 monoclonal antibody, with resolution of all signs and symptoms of chronic hemolysis.

Paroxysmal Cold Hemoglobinuria

Paroxysmal cold hemoglobinuria (PCH) is the least common type of autoimmune hemolytic anemia. It is a cold-autoantibody-mediated hemolytic disease originally associated with tertiary syphilis. With the improvements in antibiotic therapy, the incidence of tertiary syphilis and, subsequently, PCH has dramatically decreased, making both diseases rare these days. PCH is now more likely to occur in children in association with various viral illnesses, including mumps, measles, and flulike syndromes.

The cause of hemolysis in PCH is the Donath–Landsteiner IgG biphasic autohemolysin. The autoantibody requires exposure to cold temperatures to attach to the red cell membrane and activate the complement cascade. Unlike IgM cold autoantibodies, Donath–Lansteiner antibodies do not detach when the red cell returns to the warmer visceral circulation, and complement activation is complete causing intravascular hemolysis. With tertiary syphilis-related PCH, patients experience recurrent, cold-induced intravascular hemolytic crises characterized by hemoglobinuria, hemoglobinemia, fever, and musculoskeletal pain. The pediatric variant of PCH presents as a single hemolytic episode with excellent prognosis. The target epitope in almost all cases of PCH is the P red cell antigen.

Diagnosis of PCH is based on recognition of the clinical presentation and in vitro demonstration of the biphasic hemolytic process: the Donath–Landsteiner test. The patient's serum is prepared while maintaining the blood sample at 37°C to prevent absorption of antibody to red cells at lower temperature. The patient's serum is mixed with group O, P-positive red cells and fresh control serum to provide an adequate source of complement. The tube containing this mixture is first incubated at 4°C for 30 minutes, then at 37°C for 60 minutes; centrifuged; and examined for hemolysis, which indicates a positive test.

Most cases of acute PCH are self-limited, and supportive therapy suffices. Patients with chronic PCH are advised to avoid exposure to cold temperatures. Pharmacotherapy is directed against syphilis if present. Transfusion is rarely indicated in the adult setting unless there is severe hemolysis. Treatment with steroids and splenectomy has not been successful, especially splenectomy, because hemolysis is primarily intravascular and not extravascular.

Additional Reading

Blood Banking and Transfusion Medicine, Basic Principles and Practice, HILLYER, C. D., SILBERSTEIN, L. E., NESS, P. M., KENNETH, C., ANDERSON, M. D., AND ROUSH, K. S. eds., Churchill Livingstone, New York, 2003.

BRECHER, M. E., ed., *Technical Manual*, 15th ed., American Association of Blood Banks, Bethesda, MD, 2005.

HARMENING, D.: *Modern Blood Banking and Transfusion Practices*, 5th ed., FA Davis Company, 2005.

PACKMAN, C. H., Hemolytic anemia resulting from immune injury. In *Williams Hematology*, 7th ed., G. HARVEY AND D. J. KLEIN, eds., McGraw-Hill Medical, New York, 2006, pp. 729–50.

PETZ, L. D.: A physician's guide to transfusion in autoimmune haemolytic anemia. *Br. J. Haematol. 124*:712–16, 2004.

ROSSE, W. F., HILLMEN, P., AND SCHREIBER, A. D.: Immune-mediated hemolytic anemia. *Hematology* 48–62, 2004.

Case 68

The Good in "Bad" Fish Tacos

Kimberley G. Crone

A healthy 34-year-old woman presented to the local emergency department with severe vomiting and diarrhea 8 hours after eating what she thought might be a "bad" fish taco at an outdoor taco stand at the local county fair. She was given fluids and supportive care. The vomiting and diarrhea resolved within 24 hours, and during the course of her hospital stay *Clostridium botulinum* was isolated from her stool.

The patient was 28 weeks pregnant and had received no prenatal care. Her first child, born 3 years earlier, also without prenatal care, was well. She denied trauma, or other problems with pregnancy. During her hospital stay, the following laboratory test results were obtained:

Mother's blood type	O, Rh-negative
Indirect Coombs test	Positive

These test results prompted follow-up testing:

Anti-Rh IgG antibody titer	1:512 (elevated)
Father's blood type	O, Rh-positive

An ultrasound examination of the fetus was performed and showed mild fetal hepatosplenomegaly, suggestive of early hydrops fetalis. There was no polyhydramnios. At 29 weeks 2 days of gestation, amniocentesis was performed. The amniotic fluid exhibited a δ 450 bilirubin (OD_{450}) of 0.307, corresponding to a high fetal risk zone on the Liley chart. Percutaneous umbilical blood sampling was performed 4 days later. In this procedure, an ultrasound-guided needle was placed in the umbilical vein to collect a fetal blood sample. From this sample, a STAT hemogram showed fetal anemia (see results tabulated below). Packed red blood cells (25 mL) were transfused into the fetal umbilical vein, and a posttransfusion blood sample was drawn. Fetal heart tones were reassuring throughout the procedure. Afterward, the patient was admitted to the

Tietz's Applied Laboratory Medicine, Second Edition. Edited by Mitchell G. Scott, Ann M. Gronowski, and Charles S. Eby
Copyright © 2007 John Wiley & Sons, Inc.

labor–delivery floor for monitoring. Ten days later, a second percutaneous umbilical blood sampling procedure was performed. Results of the fetal testing are shown:

	Pretransfusion, SI Units	Posttransfusion, SI Units	10 Days Posttransfusion, SI Units	Reference Interval, SI Units
Fetal hemoglobin	10.5 g/dL	13.4 g/dL	3.1 g/dL	11.5–14.3
	(105 g/L)	(134 g/L)	(31 g/L)	(115–14)
Fetal hematocrit	30.1 g/dL	39.5 g/dL	8.9 g/dL	36.5–45.3
	(301 g/L)	(395 g/L)	(89 g/L)	(365–453)

Fetal monitoring indicated fetal distress significant enough for immediate delivery. A jaundiced baby boy was delivered by emergency cesarean section at 31 weeks, but initially he did not cry or show respiratory effort. The placenta was grossly unremarkable. He was resuscitated and transferred to the neonatal intensive care unit, where he received red blood cell transfusions. His neonatal serum total bilirubin was 16.3 mg/dL (reference interval 1–8 mg/dL) (278.7 mmol/L; reference interval 17.1–137 mmol/L), for which he received daily phototherapy. The infant showed slow clinical improvement and was discharged 7 weeks later.

Definition of the Disease

Hemolytic disease of the newborn is caused by a blood group incompatibility between fetus and mother.[1–4] Fetal red blood cells with surface antigens inherited from the father are destroyed once they are bound by maternal antibodies. The clinical consequences for the baby can be severe, including hydrops fetalis (fluid accumulation in body cavities) and kernicterus (staining and damage to the brain from bilirubin). Today, hemolytic disease of the newborn due to the rhesus (Rh)-group antigens is preventable with the use of immunoglobulin, such as the purified anti-Rh immunoglobulin RhoGAM®. When prevention is not possible, obstetricians work closely with the laboratory to monitor fetal health.

Blood groups are defined by their red blood cell surface carbohydrates. Although many groups have been implicated in hemolytic disease of the newborn, the rhesus (Rh) group (D antigen) is particularly important because of its high immunogenicity and opportunity for clinical intervention. ABO incompatibility, present in at least 20% of pregnancies, uncommonly causes severe disease. Most antibodies to these groups (anti-A and anti-B) are IgM class immunoglobulins—too large to cross the placenta and inflict damage on fetal cells. Additionally, fetal red blood A and B antigens are not well developed, decreasing the likelihood of binding. With the appropriate use of Rh immunoglobulin by obstetricians, ABO incompatibility is replacing Rh incompatibility as the most frequent cause of hemolytic disease of the newborn.

The clinical entity hydrops fetalis (discussed below) has immune causes (e.g., Rh or ABO incompatibility). However, 9 out of 10 cases of hydrops fetalis today have a non-immune etiology, including fetal cardiovascular defects, chromosomal anomalies, and twin–twin transfusion. Intrauterine infection and inherited metabolic diseases are other important considerations.

Pathogenesis

Although the fetal and maternal circulatory systems are normally independent, small tears can allow fetal blood to enter the maternal circulation and occur in most pregnancies. Just

1 mL of fetal blood is enough to stimulate the maternal immune system to generate specific antibodies against fetal red cell antigens. In the first pregnancy, a mother initially produces IgM class antibodies, which have a pentameric structure too large to cross the placenta. This fetus is at low risk for hemolytic disease of the newborn. By the second pregnancy, the previously sensitized (alloimmunized) mother can produce smaller IgG class antibodies, which easily cross the placenta and bind fetal red cells, marking them for destruction by the spleen.

Hemolytic disease of the newborn encompasses a spectrum of clinical manifestations, ranging from mild anemia to severe hemolysis. The severity depends on the concentration of maternal antibodies, the specificity of the antibody to fetal red cells, and the ability of the fetal spleen to destroy antibody bound red cells. The liver and spleen, sites of extramedullary hematopoeisis in the fetus, enlarge to compensate for hemolysis. Erythroblastosis fetalis describes the finding of erythroblasts (immature nucleated red cells) released prematurely into the fetal circulation. If the liver and spleen cannot produce sufficient red blood cells, consequent severe hypoxia may damage the developing heart and liver. Since the liver normally manufactures blood proteins that help maintain intravascular oncotic pressure, damage to this organ is serious. Liver damage, combined with heart failure produced by myocardial hypoxia, produces a generalized edema known as *hydrops fetalis*, carrying with it a poor prognosis.

Bilirubin, a hemoglobin breakdown product present in elevated concentrations in fetuses with hemolytic disease of the newborn, can cross the placenta and be metabolized by the mother's liver during pregnancy. Only a fraction of the bilirubin produced is excreted into the amniotic fluid. After delivery, when maternal antibodies still circulate in the infant, but before the fetal liver enzymes are fully functional, bilirubin accumulates and may result in bilirubin encephalopathy (kernicterus). Yellow bilirubin staining of the central nervous system (CNS) can be seen in the basal ganglia, thalamus, cerebellum, cerebral gray matter, and spinal cord, resulting in severe neurological impairment.

Prevention and Diagnosis

All women should receive ABO and Rh typing as part of routine care at their first prenatal visit. The patient in this case did not obtain prenatal care for her first pregnancy and would not have obtained it for the second pregnancy until she presented to the hospital with food poisoning. Some good *can* come from "bad" fish tacos!

Like the ABO system, typing for Rh involves determining the presence (+) or absence (−) of carbohydrate antigens. An indirect Coombs test detects antibodies (such as anti-Rh) in the maternal blood. In this test, maternal serum is mixed with stock Rh+ cells. If antibodies to Rh are present, they bind the cells and cause agglutination. Maternal serum anti-Rh titers are followed through the course of the pregnancy if necessary.

To prevent hemolytic disease of the newborn, one dose of purified anti-Rh immunoglobulin (RhoGAM®) is given to Rh-negative mothers in their third trimester, when transplacental hemorrhage is most likely (28–32 weeks' gestation), and again within 72 hours of delivery. Amniocentesis, spontaneous or induced abortion, ectopic pregnancy, hydatidiform mole, chorionic villus sampling, percutaneous umbilical blood sampling, or abdominal trauma—all situations where alloimmunization may occur—are other indications for RhoGAM® for the protection of a current or future pregnancy. A single dose is sufficient to neutralize the immune response to 30 mL of fetal blood, with protection lasting 12 weeks. The mechanism of action of RhoGAM® is not completely understood, but it appears to facilitate removal of fetal red blood cells from maternal circulation, preventing the ability for alloimmunization. With the successful use of RhoGAM®, hemolytic disease of the newborn affects only about 0.1% of at-risk fetuses.

Laboratory Testing

The most commonly used screening test for the presence of transplacental hemorrhage is the erythrocyte "rosette test." This test effectively demonstrates a small number of Rh+ cells in a Rh− suspension. Maternal blood is mixed with anti-Rh antibody of human origin. If fetal red cells are present, these cells will become coated with the anti-Rh antibody. The sample is then washed, and indicator Rh+ cells are added. Visible rosettes are formed with several red cells clustered around each antibody-coated Rh-positive red cell. The number of rosettes is roughly proportional to the number of D-positive red cells present in the original mixture, but a quantitative method should be employed to estimate the dose of Rh-immune globulin needed.

The Kleihauer−Betke acid elution quantifies the amount of transplacental hemorrhage. In this test, a maternal blood smear is treated with an acid and then stained. Acid dissolves adult hemoglobin, leaving only empty red cell membrane "ghosts," but has no effect on fetal hemoglobin. By counting the normal appearing fetal cells, one can estimate the amount of hemorrhage, estimated, and administer an appropriate dose of RhoGAM®.

Patients with a positive indirect Coombs test and elevated antibody titers are followed closely, and often require amniotic fluid analysis to assess fetal health. The concentration of bilirubin in the amniotic fluid is an indicator of fetal hemolysis and anemia. During normal pregnancy, amniotic fluid bilirubin peaks at ∼19−22 weeks at concentrations of 1.6−1.8 mg/L. Intrauterine hemolysis severe enough to cause erythroblastosis fetalis can increase the bilirubin concentration of amniotic fluid to ∼10 mg/L. Because the concentration of amniotic fluid bilirubin is often too low to be measured by standard chemical techniques, an alternative method using scanning spectrophotometry has been devised. The principle of this approach is based on the fact that the deviation in amniotic fluid optical density at 450 nm is due to the presence of bilirubin. As bilirubin absorbs light maximally at 450 nm, the extent to which the curve deviates from a baseline (drawn between the optical density readings at 350 and 550 nm) at this wavelength is proportional to the concentration of bilirubin in the amniotic fluid, and it is this change in absorbance that is known as the ΔOD_{450}.

First introduced into clinical practice in 1961 by Liley, the ΔOD_{450} has become the most widely used test to predict the severity of HDN. Liley constructed a graph, referred to as the "Liley chart," which is now well known and is used to predict the severity of HDN. Liley created his chart by plotting the gestational age (in weeks) on the x axis and the log of the ΔOD_{450} value on the y axis then divided the chart into three zones based on patient outcomes. Results falling within zone I (low zone) were associated with unaffected or very mildly affected infants, results in zone II (mid zone) included infants with mild to severe anemia, and results within zone III (high zone) represented the most severely affected infants, most of whom died in utero. A limitation of the Liley curve relates to the fact that it plots data only between 27 and 42 weeks of gestational age. Linear extrapolations back to 20 weeks' gestational age are currently in use; however discussion remains in the literature regarding the validity of this method.

In 1993, Queenan and colleagues reported an alternative to the extrapolated Liley chart for the clinical management of Rh-immunized pregnancies.[2,5] When ΔOD_{450} results were plotted on a linear scale relative to gestational age, ΔOD_{450} values showed a slight increasing trend from 14 to 22 weeks, leveled off until 24 weeks, and then declined to term. The authors developed their own chart with zones demarcated by the ΔOD_{450} data from pregnancies unaffected and affected by HDN. The so-called Queenan chart allows data to be plotted from 14 weeks' gestation. Unlike the Liley curve, it contains a fourth zone of fetal risk. Comparison of the two methods suggests that they overlap considerably, but that the Queenan chart may overestimate fetal risk.[5] This chart is now widely used as a tool to manage alloimmunized pregnancies in the second and third trimesters.

More recently, the use of Doppler ultrasonography to measure blood flow through the middle cerebral artery has been investigated as a noninvasive method that could potentially replace amniocentesis in the assessment of fetal anemia. While the data supporting its use are encouraging, additional studies are required before its use is widely adopted. This approach may one day be used as the principal diagnostic test in the assessment of HDN.

References

1. MAITRA, A. AND KUMAR, V.: Diseases of infancy and childhood. In *Robbins and Cotran Pathologic Basis of Disease*, 7th ed., V. KUMAR, A. K. ABBAS, AND N. FAUSTO, eds., Elsevier, Philadelphia, 2005, pp. 469–512.

2. GRENACHE, D. G.: Hemolytic disease of the newborn. In *Handbook of Clinical Laboratory Testing during Pregnancy*, A. M. GRONOWSKI, ed., Humana Press, Totowa, 2004, pp. 219–43.

3. BRACEY, R. W. AND MOISE, K. J.: Hemolytic disease of the fetus or newborn: Treatment and prevention. In *Rossi's Principles of Transfusion Medicine*, 3rd ed., T. L. SIMON, W. H. DZIK, E. L. SNYDER, C. P. STOWELL, AND R. G. STRAUSS, eds., Lippincott, Williams & Wilkins, Philadelphia, 2002, pp. 428–45.

4. OHLS, R. K. AND CHRISTENSEN, R. D.: Development of the hematopoietic system. In *Nelson Textbook of Pediatrics*, 17th ed., R. E. BEHRMAN, R. M. KLIEGMAN, AND H. B. JENSEN, eds. Saunders, Philadelphia, 2004, pp. 1599–604.

5. SPINNATO, J. A., CLARK, A. L., RALSTON, K. K., GREENWELL, E. R., AND GOLDSMITH, L. J.: Hemolytic disease of the fetus: A comparison of the Queenan and extended Liley methods. *Obstet. Gynecol.* 92:441–5, 1998.

Case 69

The Jaundiced Mother

Nathan Walk

A 31-year-old white woman sought medical attention for complaints of fatigue and jaundice. Her two children, ages 4 and 3 months, had recently recovered from respiratory syncytial virus (RSV) infections, and the patient had experienced similar symptoms. About 10 years ago, she had an episode of mild jaundice that spontaneously resolved. Evaluation at that time confirmed a mild anemia and negative serologies for hepatitis A, B, and C. Her family history is notable for an older sister who has also experienced an episode of self-limited jaundice, and a chronically anemic mother. Physical exam was notable for a well-appearing woman with normal vital signs. Sclerae were icteric, and a spleen tip was palpable 2 cm below the left costal margin. The remainder of the exam was normal.

The following laboratory tests were obtained:

Analyte	Value, Conventional Units	Reference Interval, Conventional Units	Value, SI Units	Reference Interval, SI Units
WBC	$5.2 \times 10^3/\mu L$	4.0–10.0	$5.2 \times 10^9/L$	4.0–10.0
RBC	$3.4 \times 10^6/\mu L$	4.2–5.9	$3.4 \times 10^{12}/L$	4.2–5.9
Hemoglobin	11.1 g/dL	12–16 g/dL	111 g/L	120–160
Hematocrit	31%	37–48%	0.31 volume	0.37–0.48
MCV	92 fL	80–100	Same	
MCHC	38 g/dL	30–37	380 g/L	300–370
Reticulocyte %	6.1%	0.5–1.5%	0.061 fraction	0.005–0.015
Reticulocyte count	$207 \times 10^3/\mu L$	20–90	$207 \times 10^9/\mu L$	20–90
Bilirubin, total	2.2 mg/dL	0.2–1.3	37.6 μmol/L	3.4–22.2
Bilirubin, indirect	0.7 mg/dL	<0.3	12 μmol/L	<5.1
LDH	179 U/L	110–210	3.0 μkat/L	1.9–3.6
Iron	127 μg/dL	30–160	22.7 μmol/L	5.4–28.6
TIBC	279 μg/dL	228–428	49.9 μmol/L	40.8–76.6
Ferritin	38 ng/mL	10–200	38 μg/L	0–200
Vitamin B_{12}	604 pg/mL	>250 pg/ml	445 pmol/L	>185
Haptoglobin	145 mg/dL	27–220	350 mg/L	270–2200

Peripheral smear showed frequent spherocytes and polychromasia (Fig. 69.1).

Tietz's Applied Laboratory Medicine, Second Edition. Edited by Mitchell G. Scott, Ann M. Gronowski, and Charles S. Eby

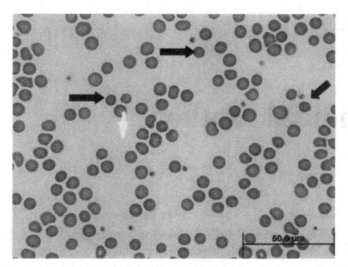

Figure 69.1 Peripheral smear (1000 × magnification) demonstrating spherocytes (darker-staining red cells without central pallor).

The history and laboratory findings were consistent with a diagnosis of hemolytic anemia due to hereditary spherocytosis. Additional tests were done to support this diagnosis and to rule out other causes of hemolytic anemia. Hemoglobin electrophoresis was normal, and direct antiglobulin test was negative. Glucose-6-phosphate (G6P) dehydrogenase (G6PD) activity was 8.9 U/g Hgb (reference interval 4.6–13.5), and flow cytometric analysis of CD59 expression was normal, eliminating a diagnosis of paroxysmal nocturnal hemoglobinuria. Finally, spherocytosis was confirmed by demonstrating increased osmotic fragility (Fig. 69.2).

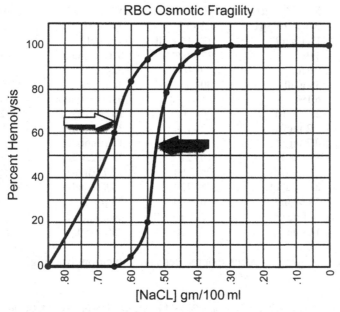

Figure 69.2 Osmotic fragility curves of unicubated red cells from a normal control ➡. The patient's red cell curve ⇨ is shifted to the left, indicating increased susceptibility to hemolysis as red cell volume increases when suspended in hypotonic saline.

Classification of hemolytic anemia is as follows:

1. Intrinsic to red cell
   a. Inherited
      i. Hemoglobin defects
         (1) Sickle cell disease
         (2) Thalassemias
      ii. Red cell membrane defects
         (1) Hereditary spherocytosis
         (2) Hereditary elliptocytosis/pyropoikilocytosis
         (3) Hereditary stomatocytosis, other rare defects
      iii. Red cell enzyme deficiencies
         (1) Glutathione metabolism: glucose-6-phosphate dehydrogenase and others
         (2) Glucose metabolism: pyruvate kinase and others
         (3) Other rare enzymes
   b. Acquired
      i. Paroxysmal nocturnal hemoglobinuria due to loss of GPI anchored anticomplement proteins.
2. Extrinsic, to red cell
   a. Immunity-mediated
      i. Autoimmune hemolytic anemia
      ii. ABO incompatible red cell transfusion
      iii. Delayed hemolytic transfusion
      iv. Drug-related immune hemolytic Anemia
   b. Non-immunity-mediated
      i. Trauma
         (1) TTP
         (2) DIC
         (3) Heart valve dysfunction
         (4) Vasculitis
         (5) Malignant hypertension
         (6) Malignancy
         (7) Marching, running
         (8) Burns
         (9) Arteriovenous malformations
      ii. Chemical
         (1) Snake, insect venoms
      iii. Infectious
         (1) Malaria
         (2) Babesiosis
         (3) Clostridium perfringes

Definition of Disease

Hereditary spherocytosis (HS) is the result of a molecular defect in one or more proteins that make up the cytoskeleton of the red blood cell (RBC) membrane. Most often, it is inherited as an autosomal dominant disorder, affecting approximately 1 in 5000 individuals of northern European ancestry. Lack of one or more of the cytoskeletal proteins destabilizes the lipid bilayer membrane. The cell membrane, not properly anchored, is lost in pieces as microvesicles are released. The remaining membrane of the RBC reforms, resulting in a smaller, denser, more spherical cell with a decreased surface area : volume ratio. Spherocytes are approximately two-thirds the diameter of a normal RBC, lack a zone of central pallor, and stain deeper red than do normal discoid erythrocytes when viewed on a Wright-stained blood smear. Spherocytes are poorly deformable; as a result, they are retained in the marrow and splenic sinusoids. There, they are exposed to a hostile environment of low pH and glucose concentration leading to red cell dehydration, increased hemoglobin concentration, further loss of cell membrane, and formation of dense "conditioned" red cells. These "conditioned" cells are even more sensitive to osmotic lysis. Ultimately, spherocytic red cells are targeted for destruction by the phagocytic action of macrophages via unknown mechanisms. It is this action by the spleen that causes the clinical manifestations of chronic hemolytic anemia, intermittent jaundice, and splenomegaly. In essence, then, two major factors are involved in HS pathophysiology: (1) an intrinsic RBC cytoskeleton defect, and (2) an intact spleen that selectively retains and destroys the abnormal erythrocytes.

The clinical features of HS have a broad range. On one end of the spectrum is a severe, transfusion-dependent anemia (<5% of cases), which usually shows an autosomal recessive inheritance pattern. A mild–moderate clinical presentation is associated with incompletely compensated anemia (~75% of cases), with a hemoglobin range of 8–15 g/dL, and reticulocyte percentages of 3–10%. These cases are associated with both autosomal dominant and recessive inheritance patterns. On the opposite end of the spectrum are patients who are not chronically anemic because of adequate bone marrow compensation (~25% of cases), and who become anemic only during periods of acute illness or stress. These cases are also inherited in both autosomal dominant and recessive patterns. The possibility of mild HS should be considered in any patient with unexplained splenomegaly, gallstones (specifically bilirubinate stones) during adolescence or young adulthood, unconjugated hyperbilirubinemia of unknown origin, severe anemia during pregnancy, or transient anemia during acute viral infections. Infection with parvovirus 19 may cause a particularly severe aplastic crisis due to its selective infection of erythroid precursors.

Differential Diagnosis

There are many causes of premature destruction of red cells, and correctly identifying the etiology requires careful review of patient and family histories, physical findings, and peripheral blood smear, combined with appropriate selection and interpretation of laboratory tests. Evidence of increased production of red cells is determined by confirming increased production of reticulocytes; immature red cells identified by staining residual RNA that disappear within days of release from the bone marrow. Reticulocyte counts, whether performed manually, or more precisely by a hematology analyzer, are often expressed as a percent of total red cell count. This is misleading when a patient is anemic, since an elevated reticulocyte percentage may not represent an absolute increase. If an absolute reticulocyte count is not provided by the laboratory, it can be calculated: reticulocyte number = RBC × reticulocyte percent/100. Typical reference interval is 20–90 × 10^3/μL. The patient in this case had an absolute reticulocyte count of 206 × 10^3/μL, indicating that her bone marrow was producing new red cells at least 2 times faster than basal rate because of shortened survival of spherocytes.

Hemolytic anemias may be classified according to whether the primary cause is intrinsic or extrinsic, immune or nonimmune, inherited or acquired, and whether hemolysis occurs primarily in the bloodstream (intravascular) or due to phagocytosis (extravascular) (see classification outline at beginning of this Discussion section). It is important to remember that spherocytes can be seen in association with hemolysis induced by splenomegaly in cirrhotic patients, in autoimmune hemolytic anemias, after being bitten by certain venomous snakes, and in clostridial sepsis. Spherocytes, in addition to schistocytes, may also be caused by mechanical, chemical, and thermal injuries to red cells.

Laboratory Diagnosis of Spherocytosis

As spherocytes on the peripheral smear are not always easily detectable in patients with mild HS, and as other laboratory features of hemolytic anemia may be nonspecific, additional testing may be helpful:

1. The mean cell hemoglobin concentration (MCHC), provided with the other red cells indices on an automated CBC report, is typically elevated in patients with HS because of loss of intracellular electrolytes and water.

2. The increased osmotic fragility of spherocytes can be quantitated. The osmotic fragility test measures in vitro lysis of erythrocytes placed in solutions of decreasing osmolarity. It can be performed on freshly collected blood, or after incubating RBCs for 18–24 hours at 37°C. Incubation "sensitizes" spherocytic red cell membranes, and increases their susceptibility to osmotic lysis. When placed in a hypotonic solution, red cells absorb water until reaching a "critical" hemolytic volume, at which point they rupture. Since spherocytes have a decreased surface area compared to a biconcave red cell, their critical hemolytic volume is reached sooner. Hence, more spherocytes lyse at a given concentration of hypotonic NaCl. Patient and normal red cells are added to separate tubes containing a range of NaCl concentrations. Following incubation, percent lysis (based on absorption of free hemoglobin at 540 nm) is plotted against NaCl concentration to generate osmotic fragility curves. Figure 69.2 shows an example of osmotic fragility curves for red cells from a normal control and a patient with mildy uncompensated HS. It is important to remember that increased osmotic fragility is not specific for HS, and can be positive when there is a different mechanism responsible for spherocyte formation such as autoimmune hemolytic anemia.

Pathogenesis

The hallmark of HS is loss of RBC membrane surface area relative to volume due to defects in the underlying cytoskeleton. The underlying cytoskeleton is composed of multiple proteins (Fig. 69.3), some of which may be deficient in hereditary spherocytosis including α or β spectrin, ankyrin, band 3, and protein 4.2. A deficiency of one or more of these proteins leads to uncoupling of the lipid bilayer from the underlying skeleton. As a result, the lipid bilayer is less well anchored and portions of it literally "bleb" off as microvesicles. The molecular basis for hereditary spherocytosis is heterogeneous, and most kindreds have unique mutations. Quantitative abnormalities in erythrocyte

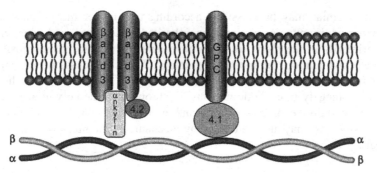

Figure 69.3   Model of red cell cytoskeleton and integral membrane proteins: α and β spectrin molecules form heterodimers that self-assemble into flexible tetramer and oligomer rods, providing shape and flexibility to the red cell membrane. Ankyrin forms the major linkage between spectrin and the membrane protein band 3. Protein 4.1 facilitates binding of spectrin to membrane protein glycophorin C (GPC), and protein 4.2 stabilizes spectrin–ankyrin–band 3 interactions.

membrane proteins in patients with HS allow for separation into subsets: (1) isolated deficiency of spectrin, (2) combined deficiencies of spectrin and ankyrin, (3) deficiency of band 3 protein, and (4) deficiency of protein 4.2.

Approximately 50% of HS patients have ankyrin mutations; these are typically transmitted in an autosomal dominant fashion, and produce mild to moderate disease. Ankyrin deficiencies are associated with a proportional decrease in spectrin, since ankyrin provides the principal linkage between spectrin and the red cell membrane. Mutations in spectrin, accounting for about 25% of patients, include defects in both the α and β spectrin chains. A mutation in β spectrin usually causes mild disease, and is inherited in an autosomal dominant fashion. Since α spectrin is normally synthesized in excess compared to β spectrin, a partial deficiency of α spectrin does not cause HS. Homozygous deficiency of α spectrin, on the other hand, produces a severe form of HS. Defects in band 3 protein present with a mild to moderate phenotype and have a dominant mode of inheritance. Mutations in protein 4.2 are relatively common in Japan, present with mild disease, and have a recessive mode of inheritance.

There are additional inherited red cell cytoskeletal disorders, defined by the dominant red cell deformity. Hereditary elliptocytosis (HE), relatively common in regions of Africa and Asia, like HS, is heterogeneous in terms of the mutated protein, severity of hemolysis, and mode of inheritance. In general, most HE patients are not anemic, and their red cells become progressively elliptical as they age as a result of autosomal dominant inheritance of mutations in α or β spectrin that interfere with assembly of spectrin dimers leading to a weakened cytoskeleton. Osmotic fragility is not increased. Hereditary pyropoikilocytosis (HPP) is a severe form of HE characterized by bizarre red cell shapes and microspherocytes, in addition to elliptocytes. The name is derived from the appearance of the red cells, which is similar to that obtained by denaturing the cytoskeleton of normal red cells after heating to 49°C. Hereditary stomatocytosis is an uncommon, incompletely understood, autosomal dominant hemolytic anemia characterized by the formation of a wide transverse slit, or stoma, of central pallor in erythrocytes. The primary defect is red cell dehydration and increase in MCHC due to net loss of intracellular potassium. Red cell membrane is not lost, and osmotic fragility is not increased. Chronic hemolysis is typically mild.

Treatment

Patients with mild forms of HS can typically be followed without specific medical intervention. Folic acid supplementation is recommended to support increased erythropoiesis due to chronic hemolysis. Patients should be advised of the signs and symptoms of cholecystitis, and surveillance ultrasounds are appropriate. Splenectomy is likely to be beneficial for patients with moderate to severe disease, which may involve growth retardation, skeletal changes due to marrow expansion, symptomatic anemia requiring transfusion, and massive splenomegaly. While splenectomy does not correct the membrane abnormality, it markedly reduces the reticuloendothelial system's scavenging and removal of spherocytic RBCs. The risks and benefits of the procedure should be carefully considered, however, and preceded by immunization against pneumococcus, *Haemophilus influenzae*, and meningococcus. In the postoperative period, patients may suffer from bleeding, infection, or pancreatitis. Longer-term risks postsplenectomy include overwhelming postsplenectomy sepsis from encapsulated bacteria and venous thrombosis.

Additional Reading

EBER, S. AND LUX, S. E.: Hereditary spherocytosis—defects in proteins that connect the membrane skeleton to the lipid bilayer. *Semin. Hematol. 41*:118–41, 2004.

HOFFMAN, R.: *Hematology: Basic Principles and Practice,* 4th ed., Churchill Livingstone, 2005 pp. 671–7.

KASPER, D. L.: *Harrison's Principles of Internal Medicine,* 16th ed., McGraw-Hill, 2005, pp. 608–9.

TSE, W., AND LUX, S.: Red blood cell membrane disorders. *Br. J. Haemotol. 104*:2–13, 1999.

Part Fifteen

Porphyrias

Cases of acute intermittent porphyria and porphyria cutanea tarda (PCT) concomitant with hemochromatosis are presented and discussed in Cases 70 and 71, respectively (both edited by MGS).

Tietz's Applied Laboratory Medicine, Second Edition. Edited by Mitchell G. Scott, Ann M. Gronowski, and Charles S. Eby
Copyright © 2007 John Wiley & Sons, Inc.

Case 70

Young Woman with Recurrent Abdominal Pain

Steven I. Shedlofsky

A 22-year-old white female presented to the emergency department with severe abdominal pain and profound generalized weakness. Milder episodes of similar abdominal pains had been occurring intermittently since age 17. When the patient was 18, an appendectomy was performed during one episode, but her appendix and terminal ileum were normal. Episodes occurred, on the average, every 3 months. Because her pain usually began 4–7 days before onset of her menstrual period and resolved with menses, a gynecological cause was suspected. However, numerous pelvic examinations; ultrasonographic examinations of her ovaries, fallopian tubes, and uterus; and even a laparoscopy revealed normal anatomy.

The patient's pains were usually dull, aching, and poorly localized and would last for hours without relief. Often there would be nausea but rarely vomiting. Frequently the patient developed abdominal distention and constipation and complained of leg weakness, but she was usually able to walk. When seen in the emergency department or office during these episodes, she was tachycardic but otherwise had a nonrevealing examination. Her stool was always negative for occult blood. Over the years, she had maintained a stable weight of 103–107 lb (47–48 kg). All of her routine laboratory studies, including complete blood counts, pancreatic enzymes, liver function tests, antinuclear antibodies, and urinalyses, were normal. The patient and her boyfriend were using condoms for contraception, and urine pregnancy tests were always negative. An upper gastrointestinal x-ray examination with a small bowel study, an endoscopic examination of her stomach and duodenum, a colonoscopy, a capsule endoscopy of her small bowel and a computed tomographic (CT) scan of her abdomen and pelvis had all been performed within the last year and were normal.

Prior to age 17, the patient never had any significant illnesses, although she had required phototherapy for neonatal jaundice. She was the eldest of four children (two sisters and one brother) who, along with her parents, were in good health. There was no history of gastrointestinal or gynecologic problems in her family, although an aunt on her father's side had periodically suffered unexplained abdominal pain.

To manage the pain, the patient would take oral meperidine and acetaminophen with some relief. Only once in the past 2 years did she have to visit the emergency department

Tietz's Applied Laboratory Medicine, Second Edition. Edited by Mitchell G. Scott, Ann M. Gronowski, and Charles S. Eby
Copyright © 2007 John Wiley & Sons, Inc.

because of dehydration due to an inability to eat or drink. The patient had been referred to a psychiatrist 2 years previously and was still seeing him occasionally. Although the psychiatrist had expressed concern about her narcotic use, he discovered no affective or thought disorder and had recommended a variety of antianxiety drugs, which the patient declined.

Just 3 days prior to the patient's current presentation, her gynecologist had prescribed trimethoprim and sulfamethoxazole for a presumed urinary tract infection. When the patient arrived in pain this time, she was complaining of much more severe abdominal pain, nausea with vomiting, bilateral leg pain with paresthesias, and generalized weakness such that she could not stand. She was a well-nourished but dehydrated young woman in obvious pain and very weak with a pulse of 125 bpm and a blood pressure of 142/105 mm Hg. Although she complained of abdominal pain, there was no localized tenderness or rebound pain. Her abdomen was distended and revealed scars from her appendectomy and laparoscopy. Neurological examination showed decreased motor strength in both legs and absent reflexes. Responses to pinprick, light touch, and proprioception were decreased.

Initial laboratory results were as follows:

Analyte	Value, Conventional Units	Reference Interval, Conventional Units	Value, SI Units	Reference Interval, SI Units
Hemoglobin (B)	13.4 g/dL	12–16	134 g/L	120–160 g/L
Hematocrit (B)	39%	37–47	0.39	0.37–0.47
Leukocyte count (B)	$9.4 \times 10^3/\mu L$	4.8–10.8	$9.4 \times 10^9/L$	4.8–10.8
MCV (B)	85 fL	80–94	Same	
Platelet count (B)	$381 \times 10^3/\mu L$	150–450	$381 \times 10^9/L$	150–450
Sodium (S)	133 mmol/L	136–145	Same	
Potassium (S)	3.6 mmol/L	3.8–5.1	Same	
Chloride (S)	97 mmol/L	98–107	Same	
CO_2, total (S)	32 mmol/L	23–31	Same	
Urea nitrogen (S)	27 mg/dL	8–21	9.6 mmol urea/L	2.9–7.5
Creatinine (S)	0.8 mg/dL	0.7–1.3	71 μmol/L	62–115
Glucose (S)	106 mg/dL	80–115	5.8 mmol/L	4.4–6.4
Calcium (S)	8.8 mg/dL	8.4–10.2	2.20 mmol/L	2.10–2.55
Phosphorus (S)	3.2 mg/dL	2.7–4.5	1.03 mmol/L	0.87–1.45
Protein, total (S)	6.6 g/dL	6.2–7.6	66 g/L	62–76
Albumin (S)	3.4 g/dL	3.5–5.0	34 g/L	35–50
AST (S)	44 U/L	16–48	0.73 μkat/L	0.27–0.80
ALT (S)	37 U/L	13–40	0.63 μkat/L	0.22–0.67
ALP (S)	88 U/L	30–100	1.46 μkat/L	0.50–1.67
GGT (S)	33 U/L	10–50	0.56 μkat/L	0.17–0.83
β-HCG pregnancy test (S)	Negative	Negative		
Urinalysis (U)	Negative for glucose, protein, bilirubin, blood, and leukocyte esterase;			
pH	5.2			
Specific gravity	1.033			

Abdominal x-ray films showed some distended loops of bowel, but no air–fluid levels or free air. The patient was admitted, and her dehydration was treated with intravenous fluids. Shortly after admission, the patient's hospitalist was contacted by the clinical laboratory and told that her urine sample had turned a deep red-wine color after standing at room temperature on the laboratory bench. The laboratory supervisor suggested ordering a semiquantitative rapid urine porphobilinogen that could be performed in the hospital laboratory. This was done and demonstrated a strongly positive result of >23 mg PBG/L (>100 μmol/L).

The hospitalist quickly obtained information on how to diagnose and treat the acute hepatic porphyrias. She stopped the patient's sulfamethoxazole and began therapy with intravenous glucose (at a rate of 12.5 g/h), meperidine (via a "patient-controlled analgesia" pump), promethazine (as need for nausea), and propranolol for the tachycardia. She also ordered intravenous hemin therapy (Panhematin, Ovation Pharmaceuticals, Deerfield, IL) at a dose of 3–4 mg/kg given mixed with a vial of human serum albumin[1] as an infusion over 15 minutes each day for 4 days. The hemin was not available until the next day. But the patient responded with some relief to hydration, carbohydrate loading, and analgesics. Her pain was markedly improved just hours after the first hemin/albumin infusion. However, her pain did not totally resolve until she started her menstrual period on admission day 4. She was then given her last infusion of hemin/albumin and discharged from the hospital.

The patient's primary care physician saw her in his clinic a week after discharge, and the patient had no symptoms. Her hypertension and constipation had resolved. Further studies were obtained to confirm the diagnosis of acute porphyria and to characterize which acute porphyria. A 24-hour urine specimen for the quantitative determination of porphyrins and porphobilinogen (PBG) was collected. (The specimen was collected with sodium bicarbonate, kept on ice, and protected from light.) Another 24-hour urine specimen for quantitative analysis of δ-aminolevulinate (ALA) was collected the next day. (The specimen bottle contained hydrochloric acid, was kept on ice, and was protected from light.) A 24-hour stool was collected and sent for quantitative porphyrins. An erythrocyte porphobilinogen deaminase activity was determined; the test results were as follows:

Analyte	Value, Conventional Units	Reference Interval, Conventional Units	Value, SI Units	Reference Interval, SI Units
24-hour urine				
(sodium bicarbonate, alkaline collection)				
Volume	750 mL			
Creatinine	945 mg/day	600–1600	8.4 mmol/day	5.3–14.1
Porphobilinogen (PBG)	12.4 mg/day	0.0–1.5	54.8 μmol/day	0.0–6.6
Uroporphyrin	64 μg/day	0–22	77 nmol/day	0–26
Heptacarboxyporphyrin	16 μg/day	0–9	20 nmol/day	0–11
Hexacarboxyporphyrin	2 μg/day	0–4	3 nmol/day	0–5
Pentacarboxyporphyrin	13 μg/day	0–3	18 nmol/day	0–4
Coproporphyrin	122 μg/day	0–60	186 nmol/day	0–92
24-hour urine				
(hydrochloric acid, acidified collection)				
Volume	625 mL			
Creatinine	956 mg/day	600–1600	8.5 mmol/day	5.3–14.1
ALA	8.4 mg/day	0.0–3.0	64 μmol/day	0–23

Analyte	Value, Conventional Units	Reference Interval, Conventional Units	Value, SI Units	Reference Interval, SI Units
Random stool specimen				
Weight	124 g			
Uroporphyrin	102 μg/100 g	<170 μg	122 nmol/100 g	<200 nmol
Coproporphyrin	152 μg/100 g	<900 μg	233 nmol/100 g	<1400 nmol
Protoporphyrin	309 μg/100 g	<1500 μg	550 nmol/100 g	<2600 nmol
Erythrocyte porphobilinogen deaminase	7.0 nmol/(s · L)	8.1–16.8	7.0 nkat/L	8.1–16.8

The elevated urinary PBG excretion confirmed that the patient had one of the *acute hepatic porphyrias*. Since the PBG excretion was much greater than the ALA excretion, lead poisoning could be ruled out as a cause of the symptoms. (In lead poisoning, ALA excretion is greater than PBG excretion.) The normal stool porphyrin studies ruled out variegate porphyria (VP) and hereditary coproporphyria (HCP) and confirmed that the patient must have acute intermittent porphyria (AIP). This diagnosis was further supported by the decreased erythrocyte PBG deaminase activity and the fact that she never experienced any photosensitivity or skin lesions in sun-exposed areas (see discussion below).

The physician surmised that the recent sulfamethoxazole therapy for the patient's urinary tract infection had induced this rather severe attack of AIP, possibly in coincidence with one of her milder, hormonally induced premenstrual attacks. Because of the diagnosis of AIP, the patient was instructed to avoid a number of potentially dangerous medications (see Website listed as Ref. 4). She continued to have mild, painful attacks 2–3 times per year, almost always prior to menses. The attacks responded to one dose of intravenous hemin that was given (without albumin) as an outpatient along with oral carbohydrate loading.

After her marriage and despite being told that AIP was a genetic disorder that had a 50% chance of being inherited by each of her children, the patient at age 26 became pregnant. However, she had no attacks during pregnancy and delivered a healthy son. She was fine until 6 months postpartum when a severe attack prompted hospitalization and a 4-day course of hemin/albumin infusions. When the patient's youngest sister also began having attacks of abdominal pain and was diagnosed with AIP, the patient decided to have a tubal ligation. By age 28, 6 years after the diagnosis of AIP was made, the patient stopped having premenstrual pain attacks and has remained in good health since. Erythrocyte PBG deaminase assays were performed on the patient again, as well as her parents, her siblings, and her son and demonstrated 50% enzymatic activity in the patient's father, and the younger sister with diagnosed AIP. The patient's other siblings and her 15-month-old son had normal activities.

Definition of Porphyrias

The Heme Pathway and the Porphyrias

The group of metabolic disorders collectively known as the *porphyrias* is a diverse group of diseases caused by defects in the heme synthetic pathway. A comprehensive review can

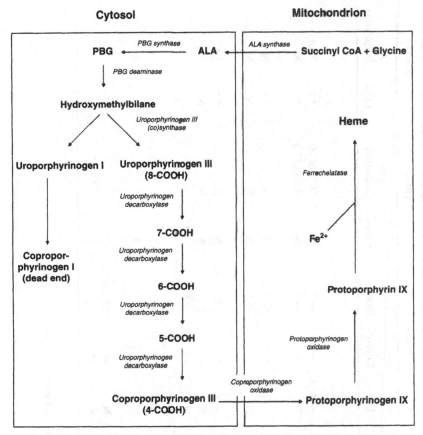

Figure 70.1 Heme metabolic pathway. Substrates are shown in bold letters and enzymes in italics. In all three acute hepatic porphyrias (AIP, VP, and HCP) there is inappropriate induction of ALA synthase. The enzyme deficiencies for each porphyria are as follows: acute intermittent porphyria (AIP)—PBG deaminase; congenital erythropoietic porphyria (CEP)—uroporphyrinogen III (co)synthase; porphyria cutanea tarda (PCT)—uroporphyrinogen decarboxylase; hereditary coproporphyria (HCP)—coproporphyrinogen oxidase; variegate porphyria (VP)—protoporphyrinogen oxidase; erythrocytic protoporphyria (EPP)—ferrochelatase.

be found elsewhere,[2] so the following brief discussion will highlight only those facts that will help reach appropriate diagnosis, avoid inducing porphyric attacks, and promote an understanding of various therapeutic measures. Figure 70.1 shows a simplified schematic of the heme pathway, and Table 70.1 summarizes the urine, feces, erythrocyte, and plasma abnormalities for diagnosing more frequently seen porphyrias.

The first important concept is that a porphyria presents either as an acute, neurologically mediated pain crisis or as a porphyrin-induced cutaneous photosensitivity reaction, depending on which heme precursors are being produced in excess. The heme precursors, δ-aminolevulinate (ALA) and porphobilinogen (PBG), are small water-soluble molecules that are rapidly excreted in the urine if overproduced; neither is photosensitizing. Porphyrins, on the other hand, are carboxylated tetrapyrroles that absorb light of 400 nm (Soret wavelength) with subsequent locally damaging release of energy. In vivo, much more heme is synthesized in the liver and marrow, although all cells must have the capacity to make heme. During heme synthesis, only the reduced porphyrinogens actually pass through the biochemical pathway. If excess porphyrinogens accumulate, they are

Table 70.1 Laboratory Findings for Diagnosis of the Most Frequently Seen Porphyrias

Porphyria type	Urine[a]				Feces			RBCs		Plasma	
	ALA	PBG	Uro	Copro	Uro	Copro	Proto	Proto[b]	PBG deaminase	PBG	Porphyrins
Acute hepatic prophyrias											
Acute intermittent porphyrias											
Manifest	↑↑	↑↑	↑↑	↑	↑↑	↑↑	→↑	N	50% of Nl	↑↑	N or →↑
Latent	↑	↑	→↑	→↑	N	N	→↑	N	50% of Nl	↑↑	N
Hereditary coproporphyia											
Manifest	↑↑	↑↑	→↑	↑↑	→↑	↑↑	→↑	N	N	↑↑	N
Latent	N	N	→↑	↑↑	N	↑	→↑	N	N	N	N
Variegate porphyria											
Manifest	↑↑	↑↑	↑	↑↑	↑	↑	↑↑	N	N	↑↑	↑↑[c]
Latent	N	N	N	↑	N	↑	↑	N	N	N	↑
Lead poisoning	↑↑	→↑	N	→↑	→↑	→↑	→↑	→↑[d]			
Porphyria cutanea tarda											
Manifest (untreated)	→↑	N	↑↑	↑↑	↑	↑[e]	N	N	N		↑↑
Manifest (treated)	N	N	→↑	→↑	→↑	→↑	N	N	N		N
Erythropoietic protoporphyria											
Manifest	N	N	N	→↑	N	→↑	↑↑	↑↑[b]			↑↑
Latent	N	N	N	N	N	N	↑	↑[b]			N

[a] Urine for ALA should be collected in acid; for PBG and porphyrins, in alkali.

[b] Erythrocyte study used to diagnose erythropoietic protoporphyria is the "free erythrocyte protoporphyrin."

[c] Simple scanning technique has unique fluorescence.[3]

[d] Although lead poisoning is not a "porphyria," abnormalities in heme precursors are seen, and erythrocytes may contain Zn–protoporphyrin.

[e] Isocoproporphyrins are characteristic in PCT.

Key: ALA = δ-aminolevulinate; PBG = porphobilinogen; Uro = uroporphyrin; Copro = coproporphyrin; Proto = protoporphyrin; N = normal; →↑ = might be mildly elevated; ↑ = elevated; ↑↑ = markedly elevated.

518

rapidly oxidized to become photosensitizing porphyrins. Porphyrins become less water-soluble as they are decarboxylated from 8-COOH (uroporphyrin) to 4-COOH (coproporphyrin) to 2-COOH (protoporphyrin). As porphyrins lose water solubility, they are excreted by the liver into bile and are found in stool rather than in urine. A high concentration of PBG in the urine will spontaneously form a red-colored tetrapyrrole, especially if the urine is exposed to light. The next important concept is that there are only three genetic *acute* porphyric disorders that have pain and neurological manifestations: acute intermittent porphyria (AIP), variegate porphyria (VP), and hereditary coproporphyria (HCP). The neuropathy responsible for the acute pain crisis in each of these disorders can also involve peripheral nerves and the central nervous system (CNS). The neuropathic manifestations are *always* associated with elevations in ALA and/or PBG. Because all these disorders are called *porphyrias*, the common and unfortunate mistake made by most clinicians is to order tests for porphyrins when the clinician really wants to know whether there is PBG overproduction. It is always best to screen for acute hepatic porphyria *during* the painful attack, since urinary PBG concentration in latent (asymptomatic) porphyria may be below the detection level of a screening test.

Because ALA has a structure similar to that of certain neurotransmitters (e.g., γ-aminobutyric acid), one theory explaining the acute neurological painful attacks of the acute porphyrias proposes that excess ALA is responsible. In general, conversion of ALA to PBG by the enzyme ALA dehydratase is very rapid, so that urinary PBG is higher than ALA in the acute porphyric attack. This is in contradistinction to lead poisoning, hereditary tyrosinemia, and homozygous ALA dehydratase deficiency in which the enzyme is inhibited (Fig. 70.1) and ALA builds up with no PBG excess. These last three disorders can also present with painful crises, but usually in childhood.

ALA production and subsequent heme biosynthesis is tightly regulated by the first and *inducible* enzyme in the heme pathway, ALA synthase. All the acute hepatic porphyrias are characterized by an inappropriate induction of ALA synthase in the liver that then leads to ALA and PBG excess. Therefore, any drug, hormone, or foreign compound that increases the need for hepatic heme (e.g., phenobarbital, sulfonamides, and phenytoin, which induce hepatic cytochromes P450) can induce ALA synthase and precipitate an attack. Hormonal changes that occur during menstrual cycles in women often affect ALA synthase activity such that many women with acute porphyria tend to have premenstrual attacks as in the case presented. For as yet unknown reasons, increasing hepatic glucose tends to blunt ALA synthase activity.

Whereas AIP presents only with neurological manifestations, VP and HCP can also have porphyrin overproduction and present with photosensitivity. This is because the enzyme defect in AIP (PBG deaminase) is a defect prior to uroporphyrinogen formation, whereas the enzyme defect in VP (protoporphyrinogen oxidase) can cause accumulation of protoporphyrin and in HCP (coproporphyrinogen oxidase) can cause accumulation of coproporphyrin. VP and HCP, like AIP, are autosomally dominant inherited disorders.

The most common porphyria to cause photosensitive skin lesions is porphyria cutanea tarda (PCT), in which there is a accumulation of 8-COOH uroporphyrinogen and 7-COOH porphyrinogen. Most cases of PCT are acquired, not genetic, and are associated with increased hepatic oxidative stress that prematurely oxidizes the reduced uro- and 7-COOH porphyrinogens, preventing further metabolism. They both accumulate, spill over into plasma (causing cutaneous photosensitivity mainly on the dorsa of the hands, arms, and face), and are overexcreted in the urine. Patients with PCT *never* have acute neurological manifestations. The hepatic oxidative stress is usually caused by alcohol use, iron overloading of the liver, smoking, and/or hepatitis C. In women, estrogen use is also associated with PCT. There are inherited (familial) forms of PCT in which mutations of uroporphyrinogen decarboxylase enzyme occurs.

The photosensitivity of VP, HCP, and PCT leads to blistering skin lesions, ulcerations, marked skin fragility, increased pigmentation, and hypertrichosis in light-exposed areas. This photosensitivity is different from that seen in erythropoietic protoporphyria (EPP), another autosomal dominant genetic defect, in which red blood cells have markedly elevated free protoporphyrin concentrations due to deficient ferrochelatase activity. EPP patients tend to present in childhood with a burning, stinging sensation during light exposure and with erythema and edema that can lead to scarring and thickening of the dermis. Although EPP patients never have acute neurological attacks, they can develop cholestatic liver failure due to hepatic accumulation of very insoluble protoporphyrin deposits.

Finally, a very rare and severe porphyria not listed in Table 70.1 called *congenital erythropoietic porphyria* (Gunther's disease), caused by a defect in uroporphyrinogen III (co)synthase, should be mentioned. These unfortunate patients produce huge amounts of excess porphyrins in bone marrow and liver that accumulate in all tissues and lead to severe photomutilation. Acute attacks do not occur.

Diagnosis of the Acute Hepatic Porphyrias and the Cutaneous Porphyrias

When a patient presents with acute, recurrent abdominal pain without clear source, especially accompanied by neurological abnormalities such as mental status changes, seizures, and peripheral neuropathies, the possibility of one of the acute hepatic porphyrias should be entertained and evaluated by qualitatively screening a fresh, random urine specimen of the patient for PBG (not porphyrins). The qualitative screening test for PBG uses p-dimethylaminobenzaldehyde (Erhlich's reagent). Whereas the classic Watson–Schwartz test and the Hoesch test are still used by some clinical laboratories, the American Porphyria Foundation recommends a rapid semiquantitative Thermo PBG test kit.[3] If the screen is positive, then therapy should be begun immediately and one should not wait for confirmatory quantitative analyses. Quantitative PBG and porphyrins can be tested on the same random urine specimen. Plasma PBG and porphyrins (qualitative and quantitative) can also be obtained if the patient is in renal failure. But only the Thermo PBG kit offers a rapid turnaround time. Alternatively, 24-hour urine collections can be undertaken either while the patient is still symptomatic or after symptoms resolve.

If clinical suspicion for an acute porphyria remains high despite a negative *qualitative* PBG test, the *quantitative* urine test may still demonstrate PBG overproduction. A quantitative determination of ALA on the same or another 24-hour urine specimen can further confirm the diagnosis and can rule out disorders in which ALA dehydratase is inhibited (e.g., occult lead poisoning). However, quantitative urine porphyrin studies often cause diagnostic confusion because of minor increases in coproporphyrin and/or uroporphyrin excretion of no clinical significance. The increases are most likely due to hepatic dysfunction causing more of these porphyrins to be excreted by the kidneys into urine rather than by the liver into bile. This confusion has often led to an inappropriate diagnosis of "acute porphyria."

Once diagnosis of an acute hepatic porphyria is made by urine PBG ($\pm$ALA) assay, then an analysis of stool for porphyrins is important to distinguish AIP from VP or HCP. A marked increase in stool protoporphyrin indicates VP, whereas an increase in coproporphyrin indicates HCP. With VP and HCP, protective measures against sun exposure may be required. AIP can also be confirmed by determining erythrocyte PBG deaminase (i.e., uroporphyrinogen-1-synthase) activity. There is considerable variability in values for PBG deaminase activity in normals and AIP patients. However, within a family, those persons exerting half the activity of the others will usually be shown to carry the defective gene.

When patients present initially with photosensitive skin lesions and skin fragility, plasma porphyrin studies, urinary qualitative screening, or quantitative analysis for porphyrins is appropriate; the tests may then be followed with quantitative stool porphyrin analysis to diagnose PCT, VP, or HCP. Diagnosis of EPP is made by analysis of erythrocyte free protoporphyrin.

Management of the Acute Hepatic Porphyrias

There are only a few important principles for managing these patients. First and most important, exacerbating drugs must be avoided.[2-4] In South Africa, where VP is relatively common, certain barbiturate sedatives have been responsible for many severe and often fatal attacks of acute porphyria. Once an attack begins, it is important to avoid fasting and administer glucose (orally or IV) at the beginning of the attack. But the best way to prevent progression of an acute attack or to prophylactically ward off recurrent attacks is to give hemin, as was done with the patient presented above. The administration of hemin (heme hydroxide) exerts a potent feedback inhibition of ALA synthase induction. For severe attacks, which can be fatal if not recognized and treated, hemin is usually given daily for 4 days. But dosing regimens for mild attacks and prophylaxis of recurrent attacks are less clear. To give hemin, which is unstable in solution and causes phlebitis, a large-bore IV needle is needed and often central lines must be inserted when peripheral veins become sclerosed. Mixing the heme with albumin improves stability. Each vial of Panhematin (Ovation Pharmaceuticals, Deerfield, IL) contains 313 mg hemin and 25 mg iron.

Because infections can precipitate attacks, the patient should be evaluated and infections treated with safe antibiotics such as penicillins, cephalosporins, or tetracyclines. Pain, nausea, anxiety, and tachycardia can be treated with meperidine, acetaminophen, phenothiazines, and propranolol (all "safe" drugs for the porphyric patient[4]). Management of seizures in porphyrics is problematic because many anticonvulsants precipitate acute porphyric attacks. Benzodiazepines appear safe, and some of the newer agents such as gabapentin and topiramate might also be safe.

As demonstrated in this case, porphyric women often have menstrually related attacks. There have been reports of some success with luteinizing hormone–releasing hormone (LH-RH) analogs in these women,[8] but generally attacks are mild and can be managed conservatively.

Although the porphyrias have diverse clinical presentations arising from defects in complex biochemical pathways, all clinicians should understand the need to check for excess PBG excretion in cases of acute pain crises and check for porphyrins *only* if there are photosensitive skin lesions present. For the acute pain crises, avoiding drugs that can exacerbate the biochemical defect and administering glucose, hemin, and appropriate pain and anxiety medications are the primary principles of management.

References

1. BONKOVSKY, H. L., HEALY, J. F., LOURIE, A. N., AND GERRON, C. G.: Intravenous heme-albumin in acute intermittent porphyria: Evidence for repletion of hepatic hemoproteins and regulatory heme pools. *Am. J. Gastroenterol.* 86:1050–6, 1991.

2. ANDERSON, K. A., SASSA, S., BISHOP, D., AND DESNICK, R.: Disorders of heme biosynthesis: X-linked sideroblastic anemia and the porphyrias. In *Metabolic and Molecular Bases of Inherited Disease*, C. SCRIVER, A. BEAUDET, W. SLY, D. VALLE, AND B. CHILDS, eds., McGraw-Hill, New York, 2001, pp. 2991–3062.

3. ANDERSON, K. A., BLOOMER, J. R., ET AL.: Recommendations for the diagnosis and treatment of acute porphyrias. *Ann. Intern. Med.* 142:439–50, 2005.

4. Website for drug safety information for the acute porphyrias: http://www.drugs-porphyria.org/eng/index2.php

Case 71

A 9-Year-Old Boy with Skin Lesions and Headaches

David Bruns and Audrey K. Bennett

A 9-year-old male presented to his physician with a 3-month history of pruritic erosive vesicular changes on the dorsum of the hands and tops of the ears in sun-exposed areas, with patchy skin thickening and hyperpigmentation. The patient also had a lifelong history of very small scarring on the face. Other symptoms included occasional headaches and stomach aches, reportedly several times a week, with no history of medications, hepatitis, excessive iron intake, increased estrogens, or exposure to chemicals. Physical examination was unremarkable except for the skin changes noted over the dorsal hands, face, and ears.

The patient's hemoglobin was increased [16.4 g/dL (164 g/L); normal range for age 11.5–15.5 g/dL (115–155 g/L)], as were serum iron, transferrin (as total iron binding capacity), urine porphyrins, and transaminases. Red blood cell (RBC) protoporphyrin and uroporphyrinogen decarboxylase (UROD) levels were normal, suggesting a diagnosis of sporadic-type porphyria cutanea tarda (PCT). Relevant laboratory data were as follows:

Analyte	Value, Conventional Units	Reference Interval, Conventional Units	Value, SI Units	Reference Interval, SI Units
	Serum Chemistry			
Serum iron	160 μg/dL	50–120	28.7 μmol/L	8.96–21.5
Transferrin (TIBC)	185 mg/dL	212–360	33.1 μmol/L	38.0–64.5
% saturation	61%	16–48	0.61	0.16–0.48
Ferritin	302 ng/mL	18–311	302 μg/L	18–311
AST	92 U/L	13–39	1.56 μkat/L	0.22–0.66
ALT	138 U/L	7–52	2.35 μkat/L	0.12–0.88
Alkaline phosphatase	238 U/L	50–380	4.05 μkat/L	0.85–6.46
	Urine Chemistry			
Total porphyrins	4484 μg/L	≤/234	6132 nmol/L	≤320
Uroporphyrins	2907 μg/L	≤46.8	3497 nmol/L	≤56.3

Tietz's Applied Laboratory Medicine, Second Edition. Edited by Mitchell G. Scott, Ann M. Gronowski, and Charles S. Eby

Analyte	Value, Conventional Units	Reference Interval, Conventional Units	Value, SI Units	Reference Interval, SI Units
Pentaporphyrin	119 µg/L	≤4.3	165 nmol/L	≤6.0
Coproporphyrin	233 µg/L	≤183	355 nmol/L	≤279
Heptacarboxyporphyrin	1226 µg/L	≤/0.9	1532 nmol/L	≤13.6

Testing was also performed for mutations of the *HFE* gene (hereditary hemochromatosis gene) on chromosome 6, by real-time PCR followed by melting curve analysis. The patient exhibited a homozygous C282Y mutation, consistent with hereditary hemochromatosis (HH). With phlebotomy treatments, the patient's skin improved, and his iron studies and liver enzymes normalized.

General Information on Porphyrias

Porphyrins are precursor molecules to heme in animals, and precursors to chlorophyll in plants.[1] The heme biosynthetic pathway contains eight enzymes, culminating in the final step of heme synthesis in which iron is inserted into protoporphyrin IX. Enzyme defects in this pathway lead to accumulation and excessive excretion of porphyrins and/or porphyrin precursors, and a compensatory increase in the activity of the rate-limiting enzyme, δ-aminolevulinate (ALA) synthase (see Fig. 70.1, Case 70). This ultimately leads to an increase in the porphyrin precursor ALA, with or without an increase in PBG, depending on the type of porphyria. Clinical presentation of porphyria is with acute neurovisceral attacks, cutaneous symptoms, or both. Acute attacks may be precipitated by events leading to increased heme requirements, including stress, infection, or exposure to medications.

Table 71.1   Classification of Human Porphyrias

Classification		Clinical presentation		Enzyme deficiency
Hepatic	Erythroid	Acute attacks	Cutaneous symptoms	
ADP		X		ALA dehydratase
AIP		X		PBG deaminase
	CEP		X	Uroporphyrinogen III synthase
PCT			X	UROD
HEP			X	UROD
HC		X	X	Coproporphyrinogen III oxidase
VP		X	X	Protoporphyrinogen oxidase
	EP		X	Ferrochelatase

Key: ADP—ALA dehydratase deficiency porphyria; AIP—Acute intermittent porphyria; ALA—5-aminolevulinic acid; CEP—congenital erythropoietic porphyria; PCT—porphyria cutanea tarda; EP—erythropoietic protoporphyria; HC—hereditary coproporphyria; HEP—hepatoerythroporphyria; PBG—porphobilinogen; UROD—uroporphyrinogen decarboxylase; VP—variegate porphyria.

In mammals, hepatic and erythropoietic tissues are the primary sites of heme biosynthesis.[1] The first enzyme in the heme synthesis pathway is ALA synthase. Two genes encode for this enzyme, one that is ubiquitous (ALA synthase-1 on chromosome 3), and one that is erythroid-specific (ALA synthase-2 on chromosome X).[1] The human porphyrias can be classified as hepatic or erythroid in type, depending on the primary site of porphyrin production,[1] subclassified according to clinical presentation with acute neurovisceral attacks, cutaneous symptoms, or both (Table 71.1). Of the hepatic forms, PCT is one of only two that present primarily with cutaneous symptoms, while the others present with acute neurovisceral attacks with or without skin lesions. The erythroid forms demonstrate only cutaneous manifestations (Table 71.1). (See also Fig. 70.1, for location of these enzymes in the heme pathway.)

Neurologic manifestations occur in the central, peripheral, and autonomic nervous systems in the acute porphyrias. The mechanism of damage to the nervous system is not well understood. The etiology of these manifestations appears to correlate with several factors, including accumulation of porphyrin and porphyrin precursors (neurotoxicity of ALA and PBG), heme deficiency in neural tissues, decrease in essential cofactors in neural tissues, and accumulation of abnormal products.[1,2]

Porphyrins and porphyrin precursors are normally excreted into urine and/or bile. Enzyme deficiency or dysfunction results in accumulation of porphyrins and/or porphyrin precursors, in a characteristic pattern in urine, feces, plasma, or red blood cells, for each porphyria. Their pattern of excretion is influenced by solubility, with decreasing solubility as the number of hydroxyl and carboxyl groups decreases.[2] Thus, uroporphyrin is excreted mainly in urine, coproporphyrin is excreted in urine and (mostly) in bile, and protoporphyrin is excreted mainly in bile and therefore is seen almost exclusively in the feces. Normally, the chief porphyrin found in urine is coproporphyrin, even though the majority of its excretion occurs in the bile. Substantial amounts of porphyrins are excreted in feces. ALA and PBG are porphyrin precursors that are excreted only into urine.

Definition of Porphyria Cutanea Tarda

Porphyria cutanea tarda (PCT) is the most common form of porphyria. Patients present clinically with cutaneous photosensitivity associated with hepatocyte damage, without acute attacks or neurologic manifestations. Both sporadic and familial forms exist, and present similarly in the fourth decade or later. Uroporphyrinogen decarboxylase (UROD) activity is decreased. The gene encoding UROD has been mapped to chromosome 1p34.[4] Evidence suggests that UROD is reversibly inactivated by an iron-dependent process, and that this is accelerated by iron overload.[5] UROD is decreased in the liver of all patients with PCT.

Sporadic type PCT (type I) accounts for 80% of cases. It is more common in males, with no family history of disease. In sporadic PCT, deficiency of UROD occurs by inactivation of this enzyme in the liver, which may be triggered by alcohol use, estrogen excess, iron overload, hepatitis C viral infection, and/or HIV infection.[1,3] The enzyme deficiency in this subtype of PCT is characterized by >50% reduction in enzymatic activity during full active disease, observed only in hepatocytes, with apparently normal enzymatic activity in erythrocytes and all other tissues. Mutations of the UROD locus have been excluded in sporadic type I PCT.

Familial-type PCT (type II) is less common than the sporadic type, and is characterized by earlier onset with no gender predilection, frequently with a positive family history of disease. In familial PCT, UROD enzymatic activity is reduced by approximately 50% in all tissues, including red blood cells and hepatocytes. A genetic mutation of the UROD gene is inherited in this form of PCT, in an autosomal dominant fashion, with incomplete penetrance, typically showing about 20% expression. There is evidence of possible complete lack of clinical manifestations in up to 90% of gene mutation carriers.[1,4,6]

Some cases of PCT are biochemically indistinguishable from sporadic type I PCT and appear clustered in families. It is unclear as to whether these cases represent a distinct disease entity. It is suspected that these cases, referred to as "type III PCT," may have an inherited defect presumed to lie outside of the UROD locus. In this so-called type III PCT, as in sporadic type I PCT, erythrocyte UROD activity and concentration are normal, while hepatic UROD activity is decreased.

Clinical Features of Porphyria Cutanea Tarda

PCT is characterized by skin lesions, without neurovisceral acute attacks. Sun exposure prompts the development of vesicles or bullae in sun-exposed skin, which heal slowly with scarring and either hypo- or hyperpigmentation, typically over the backs of the hands and on the face, neck, and legs.[1] Skin fragility is common and characteristic, seen as erosions after minimal trauma. Other lesions include milia in sites of previous bullae, hypertrichosis often in a malar distribution, and less commonly alopecia and scleroderma-like hypopigmented lesions.

PCT should be distinguished from the more severe HEP (hepatoerythropoietic porphyria), in which the skin shows more severe photosensitivity, usually beginning in early infancy.[1,3] In addition, both alleles of the UROD gene are mutated in HEP. Features favoring a diagnosis of PCT include demonstration of enzymatic activity of UROD close to 50% of normal, normal erythrocyte porphyrin concentration, and the presence of only one mutated allele of the UROD gene.[1,6]

Other forms of porphyria with cutaneous manifestations should be distinguished from PCT. CEP shows more severe clinical presentation, with early onset of symptoms in infancy, extreme cutaneous photosensitivity, and red discoloration of urine and teeth.[1,3] The skin lesions in PCT are essentially the same as in HC and VP; however, both of the latter exhibit acute attacks much as in AIP. Occasional cases of HC or VP may present with skin changes only, and distinction from PCT then must rely on laboratory evaluation of excreted porphyrins, possible red cell enzyme testing, and genetic testing.

Pathophysiology of Porphyria Cutanea Tarda

Porphyrins share the property of absorption of light at 400–410 nm wavelength. When exposed to light in this spectrum, they exhibit orange-red fluorescence of 550–650 nm.[2] In the forms of porphyria with skin lesions, absorption of light at the skin surface results in the production of reactive oxygen species, with a subsequent inflammatory response, and ensuing damage to the basement membrane and dermis by activation of metalloproteinases.[3] The result is porphyrin accumulation in the skin.

Iron overload is an important and well-known association in the pathogenesis of PCT. While increased iron is one of the triggers of clinical manifestations in PCT, exactly how this occurs is not entirely clear. Iron does not appear to directly inhibit the UROD enzyme, unless raised to very high nonphysiologic levels; however, iron does appear to be required for inactivation of the UROD enzyme.[8,9] There is some evidence that iron facilitates oxidation of uroporphyrinogen and other porphyrinogens, and that these products affect the function of the UROD enzyme.[9] In addition, induction of the enzyme ALA synthase by iron is another proposed mechanism of accumulation of porphyrinogens in PCT.[9]

Iron stores in the liver in PCT range from normal to the lower end of hemochromatosis range iron.[8] At least 80% of PCT patients show hepatic siderosis, and 65% exhibit an increase in total body iron stores. However, fewer than 25% of PCT patients meet the strict definition of hemochromatosis, and cirrhosis of the liver is unusual.[6] In terms of clinical disease, remission follows hepatic iron depletion, while iron administration may exacerbate the condition, consistent with the iron-dependent nature of PCT.

The causes of iron overload in PCT are heterogeneous. Exogenous factors such as alcohol, diet, and viral hepatitis have been shown to increase hepatic iron deposition. Another important causative factor of iron overload in PCT is HH, a genetically inherited autosomal recessive disease of increased iron absorption.

Diagnosis of PCT

The diagnosis of porphyria employs measurement of excretion of porphyrins and porphyrin precursors ALA and PBG, which accumulate in the steps preceding the enzymatic defect. When defects occur in the heme biosynthetic pathway, there is also a compensatory increase in the enzymatic activity of the rate-limiting enzyme, ALA synthase. The particular enzyme defect determines which products will accumulate. In acute forms of porphyria, there is overproduction of all the porphyrins proximal to the enzyme defect, as well as a *decrease* in activity of porphobilinogen deaminase (PBG deaminase), with a resultant increase in excretion of porphyrin precursors ALA and PBG. This decreased PBG deaminase activity may be the result of genetic defect of the enzyme as in AIP, for example, but also may be a result of inhibition of this enzyme by accumulated copro- and/or protoporphyrinogens. In nonacute porphyrias, there is overproduction of all porphyrins prior to the enzyme defect, but no overproduction of the porphyrin precursors ALA and PBG. One possible reason perhaps relates to a compensatory *increase* in activity of PBG deaminase, as opposed to the decrease seen in acute porphyrias.[2] The algorithm for diagnostic testing in porphyria varies according to the symptomatology and suspected type of porphyria, but expected findings are summarized in Table 70.1 (of Case 70).

An acute attack of abdominal pain should be initially evaluated with a urine screen for PBG and ALA. Acute attacks are characterized by increased urinary excretion of ALA and PBG (20–200 times that of normal levels).[1] If negative, consider that the patient may be between attacks, in which case testing should proceed as if positive, or repeat testing can be done during an attack. Porphyria may be latent in individuals who do not exhibit increased production of heme precursors, and assessment of red cell enzymes or mutational analysis can be helpful in this regard. For example, the RBC levels of the enzyme PBG deaminase can be measured to assist in the diagnosis of AIP. VP and HC red cell enzyme detection can be more complex, and therefore mutational analysis may eventually be the method of choice in these forms of porphyria.

If the urine screen is positive for ALA and/or PBG, confirmatory testing should follow with a quantitative PBG and ALA. If suspicious skin lesions are present, urine and fecal porphyrins distinguishes PCT (elevated urinary uroporphyrin > coproporphyrin—elevated fecal porphyrins), VP (elevated urinary ALA and PBG-elevated fecal protoporphyrin), and HC (elevated urinary ALA, PBG, and coproporphyrin-elevated fecal coproporphyrin).

Fecal copro- and protoporphyrin testing help differentiate VP (increased protoporphyrins) and HC (increased coproporphyrins). Decreased RBC PBG deaminase helps confirm AIP. Urticaria or erythema induced by sunlight merits investigation of RBC protoporphyrin, which would be elevated in EP. Some cases of iron deficiency anemia and lead poisoning exhibit elevated zinc-chelated protoporphyrin in RBCs, while the nonchelated form is present in EP. Interestingly, increased RBC zinc–protoporphyrin is seen in one very rare type of porphyria—hepatoerythropoietic porphyria—as well as being reported in some homozygous porphyrias.[1] Other cutaneous forms of porphyria may be excluded or confirmed by additional urine and feces testing as indicated.

Porphyrins exhibit a characteristic absorption of light at 400–410 nm, and orange-red fluorescence at 550–650 nm. This pattern of absorption and fluorescence varies somewhat with substitution and metal binding within the porphyrin ring. HPLC with fluorescence detection is used for porphyrin quantification in the clinical laboratory, while other detection methods include capillary electrophoresis and mass spectrometry.[2]

Hereditary Hemochromatosis and its Relationship to Porphyria Cutanea Tarda

Hereditary hemochromatosis (HH) is a common autosomal recessive inherited disorder of iron metabolism in which excess iron absorption leads to deposition of iron in multiple organs, resulting in cirrhosis, diabetes, skin "bronzing," cardiomyopathy, and/or hypogonadism. Genetic studies have linked the disease-causing gene to the HLA locus on chromosome 6, called the *HFE* gene. HH has a carrier frequency of up to one in eight people of northern European descent, although 10–15% of patients who go on to develop hemochromatosis do not appear to carry a recognized *HFE* mutation.[10] The implicated HH gene was initially called "HLA-H" because of its location within the major histocompatibility locus, but it is not thought to have immunologic function, and it later came to be known as the *HFE* gene.[10] Two of the major *HFE* mutations are single-nucleotide substitutions, including C282Y (resulting in substitution of tyrosine for cysteine at amino acid 282 in the HFE protein), and H63D (a common polymorphism). The majority of patients with clinical HH demonstrate homozygosity for the C282Y mutation (approximately 90% of northern European patients with typical HH exhibit a homozygous C282Y mutation). Other possible combinations result in a milder phenotype and less severe iron overload, including heterozygous C282Y mutations, and compound heterozygous C282Y/H63D mutations. A heterozygous H63D mutation is not definitively proved to cause clinical disease, and interestingly there is a high frequency of this allele in southern Europe, where it is seen in up to 20% of the general population. Another minor mutation in HH is the missense mutation S65C, which may cause a milder form of HH. The diagnosis of HH is based on clinical and laboratory features, including demonstration of elevated serum transferrin saturation, elevated ferritin levels, elevated hepatic iron, and histologic changes on liver biopsy including evidence of increased iron.

HFE mutations are now known to confer susceptibility to PCT,[5] and studies have demonstrated a high frequency of *HFE* mutations in PCT. It has been reported that iron status in PCT patients, as measured by serum ferritin, serum iron, and transferrin saturation, was not significantly different between patients with *HFE* mutations, versus those without *HFE* mutations.[11] It is possible that iron overload of various origins is important in precipitation of clinical disease in PCT, with *HFE* mutation as one of the most frequent causes, but that other causes of iron overload also contribute; ultimately it appears that the precise mechanism of iron overload is not as important as the fact that it is present as a precipitating factor.

Identification of the genetic mutations of HH has facilitated determination of the relationship between HH and PCT. In sporadic PCT, 53–87% of patients carry a mutant allele of the *HFE* gene, showing strong evidence of the link between these disorders.[9] The frequency and types of HH mutations in PCT have been shown to vary, depending on the population being studied. Northern European/Australian/North American British ancestry communities exhibit HH mutation frequencies different from those of southern European communities.[9] Among PCT patients, a significantly increased frequency of the C282Y mutation was identified over controls in northern Europe (Great Britain and The Netherlands), the United States (British ancestry population), and Australia. Increased frequency of both heterozygosity and homozygosity for the C282Y mutation of the *HFE* gene is seen in PCT, particularly in patients of northern European descent.[6] C282Y homozygosity is an important susceptibility factor for PCT, while heterozygosity for C282Y is less strongly associated, and has less impact on disease development. Interestingly, geographically speaking, the distribution of mutations in PCT appears similar to that of HH, with a predominance of C282Y in northern European countries, and relative predominance of H63D in Mediterranean countries.[11] Taken one step further, homozygous C282Y mutations, the most frequent HH-associated mutation in northern European countries, is found in up to 20% of PCT patients in these regions, with greater iron overload in this population than is seen in other PCT patients.[5,11] Homozygosity for the C282Y mutation was found to accelerate the clinical onset of familial, and to a lesser extent, sporadic PCT.[6]

In a study performed of PCT patients from Italy, in contrast to those of the northern European population, an increase in C282Y mutations was not detected above the general population, but the H63D mutation was found to be present in approximately half of these patients.[9] The presence of this mutation did not necessarily correlate with the iron status of these PCT patients, as measured by transferrin saturation, iron removed by phlebotomy, and hepatic iron levels.[9] Sampietro et al. propose that this finding could suggest that our standard measures of iron status may be unable to detect the mild iron metabolism abnormality caused by mutations of H63D.[9] They suggest that H63D mutation may result in hepatocellular accumulation of difficult-to-detect toxic iron metabolites, which are nonetheless capable of contributing to inactivation of the UROD enzyme.

Elder and Worwood highlight several observations on the relationship of PCT with hereditary hemochromatosis (HH). These authors state that mutations in the *HFE* gene impart susceptibility to PCT, and that the mechanism for this susceptibility appears to be related to iron metabolism and storage, and possibly the accumulation of toxic iron species, which may accelerate inactivation of the UROD enzyme.[5]

Treatment of PCT and HH

In general, all patients with PCT should have their underlying disease treated (HCV, HIV), and should avoid precipitating factors such as alcohol, medications/drugs, and iron supplementation. Avoidance of excess sunlight is advised until clinical remission is achieved. Phlebotomy remains a primary treatment, even in cases in which the serum iron or ferritin is not necessarily elevated. Urine porphyrins should be monitored until biologic remission is achieved, typically within a 6-month period of treatment. In cases where phlebotomy may be contraindicated, low-dose chloroquine therapy can be used in addition to or in lieu of phlebotomy.[1] Chloroquine complexes with porphyrins, assisting in their mobiliz-ation from the liver.[3] A low dosage of chloroquine is important in these patients because of the risk for transient but occasionally severe hepatitis, and the possibility for worsening photosensitivity in PCT patients. In patients with PCT *and* with mutations of HH, treatment guidelines are aimed at decreasing iron overload. It is recommended that homozygotes for C282Y with manifestations of PCT be treated with phlebotomy to decrease or prevent iron overload. In both HH and in PCT, transferrin saturation should be kept below 55% and serum ferritin, below 100 μg/L.[5] In PCT, because of an increased risk for liver disease and hepatic carcinoma, appropriate surveillance is indicated. Finally, due to an established association, testing for *HFE* gene mutations is valuable in patients with PCT, particularly in populations of high prevalence of HH. Family screening for hemochromatosis should also be considered in these cases.

References

1. NORDMANN, Y. AND PUY, H.: Human hereditary hepatic porphyrias. *Clin. Chim. Acta 325*:17–37, 2002.
2. HRISTOVA, E. N. AND HENRY, J. B.: Metabolic inter-mediates, inorganic ions, and biochemical markers of bone metabolism. In *Clinical Diagnosis and Manage-ment by Laboratory Methods*, 20th ed., J. B. HENRY, ed., WB Saunders, Philadelphia, pp. 191–4, 2001.
3. BADMINTON, M. N. AND ELDER, G. H.: Management of acute and cutaneous porphyrias. *Int. J. Clin. Pract. 56*:272–8, 2002.
4. BYGUM, A., CHRISTIANSEN, L., PETERSEN, N. E. ET AL.: Familial and sporadic porphyria cutanea tarda: Clinical, biochemical, and genetic features with emphasis on iron status. *Acta Dermato-venereologica, 83*:115–20, 2003.
5. ELDER, G. H. AND WORWOOD, M.: Mutations in the hemochromatosis gene, porphyria cutanea tarda, and iron overload. *Hepatology 27*:289–91, 1998.
6. BRADY, J. J., JACKSON, H. A., ROBERTS, A. G. ET AL.: Co-inheritance of mutations in the uroporphyrinogen decarboxylase and hemochromatosis genes accelerates the onset of porphyria cutanea tarda. *J. Invest. Dermatol. 115*:868–74, 2000.
7. CHRISTIANSEN, L., GED, C., HOMBRADOS, I. ET AL.: Screening for mutations in the uroporphyrinogen decar-boxylase gene using denaturing gradient gel electro-phoresis. Identification and characterization of six novel mutations associated with familial PCT. *Hum. Mut. 14*:222–32, 1999.
8. ROBERTS, A. G., WHATLEY, S. D., MORGAN, R. R. ET AL.: Increased frequency of the haemochromatosis Cys282Tyr mutation in sporadic porphyria cutanea tarda. *Lancet 349*:321–3, 1997.
9. SAMPIETRO, M., FIORELLI, G., AND FARGION, S.: Iron overload in porphyria cutanea tarda. *Haematologica 84*:248–53, 1999.
10. GRODY, W. W. AND NOLL, W. W.: Molecular diagnosis of genetic diseases. In *Clinical Diagnosis and Manage-ment by Laboratory Methods*. 10th ed., J. B. HENRY, ed., Saunders, Philadelphia, p. 1387, 2001.
11. DEREURE, O., AGUILAR-MARTINEZ, P., BESSIS, D. ET AL.: HFE mutations and transferrin receptor poly-morphism analysis in porphyria cutanea tarda: A pro-spective study of 36 cases from southern France. *Br. J. Dermatol. 144*:533–9, 2001.

Part Sixteen

Pharmacogenomics

Cases of CYP3A4 and 5A (CsA metabolism), pain management for CYP2D6, and factor V plus CYP2c9 are presented and discussed in Cases 72, 73, and 75, respectively (all edited by MGS); a case of thiopurine methyltransferase (TPMT) is presented and discussed in Case 74 (edited by CSE).

Tietz's Applied Laboratory Medicine, Second Edition. Edited by Mitchell G. Scott, Ann M. Gronowski, and Charles S. Eby
Copyright © 2007 John Wiley & Sons, Inc.

Case 72

Personalized Medicine for a Renal Transplant Patient

Paul J. Jannetto

A 35-year-old intellectually challenged African-American male was referred to the transplant clinic for pretransplant evaluation. The patient had end-stage renal disease (ESRD) due to tubular sclerosis. Tuberous sclerosis or tuberous sclerosis complex (TSC) is a rare, autosomal dominant disease that causes benign tumors to grow in the brain and other vital organs such as the kidneys, heart, skin, and eyes.[1] It commonly affects the central nervous system and results in a combination of symptoms including seizures, developmental delay, skin abnormalities, and kidney disease. The incidence of TSC has been cited to be 1 in 10,000 with 50–84% of the cases being sporadic.[2,3] TSC is caused by mutations in one of two tumor suppressor genes (TSC1 and TSC2).[4] Although a peripheral lymphocyte genetic test exists for mutations in TSC1 and 2, TSC is still diagnosed primarily by a careful clinical exam along with computed tomography (CT) or magnetic resonance imaging (MRI) of the brain. Some of the first clinical signs of TSC include seizures, delayed development, and/or white patches on the skin (hypomelanotic macules).[1,2] Currently, there is no cure for TSC, but medications can be used to treat the symptoms (i.e., antiepileptic drugs for the seizures).

On physical examination, the patient had hypopigmented macules (ash-leaf spots) located on the face, trunk, and buttocks. The patient also had a retinal phacoma, a grayish yellow plaque, in his retina. Extraocular movements were normal without nystagmus. There was also truncal ataxia. He could take a few steps with guidance, but otherwise could not ambulate independently. Overall, the patient was alert, active, and in no acute distress. Currently, the patient lives with his mother, who is his primary caregiver. The patient is unable to work or drive but has been seizure-free for several years, due to successful control with multiple medications (phenytoin, carbamazepine, and lorazepam). For the past several years, the patient has been on dialysis for ESRD. The final assessment showed a 35-year-old mentally retarded male with ESRD due to TSC. It was also evident that the patient had a strong family support system that could provide transportation and ensure that the patient took his prescription medications.

Tietz's Applied Laboratory Medicine, Second Edition. Edited by Mitchell G. Scott, Ann M. Gronowski, and Charles S. Eby

Initial predialysis laboratory tests included a chemistry profile, complete blood count, prothrombin time, hepatitis panel, HIV, cytomegalovirus antibody, and syphilis. Results are shown below:

Analyte	Value, Conventional Units	Reference Interval, Conventional Units	Value, SI Units	Reference Interval, SI Units
BUN	89 mg/dL	6–20	4.9 mmol/L	0.3–1.1
Creatinine	9.2 mg/dL	0.6–1.2	813 μmol/L	53–106
Na	136 mmol/L	133–145	Same	
K	4.9 mmol/L	3.5–5.1	Same	
Cl	109 mmol/L	98–112	Same	
HCO_3	21 mmol/L	21–31	Same	
Glucose	81 mg/dL	70–110	4.5 mmol/L	3.9–6.1
Hgb/Hct	8.3 g/dL,/25%	13–17/42–52	83 g/L/0.25	130–170/0.42–0.52
WBC	$12.2 \times 10^3/\mu L$	$4–10 \times 10^3$	$12.2 \times 10^9/L$	4–10
Platelet	$371 \times 10^3/\mu L$	150–350	$371 \times 10^9/L$	150–350
Protime/INR	12.6 s/1.2	9.3–12.5/0.8–1.2		
HBsAg	Nonreactive	Nonreactive		
HBcAb	Nonreactive	Nonreactive		
HCV-Ab	Nonreactive	Nonreactive		
HIV-1/HIV-2 Ab	Nonreactive	Nonreactive		
HTLV-1 Ab	Nonreactive	Nonreactive		
CMV-Ab	Nonreactive	Nonreactive		
RPR	Nonreactive	Nonreactive		

After a thorough medical history, physical examination, and laboratory tests (including HLA typing), the patient was placed on the national kidney waiting list. A renal cadaveric transplant was performed, and the patient was placed on immunosuppressive [cyclosporine A (CsA) 700 mg bid, prednisone 25 mg qd, and mycophenalate mofetil 1500 mg bid], antibiotic (sulfamethoxazole/trimethoprim-1 qd), antiviral (acyclovir 200 mg qid) (because of the negative CMV titers), and antifungal (fluconazole 100 mg) therapy. Follow-up laboratory testing was performed:

Analyte	Value, Conventional	Reference Interval, Conventional	Value, SI Units	Reference Interval, SI Units
BUN	8 mg/dL	6–20	0.4 mmol/L	0.3–1.1
Creatinine	1.1 mg/dL	0.6–1.2	97.2 μmol/L	53–106
Na	138 mmol/L	133–145	Same	
K	4.5 mmol/L	3.5–5.1	Same	
Cl	108 mmol/L	98–112	Same	
HCO_3	23 mmol/L	21–31	Same	
Glucose	102 mg/dL	70–110	5.7 mmol/L	3.9–6.1
CsA	683 ng/mL	50–200	683 μg/L	50–200

Over the course of the next month, the CsA dosage had to be continually adjusted according to the patient's CsA level and creatinine, which increased from 1.0 to

1.4 mg/dL. The CsA dosage and trough concentrations are shown below:

CsA Dosage, mg	Value, Conventional Units	Reference Interval, Conventional Units	Value, SI Units	Reference Interval, SI Units
600 mg bid	551 ng/mL	50–200	551 μg/L	
500 mg bid	333 ng/mL	50–200	333 μg/L	
300 mg bid	191 ng/mL	50–200	191 μg/L	

CsA is a potent immunosuppressive agent, with a narrow therapeutic index (range between efficacy and toxicity).[5] The effectiveness of CsA is due primarily to the parent drug through specific and reversible inhibitions of lymphocyte proliferation and activation by its inhibition of the phophatase calcineurin. Normally calcineurin dephosphorylates the cytosolic transcription factor NFATC, which then enters the nucleus and enhances transcription of the cytokine, IL-2. Due to extensive inter- and intrapatient variability in cyclosporine absorption, distribution, and metabolism, clinical monitoring of cyclosporine exposure is mandated for drug administration. Inadequate CsA exposure is a key factor for acute organ rejection in organ transplant patients, and may also play an important role in chronic rejection and graft failure. On the other hand, overexposure to CsA causes increased adverse effects such as renal toxicity, which also leads to graft failure.

The patient's new kidney was relatively swollen with prominent corticomedullary differentiation, but hemodynamics appeared normal. Because of an increase in the baseline creatinine (from 1.0 to 1.4 mg/dL) and concern for nephrotoxicity, a renal biopsy was performed. A suitable site for percutaneous sonographically guided renal biopsy was marked over the upper pole of the transplant. Several cores of firm white-tan tissue from 1.5 cm down to 0.3 cm in length and less than 0.1 cm in diameter were collected. Microscopic examination showed interstitial fibers with some vascular changes. In addition, tubular atrophy and focal glomerular sclerosis were noted. Viral inclusions, organisms, or malignancy were not identified. The observed nephrotoxicity was likely due to the cyclosporine therapy. As a result, the cyclosporine dosage was further decreased to 200 mg bid.

In the end, the kidney transplant was successful and continues to work well. Additional laboratory results (chemistry panels, complete blood count, liver function tests) all were within referenced limits. However, an IRB-approved research study was being conducted at the transplant clinic to correlate the role of genetic polymorphisms in cytochrome P450 (CYP) genes CYP3A4 and CYP3A5 to see if they correlate to CsA concentrations and dosages. Previous studies have suggested that the large interindividual variability in CsA pharmacokinetics is due to polymorhpisms in these genes as CsA is extensively metabolized by these two genes.[6,7] Therefore, this patient was genotyped for CYP3A4/CYP3A5 polymorphisms. The patient's CYP3A4/CYP3A5 genotype was *1B/*1B and *3/*3, respectively.

Role of "Personalized Medicine" in Therapeutic Drug Dosing

In this patient reversible CsA-induced renal toxicity was noted on biopsy and was suggested by slightly increasing creatinine values and higher than therapeutic CsA trough concentrations. The higher CsA concentration were somewhat unexpected as the patient was given standard CsA dosing in the early days posttransplant. Even before results of his CYP3A genotyping were known, the appropriate therapeutic drug monitoring (TDM) and change in CsA dosing was done, which likely prevented any permanent damage from CsA toxicity. In some sense such TDM and changes in dosing represents a simple form of "personalized medicine" in which the laboratory plays a large role. Today, as more is learned about the genetic basis for heterogeneity in drug response and metabolism, medicine is looking forward to true personalized medicine where genetic testing can help predict proper drug dosing and the expected response to a drug for an individual.

There are four CYP3A genes (A4, A5, A7, and 43) in a 231-kb locus on chromosome 7q 21–22.1. The CYP3A4 and A5 enzymes are responsible for the metabolism of up to 60% of all oxidatively metabolized drugs and are the most abundant cytochrome P450 enzymes in the liver. Like many of the cytochromes, there are many polymorphisms of the CYP3A4 and CYP3A5 genes. Over 40 and 20 alleles have been described for CYP3A4 and CYP3A5, respectively. The different alleles for each of these genes can result in increased, decreased, or no metabolism of a particular drug or can have no affect. Laboratory testing to identify which allele(s) an individual expresses combined with knowledge of how different allelic forms of a cytochrome P450 enzyme metabolizes a particular drug is the basis of personalized medicine. The alleles of this patient, 3A4*1B and 3A5*3, are both associated with decreased metabolism of CsA, although this has been questioned for 3A4*1B in one study.[8] In this case knowledge of the patient's CYP3A4/CYP3A5 genotype at the time of transplant may have resulted in a lower starting dosage of CsA and minimization of the renal toxicity observed.

Among the more important clinical drugs metabolized by CYP3A enzymes are macrolide antibiotics, benzodiazepines, calcineurin inhibitors, (e.g., CsA and FK506), HIV protease inhibitors, some antihistamines, calcium channel blockers, and many of the HMG CoA reductase inhibitors (statins).[9] In addition, other common clinical drugs can either induce or inhibit CYP3A activity. Inducers include two drugs that this patient was receiving, carbamazepine and phenytoin, as well as phenobarbital, rifampin, and St. John's wort. Inhibitors of CYP3A activity include amiodarone, verapamil, ketoconazole, and grapefruit juice (mainly in the gut epithelium). The 3A4*1B allele, also called CYP3A4-V, is the result of an A → G change in positions −392 of the 5′ regulatory element in the promoter region of the gene. The CYP3A5*3 allele is the result of a splicing defect leading to a truncated protein with very low or no activity.[9] The CYP3A4*1B allele is found in 53% of African-Americans and only 9% of Caucasions. The CYP3A5*3 allele is present in 27% of African-American and almost 90% of Caucasions.[9]

This patient's CYP3A genotyping results were consistent with decreased metabolism of CsA. In light of the other drugs the patient was receiving, namely, carbamazepine and phenytoin, which induce CYP3A activity, these results must be "personalized" for the individual patient in accordance with genotyping, concomitant drugs, and standard TDM values for CsA.

In summary, this individual had severly decreased CYP3A activity and was at an increased risk for toxicity from any medication (i.e., CsA) metabolized by these enzymes. Therefore, the patient's CYP3A4/CYP3A5 genotype provided a rational explanation for the elevated (toxic) CsA concentrations seen when the patient was started on the standard dose of CsA. In the end, the patient's CsA initial dosage had to be reduced by 62% to achieve therapeutic concentrations. In the future, transplant patients' CsA dosages might be influenced by their CYP3A4/CYP3A5 genotypes. Such personalized medicine has the potential to minimize toxicity and maximize clinical efficacy by decreasing the length of time required to achieve therapeutic concentrations.

References

1. LENDVAY, T. S. AND MARSHALL, F. F.: The tuberous sclerosis complex and its highly variable manifestations. *J. Urol. 169*:1635–42, 2003.

2. JOZWIAK, S., SCHWARTZ, R. A., JANNIGER, C. K., MICHALOWICZ, R., AND CHMIELIK, J.: Skin lesions in children with tuberous sclerosis complex: Their prevalence, natural course, and diagnostic significance. *Int. J. Dermatol. 37*:911, 1998.

3. JONES, A. C., SHYAMSUNDAR, M. M., THOMAS, M. W. ET AL.: Comprehensive mutation analysis of TSC1 and TSC2- and phenotypic correlations in 150 families with tuberous sclerosis. *Am. J. Hum. Genet. 64*:1305, 1999.

4. CRINO, P. B. AND HENSKE, E. P.: New developments in neurobiology of the tuberous sclerosis complex. *Neurology 53*:1384, 1999.

5. KEEVIL, B. G., TIERNEY, D. P., COOPER, D. P., MORRIS, M. R., MACHAAL, A., AND YONAN, N.: Simultaneous and rapid analysis of cyclcosporin A and creatinine in finger prick blood samples using liquid chromatography tandem mass spectrometry and its application in C2 monitoring. *Ther. Drug Monit. 24*:757–67, 2002.

6. ZHANG, Y. AND BENET, L. Z.: The gut as a barrier to drug absorption: Combined role of cytochrome P450 3A and P-glycoprotein. *Clin. Pharmocokinet. 40*:59–168, 2001.

7. KUEHL, P., ZHANG, J., LIN, Y. ET AL.: Sequence diversity in CYP3A promoters and characterization of the genetic basis of polymorphic CYP3A5 expression. *Nat. Genet. 4*:383–91, 2001.

8. VON AHSEN, N., RICHTER, M., GRUPP, C., RINGE, B., OELLERICH, M., AND ARMSTRONG, V. W.: No influence of the MDR-1 C345T polymorphism or a CYP3A4 promoter polymorphism (CYP3A4-V allele) on dose-adjusted cyclosporine A trough concentrations or rejection incidence in stable renal transplant recipients. *Clin. Chem. 47*:1048–52, 2001.

9. www.ncbi.nlm.nih.gov/entrez/dispomim.cgi?id = 124010.

Case 73

Personalized Medicine for Pain Management

Paul J. Jannetto and Nancy C. Bratanow

A 48-year-old white male presented to the pain management clinic with a history of chronic sinus pain. The pain was a result of severe chronic frontal sinusitis that was refractory to medical management, including three previous endoscopic sinus surgeries and frontal sinusotomy.

Chronic sinusitis is one of the most prevalent chronic illnesses that can affect people of all age groups. In the United States, chronic sinusitis affects approximately 32 million people each year and accounts for 11.6 million visits to physicians' offices.[1] Chronic sinusitis is defined as a sinus infection that persists for more than 3 months.[1] Common symptoms of chronic sinusitis include nasal congestion, cough, postnasal drip, facial tenderness, and pressure. Most cases are continuations of unresolved acute sinusitis. Allergic and nonallergic rhinitis, anatomic obstruction in the osteomeatal complex, and immunologic disorders are known risk factors.[1] The diagnosis of sinusitis is usually confirmed using imaging techniques such as ultrasonography, computed tomography, or magnetic resonance imaging. Medical treatment usually consists of antibiotics, decongestants, and pain medications. However, persistent frontal pain and edema may indicate disease progression and require surgical intervention. The most common and effective surgical treatment for chronic frontal sinusitis is considered to be an osteoplastic flap with obliteration.[2] Numerous bacterial pathogens have been defined in acute and chronic frontal sinusitis. *Streptococcus pneumoniae*, *Haemophilus influenzae*, and *Moraxella catarrhalis* are predominant in acute sinusitis, while anaerobic bacteria and *Staphylococcus aureus* are more common in chronic sinusitis.[3] Because of its persistent nature, chronic sinusitis can reduce the quality of life and productivity of the affected person. In fact, chronic sinusitis is associated with exacerbation of asthma and serious complications such as brain abscess and meningitis, which can produce significant morbidity and mortality.[1]

Currently, the patient was post–major surgery (osteoplastic flap and fat obliteration of the sinuses) with subsequent recurrent infection and fungal sinusitis. The patient had suffered moderate to severe frontal and maxillary sinus pain (8 out of 10 on the visual analog scale) for years. The patient described the pain as severe pressure with burning, throbbing, and sharp stabbing sensations. Initially, he was managed with Neurontin (gabapentin), tramadol, and Bextra (valdecoxib), but his pain continued to escalate and caused functional impairment. Ultimately, it was so severe that he was unable to focus on his job as a mechanics inspector. As a result, he was prescribed transdermal fentanyl (Duragesic 25 μg/h q72 h). The patient's dosage was continually increased over the course of several months from 25 to 50, 75, and then 100 μg/h with minimal pain relief.

During this time, his underlying problem continued to escalate and surgery was again considered. He was repeatedly treated with numerous antibiotics, and eventually hydromorphone (Dilaudid 4 mg every 4–6 hours as needed) was added to assist with the pain management. After 2 weeks, the patient reported no additional pain relief. As a result, a trial of tramadol (25 mg/day) was initiated and titrated up to 25 mg every 5–6 hours. However, the patient's pain continued to escalate. The patient sought relief in any way, journeying to ENT specialist consultants in two other states. Diagnostic studies revealed persistent infection. Attempts were made to alleviate his pain with other breakthrough-type medications, including oxycodone, Actiq (oral transmucosal fentanyl citrate), and immediate-release morphine. Methadone was even substituted for the fentanyl patch. Other pharmacotherapy interventions that were tried included neuromodulators like Itrileptal (oxcarbazepine), Gabitril (tiagabine), clonazepam, Keppra (levetiracetam), Zoloft (sertraline), and Paxil (paroxetine). In addition, orbital nerve blocks were attempted without success.

Over time, the patient experienced episodes of obvious frontal swelling, with scans confirming recurrent infections. The patient had repeated ENT surgeries performed, and subsequently felt more of a "burning"-type pain. The patient was also seen over time by other consultant pain practitioners and was being followed by his internist. Investigational studies were obtained throughout his course. There were occasional small episodic increases in his white blood cell count related to infections and one solitary occurrence of an elevated glucose. The results of the general laboratory screens, metabolic panels, and liver function tests were as follows:

Analyte	Value, Conventional Units	Reference Interval, Conventional Units	Value, SI Units	Reference Interval, SI Units
Na	140 mmol/L	136–145	Same	
K	4.5 mmol/L	3.5–5.1	Same	
Cl	107 mmol/L	100–108	Same	
HCO$_3$	26 mmol/L	22–31	Same	
Glucose	159 mg/dL	70–110	8.8 mmol/L	3.9–6.1
BUN	9 mg/dL	8–20	0.5 mmol/L	0.4–1.1
Creatinine	0.9 mg/dL	0.7–1.3	79.6 μmol/L	61.9–114.9
Calcium	9.9 mg/dL	8.5–10.5	2.5 mmol/L	2.1–2.6
RBC	4.71 × 10^6/μL	4.20–5.70	4.71 × 10^{12}/L	4.2–5.7
Hgb	14.4 g/dL	13–17	144 g/L	130–170 g/L
Hct	43.3%	39.0–51.0	0.43	0.39–0.51
WBC	6.3 × 10^3/μL	4–10 × 10^3	6.3 × 10^9/L	4–10 × 10^9
Platelet	241 × 10^3/μL	150–400	241 × 10^9/L	150–400 × 10^9
AST	41 U/L	10–45	0.7 μkat/L	0.17–0.77
ALT	65 U/L	13–40	1.1 μkat/L	0.22–0.68
Alkaline phosphatase	43 U/L	42–121	0.7 μkat/L	0.71–2.1
Total bilirubin	0.4 mg/dL	0.2–1.2	6.8 μmol/L	3.4–20.5
Albumin	4.2 g/dL	3.2–5.5	42 g/L	32–55
Total protein	7.2 g/dL	6.2–8.0	72 g/L	62–80
TSH	0.8 mIU/mL	0.4–4.9	Same	
Thyroxine, free	1.1 ng/dL	0.7–1.5	14.2 pmol/L	9.0–19.3

Urine drug testing was also periodically performed and confirmed compliance. The results of the urine drug of abuse panel are shown below:

Analyte	Value	Positive Cutoff Concentration, ng/mL
Amphetamine/ methamphetamine	Negative	1000
Barbiturates	Negative	200
Benzodiazepines	Negative	200
Cannabinoids	Negative	25
Cocaine	Negative	300
Opiates	Negative	300

In addition, other diagnostic testing was performed and included numerous scans (MRI and MRA of the brain with and without contrast) to demonstrate the infections and surgical changes. An EKG was also obtained and showed a sinus arrhythmia, so it was decided not to pursue the option of mexilitene.

Eventually it became known that the patient was receiving opioid medications from other physicians. He was informed of the situation and offered several options, including counseling and detoxification programs, but chose to seek another physician. He did return to the practice briefly, but subsequently failed to return after another scheduled operation.

Prior to leaving the practice, the patient entered into an IRB-approved research study on pharmacogenomic testing for chronic pain patients. As a result, the patient had a blood sample drawn for therapeutic drug management and genetic analysis of cytochrome P450 2D6 (*CYP2D6*) polymorphisms. The patient's steady-state serum concentration (Css) of tramadol and *O*-desmethyltramadol were 340 and 42 μg/L, respectively. Tramadol is extensively metabolized to *O*-desmethyltramadol, an active metabolite, by *CYP2D6*.[4] The patient was genotyped for the some of the most prevalent *CYP2D6* polymorphisms (*3, 4, 5, 6, 7, and 8). According to the patient's genotype (*1/*5), he was heterozygous for *CYP2D6**5 (the gene deletion), making him an intermediate metabolizer.

CYP2D6 is a mixed-function oxidase that is part of the cytochrome P450 family of enzymes. It is part of the xenobiotic class of these enzymes in that it oxidizes dietary toxins and many drugs. Of the cytochroms P450, CYP2D6 is among those with the greatest amount of phenotypic variability. Over 80 allelic variants have been described, and these polymorphisms can have normal, increased, decreased, or absent enzymatic activity. Increased activity is present when multiple copies of the gene are present. Currently, there is an FDA-approved gene chip assay available that will detect the presence of 27 of the most common allelic variations for CYP2D6. Among the more common allelic variations with no activity are CYP2D6*3, *4, and *5, while CYP2D6*9, *10, and *17 are three of the more common variations with decreased activity. This patient was heterozygous for CYP2D6*5 (a gene deletion) making him an intermediate metabolizer with decreased CYP2D6 activity. About 10% of the U.S. Caucasian population and 2% of Asians and African-Americans are poor metabolizers of CYP2D6.

CYP2D6 is responsible for the metabolism of approximately 25% of all medications. Among the drugs metabolized by CYP2D6 (and some examples) are antiarrythmics (flecainide, mexiletine), antipsychotics (haloperidol, risperidone), β-blockers (metoprolol, propranolol), opiates (codeine, tramadol), selective-serotonin-reuptake inhibitors (fluoxetine, paroxetine), and tricyclic antidepressants (amitriptyline, imipramine). CYP2D6 is also induced by a variety of drugs, including dexamethasone and rifampicin.

It should be obvious from the preceding list of substrates and common drugs that knowledge of 2D6 allele status may be important in directing therapy with such common drugs as antidepressants and opiates. This patient had decreased *CYP2D6* activity and might be at a greater risk for toxicity, since he could not metabolize tramadol as efficiently as someone who was an extensive metabolizer. This was clearly evident by the steady-state concentrations (Css) of tramadol and *O*-desmethyltramadol. Typically, a patient receiving 200–400 mg/day of tramadol has an average Css of 365 µg/L.[5] However, this patient was taking only one-fourth to one-half of that dosage (100 mg/day), but had a similar Css (340 µg/L). Therefore, insight into the patient's genetic makeup provided a better understanding and rationale for the insufficient pain relief that he experienced with the attempted therapeutic measures. It also supports the frequent incidents of side effects he reported.

Furthermore, the genotype might help explain the patient's-opioid seeking behavior. Drug addiction is a complex disease caused by numerous factors, including genetics. Polymorphisms in genes that are involved in the absorption, biotransformation, and physiological processes (i.e., intracellular signal transduction pathways) may affect an individual's vulnerability to develop addiction.[6] It has been hypothesized that individuals with an inability to metabolize oral opioids into more active metabolites (poor metabolizers of *CYP2D6*) may be protected from opioid dependence.[7] However, this patient was an intermediate, not a poor, metabolizer of *CYP2D6*. This case presents an example of how personalized medicine and the use of pharmacogenomics in pain management might be useful in the future to select the appropriate pharmacotherapy and dosages to minimize side effects, and how it might also predict who may be at risk for addiction.

References

1. BAJRACHARYA, H. AND HINTHORN, D.: *Sinusitis, Chronic. Medicine.* http://www.emedicine.com/med/topic2556.htm (accessed June 2005).
2. BROOK, I.: Acute and chronic frontal sinusitis. *Curr. Opin. Pulm. Med. 9*:171–4, 2003.
3. Brook, I.: Microbiology and management of sinusitis. *J. Otolaryngol. 25*:249–56, 1996.
4. Product Information: *Ultram(R), Tramadol Hydrochloride.* Ortho-McNeil Pharmaceutical, Raritan, NJ, (PI revised Dec. 1999) reviewed March 2000.
5. BASELT, R. C.: *Disposition of Toxic Drugs and Chemicals in Man*, 6th ed., Biomedical Publications, Foster City, CA, 2002.
6. LICHTERMANN, D., FRANKE, P., MAIER, W., AND RAO, M. L.: Pharmacogenomics and addiction to opiates. *Eur. J. Pharm. 410*:269–79, 2000.
7. TYNDALE, R. F., DROLL, K. P., AND SELLERS, E. M.: Genetically deficient CYP2D6 metabolism provides protection against oral opiate dependence. *Pharmacogenetics 7*:375–9, 1997.

Case 74

A Man with Colitis and Pancytopenia

Alison Woodworth

A 32-year-old Caucasian male presented to the emergency department with complaints of bloody diarrhea 20 times per day and dehydration. A CBC was notable for anemia with normal white blood cell and platelet counts. Past medical history was significant for Crohn's disease diagnosed at age 20 involving the small and large intestines. He underwent ileocecal resection, and had been asymptomatic and required no therapy for the past 5 years. During his 2-day hospital course, anemia and dehydration were corrected, the diarrhea resolved, and immunosuppression with prednisone and azathioprine was started to treat a flare of inflammatory bowel disease.

Three weeks later, he returned to the gastroenterology clinic for a follow-up appointment during which he complained of fevers, chills, and rectal pain for the past 3 days. On physical examination he was diaphoretic, febrile (39.8°C), and tachycardic, and experienced pain with movement. No lymphadenopathy was appreciated, and lung and heart exams were normal. His abdomen was mildly tender with hypoactive bowel sounds. No ascites or peripheral edema was noted.

Laboratory data included the following:

Analyte	Value, Conventional Units	Reference Interval, Conventional Units	Value, SI Units	Reference Interval, SI Units
WBC	$0.6 \times 10^3/\mu L$	3.8–9.8	$0.6 \times 10^9/L$	3.8–9.8
Neutrophil count	$0.0 \times 10^3/\mu L$	1.7–6.7	$0.0 \times 10^9/L$	1.7–6.7
Lymphocyte count	$0.6 \times 10^3/\mu L$	0.9–3.2	$0.6 \times 10^9/L$	0.9–3.2
Monocyte count	$0.0 \times 10^3/\mu L$	0.2–0.9	$0.0 \times 10^9/L$	0.2–0.9
Hemoglobin	8.2 g/dL	13.8–17.2	82 g/L	138–172
Hematocrit	23%	41–50	0.23 volume	0.41–0.50
Platelets	$42 \times 10^3/\mu L$	140–440	$42 \times 10^9/L$	140–440
Sodium	145 mmol/L	135–145	Same	
Potassium	3.5 mmol/L	3.3–4.9	Same	

Tietz's Applied Laboratory Medicine, Second Edition. Edited by Mitchell G. Scott, Ann M. Gronowski, and Charles S. Eby

Analyte	Value, Conventional Units	Reference Interval, Conventional Units	Value, SI Units	Reference Interval, SI Units
Chloride	106 mmol/L	97–110	Same	
CO_2, total	29 mmol/L	22–32	Same	
Glucose	98 mg/dL	65–199	5.4 mmol/L	3.6–11.0
Urea nitrogen	19 mg/dL	8–25	6.8 mmol/L	2.9–9.0
Creatinine	1.3 mg/dL	0.7–15	114.9 µmol/L	62–133
Protein, total	7.0 g/dL	6.8–8.5	70 g/L	68–85
Albumin	3.6 g/dL	3.6–5.0	36 g/L	36–50
AST	37 IU/L	11–47	0.63 µkat/L	0.19–0.80
ALT	50 IU/L	7–53	0.85 µkat/L	0.12–0.90
Bilirubin	0.4 mg/dL	0.3–1.1	6.8 µmol/L	5.1–18.8

Chest x-ray showed no active disease. Blood cultures were positive for *Esherichia coli* and *Streptococci viridans*. Urine cultures were negative. A bone marrow biopsy and aspirate were markedly hypocellular (<10% cellularity, normal for 30-year-old adult ∼70%) without features of myelodysplasia or a myeloid or lymphoid malignancy.

Differential Diagnosis

Bone marrow failure syndromes are characterized by inadequate production of red cells, white cells, and platelets, leading to various combinations and severities of peripheral blood cytopenias. Typically, the bone marrow is hypocellular, as in this case, but a cellular bone marrow is encountered with clonal disorders including myelodysplastic syndrome, some acute leukemias and lymphomas, and paroxysmal nocturnal hemoglobinuria, secondary conditions such as bone marrow infiltration by metastatic cancer, sarcoidosis, or granulomas due to infections, and ineffective hematopoiesis due to longstanding folate or B_{12} deficiency.

The differential for pancytopenia and a hypocellular bone marrow includes constitutional and acquired aplastic anemia, starvation, hypothyroidism, and rarely, hematopoietic malignancies, most commonly myelodysplastic syndrome. Acquired aplastic anemia may be idiopathic or secondary to environmental toxins (benzene), radiation exposure, acute viral infection, or an idiosyncratic reaction to certain medications including nonsteroidal analgesics, antithyroid and psychotropic drugs, penicillamine, and gold salts. Finally, pancytopenia is a potential side effect of myelosuppressive chemotherapy agents. Based on the temporal association and the bone marrow findings, the diagnosis for this patient was azathioprine-induced bone marrow suppression.

Azathioprine therapy was immediately discontinued. He required many transfusions of red cells and platelets during his hospital stay. His blood cell counts slowly recovered with antibiotic, vitamin, granulocyte–monocyte colony stimulating factor, and erythropoietin therapies. He was discharged on hospital day 38.

Thiopurine Metabolism and Toxicity

Thiopurine drugs such as 6-mercaptopurine (6-MP), azathioprine (AZA), and 6-thioguanine (6-TG) are used as both chemotherapeutic agents to treat leukemias and immunosuppressive agents to treat inflammatory bowel disease, rheumatic and hematologic autoimmune diseases, and following solid organ transplant. Thiopurine drugs are inactive and require metabolism of the prodrug to thioguanine nucleotides (TGN) for cytotoxic and immunosuppressive action. TGNs are formed after a series of enzymes modify the prodrug (Fig. 74.1) beginning with hypoxanthine guanine phosphoribosyl transferase (HGPRT). While the exact mechanism of the effects of these drugs is unknown, theories include TGN incorporation into and interference with DNA and RNA synthesis and chromosomal replication, inhibition of T and B cell proliferation, and interference with natural-killer (NK) cell cytotoxicity.[4,5]

There is a delayed onset of therapeutic action of the thiopurines (about 17 weeks in Crohn's disease patients), and the clinical response rate varies among different

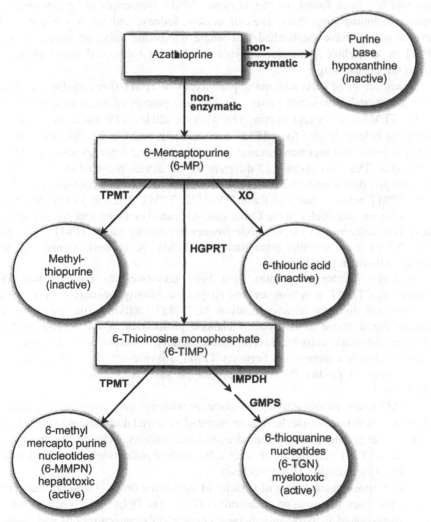

Figure 74.1   Metabolism of azathioprine and 6-mercaptopurine. A series of competing enzymatic pathways result in formation of either inactive metabolites or hepato or myelotoxic metabolites (TPMT—thiopurine methyltransferase; XO—xanthine oxidase, HGPRT—hypoxanthine guanine phosphoribosyltransferase; IMPDH—inosine monophosphate dehydrogenase; GMPS—guanine monophosphate synthase).

diseases. Side effects of the thiopurines include allergic reactions, nausea, acute pancreatitis, bone marrow suppression, hepatotoxicity, and infections. Thiopurine toxicity leading to withdrawal of patients from the drug occurs in 10–28% of patients.[5,6] Symptoms of severe and potentially life-threatening bone marrow suppression, affecting about 1.4–5% of patients, usually occur within the first 30 days.[5] Patients with a deficiency of thiopurine S-methyltransferase enzyme (TPMT) activity are particularly at risk.

Pharmacogenetics of TPMT

Thiopurine S-methyltransferase (TPMT) is a cytosolic enzyme that catalyzes the S-methylation of thiopurine drugs to inactive, nontoxic metabolites. Thus far no natural substrate has been found for this enzyme. TPMT transcripts are expressed in various tissues, including lung, liver, skeletal muscle, kidney, and red and white blood cells. Several studies have established that single nucleotide polymorphisms (SNPs) in the TPMT gene leading to inactive enzyme are the major cause of hematopoietic toxicity due to thiopurine drugs.

There are three main enzymatic phenotypes of TPMT (low, medium, and high) that show a trimodal inheritance pattern. Eighty-nine percent of the population have normal to high TPMT activity representing two wildtype alleles, 11% have intermediate activity indicating heterozygosity for a TPMT mutant allele, and 1 in 300 (0.3%) have low or no TPMT activity and represent homozygous or compound heterozygotes for TPMT polymorphisms. There are at least 23 different TPMT alleles reported in the literature, with the wildtype designated as TPMT*1. At least 22 alleles have been associated with low or no TPMT activity, but 3 of these (TPMT*2, TPMT*3A, and TPMT*3C) account for 95% of the mutant alleles in the Caucasian, African-American, and Asian populations.[2,4] There is a difference in variant allele frequencies among races. TPMT*3A is present in about 5% of the Caucasian population, and TPMT*3C is most common in Asian and African-American populations.

A large number of studies have been performed to evaluate the correlation between the TPMT genotype and its enzymatic activity/phenotype (Fig. 74.2). Both in vitro and in vivo characterization of TPMT activities of the most common mutants listed above demonstrate enhanced proteolysis of the variant proteins, thus reducing enzymatic activity. Several studies among different populations have demonstrated a >98% concordance between TPMT enzyme activity and genotype.[1] Using the genotype to predict the TPMT phenotype yielded >90% sensitivity and >95% specificity.

TPMT genotype and activity also correlate with myelotoxicity. Several studies among different patient populations have demonstrated a skewed distribution of TPMT genotypes in patients experiencing thiopurine drug-induced toxicity. Whereas an unselected population has a TPMT variant rate of ~10%, 60–70% of patients who develop myelotoxicity have one or two mutant TPMT alleles.[2]

The proposed mechanism of toxicity of thiopurine drugs is through incorporation of drug metabolites, thioguanine nucleotides (TGN), into DNA and RNA, and many studies have demonstrated an association between higher TGN concentrations and mutant TPMT alleles.[1,2] These data suggest that physicians can identify patients who are at increased risk for adverse drug reactions to thiopurine drugs by genotyping or phenotyping the TPMT gene or enzyme prior to prescribing the drug.

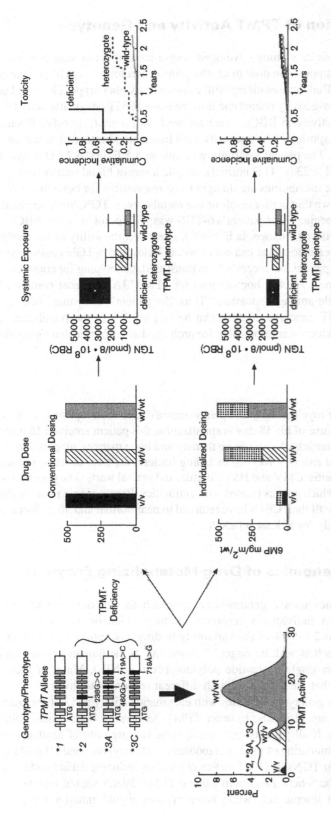

Figure 74.2 Genetic polymorphism of thiopurine methyltransferase and its role in determining response to thiopurine medications (azathioprine, mercaptopurine, thioguanine). The left panels depict the predominant TPMT mutant alleles causing autosomal codominant inheritance of TPMT activity in humans. As depicted in the subsequent top three panels, when uniform (conventional) dosages of thiopurine medications are administered to all patients, TPMT-deficient patients accumulate markedly higher (10-fold) cellular concentrations of active thioguanine nucleotides (TGNs), and heterozygous patients accumulated about twofold higher TGN concentrations, translating into a significantly higher frequency of hematopoietic toxicity (far right panels). As depicted in the bottom three panels, when genotype-specific dosing of thiopurines is administered, comparable cellular TGN concentrations are achieved, and all three TPMT phenotypes can be treated without acute toxicity. (Reproduced with permission from Evans, W. E.: Thiopurine 5-methyl transferase: a genetic polymorphism that affects a small number of drugs in a big way. *Pharmacogenetics* 12(6):421–3, 2002).

547

Determination of TPMT Activity and Genotype

The patient in this case study developed severe pancytopenia after 3 weeks of taking a typical immunosuppressive dose of azathioprine. Therefore, it was likely that he possessed one or two TPMT alleles associated with a low-activity phenotype. The "gold standard" for diagnosis of a low-activity phenotype is to measure TPMT enzymatic activity in red blood cells (RBCs). Activity in RBCs correlates well with activity in other tissues. However, results are often spurious when patients have had a blood transfusion within 30–60 days of measurement. The patient's activity was low, at 3.5 EU (<6.7 EU is low, 6.7–23.6 is intermediate, and >23.6 EU is normal), despite a recent blood transfusion.

Azathioprine metabolites are thought to be responsible for bone marrow suppression. Studies have shown that higher levels of one metabolite, 6-TGN, are associated with development of leukopenia.[2,6] The patient's 6-TGN was 1673 pmol/8×10^8 RBC (normal 230–400 and higher risk of leukopenia if >400). However, the utility of measuring 6-TGN is controversial since cytopenias can occur without elevated 6-TGN concentrations.

Because the patient had recently been transfused, genotyping for common TPMT SNPs was also performed. He was homozygous for TPMT*3A, the most common low-activity polymorphic allele among Caucasians. Thus, the patient's enzymatic activity, metabolite levels, and TPMT genotype confirm that he is 1 of 300 in the population that has low TPMT activity, which was responsible for prolonged and life-threatening myelosuppresion.

Treatment

The treatment for myelotoxicity and pancytopenia due to azathioprine toxicity is supportive care. Over the course of his 38-day hospitalization, this patient received 16 units of red cells and 19 units of platelets. Azathioprine therapy and bone marrow suppression are associated with an increased risk of infection, including bacteremia, liver abscess, pneumonia, septic phlebitis and arthritis, CMV and HSV viremia, and genital warts. The patient developed bacterial sepsis for which he was treated with antibiotics. Pancytopenic patients should receive supportive care until their CBCs have returned to near normal and after discharge should be monitored monthly for at least 6 months.

Pharmacogenomics of Drug-Metabolizing Enzymes

Pharmacogenomics uses a genomewide approach to elucidate the inherited basis for differences in an individual's response to drugs. Genetic variation is estimated to account for about 20–95% of the variability in drug absorption, distribution, and metabolism, and interaction with its target.[2] Sequencing of the human genome has uncovered about 1.4 million single-nucleotide polymorphisms (SNPs). Many of these encode for variant proteins that are associated with different responses to drugs.

Since TPMT genotype correlates with enzymatic activity and in turn azathioprine toxicity, physicians are beginning to order TPMT genotyping before prescribing thiopurine drugs (Fig. 74.2). If all patients receive the same starting dose of azathioprine, there will be moderate accumulation of toxic metabolites in heterozygotes and 10-fold higher concentrations of cellular TGNs in TPMT-deficient patients, inducing earlier and more severe toxicity. Patients who inherit two nonfunctional TPMT alleles should receive 5–10% of the standard dose of thiopurines, while heterozygotes should initially receive 70% of the dose, thus reducing TGN accumulation and hematotoxicity.[2] There is also evidence in the pediatric leukemia population that outcome is related to thiopurine dose intensitivity; higher doses should be given to TPMT wildtype patients because better event-free survival or early treatment response was seen in intermediate- or low-TPMT-activity patients.[1]

Currently, manufacturers recommend a complicated laboratory monitoring scheme to reduce the risk of toxicity when patients start a thiopurine drug: baseline CBC and liver chemistries, weekly monitoring of CBC for 4 weeks, biweekly for 2 weeks, and monthly for the remainder of treatment.[5,6] Prior knowledge of TPMT status may permit less intense monitoring, making treatment more convenient and less costly for patients.

More than 30 families of enzymes are involved in drug metabolism, and SNPs that affect function have been identified for most of them. For example, two SNPs in the cytochrome P450 2C9 enzyme reduce the rate of warfarin metabolism, are associated with higher rates of bleeding complications during initiation of warfarin therapy, and lower maintenance warfarin doses (see Case 75).

Irinotecan is a chemotherapeutic drug that is being used to treat colon, lung, rhabdomyosarcoma, and neuroblastoma cancers. Irinotican is converted to an activate metabolite, SN-38, which inhibits topoisomerase I. SN-38 is eliminated through hepatic glucuronidation by UDP–glucuronyltransferase 1A1 (UGT1A1). Toxicities such as diarrhea and leukopenia are associated with increased levels of SN-38.[1,3] Treatment efficacy and toxicity of irinotecan has been associated with polymorphisms in UGT1A1. In particular, the UGT1A1*28 allele has been associated with increased risk of toxicity during irinotecan therapy, suggesting that determination of UGT1A1 genotype prior to irinotecan therapy may reduce toxicity by up to 50%.[1,3]

Conclusion

Adverse drug reactions may be responsible for greater than 100,000 deaths and about 5% of hospital admissions per year.[1] Genetic polymorphisms may be involved in many of these reactions. Therefore, pharmacogenomic evaluation of SNPs present in enzymes involved in drug pharmacokinetics and pharmacodynamics prior to treatment may help reduce toxicity and death as well as costly hospital admissions. Introduction of individualized drug therapy based on pharmacogenomic data, as in the case of TPMT, may promote more cost-effective and efficient patient care.

References

1. EICHELBAUM, M., INGELMAN-SUNDBERG, M., AND EVANS, W. E.: Pharmacogenomics and individualized drug therapy. *Ann. Rev. Med. 57*:119–137, 2006.
2. EVANS, W. E.: Pharmacogenetics of thiopurine S-methyltransferase. *Ther. Drug Monit. 26*:186–191, 2004.
3. MARSH, S. AND MCLEOD, H. L.: Pharmacogenetics of irinotecan toxicity. *Pharmacogenomics 5*:835–43, 2004.
4. MCCLEOD, H. L. AND SIVA, C: The thiopurine S-methyltransferase gene locus—implications for clinical pharmacogenomics. *Pharmacogenomics 3*: 89–98, 2002.
5. SANDERSON, J., ANSARI, A., MARINAKI, T., AND DULEY, J.: Thiopurine methyltransferase: Should it be measured before commencing thiopurine drug therapy? *Ann. Clin. Biochem. 41*:294–302, 2004.
6. SU, C. AND LICHTENSTEIN, G. R.: Treatment of inflammatory bowel disease with azathioprine and 6-mercaptopurine. *Gastroenterol Clin North Am. 33*:209–34, 2004.

Case 75

A 46-Year-Old Female with a Painful, Swollen Right Calf

Syamal Bhattacharya, Bradley D. Freeman, and Barbara A. Zehnbauer

A 46-year-old obese Caucasian woman presented to her general internist with recent onset of flushed skin and sweating. Over the previous 6 months she has noticed her hair thinning and complained of increasing irritability. She described occasional alcohol use and a 30-year history of 1 pack per day of tobacco use. The physician diagnosed early-onset menopause and discussed options for symptom management and prevention of osteoporosis. Conjugated estrogen therapy was initiated. Eight weeks later, the patient came to the emergency department with pain, redness, and swelling of the right calf. Venous Doppler studies confirmed deep venous thrombosis. Laboratory investigations characterized her coagulation status, and genetic tests for *F5* (factor V) and *F2* (prothrombin) mutations, associated with heritable predisposition to venous thrombosis, were performed:

Analyte	Value, Conventional Units	Reference Interval, Conventional Units	Value, SI Units	Reference Interval, SI Units
Hemoglobin	14.5 g/dL	12.0–15.0	145 g/L	120–150
Hematocrit	38.2%	37.0–47.0	0.38	0.37–0.47
Red blood cells	$4.4 \times 10^6/\mu L$	4.2–5.2	$4.4 \times 10^{12}/L$	4.2–5.2
Platelet count	$223 \times 10^3/\mu L$	150–450	$223 \times 10^9/L$	150–450
Prothrombin	12.2 s	10.5–15.0	Same	
Partial thromboplastin time	29s	23–35	Same	
Protein C	129%	60–132%	Same	
Protein S	136%	70–140%	Same	
Antithrombin III	114%	80–140%	Same	
Homocysteine	6.2 μmol/L	0.0–20.0	Same	
Antiphospholipid antibody	Negative	Negative	Same	

Anticoagulation therapy was initiated with systemic heparinization and warfarin following hospital admission. International Normalized Ratio (INR) obtained 1 week

Tietz's Applied Laboratory Medicine, Second Edition. Edited by Mitchell G. Scott, Ann M. Gronowski, and Charles S. Eby
Copyright © 2007 John Wiley & Sons, Inc.

following warfarin initiation was therapeutic at 2.7 (target range 2.0–3.0). At a follow-up office visit, results of the genetic screening were reviewed:

F5 NM_000130.2: c.1517G > A (factor V Leiden, 1691G > A)   G/A; heterozygous for variant allele

F2 AF478696.1: g.21538G > A (prothrombin, 20210G > A)   G/G; no variant detected

The patient was informed that her deep venous thrombosis was likely the result of multiple factors: cigarette smoking, obesity, estrogen replacement therapy, and the factor V Leiden mutation. The patient was counseled about overall risk of venous thrombotic events and the increased risk conferred by her factor V Leiden genotype. The patient was also educated about the signs and symptoms of pulmonary embolism.

Three weeks later, the patient returned to her physician complaining of dark, tarry stools. On physical exam, the physician noticed bruising on her legs and forearms. An INR of 8.3 was recorded. The patient was admitted to the hospital and treated with fresh-frozen plasma and vitamin K to reverse the clotting deficiency. Endoscopy confirmed the presence of a duodenal ulcer that was not actively bleeding. Proton pump inhibitor therapy was initiated to suppress gastric acid. In order to determine a basis for the excessive effect of warfarin therapy, additional genetic tests were performed. The patient was found to be heterozygous [CYP2C9*1/CYP2C9*2] for a variant allele (2C9*2) associated with a functional deficiency in this cytochrome P450 enzyme, which metabolizes warfarin. CYP2C9*2 contains a single-nucleotide sequence variation that produces a substitution of cysteine for arginine at amino acid position 144. The CYP2C9*2-encoded enzyme demonstrates only about 12% of wildtype [CYP2C9*1] enzymatic activity.

Definition of the Disease

Factor V is critical in the coagulation cascade, binding to activated factor X to form the prothrombin activation complex. This step in the cascade is a positive feedback resulting in a rapid increase in available activated thrombin to yield crosslinked fibrin clots for hemostasis. A negative feedback signal that prevents excess coagulation is provided by activated protein C, which degrades factor V in the normal patient. Low protein C activity will lead to a higher risk and incidence of thrombotic events. In this patient protein C activity was normal. The factor V Leiden (FVL) allele contains a single nucleotide missense mutation in exon 10 of the factor V gene (G to A at nucleotide 1691, which produces a glutamine substitution for the normal arginine at amino acid position 506). This mutation renders the protein resistant to degradation by activated protein C, allowing the clotting cascade to continue unchecked, producing a hypercoaguable state in the patient. Studies have shown that 5–10% of the white population of the United States carry this mutation, with smaller percentages found in African-American and Hispanic American populations. The mutation is almost never detected in the indigenous African or Asian population. FVL predisposes the patient to many complications including primary venous thrombosis and thromboembolism resulting in pulmonary embolism. Patients heterozygous for FVL mutation have a 4–7-fold increased annual relative risk of thrombosis. The annual relative risk of venous thrombosis in individuals homozygous for FVL is up to 80-fold. FVL variant has also been implicated as a cause of fetal loss. FVL has *not* been linked to either arterial emboli (secondary to atrial fibrillation or prosthetic valves) or secondary venous thrombosis from trauma or elective surgery. Preventive measures and avoidance of risky behaviors may prove beneficial for carriers of the FVL variant. Smoking, obesity, hormone replacement therapy, estrogen-containing oral contraceptives, and prolonged inactivity may further increase risk of venous thrombotic events in this population.

The patient in this case was not only a FVL heterozygote but also a cytochrome P450 2C9*1/2C9*2 heterozygote. This mutation in CYP2C9 decreases warfarin metabolism, resulting in prolonged, increased concentrations of the drug, a rise in the INR, decreased coagulation, and increased risk for bleeding. Complications can range from easy bruising and hemorrhage after surgery or minor trauma, to spontaneous, life-threatening gastrointestinal or cerebral bleeding. Immediate treatment includes fresh-frozen plasma and vitamin K replacement and transfusion if warranted.

Recent studies also demonstrate that heritable variations in the vitamin K epoxide reductase complex subunit 1 gene (*VKORC1*) influence the pharmacodynamic response to warfarin.[7] These alleles may contribute to as much as 25% of the observed variation in the anticoagulation activity of warfarin.[8] Both regulatory and coding region base changes, with effects ranging from increased warfarin sensitivity to warfarin resistance, have been described.[8] These polymorphisms also exhibit significantly different allele frequencies among Asian, Caucasian, and African-American patients contributing further to population differences in warfarin dosing required to achieve anticoagulation.[9]

Differential Diagnosis of Hypercoaguability

There are many important causes of hypercoagulation, some are inherited and others are acquired. Heritable causes of hypercoagulation include common polymorphisms of the *F5* and *F2* genes (factor V Leiden and prothrombin G20210A, respectively) and more rare mutations in proteins C, S, antithrombin III, and 5,10-methylenetetrahydrofolate reductase (*MTHFR*). In this patient the protein S and antithrombin II activities were normal. The normal homocysteine values are consistent with normal activity of the MTHFR protein. Acquired causes are numerous, including hypercoaguability of malignancy, antiphospholipid antibody, chronic medical illness, paroxysmal nocturnal hemoglobinuria, pregnancy, surgery, smoking, estrogen-containing oral contraceptives, and hormone replacement therapy.

Clinical geneticists[1,2] and molecular pathologists[3,4] recommend the following criteria to consider genetic testing for FVL:

- Patients with first venous thrombosis (VTE) at a young age (<45–50 years of age)
- Patients with a strong family history of VTE in first-degree relatives
- VTE during pregnancy or postpartum period
- VTE during oral contraceptive therapy, hormone replacement, or methotrexate therapy
- Female smokers age <50 with a myocardial infarction
- VTE in an unusual site (cerebral, mesenteric, portal, or hepatic veins)
- Recurrent VTE
- Idiopathic VTE unrelated to surgery or trauma.

Treatment of VTE in FVL

Anticoagulation therapy of a patient with FVL mutation does not differ from the therapy of the standard patient. Anticoagulation induction with low-molecular-weight heparin concurrent with gradual warfarin therapy is the initial step. When the INR value is between 2 and 3, heparin can be discontinued. Gradual induction of the warfarin therapy is recommended to reduce the risk of necrosis. Warfarin-associated skin necrosis is believed to be caused by the depletion of antithrombin III before other vitamin K–dependent clotting factors are consumed, thereby inducing a paradoxical hypercoagulable state. Prophylactic heparin or warfarin anticoagulation may be warranted in FVL carriers who are immobilized because of surgery or prolonged illness. Postoperatively, these patients should be encouraged to ambulate as soon as possible.

Currently, warfarin therapy is often initiated in the inpatient setting to allow dose titration, INR monitoring, and systemic heparinization. While the patient is discharged from the hospital once a therapeutic INR is achieved, it requires to accurate determination of the optimal maintenance dose of warfarin takes 1–2 weeks. Many patients, however, are unusually warfarin-sensitive, and may become dangerously anticoagulated after standard dosing. Rapid genetic screening allows the identification and appropriate dosing of the warfarin-sensitive (or -resistant) patient. Such customized dosing could shorten the length of stay, lessen the cost, and decrease the morbidity associated with warfarin initiation.[5,6]

References

1. GRODY, W. W., GRIFFIN, J. H., TAYLOR, A. K. ET AL.: American College of Medical Genetics consensus statement on factor V Leiden mutation testing. *Genet. Med.* *3*:139–48, 2001.

2. REICH, L. M., BOWER, M., AND KEY, N. S.: Role of the geneticist in testing and counseling for inherited thrombophilia. *Genet. Med.* *5*:133–43, 2003.

3. College of American Pathologists Consensus Conference XXXVI.: Diagnostic issues in thrombophilia. *Arch. Pathol. Lab. Med. 126*, 2002.

4. PRESS, R. D., BAUER, K. A., KUJOVICH, J. L. ET AL.: Clinical utility of factor V Leiden (R506Q) testing for the diagnosis and management of thromboembolic disorders. *Arch. Pathol. Lab. Med. 126*:1304–18, 2002.

5. FREEMAN, B. D., ZEHNBAUER, B. A., MCGRATH, S. D., BORECKI, I., AND BUCHMAN, T G.: Cytochrome P450 polymorphisms are associated with reduced warfarin dose. *Surgery 128*:281–5, 2000.

6. TABRIZI, A. R., ZEHNBAUER, B. A., BORECKI, I. B., MCGRATH, S. D., BUCHMAN, T. G., AND FREEMAN, B. D.: The frequency and effects of cytochrome P450 (*CYP*) *2C9* polymorphisms in patients receiving warfarin. *J. Am. Coll. Surg. 194*:267–73, 2002.

7. ROST, S., FREGIN, A., IVASKEVICIUS, V., CONZELMANN, E., HORTNAGEL, K., PELZ, H.-J., LAPPEGARD, K., SELFRIED, E., SCHARRER, I., TUDDENHAM, E. G. D., MULLER, C. R., STROM, T. M., AND OLDENBURG, J.: Mutations in *VKORC1* cause warfarin resistance and multiple coagulation factor deficiency type 2. *Nature 427*:537–41, 2004.

8. RIEDER, M. J., REINER, A. P., GAGE, B. F., NICKERSON, D. A., EBY, C. S., MCLEOD, H. L., BLOUGH, D. K., THUMMEL, K. E., VEENSTRA, D. L., AND RETTIE, A. E.: Effect of *VKORC1* haplotypes on transcriptional regulation and warfarin dose. *N. Engl. J. Med. 352*:2285–93, 2005.

9. TAKAHASHI, H., WILKINSON, G. R., NUTESCU, E. A., MORITA, T., RITCHIE, M. D., SCORDO, M. G., PENGO, V., BARBAN, M., PADRINI, R., IEIRI, I., OTSUBO, K., KASHIMA, T., KIMURA, S., KIJIMA, AND S., ECHIZEN, H.: Different contributions of polymorphisms in *VKORC1* and *CYP2C9* to intra- and inter-population differences in maintenance dose of warfarin in Japanese, Caucasians, and African-Americans. *Pharmacogenet. Genom. 16*:101–10, 2006.

Part Seventeen

Toxicology

A case of drug abuse analyzed by forensic toxicology is presented and discussed in Case 76; a case of opioids intoxication, diversion, and pharmacogenomics also analyzed by forensic toxicology, is reported and discussed in Case 77; and a case involving metabolic acidosis of unknown etiology is the topic of Case 78 (all three cases edited by MGS).

Tietz's Applied Laboratory Medicine, Second Edition. Edited by Mitchell G. Scott, Ann M. Gronowski, and Charles S. Eby
Copyright © 2007 John Wiley & Sons, Inc.

Case 76

A Case of Mixed Club Drugs Abuse

Susan B. Gock, Run-Zhang Shi, Jeffrey M. Jentzen, and Steven H. Wong

The decedent was a 24-year-old white female with no known significant medical history other than occasional alcohol and marijuana use. She had driven from another state with several friends to attend the Grateful Dead concert at a popular outdoor concert venue in Wisconsin. According to friends, she had remained sober throughout the concert and drove the group to a hotel where they checked in during the early morning hours after the concert. The decedent went to the bathroom and locked the door. That morning she was found floating on her back in the bathtub full of water by one of her friends. Attempts to resuscitate at the scene were made by paramedics, but she expired despite these efforts. A needle puncture mark was present in her right antecubital fossa.

Paraphernalia found at the scene included an insulin syringe and two other syringes, a ziplock bag containing a brown powdery substance, a separate bag containing 21 white pills, a bag containing white rocklike substances, an empty pink plastic container, and rolling papers. Autopsy findings showed recent injection site, right antecubital fossa, and there was no evidence of drowning.

Toxicology Lab Results

Analyte	Specimen	Result
Ethyl alcohol	Subclavian (SC) blood	Negative
Carbon monoxide	SC blood	2.9%

Drug Screens by Gas Chromatography/Mass Spectrometry (GC/MS)

Analyte	Specimen	Result
Acidic/neutral drugs	SC blood	None detected
Basic drugs		
Methylenedioxy-methamphetamine (MDMA)	SC blood	Positive
Ketamine	SC blood	Positive
Oxycodone	SC blood	Positive
Diazepam	SC blood	Positive

Tietz's Applied Laboratory Medicine, Second Edition. Edited by Mitchell G. Scott, Ann M. Gronowski, and Charles S. Eby
Copyright © 2007 John Wiley & Sons, Inc.

Analyte	Specimen	Result
Diphenhydramine	Syringe contents	Positive
Acetylated codeine	Syringe contents	Positive
Heroin	Syringe contents	Positive
Cocaine	White substance, baggy 1	Positive
THC (Δ^9-tetrahydrocannabinol)	Brown substance, baggy 2	Positive
Diazepam	White pills	Positive

Blood Drug Screens by Radioimmunoassay

Analyte	Specimen	Result
Opiates	SC blood	Positive
Benzodiazepines	SC blood	Positive
Cannabinoids	SC blood	Positive
Methamphetamines	SC blood	Positive
Unconjugated morphine	SC blood	Positive

Analyte Quantification

Analyte	Specimen	Result	Method
MDMA (Ecstasy)	SC blood	1.49 mg/L	GC/MS
MDA[a] (MDMA metabolite)	SC blood	ND[b]	GC/MS
Oxycodone	SC blood	0.13 mg/L	GC/MS
Ketamine	SC blood	0.22 mg/L	GC/FID[c]
Diazepam	SC blood	0.07 mg/L	GC/ECD[d]
Nordiazepam (Diazepam metabolite)	SC blood	0.02 mg/L	GC/ECD
Morphine	SC blood	0.26 mg/L	GC/MS
Codeine	SC blood	0.012 mg/L	GC/MS
6-Monoacetyl morphine	Vitreous fluid	0.046 mg/L	GC/MS

[a]MDA: methylenedioxyamphetamine.
[b]ND: not detected.
[c]FID: flame ionization detector.
[d]ECD: electron capture detector.

This fatality was the result of mixed "club drug" use. The use of postmortem forensic toxicology laboratory findings was essential to the investigation and for certifying the cause of death. This young lady's death illustrates the dire consequences of the present popularity of club drug abuse. Obtaining the complete picture of club drug abuse as demonstrated in this case calls for an extensive list of forensic toxicology detection and quantification techniques and methods.[1] The final diagnosis of mixed drug toxicity (heroin, oxycodone, ketamine, and MDMA) for the case reported here was made on the basis of forensic toxicology studies, drug paraphernalia found at the scene, and recent injection site (right antecubital fossa). There was no evidence of drowning.

The term "club drugs" describes illicit recreational drugs that have gained popularity in recent years at nightclubs, large dance parties ("raves") and rock concerts. Club or rave drugs include stimulants, depressants, and hallucinogenic substances, frequently taken for their psychedelic and/or euphoric effects to enhance dancing, auditory, and visual perceptions. Drugs in this class include lysergic acid diethylamide (LSD), γ-hydroxybutyrate

(GHB), ketamine, flunitrazepam (Rohypnol), and methylenedioxymethamphetamine (MDMA, "Ecstasy"). MDMA is the most prominent member of the methylenedioxy-substituted amphetamines (hallucinogenic amines) to have gained popularity for illicit recreational drug use. This class of club drugs is also referred to as "dissociative anesthetics" because of their original development as potential anesthetics and the dissociative, out-of-body feeling they produce. At normally taken doses of 100–150 mg, MDMA effects include mild to moderate central nervous system (CNS) stimulation as well as enhanced feelings of empathy, closeness, and response to intimate touch. Ketamine hydrochloride ("special K") produces similar dreamy, hallucinogenic feelings. Typical ketamine doses are 100 mg, and effects are noticed within 5 minutes if snorted or in 10–20 minutes if swallowed. Ketamine is odorless and tasteless and thus can be given to unsuspecting victims and, like Rohypnol, has been used as a "date rape" drug. Club drugs are often taken in combination with each other, with alcohol, or with other drugs. The fact that these drugs can be taken orally in various convenient forms (small pills, powders, or liquid) and their relatively low cost is driving their popularity among young people.[2] For the year 2002, club drugs were implicated in approximately 1.2% of all drug-abuse-related ER visits reported to DAWN (Drug Abuse Warning Network), with some of these visits involving multiple club drugs being used in combination with alcohol, marijuana, cocaine, and heroin.

There is no legitimate, approved therapeutic use for MDMA in the United States. MDMA is manufactured in clandestine laboratories, primarily in western European countries, where the precursor chemicals are easier to obtain than in the United States. Most frequently, MDMA is administered orally in tablet or capsule form in doses of 100–150 mg. The onset of action following oral administration is 30–60 minutes, and the half-life is approximately 7 hours. MDMA undergoes N-demethylation to the active metabolite MDA, which is the only metabolite usually detected in the blood of MDMA users. About 65% of the dose is eliminated in the urine as parent drug and 7% as MDA. Mono- and dihydroxy metabolites are excreted in the urine as conjugates and make up the remaining metabolites found in urine. Ketamine HCl is used legitimately as a veterinary and, occasionally, a human anesthetic. The most common source of ketamine for use as a club drug is diverted or stolen veterinary products. Ketamine is structurally similar to another common club drug, phencyclidine (PCP or "angel dust") that was also originally developed as an anesthetic. These drugs act by disrupting the function of the glutamate receptor, which plays a major role in the perception of pain and in expressing emotion.

Analysis of postmortem specimens for the presence of club drugs such as MDMA and MDA typically involves extraction of the drugs from tissues such as liver, muscle, and brain, as well as from urine, central blood, peripheral blood, and vitreous humor. Varying degrees of putrefaction and postmortem redistribution of drugs further complicate the analysis. Peripheral blood and vitreous humor have been reported to provide the best estimate of the blood drug concentration at the time of death.[3]

Analytical techniques available for initial screening, confirmation, and quantification of club drugs such as MDMA and ketamine in forensic specimens may include thin-layer chromatography (TLC), HPLC, gas chromatography (GC), GC/MS, and immunoassays. TLC is a common initial screening technique capable of detecting a broad spectrum of drugs in urine. Identification is based on the rate of flow (Rf) value and the color characteristics following exposure to specific staining reagents. The Toxi-Lab A system can be used for the detection of ketamine and MDMA in urine, and has the ability to differentiate sympathomimetic amines such as ephedrine, pseudoephedrine, and phenylpropanolamine from illicit dugs such as amphetamine, methamphetamine, MDMA, and MDA. More sensitive methods such as GC, HPLC, GC/MS are usually used for detection and quantification of drugs in postmortem blood samples and tissues.

Immunoassays may also be applied to forensic drug screens for the presence of MDMA and related metabolites. Immunoassays for the detection of amphetamine and methamphetamine have variable degrees of cross-reactivity with MDMA, MDA, and other structurally related over-the-counter sympathomimetic amines such as pseudoephedrine and ephedrine. Antibody cross-reactivity in commercially available immunoassays is variable and is dependent on both the concentration of the structurally related analyte present in the specimen and the source of the antibodies used. In general, greater cross-reactivity occurs with polyclonal-antibody-based assays in comparison to monoclonal-antibody-based assays. Monoclonal antibody should be used when high selectivity is desired.

Postmortem specimens often pose a problem to immunoassays used for the detection of MDMA and metabolites in urine or blood because of decomposition occurring during the postmortem interval. This may result in the production of biogenic amines such as β-phenethylamine or tyramine that have the potential to produce a false-positive result in amphetamine immunoassays due to antibody cross-reactivity with these analytes. Because of the lack of specificity associated with immunoassays for the detection of MDMA and metabolites present in postmortem samples, confirmation of positive immunoassay results should always be made using an alternate analytical methodology. GC/MS analysis with selective ion monitoring is the analytical method of choice routinely utilized for drug confirmation and quantification in the forensic toxicology lab.

References

1. B. Levine, ed.: *Principles of Forensic Toxicology*, AACC Press, 2nd ed., 2003.
2. Skrinska, V. A. and Gock, S. B.: Measurement of 3,4-MDMA and related amines in diagnostic and forensic laboratories. *Clin. Lab. Sci. 18*:119–23, 2005.
3. Pelissier-Alicot, A. L., Gaulier, J. M., Champsaur, P., and Marquet, P.: Mechanisms underlying postmortem redistribution of drugs: A review. *J. Anal. Toxicol. 27*:533–44, 2003.

Case 77

A 43-Year-Old Male with Chronic Pain

Run-Zhang Shi, Susan B. Gock, Jeffrey M. Jentzen, and Steven H. Wong

This is a 43-year-old male who had a medical history of chronic pain related to reflux sympathetic dystrophy and narcotic dependence. On the day of his demise, the decedent drove to a drive-thru prescription center at a major chain store, where he was to pick up a prescription for oxycodone. He never did pick up his medication, and one of the store employees found him unresponsive and slumped over the steering wheel in the store parking lot. An emergency medical team was unable to resuscitate him.

The decedent had a medical history of peripheral neuropathy, reflux sympathetic dystrophy syndrome, anxiety, depression, and panic disorder. There was no suicidal ideation known; however, there was worsening of depression, and the decedent became increasingly withdrawn. He had been taking narcotic painkillers for a very long time and required increasingly higher doses to ease his pain, according to one of his physicians. Information from the pharmacy showed that the decedent had multiple prescriptions filled over the last few months. His long history of chronic pain problems resulted in his taking several narcotic medications simultaneously that were prescribed by different physicians. The decedent was having difficulty lately with his insurance coverage, and this latest prescription would be costly. A 300-pill bottle of methadone was found at his residence that was prescribed 8 days earlier, and only 50 pills remained.

In the 3-month period leading up to his death, the decedent was prescribed multiple medications with alarming quantities (Table 77.1). A large amount of cash (>$1000) was found with the decedent at the scene.

Tietz's Applied Laboratory Medicine, Second Edition. Edited by Mitchell G. Scott, Ann M. Gronowski, and Charles S. Eby
Copyright © 2007 John Wiley & Sons, Inc.

Table 77.1 Prescription and OTC Medication Record

Trade name	Chemical (generic) name	Dose, mg	Amount	Trade name	Chemical name	Dose, mg	Amount
Prilosec	Omeprazole	20	200	Roxicodone	Oxycodone	30	1299
Topamax	Topiramate	25	75	Methadose	Methadone	10	1530
Xanax	Alprazolam	0.5	840	Provigil	Modafinil	200	120
Demerol	Meperidine	50	360	Paxil	Paroxetine	20	30
Roxanol	Morphine	100	1920	Allegra-D	Fexofenadine	—	30
OxyContin	Oxycodone	80	3225	Zithromax	Azithromycin	—	6
Duragesic	Fentanyl	100	20				

Vitreous Humor Electrolytes

Analyte	Value, Conventional Units	Expected Values, Conventional Units	Value, SI Units	Expected Values, SI Units
Na	134 mmol/L	130–155	Same	
K	5.9 mmol/L	(varies with postmortem time)	Same	
Cl	123 mmol/L	105–135	Same	
Glucose	37 mg/dL	<200	2.1 mmol/L	<11.1
Urea nitrogen	10 mg/dL	7–19	3.6 mmol/L	2.5–6.8

Toxicology Result[1]

Analyte	Specimen	Result
Ethyl alcohol	Subclavian (SC) blood	None detected
Carbon monoxide	SC blood	2.5%

Blood Toxicology Screening by GC/MS

Analyte	Specimen	Result
Acidic/neutral drugs	SC blood	None detected
Basic drugs		
Diphenhydramine	SC blood	Positive
Methadone and metabolite (2-ethylidine 1,5-dimethyl-3,3-diphenylpyrrolidine, EDDP)	SC blood	Positive

Liver Toxicology Screening by GC/MS

Analyte	Specimen	Result
Basic drugs		
Diphenhydramine	Tissue	Positive
Methadone and metabolite	Tissue	Positive

Blood Immunoassay Screening

Cocaine metabolite	SC blood	Negative
Opiates	SC blood	Negative
Benzodiazepines	SC blood	Negative
Cannabinoids	SC blood	Negative
Metamphetamine	SC blood	Negative
Fentanyl	SC blood	Negative

Urine Drug Screening by Immunoassay, TLC, GC/MS

Methadone	Urine	Positive
Methadone metabolite (EDDP)	Urine	Positive
Diphenhydramine and metabolite	Urine	Positive
Opiates	Urine	Positive

Gastric Fluid Screening by Immunoassay, TLC, GC/MS

Methadone	Gastric Fluid	Positive

Analyte Quantification

Analyte	Specimen Source	Result	Method
Salicylate	SC[a] blood	None detected	GC/FID[b]
Methadone	SC blood	13.8 mg/L	GC/FID
Methadone (repeat)	SC blood	12.7 mg/L	GC/FID
Methadone	Vitreous humor	1.10 mg/L	GC/FID
Methadone	Bile fluid	13.9 mg/L	GC/FID
Methadone	Liver tissue	82.3 mg/kg	GC/FID
Methadone	Gastric fluid	0.43 mg	GC/FID
Diphenhydramine	SC blood	0.87 mg/L	GC/FID
Diphenhydramine	Liver tissue	5.53 mg/kg	GC/FID
Total morphine	Urine	533 μg/L	GC/MS
Total codeine	Urine	ND	GC/MS
Total morphine	Bile fluid	557 μg/L	GC/MS
Total codeine	Bile fluid	None detected	GC/MS
Methadone	SC blood	7.90 mg/L	GC/MS
EDDP	SC blood	2.90 mg/L	GC/MS
Methadone	Liver tissue	70.0 mg/kg	GC/MS
EDDP	Liver tissue	11.0 mg/kg	GC/MS
Topiramate	SC blood	1.7 mg/L	FPIA[c]

[a]SC—subclavian.

[b]GC/FID—gas chromatography/flame ionization detector.

[c]FPIA—fluorescent polarization immunoassay.

CYP450 2D6 Genotyping

Mutation	Result	Method
CYP450 2D6*3	WT[a]	LC PCR[b]
CYP450 2D6*4	HT[c]	LC PCR
CYP450 2D6*5	WT	LC PCR

[a]Wildtype (WT)—no detectable variant on either allele.

[b]LC PCR—long-chain polymerase chain reaction.

[c]Heterozygous (HT)—variant present on only one of the two alleles.

The Problem

With increasing use of opioids in pain management, opioid abuse, and diversion of pre-scribed drugs to illegitimate use are on the rise. Diversion of these important pain manage-ment medications from medical use to illegal market and abuse is overshadowing their legitimate use. Compared to other forms of substance abuse, prescription drug abuse tends to be a "closet" offense and often is not recognized until overdose mishaps occur or the users begin to exhibit cognitive or functional impairment. This forensic case high-lights the problems associated with prescription opioid abuse.

Nonmedical use and abuse of prescription opioids are on the rise in this country, with the illicit use of several widely prescribed opioids such as methadone and oxycodone increasing disproportionately more than their legal medical use. Although most patients use medications as instructed by their physicians, abuse of and addiction to prescription drugs are public health problems for many Americans. Healthcare providers such as primary care physicians, nurse practitioners, and pharmacists, as well as patients them-selves, can all play a critical role in the prevention and detection of prescription drug abuse.

Discussion of Case Presented Here

This case illustrates opioid drug abuse in a patient and the breakdown of detection and pre-vention mechanisms played in part by physicians and the patient, leading to the patient's death. Possible drug diversion is also suggested by the staggering amount of opioid medi-cations prescribed over a short period of time and the large sum of cash found in the dece-dent's possession.

The toxicology analysis showed a high level of methadone in the decedent's postmor-tem blood samples. In addition, the over-the-counter drug diphenhydramine (benadryl) and other opiates were present, but no street drugs were found. Of note is the fact that the blood immunoassay was negative for opiates despite the high concentration of metha-done in the blood. This is because the immunoassay does not cross-react with methadone. On the other hand, the urine was positive for opiates, due to the presence of conjugated morphine in the patient's urine from some other opioid analgesics that the decedent had in his possession. Considering the history of opioid drug abuse, the final cause of death in this case was determined to be methadone toxicity, with the manner of death deemed accidental.[2]

The decedent's CYP2D6 genotype showed him to be a heterozygote for the *CYP2D6*4* allele, which is a result of substitution mutation of nucleic acid $G > A$ at nucleotide 1846, which results in a splicing defect and no enzymatic activity. Since only one allele was affected, the decedent was categorized as a person with impaired CYP2D6 enzymatic activity. CYP2D6 is important in the metabolism of methadone and oxycodone; therefore, in addition to his obvious abuse of prescription painkillers, his genetic composition may have been a factor in the cause of the toxicity leading to his death.

Pharmacogenetics is the study of the impact of heritable traits on effects and disposi-tion of drugs, which may serve as an adjunct for certifying opioid fatalities. Methadone is frequently prescribed for the relief of moderate to severe pain, in addition to its illicit use as an opioid. Methadone is metabolized to inactive metabolites (EDDP, etc.), primarily by cytochrome P450 (CYP) 3A4, secondarily by CYP2D6, and to a small extent by CYP1A2 enzymes. CYP3A4 is the most abundant drug-metabolizing enzyme in the human body, carrying as much as 30-fold variation in terms of amount and activity. CYP3A4 is encoded by a polymorphic gene with main mutation (*1B) at an allelic frequency of about 5.5%. However, the correlation of mutation of CYP3A4 *1B with enzymatic activity is currently unclear.

On the other hand, the correlation of mutation in the CYP2D6 gene and its enzymatic activity has been established. By detecting mutations of the CYP2D6 gene, it was hypothesized that this methadone fatality may be due partially to poor drug metabolism caused by the nonfunctioning *4 CYP2D6 allele. In this case the decedent's mutation in his CYP2D6 gene reduces his CYP2D6 enzymatic activity 20–80% of wildtype enzymatic activity and is deemed to have impaired metabolism of drugs that are CYP2D6 substrates. Other CYP2D6 alleles that lack enzymatic activity include *3 and *5, while *9, *10, and *17 alleles have decreased activity. Taken together, pharmacogenetics may serve as an adjunct in determination of the cause and manner of death in this case and in investigating other similar deaths.[3,4] For a heterozygote-impaired metabolizer such as the decedent's, not only are parent drugs metabolized at a decreased rate; production of more potent metabolites is decreased as well, leading patients to take more drugs for pain relief. For more discussion of CYP2D6, see Case 73.

In addition to the heterozygote CYP2D6*4 status, the possibility of drug–drug interactions of methadone and other medications is likely in this case, indicated by the large number of comedications the decedent consumed over the time period when methadone was abused (e.g., concomitant use of methadone, alprazolam, and oxycodone). Pharmacotherapy is increasingly complicated by the use of multidrug regimens that may result in clinically important drug interactions. In particular, some drugs are inhibitors of specific CYP enzymes and therefore could inhibit the metabolism of drugs that are substrates of these CYP enzymes, while others may serve as inducers of CYP enzymes in that enzymatic activity is induced over time, resulting in rapid metabolism of substrate drugs. Coadministrated drugs that share the same enzyme pathway for metabolism may compete with each other, resulting in diminished metabolism for one drug.

The illegal diversion of pain management medication may result in significant cost in terms of lives lost, increase in crime, misery associated with addiction, substantial increase of medical cost for society as a whole, and medical fraud, among many others. The roles of primary care physicians, pharmacists, and close relatives as well as patients themselves, need to be evaluated further to formulate better management and prevention strategies.

References

1. LEVINE, B., ed.: *Principles of Forensic Toxicology*, 2nd ed., AACC Press, 2003.
2. DRUMMER, O. H.: Postmortem toxicology of drugs of abuse. *Forens. Sci. Int. 142*:101–13, 2004
3. KREEK, M. J., BART, G., LILLY, C., LAFORGE, K. S., AND NIELSEN, D. A.: Pharmacogenetics and human molecular genetics of opiate and cocaine addictions and their treatments. *Pharmacol. Rev. 57*:1–26, 2005.
4. GARCIA-MARTIN, E., MARTINEZ, C., PIZARRO, R. M. ET AL.: CYP3A4 variant alleles in white individuals with low CYP3A4 enzyme activity. *Clin. Pharmacol. Ther. 71*:196–204, 2002.

Case 78

Metabolic Acidosis of Unknown Origin Among Burn Patients

Deborah Chute and David Bruns

A 33-year-old man was brought to the emergency department after being dragged by fire-fighters from his home during a house fire, where he sustained 56% body surface area second- and third-degree burns. The burns involved primarily his extremities, back, and posterior head. CT scanning showed no evidence of other trauma. He had no significant past medical history, and toxicology testing on admission was negative for alcohol or other drugs. Initial laboratory tests, including a chemistry panel, CBC, and urinalysis were normal. Aggressive fluid resuscitation was instituted, and he was admitted to the burn unit for specialized care.

On day 9 in the burn unit, he was noted to have decreased responsiveness with confusion and lethargy. On physical examination, his chest and heart were normal. His abdomen was normal, and by report his bowels were moving normally. Skin examination showed extensive burn injuries with recent debridement, and no evidence of infection. Intact skin showed good tissue perfusion. A Foley catheter was in place and showed minimal dark brown urine. His medications included topical antibacterial cream for his burns (Furacin Soluble Dressing), Colace, morphine, and IV ranitidine.

Laboratory tests included a chemistry panel, serum osmolality, and ABG; urinalysis showed granular casts, few red blood cells, no ketones, no bacteria, and no crystals:

Analyte	Value, Conventional Units	Reference Interval, Conventional Units	Value, SI Units	Reference Interval, SI Units
Sodium	148 mmol/L	135–148	Same	Same
Potassium	4.1 mmol/L	3.5–5.0	Same	Same
Chloride	85 mmol/L	95–107	Same	Same
CO_2, total	6 mmol/L	21–31	Same	Same
Blood urea nitrogen	89 mg/dL	7–18	32 mmol/L	2.5–6.4
Creatinine	6.9 mg/dL	0.7–1.4	610 µmol/L	6–120
Glucose	108 mg/dL	70–105	6.0 mmol/L	3.9–5.8
Calcium (total)	15.1 mg/dL	8.4–10.5	3.78 mmol/L	2.1–2.63
Ionized calcium	4.2 mg/dL	4–5	1.05 mmol/L	1.0–1.25

Tietz's Applied Laboratory Medicine, Second Edition. Edited by Mitchell G. Scott, Ann M. Gronowski, and Charles S. Eby
Copyright © 2007 John Wiley & Sons, Inc.

Analyte	Value, Conventional Units	Reference Interval, Conventional Units	Value, SI Units	Reference Interval, SI Units
Calculated AG	57 mmol/L	10–14	Same	Same
Measured osmolality	355 mOsmol/kg	280–300	Same	Same
Calculated osmolality	334 mOsmol/kg	280–300	Same	Same
Osmolal gap	21 mOsmol/kg	± 13	Same	Same
pH	7.26	7.35–7.45		

The findings of severe acidemia and an elevated anion gap suggested the presence of a high-anion-gap metabolic acidosis. Further testing demonstrated that serum lactate and ketones were within the reference interval. The renal failure and the high osmolal gap led to consideration of a toxic exposure. Testing for ethylene glycol, methanol, and ethanol revealed a low concentration of ethylene glycol:

Ethylene glycol	1.3	mmol/L
Methanol	0	mmol/L
Ethanol	0	mmol/L

Despite therapy with bicarbonate and dialysis, the patient became progressively obtunded and acidotic, developed multisystem organ failure, and died on day 12. Autopsy demonstrated acute tubular necrosis of the proximal tubules of the kidney, suggesting a toxic injury.

During the next few months, 8 additional burn unit patients showed a similar constellation of findings, including high-anion-gap metabolic acidosis, serum osmolal gap elevation, renal failure, and elevated total serum calcium; two of them died. On review, the only factor in common for all patients was presence in the burn unit and use of the antimicrobial burn cream Furacin Soluble Dressing (FSD).

Analysis of the contents of FSD showed that it contained 99.8% polyethylene glycol (63% PEG-300, 32% PEG-4000, and 5% PEG-1000) and trace amounts (approximately 0.01%) of ethylene glycol, in addition to nitrofurazone (0.2%), the active ingredient. Retrospective analysis of the three deceased burn patients' urine and serum by tandem mass spectrometry demonstrated diacid and hydroxyl acid metabolites of polyethylene glycol. Demonstration of toxicity of polyethylene glycol in an animal model for open-wound toxicity led to an FDA warning and additional studies on the toxicity of polyethylene glycol.

Definition of Disease

Toxic alcohol exposures include intoxication with methanol, ethylene glycol, and isopropanol. Intoxication by polyethylene glycol (PEG) through skin burns was not previously reported before this case series in 1982, but PEG could be considered a toxic alcohol. Toxic exposure due to ethylene glycol (1,2-ethanediol) is unfortunately a common cause of high-anion-gap metabolic acidosis, and shows similar features to this case. Ethylene glycol's molecular structure is similar to that of ethanol (Fig. 78.1). While ethylene glycol is not toxic in itself, it is metabolized by alcohol dehydrogenase (ADH) and aldehyde dehydrogenase (ADHG) in the liver to glycolic acid, oxalic acid, and formic acid, which are toxic to the kidney and cause a severe metabolic acidosis.

HOCH$_2$—CH$_2$OH   CH$_3$CH$_2$OH   HOCH$_2$-(CH$_2$—O—CH$_2$)$_n$-CH$_2$OH

(Ethylene glycol)   (Ethanol)   (Polyethylene glycol)

$\downarrow$ ADH

HOCH$_2$CHO

(Glyoxal)

$\downarrow$ ADHG

HOCH$_2$—COOH $\rightarrow$ OCH—COOH $\rightarrow$ 2 HCOOH

(Glycolic acid)   (Glyoxilic acid)   (Formic acid)

$\downarrow$

HOOC—COOH

(Oxalic acid)

Figure 78.1 Pathway leading to metabolic acidosis in ethylene glycol poisoning.

Direct measurement of ethylene glycol in the serum requires gas chromatography or high-performance liquid chromatography and is not routinely available in most institutions. In these instances, rapid laboratory diagnosis of ethylene glycol intoxication includes calculation of the serum osmolal and anion gaps.

The osmolal gap is important in the diagnosis of ethylene glycol toxicity as it can be used as a surrogate marker for the serum concentrations. The osmolal gap is the difference between the calculated serum osmolality and the measured osmolality. Osmolality is calculated by one of several equations, one of which is (in SI units)

$$\text{Calculated osmolality} = 2\text{Na}^+ + [\text{glucose mmol/L}] + [\text{BUN mmol/L}] + [\text{ethanol mmol/L}]$$

or in conventional units:

$$\text{Calculated osmolality} = 2\text{Na}^+ + \frac{[\text{glucose mg/dL}]}{18} + \frac{[\text{BUN mg/dL}]}{2.8} + \frac{[\text{ethanol mg/dL}]}{4.3}$$

It is important to remember that the measurement of osmolality must be performed by freezing-point depression, as those techniques that use boiling-point elevation will also volatilize the toxic alcohols and give a falsely low serum osmolality. Once the osmolal gap is determined, the serum ethylene glycol concentration can be estimated by multiplying the osmolal gap by a conversion factor of 5 (methanol conversion = 2.6, isopropyl alcohol conversion = 5.9).

The anion gap is also useful as supportive evidence for toxic alcohol exposures, particularly ethylene glycol and methanol. It is the difference between serum anions and cations that are commonly measured (sodium, chloride, and bicarbonate):

$$\text{Anion gap} = \text{Na}^+ - (\text{Cl}^- + \text{HCO}_3^-)$$

Some prefer to add the concentration of potassium to that of sodium; in that case, the reference interval is increased. An increased anion gap is suggestive of a metabolic acidosis with an excess of unmeasured anions, which in the case of ethylene glycol toxicity are the glycolic acid and formic acid anions.

Differential Diagnosis of Metabolic Acidoses

Metabolic acidosis can be caused by a variety of processes and is produced by three major mechanisms: increased acid generation, loss of bicarbonate, and diminished acid excretion. In health, the anion gap largely reflects the negative charges on albumin and other plasma proteins. However, a fall in unmeasured cations or an increase in unmeasured anions will increase the anion gap. Depending on the mechanism underlying the acidosis, the anion gap can be normal or elevated in a metabolic acidosis.

In normal anion gap metabolic acidosis (also known as *hyperchloremic metabolic acidosis*), the loss of bicarbonate is equal to the increase in serum chloride concentration. The most common causes of this type of metabolic acidosis are diarrhea, early renal failure, hypoaldosteronism, and renal tubular acidosis. Other less common causes include carbonic anhydrase inhibitor use and ureteral diversion surgery.

In increased anion gap metabolic acidosis, there is typically an increase in unmeasured anions related to the acid that produces H^+, causing the acidemia. The most common causes of increased anion gap metabolic acidosis are lactic acidosis, ketoacidosis (due to diabetes mellitus, starvation, or alcohol) and chronic renal failure. Ingestions of toxic substances are less common causes, but important differential diagnostic considerations. Aspirin and toxic alcohols, including methanol and ethylene glycol, are the most common culprits. Isopropanol, while considered a toxic alcohol, does not increase the anion gap, but will increase the osmolal gap.

Increase of the serum osmolality, with an increased osmolal gap, is seen when there is an increase in solutes not typically measured in the serum. Common causes of an increased osmolal gap include ketoacidosis, lactic acidosis, and chronic renal failure. Less common causes include toxic alcohol ingestion, formaldehyde/paraldehyde ingestion, mannitol use, and severe hyperproteinemia/hyperlipidemia.

The combination of acidosis with elevated anion and osmolal gaps leads to a differential diagnosis of ketoacidosis, lactic acidosis, chronic renal failure, toxic alcohol ingestion, salicylate ingestion, and formaldehyde/paraldehyde ingestion. In this case, the absence of urine ketones or serum lactate, and a history of prior normal renal function, led the laboratory physicians to consider the diagnosis of toxic alcohol intoxication.

The differential diagnosis of toxic alcohol intoxication includes ethylene glycol, methanol, and isopropyl alcohol, although as this case demonstrates, unusual toxic exposures may show similar findings. Discrimination between these is facilitated by knowledge of any recent exposures and the clinical signs and symptoms of the patient. However, confirmation by laboratory testing is important for diagnosis and treatment decisions.

Ethylene glycol is commonly present in antifreeze and de-icing substances. As described above, its toxicity is related primarily to the toxic metabolites glyoxilic acid, oxalic acid, and formic acid. A high-anion-gap metabolic acidosis, an elevated osmolal gap, renal failure, and urine calcium oxalate crystals characterize toxicity due to ethylene glycol. In addition, many antifreezes contain a fluorescent dye, which is excreted in the urine, and will cause fluorescence of the urine under Wood lamp examination. Of note, elevation of the osmolal gap can be absent, due to the higher molecular weight of ethylene glycol and rapid turnover to toxic metabolites, and should not preclude this diagnosis.

Methanol is commonly found in antifreeze and glass cleaners. Methanol toxicity is mediated primarily by formic acid, its primary metabolite. Methanol ingestion leads to a high-anion-gap metabolic acidosis with an elevated osmolal gap and renal failure. It does not typically produce oxalate crystals in the urine.

Isopropyl alcohol is prevalent in rubbing alcohol and hair products. Toxicity is due to itself and its primary metabolite acetone. Isopropyl alcohol ingestion typically causes an elevation of the osmolal gap without metabolic acidosis, and is accompanied by elevations in serum acetone levels.

An interesting finding in this case was an elevation in total serum calcium, with decreased ionized calcium. Ethylene glycol and methanol intoxication typically cause hypocalcemia, and monitoring of this electrolyte is important to prevent cardiac arrhythmia. In health, approximately 40% of calcium is protein-bound, 10% is bound to organic and inorganic anions, and the remaining 45% is the physiologically active free calcium. In this case, the two alcohol groups of polyethylene glycol were metabolized to carboxylic acids, thus producing diacid metabolites. The diacid metabolites of low-molecular-weight PEGs are known binders of calcium that have been used as phosphate substitutes in detergents. Binding of calcium by these metabolites in plasma decreased free calcium, which led to increased secretion of parathyroid hormone and mobilization of calcium from bone, and, thus, increased total serum calcium. As the physiologically active free calcium was decreased, monitoring of this fraction was necessary to prevent cardiac arrhythmia.

While this case is unusual, it emphasizes the need to maintain a broad differential and think chemically when dealing with difficult cases and to be vigilant for unusual discrepancies and to follow these up with appropriate testing. The first cases were investigated in 1982 by a clinical pathology resident and one of the authors (DB).

Treatment

Treatment of toxic alcohol exposures, particularly methanol and ethylene glycol poisoning, is directed primarily to prevent the formation of the toxic metabolites. Since alcohol dehydrogenase is the rate-limiting step in this metabolism, classically, intravenous ethanol administration has been used to overwhelm ADH and thus prevent accumulation of toxic metabolites. This therapy is more complex than might be imagined, requiring a rapid infusion of ethanol followed by a continuous infusion to maintain a therapeutic plasma ethanol concentration. A pitfall is administration of a maintenance infusion without an initial "bolus." This will lead to a complaint that the laboratory assay for ethanol cannot detect ethanol as, indeed, a maintenance infusion rate is enough just to balance the rate at which the liver metabolizes ethanol. Blood or plasma ethanol will remain far below the therapeutic target range. Recently the FDA approved a medication, fomepizole [4-methylpyrazole (4MP)], which is a competitive antagonist of ADH and does not cause sedation, respiratory depression, and hypoglycemia seen with ethanol administration. Moreover, a single dose can be given while investigations are under way in suspicious cases, a feature that proves especially handy when treating patients in outlying hospitals without facilities for toxicological investigations.

Additional treatment should include aggressive fluid replacement to maintain urine output and prevent crystal deposition in the kidney tubules, bicarbonate to treat acidosis, cofactor repletion (folic acid, pyridoxine, and thiamine), and dialysis in severe cases to enhance clearance of the parent molecules and toxic metabolites.

References

1. Bruns, D. E., Herold, D. A., Rodeheaver, G. T., and Edlich, R. F.: Polyethylene glycol intoxication in burn patients. *Burns* 9:49–52, 1982.

2. Church, A. S. and Whitting, M. D.: Laboratory testing in ethanol, methanol, ethylene glycol, and isopropanol toxicities. *J. Emerg. Med. 15*:687–92, 1997.

Part Eighteen

Lipid Disorders

Cases of coronary heart disease (CHD), Tangier disease, abetalipoproteinemia, and sitosterolem are presented and discussed in Cases 79, 80, 81, and 82, respectively (all edited by MGS).

Tietz's Applied Laboratory Medicine, Second Edition. Edited by Mitchell G. Scott, Ann M. Gronowski, and Charles S. Eby
Copyright © 2007 John Wiley & Sons, Inc.

Case 79

The Family Reunion Party

Veronica Luzzi

A 59-year-old woman presented to the emergency department with a 10-hour history of chest pain, nausea, and headache. The pain initiated after a family reunion party and persisted into the evening even after rest. Initially, the patient thought the symptoms were due to the large meal and late hours of the party. The medical history revealed hypertension, type II diabetes, and 30 years of smoking. The patient was not taking any medications at the time except for aspirin and a "medicinal" herbal tea.

The patient's vital signs showed a blood pressure of 190/125 mm Hg, a pulse of 90 beats/min, a respiratory rate of 22 breaths/min, and a normal body temperature. The patient weighed 220 lb (100 kg) and was 5 ft 3 in. in height. An electrocardiogram revealed characteristic changes consistent with myocardial infarction showing an elevated ST segment. The patient was immediately taken to the catheterization laboratory. The catheterization procedure showed a partial occlusion of the left coronary artery. A coronary angioplasty was performed.

Laboratory tests on admission included TnI, routine chemistries, and lipids. Results of these tests are shown below:

Analyte	Value, Conventional Units	Reference Interval, Conventional Units	Value, SI Units	Reference Interval, SI Units
TnI	15 ng/mL	0.0–0.2	15 µg/L	<0.2 µg/L
Sodium	137 mmol/L	135–145	Same	
Potassium, plasma	4.1 mmol/L	3.3–4.9	Same	
Chloride	102 mmol/L	97–110	Same	
Carbon dioxide	28 mmol/L	22–32	Same	
Anion gap	7 mmol/L	0–16	Same	
Glucose	112 mg/dL	65–199	Same	
Urea nitrogen	3 mg/dL	8–25	1.1 mmol/L	2.9–8.9
Creatinine	0.8 mg/dL	0.7–1.5	70.7 µmol/L	62–133
Calcium	8.8 mg/dL	8.6–10.3	2.2 mmol/L	2.2–2.6
Plasma protein	5.9 g/dL	6.5–8.5	59 g/L	65–85
Albumin	3.0 g/dL	3.6–5.0	30 g/L	36–50
Bilirubin	1.2 mg/dL	0.3–1.1	20.5 µmol/L	5.1–18.8
Alkaline phosphatase	132 IU/L	38–126	2.2 µkat/L	0.6–2.1

Tietz's Applied Laboratory Medicine, Second Edition. Edited by Mitchell G. Scott, Ann M. Gronowski, and Charles S. Eby
Copyright © 2007 John Wiley & Sons, Inc.

Analyte	Value, Conventional Units	Reference Interval, Conventional Units	Value, SI Units	Reference Interval, SI Units
Aspartate transaminase (AST, SGOT)	30 IU/L	11–47	0.5 μkat/L	0.19–0.80
Alanine transaminase (ALT, SGPT)	23 IU/L	7–53	0.4 μkat/L	0.12–0.90
Triglycerides	187 mg/dL	0–199	4.8 mmol/L	0–5.2
Cholesterol	306 mg/dL	0–199	7.9 mmol/L	0–5.2
HDL cholesterol	40 mg/dL	40–199	1.0 mmol/L	1.0–5.2
LDL cholesterol	229 mg/dL	0–129	5.9 mmol/L	0–3.3

The patient was discharged after 4 days of hospitalization. Her 10-year risk of recurring coronary heart disease (CHD) according to the Framingham point score was calculated to be 27%. Based on this observation, the patient was instructed to follow therapeutic changes in lifestyle and diet, and was prescribed atorvastatin, niacin, clofibrate, and an angiotensin-converting enzyme (ACE) inhibitor. The patient was asked to schedule a follow-up visit with her cardiologist in 1 month.

Definition of the Disease

Coronary heart disease is the number one cause of death in men and women in the United States. This disorder is characterized by the hardening and narrowing of the lumen of the coronary arteries and the development of unstable plaques in the arterial endothelium.[1] As a consequence of plaque rupture and occlusion of these arteries, there is a decrease of blood flow to the heart (see also Case 1). The symptoms associated with CHD can vary according with the severity of the obstruction of blood flow to cardiac muscle. In the initial stages of CHD there are no symptoms. As the disease progresses, chest pain or angina pectoris may be present. In the early stages of CHD, the angina consists of chest pressure with mild burning, heaviness, and shortness of breath on exertion. As the disease progresses, the severity of these symptoms will increase and even occur at rest, indicating the presence of unstable angina. Myocardial infarction may occur with or without being preceded by unstable angina (see also Case 1).

Differential Diagnosis

The differential diagnosis of CHD is often performed in the emergency department. Dyspnea, one of the most common symptoms of CHD, is also present in other disorders.[2] Among disorders to be considered and ruled out in the differential diagnosis of CHD are congestive heart failure, cardiomyopathy, arrhythmias, asthma, trauma, metabolic conditions, and chronic obstructive pulmonary disease. Physical examination and patient history are often the first clue in the differential diagnosis. However, clinicians often use the electrocardiogram, chest radiographs, and laboratory tests to aid in identifying the cause of the dyspnea.

The electrocardiogram can show abnormal cardiac electrical patterns, heart rate and rhythms, or evidence of ischemia, injury, or infarction. Chest radiographs may reveal pulmonary obstruction, edema, or trauma. Cardiac-specific biomarkers, such as cardiac troponin I, are the mainstay of diagnosing MI, and negative serial troponin I values can be used to rule out MI (see Cases 1 and 2), while a negative B-type natriuretic peptide result can be used to help rule out congestive heart failure.

Pathogenesis

CHD is the result of a variety of interacting factors that lead to the formation of an unstable atherosclerotic plaque in the coronary artery endothelium. These include age, hypercholesterolemia, smoking, hypertension, and diabetes, among many others. Although atherosclerotic plaques have been found in children as young as 3 years of age, CHD is most prevalent in the adult population[3] (also see Case 1). The risk of CHD has been directly correlated with increased serum cholesterol concentrations. Because of their role in cholesterol transport, low-density lipoprotein (LDL) and high-density lipoprotein (HDL) play a pivotal role in the pathogenesis of this disease. LDL is responsible for transporting cholesterol to the peripheral tissues. An increase in the LDL cholesterol correlates with increased plaque formation in the endothelial wall. As HDL transports cholesterol from the peripheral tissues to the liver, it has the opposite effect of LDL, and higher concentrations of HDL negatively correlate with the risk of CHD. Cigarette smoking is considered a risk factor for CHD because it promotes LDL oxidation and enhances platelet activation. Both of these events have been found to promote plaque disruption. Hypertension is another factor that causes a disruption in the atherosclerotic plaque. Angiotensin II activates inflammatory molecules that in turn will disrupt the homeostasis in the endothelial wall. In diabetes, glycated macromolecules can promote oxidative stress in the endothelial wall and increase the production of inflammatory molecules.

Treatment and Prevention

An estimated 1.2 million new or recurrent MI were reported in the United States in 2004. The most common treatments for existing CHD and for prevention of CHD consist of elimination of the factors contributing to the pathogenesis. Thus, decreasing blood pressure, improving glycemic control, antiplatelet therapy with aspirin and/or clopidogrel, lifestyle changes, such as quitting smoking and losing weight, are all part of the arsenal to treat and prevent, CHD. In acute settings or when evidence of significant coronary artery blockage is present, invasive treatments include coronary artery bypass surgery and interventional catherization and stent placement. However, such treatments are expensive and carry significant risk. The goal of treatment is to minimize risk and prevent the occurrence of acute events.

One of the most visible treatment and prevention strategies for CHD has targeted decreasing high blood cholesterol and LDL-C. The National Cholesterol Education Program (NECP) Expert Panel in Detection, Evaluation, and Treatment of High Blood Cholesterol in Adults published their third report (ATP III) in 2001.[4] This report constitutes the guidelines for cholesterol testing and CHD risk management and is the third in a series that identifies LDL cholesterol as the primary target for therapy. The most common approach for lowering LDL is the use of 3-hydroxy-3-methylglutaryl coenzyme A (HMGCoA) inhibitors (statins), but other therapies include bile acid sequestrants, nicotinic acid, fibric acid, and diet. The LDL-lowering therapy is tailored according to the patient's overall risk of CHD. Assessment of the overall risk for CHD is the first step in patient management. In individuals without current CHD, the number of risk factors present should be determined and the 10-year risk of CHD calculated using the Framingham scoring system.[5] The Framingham scoring system assigns points according to the risk factors present in a patient, and these points are added up to determine a final 10-year risk. The risk factors included in this assessment are cigarette smoking, hypertension (systolic >140 mm Hg), HDL cholesterol <40 mg/dL (1.0 mmol/L), diabetes, family history of premature CHD, and age. Reflecting its protective nature, a concentration of HDL >60 mg/dL (1.6 mmol/L) subtracts one point from the risk score.

There are three risk categories: (1) current CHD or CHD risk equivalent score giving a 10-year risk greater than 20%, (2) two or more risk factors but with a 10-year risk lower than 20%, and (3) one to two risk factors. The LDL goal, the need for therapeutic life changes, and the concentration of the drug used in the therapy will depend on the risk category for each patient. The LDL goal in the 2001 ATP III report for risk categories 1, 2, and 3 were <100, <130, and <160 mg/dL (2.6, 3.4, and 3.9 mmol/L), respectively.[4]

In order to assess this risk, the laboratory must measure LDL cholesterol, total cholesterol, and HDL cholesterol. The reference method to obtain LDL cholesterol values is the β-quantification. In this procedure, β-lipoproteins [LDL, IDL, and Lp(a)] are separated from the non-β (VLDL and HDL) by combining ultracentrifugation at 105,000g at plasma density ($d = 1.006$ kg/L) for 18 hours at 10°C and heparin sulfate precipitation. After ultracentrifugation, VLDL is found in the top of the tube and is removed with a tube slicer. The bottom fraction contains HDL, LDL, IDL, and Lp(a) particles, and heparin sulfate is used to precipitate LDL, IDL, and Lp(a) away from HDL in an aliquot of the bottom fraction. Cholesterol is then measured using the Abell–Kendall method in an untreated aliquot to determine total cholesterol, in the bottom fractionated aliquot to measure HDL, LDL, and IDL, and in the bottom heparin–sulfate fractionated aliquot to measure HDL. In the Abell–Kendall method cholesterol is hydrolyzed, extracted with hexane, and treated with the Liebermann–Burchard reagent to produce a colored product that can be detected at 620 nm. LDL cholesterol is calculated by subtracting the HDL cholesterol from the cholesterol measured in the untreated bottom fraction. Newer direct homogeneous cholesterol methods that use a variety of physicochemical lipoprotein properties to separate the LDL from the non-LDL fraction are currently available (Roche Diagnostics, Genzyme Diagnostics, Equal Diagnostics, etc.). The NCEP expert panel requires manufacturers of these homogeneous cholesterol assays to consistently demonstrate cholesterol concentration values within 3% of the reference method for use in determining the risks for CHD.[6] In addition, clinical laboratories can participate in the Lipid Standardization Programs (LSP) such as the one directed by the Centers for Disease Control and Prevention to periodically compare their cholesterol values with the reference method. If the method used to measure cholesterol deviates by >3% from the reference method, errors in the calculation of future risk may alter the treatments chosen for a given patient.

Since mid-1990s large clinical endpoint studies using various HMG-CoA reductase inhibitors ("statins") demonstrated a reduction in the relative risk of myocardial infarction and/or CHD death by 23–37% in primary and secondary prevention, respectively. Statins lower LDL cholesterol by inhibiting HMG-CoA reductase and are the most widely LDL-lowering drug used. Newer evidence is also being gathered to determine whether statins may also aid in reduction of inflammation. The JUPITER clinical trial (*justification for the use of statins in primary prevention: an intervention trial evaluating rosuvastatin*) is assessing whether statin therapy should be given to low-risk individuals who present with high concentrations of inflammatory markers such as high-sensitivity C-reactive protein.[7]

Other drugs that affect lipoprotein metabolism are bile acid sequestrants, nicotinic acid, and fibric acids. All of these drugs reduce high LDL cholesterol by varying amounts, and have the additional benefit of increasing HDL cholesterol. Unfortunately, statins and any of the combination therapy have several side effects and contraindications. Common side effects are myopathy, gastrointestinal distress, flushing, and hyperglycemia. Chronic liver disease and peptic ulcer are some of the contraindications.

More recent randomized clinical control trials have confirmed the treatment algorithm from the ATP III expert panel and introduce additional guidelines for high- and moderate-risk patients.[8] The LDL cholesterol goal for very high-risk patients has recently been changed to <70 mg/dL. If triglycerides are high and HDL is low, fibrate or nicotinic acid should be added to the LDL-lowering therapy. The therapy should be tailored to achieve a 30–40% reduction in LDL cholesterol. In addition, individuals with obesity, physical inactivity, elevated triglycerides, low HDL cholesterol, or metabolic syndrome should be advised to follow a therapeutic life change regardless of their LDL-cholesterol concentrations.

References

1. RIFAI, N., WARNICK, G. R., AND DOMINICZAK, M. H., eds.: *Handbook of Lipoprotein Testing*, 2nd ed., AACC Press, Washington, DC, 2000.

2. MAHLER, D. A., ed.: *Dyspnea*. Futura Publishing, Mount Kisco, NY, 1990.

3. ZAMAN, A. G., HELFT, G., WORTHLEY, S. G., AND BADIMON, J. J.: The role of plaque rupture and thrombosis in coronary artery disease. *Atherosclerosis 149*:251–66, 2000.

4. Expert Panel in Detection, Evaluation, and Treatment of High Blood Cholesterol in Adults: Executive Summary of the Third Report of the National Cholesterol Education Program. *JAMA 285*:2486–97, 2001.

5. WILSON, P. W. F., GARRISON, R. J., ABBOTT, R. D., AND CASTELLI, W. P.: Factors associated with lipoprotein cholesterol levels: The Framingham Study. *Arteriosclerosis 3*:273–81, 1983.

6. NIH: *Recommendations on Lipoprotein Measurement from the Working Group on Lipoprotein Measurement*, National Institutes of Health Publication 95–3044, U.S. Government Printing Office, Washington, DC, 1995, p. 186.

7. MORA, S. AND RIDKER, P. M.: Justification for the use of statins in primary prevention: An intervention trial evaluating rosuvastatin (JUPITER)—can C-reactive protein be used to target statin therapy in primary prevention? *Am. J. Cardiol. 97*:33A–41A, 2006.

8. GRUNDY, S. ET AL: Implications of recent clinical trials for the National Cholesterol Education Program Adult Treatment Panel III guidelines. *Circulation 110*:227–39, 2004.

Case 80

A 5-Year-Old Boy with Yellow-Orange Tonsils: Hypoalphalipoproteinemia

Raffick A. R. Bowen and Alan T. Remaley

A 5-year-old boy presented with a history of chronic tonsillitis, which was treated by tonsillectomy. During gross inspection of the resected tonsils, it was noted that they did not have the normal appearance of inflamed tonsils. They were enlarged but were yellow-orange in color. Histologic examination revealed the presence of many macrophages, which contained numerous small intracellular droplets that stained positive for neutral lipids.

On physical examination, the patient was observed to have mild hepatosplenomegaly, but otherwise was apparently healthy with normal growth and development. Interestingly, an examination of the patient's 4-year-old sister showed that she also had abnormally enlarged yellow-orange tonsils.

Routine laboratory tests were all within normal limits except for the complete blood count and serum lipoproteins. The patient had normal red blood cell and leukocyte counts, but numerous "target" red blood cells were observed by a microscopic examination of the blood smear. The following are the results of a lipoprotein analysis on fasting serum:

Analyte	Value, Conventional Units	Reference Interval, Conventional Units	Value, SI Units	Reference Interval, SI Units
Cholesterol, total	70 mg/dL	108–187	1.81 mmol/L	2.8–4.8
HDL-C	1 mg/dL	35–82	0.025 mmol/L	0.91–2.12
Trigylcerides	180 mg/dL	32–116	2.02 mmol/L	0.36–1.31
ApoA-I	<5 mg/dL	104–167	<1.04 g/L	1.04–1.67
ApoB	62 mg/dL	51–80	6.2 g/L	6.2–8.0
LDL-C	70 mg/dL	38–140	1.81 mmol/L	0.98–3.62

Tietz's Applied Laboratory Medicine, Second Edition. Edited by Mitchell G. Scott, Ann M. Gronowski, and Charles S. Eby
Copyright © 2007 John Wiley & Sons, Inc.

Although there were several abnormalities on the lipoprotein analysis, the most remarkable finding was the very low total cholesterol and the near absence of HDL (HDL-C) and apolipoprotein A-I (apoA-I), the main protein component of HDL. An analysis of the patient's younger sibling also revealed a very low HDL-C value of 3 mg/dL. In addition, both parents, who were distantly related, had about half the normal serum concentration of HDL-C. A skin biopsy was performed on the patient, and a primary culture of skin fibroblasts was established. A cholesterol efflux assay was performed on the cells, and they were found to be completely defective in effluxing cholesterol to apoA-I added to the cell culture media, thus establishing the diagnosis of Tangier disease.

Definition of the Disease

Tangier disease is a rare autosomal recessive disorder of HDL metabolism that was first described in 1961 from patients who resided on Tangier Island, a small island in the Chesapeake Bay.[1] The main biochemical feature of Tangier diseases is a marked decrease in HDL-C and apoA-I. Enlarged yellow-orange tonsils is a clinical hallmark for the disease and is due to accumulation of cholesteryl esters in various cell types.[2] The main cell affected in Tangier disease is macrophages. Organs and tissues rich in macrophages, such as the tonsils, liver, spleen, and lymph nodes, are, therefore, often enlarged because of the intracellular accumulation of cholesteryl esters in macrophages. Similarly, macrophages in the vascular wall also accumulate excess cholesterol, which accounts for the main clinical sequel of Tangier disease, namely, coronary artery disease. Excess lipid accumulation in other cell types and organs accounts for the other manifestations of Tangier disease. For example, adult Tangier patients often develop peripheral neuropathy, most likely because of lipid accumulation in Schwann cells.

The other laboratory abnormality observed in this case was the presence of numerous target cells on the blood smear. Red blood cells rapidly exchange cholesterol in their plasma membranes with lipoproteins, and when there is an abnormal level of plasma lipoproteins, red cells can form abnormal cell shapes because of an imbalance between the membrane lipid content and intracellular hemoglobin content. Splenomegaly, which also develops in Tangier disease patients from lipid accumulation, can also alter red cell shape and can cause thrombocytopenia.

There are several different genetic disorders and various conditions (see discussion below) that can cause hypoalphalipoproteinemia, which is the general term for low HDL-C. As in the case presented above, the diagnosis of Tangier disease can be made by measuring the ability of fibroblasts to give up, or efflux, cholesterol to apoA-I. Because most peripheral cells cannot catabolize cholesterol, they maintain their homeostasis by the reverse cholesterol transport pathway, the pathway; in which excess cholesterol is transported by HDL to the liver for excretion in the bile. The first step in this pathway is the efflux of cholesterol onto extracellular apoA-I, which results in the formation of nascent HDL. Approximately half of the effluxed cholesterol is transported back to the liver directly on HDL, and the other half is returned to the liver after first being transferred from HDL by cholesterol ester transfer protein (CETP) to LDL, which is taken up by hepatic LDL receptors.

The genetic defect in Tangier disease is caused by mutations in the ABCA1 transporter. The ABCA1 transporter is a member of a large family of ATP-binding cassette (ABC) transporters, which transfer a wide variety of ligands across membranes in an

ATP-dependent manner.[3] The exact substrate for the ABCA1 transporter is not known, but it facilitates the first step in the reverse cholesterol transport pathway by promoting the efflux of cholesterol and phospholipid to lipid-free or lipid-poor apoA-I in the extracellular space.[4] Macrophages are apparently heavily dependent on this pathway and will readily accumulate excess cholesterol in the absence of the ABCA1 transporter. In addition to cholesterol, other lipophilic substances, such as the chromogenic carotenoids and retinyl esters, also accumulate in cells with a defective ABCA1 transporter, which accounts for the yellow-orange color of the affected tissues in Tangier disease.

The other consequence of defective ABCA1 transport is that it alters the level of various serum lipoproteins and apolipoproteins. ApoA-I is particularly affected because the lipidation of apoA-I by the ABCA1 transporter delays its catabolism. ApoA-I is relatively small in size, less than 28 kDa, and is readily filtered by the kidney, unless it acquires lipid from cells via the ABCA1 transporter. HDL-C is decreased simply because of the lack of apoA-I and the decreased formation of nascent HDL by the ABCA1 transporter. Patients with Tangier disease frequently have modestly decreased total cholesterol and LDL-C. This occurs because normally a large proportion of the cholesterol on LDL is from the CETP-mediated transfer from HDL. One potential beneficial consequence of the low LDL-C is that it most likely ameliorates the risk for coronary artery disease in these patients. Serum triglycerides are also often indirectly altered in Tangier disease patients. The level of triglyceride, however, is highly variable and can range from normal to moderately elevated, possibly due to decreased lipolysis by lipoprotein lipase from reduced levels of apoC-II, the main lipoprotein lipase activator.

Differential Diagnosis

It is important in the differential diagnosis of hypoalphalipoproteinemia and in the management of patients with low HDL-C to distinguish between rare cases with a profound decrease in HDL-C (<10 mg/dL) from more common cases, in which there is only a modest decrease in HDL-C. Patients with a marked reduction in HDL-C such as the one presented here often have a genetic disorder in HDL metabolism, whereas patients with only a modest HDL-C decrease often have elevated serum triglycerides and/or other secondary causes for low HDL.

The primary genetic causes of hypoalphalipoproteinemia besides Tangier disease include deletions and or mutations in the apo-AI gene and lecithin:cholesterol–acyltransferase (LCAT) deficiency. Because apoA-I is the main structural protein on HDL, deletions or structural defects in the apoA-I gene often affect the level of HDL. Familial apolipoprotein AI deficiency is due to deletion of the apoA-I gene, and these patients have no detectable apoA-I. These patients also typically have corneal opacities due to lipid accumulation and may have cutaneous or planar xanthomas. Like Tangier disease patients, they are at an increased risk of developing premature coronary atherosclerosis, but typically develop more severe atherosclerosis and at an earlier age. In addition to gene deletions, many point mutations in apo-AI have been described that alter the structure of apoA-I, leading to increased catabolism and low HDL-C. Some forms of apoA-I mutants will spontaneously self-aggregate and can cause systemic amyloidosis.

LCAT plays a key role in HDL metabolism by converting free cholesterol on HDL to cholesteryl esters, which promotes reverse cholesterol transport by trapping on HDL any cholesterol that has effluxed from cells. Patients homozygous for LCAT deficiency have low HDL-C and develop corneal opacities from lipid accumulation but do not appear to have a significantly increased risk for coronary artery disease. Because of the decreased content of cholesteryl esters in lipoproteins, they do form abnormal-shaped lipoproteins, which accumulate in the glomerulus, causing renal insufficiency. Heterozygous patients with only a partial deficiency of LCAT, which is sometimes called "Fish-eye disease," usually just have corneal opacities and only have a modest decrease in HDL-C.

There are many secondary causes of hypoalphalipoproteinemia, such as obesity, sedentary lifestyle, cigarette use, and low-fat diets. Low HDL-C is also often associated with diabetes, end-stage renal disease, and uremia. Hypertriglyceridemia from almost any cause also lowers HDL, due to the enrichment of triglycerides on HDL, which alters the physical properties of HDL and leads to its increased catabolism. Finally, certain medications, such as β-blockers, thiazide diuretics, retinoids, probucol, androgenic steroids, and many progestational drugs, can also lower HDL.

Treatment

Besides symptomatic relief for any of the complications of Tangier disease, there is no specific treatment. The main concern in the management of these patients is to reduce their risk for developing coronary artery disease. Following the general lifestyle changes recommended by the National Cholesterol Education Program, such as exercise, low-fat diets, weight reduction, and smoking cessation, is likely to be beneficial for these patients. Treatment for other conditions, such as hypertension and diabetes, which also promote coronary artery disease, is also important. In general, the current drugs used for treating dyslipidemias do not work as well in raising HDL as they do in lowering LDL, and in many cases, Tangier disease patients will often not respond to the drugs that do raise HDL, such as niacin and the statin drugs.

Although there is no currently approved drugs for increasing the expression or function of the ABCA1 transporter, elucidation of the genetic defect in Tangier disease and subsequent studies with ABCA1 transgenic mice suggest that such an approach most likely would be useful for reducing the risk of coronary artery disease in the general population. Recent studies in humans, involving the intravenous infusion of lipid-poor apoA-I, have also shown that this may also be a viable approach for quickly mobilizing excess cholesterol from atherosclerotic plaques, in patients with a normally functioning ABCA1 transporter.[5]

References

1. ASSMANN, G., VON ECKARDSTEIN, A., AND BREWER, J. B. JR.: Familial analphalipoproteinemia: Tangier disease. In *The Metabolic and Molecular Bases of Inherited Disease*, 8th ed., C. R. SCRIVER, A. L. BEAUDET, W. S. SLY, ET AL., eds., McGraw-Hill, New York, 2001, pp. 2937–60.

2. FREDRICKSON, D. S., ALTROCCHI, P. H., AVIOLI, L. V. ET AL.: Tangier disease—combined clinical staff conference at the National Institute of Health. *Ann. Intern. Med.* 55:1016–31, 1961.

3. STEFKOVA, J., POLEDNE, R., AND HUBACEK, J. A: ATP-binding cassette (ABC) transporters in human

metabolism and diseases. *Physiol. Res.* 53:235–43, 2004.

4. BREWER, H. B. JR., REMALEY, A. T., NEUFELD, E. B., BASSO, F., AND JOYCE, C.: Regulation of plasma high-density lipoprotein levels by the ABCA1 transporter and the emerging role of high-density lipoprotein in the treatment of cardiovascular disease. *Arterioscler. Thromb. Vasc. Biol.* 24:1755–60, 2004.

5. NISSEN, S. E., TSUNODA, T., ET AL.: Effect of recombinant ApoA-I Milano on coronary atherosclerosis in patients with acute coronary syndromes: A randomized controlled trial. *JAMA* 290:2292–300, 2003.

Case 81

Worsening Diarrhea in a 5-Year-Old Girl

Masako Udewa and Alan T. Remaley

A 5-year-old girl was brought to her physician for worsening of diarrhea. She was having about six to seven bowel movements of foul-smelling stools per day. The diarrhea seemed to worsen with ingestion of fatty food. The mother described that since infancy, her daughter had failure to thrive, chronic diarrhea, and malabsorption. She was tentatively diagnosed with celiac disease at 18 months of age without a biopsy. A gluten-free diet was started but did not appear to relieve her diarrhea. There was no family history of celiac disease.

On physical examination, she was noted to be below the fifth percentile for height and weight. The abdomen was mildly distended with the liver edge palpable approximately 2 cm below the right costal margin. The spleen could not be palpated. The deep tendon reflexes were slightly diminished, but present. Her gait was wide-based.

Laboratory tests included a comprehensive serum chemistry panel and complete blood count. All results were within normal limits except AST and ALT, which were mildly elevated. The blood smear showed a moderate amount of acanthocytes. An ultrasound of the abdomen showed hepatomegaly, with increased echogenicity consistent with fatty infiltration.

The patient returned for another visit a month later. On further questioning, the mother revealed that her daughter seemed to be less coordinated than her 4-year-old cousin. She also noted that her daughter had difficulties with fine-motor skills. No bleeding problem or easy bruising was reported. The following additional laboratory blood tests were performed:

Analyte	Value, Conventional Units	Reference Interval, Conventional Units	Value, SI Units	Reference Interval, SI Units
Cholesterol, total	25 mg/dL	108–187	0.648 mmol/L	2.8–4.8
HDL-C	28 mg/dL	35–82	0.725 mmol/L	0.91–2.12
Triglycerides	<1 mg/dL	32–116	<0.01 mmol/L	0.36–1.31
ApoA-1	50 mg/dL	104–167	0.5 g/L	1.04–1.67

Analyte	Value, Conventional Units	Reference Interval, Conventional Units	Value, SI Units	Reference Interval, SI Units
ApoB	<35 mg/dL	51–80	<0.35 g/L	0.51–0.8
LDL-C	10 mg/dL	38–140	0.259 mmol/L	0.98–3.62
Vitamin A	32 μg/dL	36–120	1.12 mmol/L	1.26–4.21
Vitamin E	0.5 μg/mL	3–9	1.16 μmol/L	7–21
Prothrombine time	15 s	11–15	15 s	11–15

Lipoprotein analysis showed that total cholesterol, triglyceride, and low-density lipoprotein (LDL) were all extremely low. Prothrombin time (PT) was slightly elevated. Vitamin K and vitamin D levels were normal; however, vitamins A and E were all abnormally low. Both of her parents' lipoprotein profiles were normal. Stool fat excretion was measured to be significantly elevated at 15 g/day (reference range <7 g/day). Tests for antigliadin, antireticulin, and antiendomysial antibodies were all negative.

Inconsistent with celiac disease, the duodenum was found by endoscopy to have normally formed villi, but it had an unusual white frosting appearance. On histologic examination, numerous Oil Red stain–positive vacuoles were observed in the villi consistent with the intracellular fat accumulation that occurs in abetalipoproteinemia. Because of the suspected diagnosis, the patient was referred to an ophthalmologist, who also observed pigmentary degeneration of the retina. The patient was started on a low-fat diet, which considerably improved her diarrhea. High-dose oral supplementation of vitamins A and E was also started. She was recommended to return for periodic monitoring of her eyes, to be followed by coagulation and liver function tests.

Definition of the Disease

Abetalipoproteinemia is an autosomal recessive disorder due to a defect in the assembly and secretion of β-lipoproteins in the small intestine and to a lesser extent in the liver, leading to decreased levels of serum triglyceride, very low density lipoprotein–cholesterol (VLDL-C), and LDL-C.[1-3] Absence of apoB-containing lipoproteins with β-electrophoretic mobility is the hallmark of the disease and also forms the basis for the name of the disease. Because of the defect in the secretion of lipoproteins, lipid accumulates in the enterocytes and hepatocytes and also results in fat malabsorption and fat-soluble vitamin deficiencies. The abnormal serum lipoprotein level causes secondary alterations in the red cell lipid composition, which causes the formation of acanthocytes.

Almost all clinical manifestations of abetalipoproteinemia are due to fat-soluble vitamin deficiencies.[1] Progressive pigmentary degeneration of the retina and the debilitating spinocerebellar disease that can develop are secondary to the defective transport of vitamin E in blood. Similar findings are also found in patients with isolated vitamin E deficiency. Nightblindness due to vitamin A deficiency and occasionally coagulation abnormalities due to vitamin K deficiency are the other consequences of fat-soluble vitamin deficiency. Obligate heterozygote parents of patients with abetalipoproteinemia typically have a normal level of fat-soluble vitamins and serum lipoproteins.

The genetic defect in abetalipoproteinemia is due to mutations in the microsomal triglyceride transfer protein (MTP).[2] MTP is a heterodimeric lipid transfer protein that is composed of protein disulfide isomerase and a unique large subunit, which transfers triglyceride, cholesteryl esters, and phopholipids between the endoplasmic reticulum membrane and nascent lipoproteins.[4] MTP affects the concentration and availability of fat soluble vitamins by altering the level of serum lipoproteins, which transport these vitamins. In addition, MTP deficiency particularly affects vitamin E and A levels because MTP also plays a role in the absorption and packaging of these vitamins onto lipoproteins in the intestine. Vitamin D levels are often normal or only slightly decreased because this vitamin is transported mainly in serum by the vitamin D binding protein.

Differential Diagnosis

The differential diagnosis of hypocholesterolemia includes disorders of cholesterol biosynthesis and of lipoprotein metabolism. Smith–Lemli–Opitz syndrome, the most common disorder of cholesterol biosynthesis, can be differentiated from the disorders of lipoprotein metabolism by elevated 7-dehydrocholestrol, a cholesterol precursor that accumulates in this disorder. Besides abetalipoproteinemia, low-apoB-containing lipoprotein can also be observed in familial hypobetalipoproteinemia, and chylomicron retention disease, which are due to other defects in lipoprotein assembly and secretion. Familial hypobetalipoproteinemia is caused primarily by mutations in the apoB gene, leading to the production of truncated apoB, which can be observed by SDS-PAGE (sodium dodecyl sulfate–polyacrylamide gel electrophoresis) gel electrophoresis. In chylomicron retention disease, there is a specific defect in chylomicron formation and secretion, which leads to a much greater reduction of chylomicrons relative to LDL than what is typically observed in abetalipoproteinemia. Abetalipoproteinemia can also be differentiated from familial hypobetalipoproteinemia by the lipoprotein profiles of parents.[5] In familial hypobetalipoproteinemia, the parents usually have partially decreased apoB-containing lipoproteins, whereas in abetalipoproteinemia and chylomicron retention disease, which are autosomal recessive disorders, they are usually normal.

Most patients with abetalipoproteinemia, however, initially come to medical attention as infants because of failure to thrive and diarrhea. Thus, they are often misdiagnosed as having celiac disease or cystic fibrosis. Abetalipoproteinemia can often be differentiated from these more common diseases by a careful medical history and the presence and/ or absence of the various clinical findings that are unique to these diseases. The finding of fat-laden but normal-size villi via endoscopic examination and a normal sweat chloride test can also be used to rule out celiac disease and cystic fibrosis, respectively.

Treatment

Treatment with a low-fat diet limiting fat to 5 g per day for children and up to 15 g per day for adults significantly ameliorates steatorrhea. Supplementation with high-dose vitamin E and vitamin A are required for life. Early intervention with vitamin A and E supplementation has been shown to retard the progression of the ophthalmological and neurological complications of this disease. Vitamin A supplementation, however, should be closely monitored to avoid toxicity. Vitamin K supplementation should be considered in patients with demonstrated coagulopathy.

References

1. KANE, J. P. AND HAVEL, R. J.: Disorders of the biogenesis and secretion of lipoproteins containing the B apolipoproteins. In *The Metabolic and Molecular Basis of Inherited Disease*, 8th ed., McGraw-Hill, New York, 2001, pp. 2717–52.

2. WETTERAU, J. R., AGGERBECK, L. P., BOUMA, M. E. ET AL.: Absence of microsomal triglyceride transfer protein in individual with abetalipoproteinemia. *Science* 258:999–1001, 1992.

3. BERRIOT-VAROQUEAUX, N., AGGERBECK, L. P., SAMSON-BOUMA, M.-E., AND WETTERAU, J. R.: The role of the microsomal triglyceride transfer protein in abetalipoproteinemia. *Ann. Rev. Nutr. 20:*663–97, 2000.

4. HUSSAIN, M. M., SHI, J., AND DREIZEN, P.: Microsomal triglyceride transfer protein and its role in apoB-lipoprotein assembly. *J. Lipid Res. 44:*22–32, 2003.

5. SCANU, A. M., AGGERBECK, L. P., DRUSKI, A. W., LIM, C. T., AND KAYDEN, H. J.: A study of the abnormal lipoproteins. *J. Clin. Invest. 53:*440–53, 1974.

Case 82

A 4-Year-Old Girl with Yellow Xanthomas and Arthritis

Robert D. Shamburek and Alan T. Remaley

A 4-year-old girl was seen by a pediatrician because of yellow streaks on her knuckles, first noted by her mother. On physical exam, she was found to have planar xanthomas at the first proximal interphalangeal and metaphalangeal joints of the hand, and in the elbow, knee, and inner gluteal creases. Her Achilles tendons were also thickened.

Laboratory tests were largely normal except for the results of the following serum lipoprotein panel, which showed marked hypercholesterolemia:

Analyte	Value, Conventional Units	Reference Interval, Conventional Units	Value, SI Units	Reference Interval, SI Units
Cholesterol, total	576 mg/dL	108–187	14.9 mmol/L	2.8–4.8
HDL-C	40 mg/dL	35–82	1.03 mmol/L	0.91–2.12
LDL-C	522 mg/dL	38–140	14.3 mmol/L	0.98–3.62
Trigylcerides	101 mg/dL	32–116	1.13 mmol/L	0.36–1.31

The patient was treated with a low-fat diet and statin drug to block endogenous cholesterol biosynthesis, but it caused only a modest decrease in her serum cholesterol concentration. However, she did show a relatively good response to cholestyramine, a bile-acid-binding resin that decreases cholesterol absorption from the intestine. Total cholesterol had fallen below 250 mg/dL. The planar xanthomas progressively disappeared over the next several years, but she continued to have thickened Achilles tendons and developed an eye arcus. At age 11, she was seen for severe joint pain in her knees and elbows, but no diagnosis was made. During her teenage years, she had persistent migratory arthritis in her hips, wrists, knees, and elbows and was told that she might have juvenile rheumatoid arthritis. At age 30, she developed mild chest pain, and a cardiac catheterization showed 50–74% stenosis in the distal left anterior descending artery and in the middle right coronary artery. In addition to cholestyramine and a statin, she was also started on ezetimibe, which is a specific drug inhibitor of cholesterol absorption, and total serum cholesterol dropped to 162 mg/dL (4.21 mmol/L).

Tietz's Applied Laboratory Medicine, Second Edition. Edited by Mitchell G. Scott, Ann M. Gronowski, and Charles S. Eby
Copyright © 2007 John Wiley & Sons, Inc.

A skin biopsy was performed and was used to demonstrate the presence of normal LDL receptor activity, thus ruling out familial hypercholesterolemia. Plasma was then analyzed by gas chromatography/mass spectroscopy and revealed a >10-fold increase in the level of the plant sterol, sitosterol, thus establishing the diagnosis of sitosterolemia.

Definition of the Disease

Sitosterolemia is a rare autosomal recessive lipid disorder characterized by the increased intestinal absorption of all sterols and diminished biliary sterol excretion, leading to an accumulation of cholesterol and other sterols in various tissues.[1-4] While exact incidence of the disease is not known, founder populations have been identified in Amish (Pennsylvania Dutch), Finnish, and Japanese populations. The hallmark biochemical feature is elevated sitosterol, a major plant sterol, which is abundant in the diet. The disorder was previously called *phytosterolemia*, because all plant sterols accumulate in this disorder, but even sterols from other dietary sources, such as shellfish, will also accumulate in these patients.[5]

Sitosterolemia is caused by a defect in a member of the ATP-binding cassette (ABC) family of transporters that is expressed in the small intestine and liver. The defect involves gene mutations in either one of two heterodimeric half-transporters for ABCG5 and ABCG8, which are on chromosome 2p21. ABCG5 and ABCG8 are located both on the apical membrane of the intestinal mucosa cells and the canalicular membranes of the liver. In the intestine, they pump cholesterol and other noncholesterol sterols out of the enterocyte and back into the intestinal lumen, thus decreasing net sterol absorption. The hepatic transporters deplete sterols in the blood by excreting them into the bile. Normally, approximately 50% of dietary cholesterol is absorbed, whereas less than 5% of dietary noncholesterol sterols is usually absorbed. Cholesterol and noncholesterol sterols are initially taken up into the enterocyte by the sterol influx transporter, Niemann–Pick C1-like 1 protein (NPC1L1). The sterols are normally then either pumped back into the intestinal lumen by ABCG5 and ABCG8 transporters or packaged into chylomicrons and secreted into the circulation. The ABCG5 and ABCG8 transporters may have a preference for noncholesterol sterols because when these transporters are defective, there is a much greater increase in the overall absorption of noncholesterol sterols relative to the increase in cholesterol absorption.

The hyperabsorption of cholesterol and noncholesterol sterols results in their tissue accumulation, leading to tuberous and tendinous xanthomas, at an early age. In addition, the Achilles tendons are frequently thickened as a result of lipid accumulation, and an eye arcus from lipid infiltration into the cornea can occur. The mechanism for arthralgias and arthritis is not completely understood but may also be the result of inflammation triggered by sterol accumulation in the joints. Episodic hemolysis and thrombocytopenia may be seen because of altered lipid cell membrane content. Finally, premature atherosclerosis can occur even in childhood because of hypercholesterolemia.

Differential Diagnosis

The typical laboratory test for measuring plasma cholesterol involves a coupled enzyme reaction, using cholesterol oxidase. Cholesterol oxidase recognizes the 3β-hydroxyl group on the A ring of cholesterol. Many other sterols, however, such as sitosterol, also have a hydroxyl group in the same position; thus the standard enzymatic test for cholesterol is nonspecific. Noncholesterol sterols can be differentiated from cholesterol only by sterol analysis by either gas chromatography–mass spectrometry or by high-performance liquid chromatography. Serum sitosterol concentrations are normally <1 mg/dL (<0.023 mmol/L) but in sitosterolemia concentrations can range from 20 to 65 mg/dL. (From 0.48 to 1.56 mmol/L.)

Patients with sitosterolemia are frequently misdiagnosed as having familial hypercholesterolemia due to the clinical resemblance with elevated LDL cholesterol, xanthomas, and premature atherosclerosis. Differentiating the two is important because of differing treatments. One clue to differentiating the two disorders is that the clinical symptoms, such as the xanthomas and atherosclerosis, may be disproportionately severe relative to the level of serum cholesterol in sitosterolemia patients. A second clue for sitosterolemia is the presence of recurrent severe migratory arthritis, which often occurs in knees, hands, and elbows and may first present in childhood. Another finding in favor of sitosterolemia is the remarkable lowering of serum cholesterol in response to therapies aimed at decreasing cholesterol absorption, such as low fat diet, bile acid resins, or ezetimibe. Finally, the parents of sitosterolemia patients usually have normal serum lipid values, whereas even in the heterozygous state, familial hypercholesterolemia is usually associated with at least a modest elevation of serum cholesterol.

One reason that sitosterolemia patients can be misdiagnosed is the rarity of this disease versus the relatively high occurrence of the autosomal dominant familial hypercholesterolemia (FH). FH is most commonly a result of mutations in the LDL receptor gene that prevents the uptake of LDL-C via binding to apolipoproteins B-100. This prevents removal of LDL-C from the circulation; furthermore, the lack of hepatocyte uptake of LDL-C prevents the normal negative feedback of cholesterol synthesis. Over 420 different mutations of the LDL receptor have been described and divided into five classes of mutations ranging from absence of the receptor to "defective" receptors with up to 25% of normal receptor activity. The prevalence of homozygote FH patients is about one in a million, whereas FH heterozygote prevalence is 1 case per 500 persons in the United States and can be up to 1 case per 67 persons in some populations such as Ashkenazi Jews.

Homozygotes generally have total cholesterol values >600 mg/dL and face the risk of sudden death at a very early age. Heterozygotes with 50% normal LDL receptors and 50% defective receptors generally have total and LDL cholesterol values about twice the population averages. Heterozygotes generally respond well to statin therapy (unlike our sitosterolemia patient here) but depending on the class of their mutations may require additional cholesterol-lowering therapy.

Treatment

A modified diet is one of the major approaches for treating sitosterolemia. The main dietary sources of sitosterol are seeds, nuts, oils, fat-rich vegetables, and fruits. Avoiding foods rich in plant sterols can decrease the hypercholesterolemia by as much as 50%. Bile acid binding resins, which inhibit sterol absorption by decreasing bile acid reabsorption in the ileum, can also considerably reduce (25–50%) hypercholesterolemia and can be a diagnostic clue to the presence of the disorder. Ezetimibe, a relatively new drug that selectively inhibits the NPC1L1 sterol influx transporter, is also often very effective in decreasing the hypercholesterolemia in these patients. In contrast, these patients often show a relatively poor response to statin drugs.

References

1. BERGE, K. E.: Sitosterolemia: A gateway to new knowledge about cholesterol metabolism. *Ann. Med. 35*:502–11, 2003.
2. BERGE, K. E., TIAN, H., GRAF, G. A. ET AL.: Accumulation of dietary cholesterol in sitosterolemia caused by mutations in adjacent ABC transporters. *Science 290*:1771–5, 2000.
3. BHATTACHARYYA, A. K. AND CONNOR, W. E.: Beta-sitosterolemia and xanthomatosis. A newly described lipid storage disease in two sisters. *J. Clin. Invest. 53*:1033–43, 1974.
4. SALEN, G., SHEFER, S., NGUYEN, L., NESS, G. C., TINT, G. S., AND SHORE, V.: Sitosterolemia. *J. Lipid Res. 33*:945–55, 1992.
5. GREGG, R. E., CONNOR, W. E., LIN, D. S., AND BREWER, H. B., JR.: Abnormal metabolism of shellfish sterols in a patient with sitosterolemia and xanthomatosis. *J. Clin. Invest. 77*:1864–72, 1986.

Part Nineteen

Autoimmune Diseases

Cases of rheumatoid arthritis, systemic leepus erythematosus (SLE), and celiac disease are reported and discussed in Cases 83, 84, and 85, respectively (all edited by CSE).

Tietz's Applied Laboratory Medicine, Second Edition. Edited by Mitchell G. Scott, Ann M. Gronowski, and Charles S. Eby
Copyright © 2007 John Wiley & Sons, Inc.

Case 83

Woman with Morning Stiffness and Tender, Swollen Joints

Liron Caplan and Sterling G. West

This 35-year-old previously healthy female noted the onset of swelling and aching in her left wrist for one week's duration. After failing a trial of acetaminophen and ibuprofen, she was diagnosed with a sprain and prescribed an alternate nonsteroidal antiinflammatory drug (NSAID) by her primary care physician. This, too, proved ineffective, and she began to experience generalized fatigue with morning stiffness lasting 2–3 hours. The physician's repeat examination revealed minimal swelling of the wrists bilaterally, but was otherwise nonfocal. He performed bilateral hand and wrist radiographs, which were read as "normal," and the patient was given a prescription for an alternate NSAID. The following laboratory values were obtained:

Analyte	Value, Conventional Units	Reference Interval, Conventional Units	Value, SI Units	Reference Interval, SI Units
Sodium	142 mmol/L	135–145	Same	
Potassium	4.2 mmol/L	4.0–5.3	Same	
Chloride	103 mmol/L	98–107	Same	
CO_2, total	23 mmol/L	20–28	Same	
Calcium, total	8.8 mg/dL	8.5–10.5	2.20 mmol/L	2.12–2.62
Urea nitrogen	14 mg/dL	5–18	5.0 mmol/L	1.8–6.4
Creatinine	0.8 mg/dL	0.7–1.2	71 μmol/L	62–106
Glucose	98 mg/dL	70–110	5.4 mmol/L	3.9–6.1
Protein, total	7.0 g/dL	6.0–8.0	70 g/L	60–80
Albumin	3.0 g/dL	3.5–5.0	30 g/L	35–50 g/L
Bilirubin, total	0.5 mg/dL	0.2–1.2	9 μmol/L	3–21
ALP	48 U/L	35–120	0.8 mkat/L	0.6–2.0
AST	35 U/L	10–42	0.6 mkat/L	0.2–0.7
Hematocrit	35%	37–44	0.35 volume	0.37–0.44
Hemoglobin	11.6 g/dL	12–16	116 g/L	120–160
WBC	$7.7 \times 10^3/\mu L$	4–11	$7.7 \times 10^9/L$	4–11

Tietz's Applied Laboratory Medicine, Second Edition. Edited by Mitchell G. Scott, Ann M. Gronowski, and Charles S. Eby
Copyright © 2007 John Wiley & Sons, Inc.

Analyte	Value, Conventional Units	Reference Interval, Conventional Units	Value, SI Units	Reference Interval, SI Units
ANA	1 : 40	<1 : 40	Same	
Rheumatoid factor	65 U/mL	<20 U/mL	Same	
Erythrocyte sedimentation rate	42 mm/h	<20 mm/h	Same	

The physician noted the abnormal laboratory results and informed his patient, who now reported pain in her hands and feet that improved through the course of the day. He prescribed her prednisone 5 mg daily and also referred her to a rheumatologist, requesting that she be seen promptly. At her initial consultation 10 days later, she endorsed continued pain and swelling of the second and third knuckles of both hands, as well as her wrists. However, the warmth and stiffness of her joints had improved somewhat since starting the glucocorticoid therapy.

The rheumatologist elicited no history of oral ulcers, neuropsychiatric disease, chest pain, back pain, dry mouth, dry eyes, or lower extremity edema. There were no acknowledged episodes of prior intravenous drug use, transfusions, or tattoos on the part of the patient. The physical examination was significant for diminished bilateral hand grip strength and range of motion, but equivocal for the presence of synovitis. No effusions or skin lesions were present. The cardiac, pulmonary, neurologic, and abdominal examination demonstrated no abnormalities.

To clarify the patient's status, the rheumatologist ordered magnetic resonance imaging of the hands and wrists, a C-reactive protein (CRP) level, and an anticyclic citrullinated peptide antibody (anti-CCP) concentration. She also empirically increased the patient's prednisone to 15 mg for one week, as a diagnostic trial to refine the potential role for long-term immunosuppression. The patient completed a health assessment questionnaire (HAQ) at the request of the rheumatologist. Imaging confirmed mild synovitis involving the wrists bilaterally, in addition to a number of metacarpal–phalangeal (MCP) joints. Laboratory results were as follows:

Analyte	Value, Conventional Units	Reference Interval, Conventional Units	Value, SI Units	Reference Interval, SI Units
CRP	6.5 mg/dL	<0.3 mg/dL	65 mg/L	<3.0 mg/L
Anti-CCP	72 IU/mL	<5 IU/mL	Same	

These findings supported the diagnosis of rheumatoid arthritis (RA), which was further bolstered by the patient's moderate clinical response to the increase glucocorticoid dosage.

Definition of the Disease

Pathophysiology

Rheumatoid arthritis refers to a systemic inflammatory disorder of undetermined cause that chronically affects synovial joints in a symmetric distribution. Infiltration of inflammatory cells (particularly mononuclear cells) into the synovium is associated with proliferation of these joint lining tissues, ultimately leading to destruction of adjacent cartilage and bone, as well as ligamentous laxity. A number of haplotypes, including specific HLA-DR4 alleles, confer susceptibility to RA. In addition, environmental factors may potentiate the risk of developing rheumatoid arthritis.

While the primary etiology of rheumatoid arthritis remains obscure, defects have been described in both humoral and cellular immunity. Ongoing research suggests a potential role for T cells, B cells, neutrophils, macrophages, synoviocytes, mast cells, and dendritic cells, with corresponding abnormalities in the cytokine profile elaborated by these cells. Tumor necrosis factor-α (TNF-α), interleukin-1 (IL-1), various cellular adhesion molecules, and matrix metalloproteinases (MMP) have all been implicated; therapies evaluating these molecular targets are actively being sought. Synovial angiogenesis is also abnormal in RA, although this is unlikely to be a primary defect.

Clinical Features

Synovitis represents the cardinal feature of rheumatoid arthritis, and the onset of disease classically occurs over weeks (to months). There is a recognized gender bias, with women accounting for 60–80% of cases in most series. Incidence rates increase rapidly from age 30 to 50, and continue to increase until age 70.

Joint involvement is polyarticular and symmetric, initially affecting smaller peripheral joints, such as the metacarpal–phalangeal, metatarsal–phalangeal, and proximal interphalangeal joints. The ankles and wrists are often involved, but the distal interphalangeal joints are spared. The joints of the lower back are also spared. Patients typically endorse morning stiffness for more than one hour that improves throughout the day and with activity. Similarly, prolonged inactivity (e.g., sitting) may provoke stiffness—a symptom termed the "gel phenomenon." Afflicted joints tend to be warm and tender with diminished range of motion, but without much erythema. Grip strength is diminished.

Extraarticular manifestations are not uncommon and include rheumatoid nodules (firm subcutaneous masses on extensor surfaces and over joints), interstitial lung disease, episcleritis, scleritis, accelerated atherosclerosis, vasculitis, and constitutional symptoms (fatigue). In addition, there appears to be an elevated incidence of lymphoproliferative malignancies. Most studies have found an increased mortality rate associated with rheumatoid arthritis, principally resulting from cardiovascular disease.

Radiographs of the hands and feet may exhibit periarticular osteopenia and soft tissue swelling, erosive changes located at the margin of the articulations, and joint space narrowing. Longstanding or aggressive disease may result in deformities such as ulnar deviation of the fingers and subluxation of the MCPs.

Diagnosis

Classification criteria have been developed for rheumatoid arthritis (Table 83.1). These criteria have been applied primarily to clinical trials, although they offer a framework

Table 83.1   Adapted Version of the ARA Classification Criteria for RA

Criterion	Comment
Three or more arthritic joints[a]	Simultaneous soft tissue swelling or fluid observed by physician in PIP, MCP, wrist, elbow, knee, ankle, or MTPs; not merely arthralgias
Rheumatoid factor	Abnormal levels by a method that identifies positives in <5% of normal controls
AM (morning) stiffness[a]	In and around joints, of at least 1 hour duration before maximal improvement
Symmetric arthritis[a]	Simultaneous bilateral involvement of at least one of the prescribed joints (see first criteria, above, for "prescribed" joints)
Hand joint arthritis[a]	At least one swollen wrist, MCP, or PIP
Rheumatoid nodules	Subcutaneous nodules (located on bony prominence, extensor surface, or juxtaarticular), observed by physician
X-ray changes	Erosions or unequivocal juxtaarticular bony decalcification on hand and wrist films

[a]These criteria must be present for 6 weeks' duration. At least 4 of 7 must be present.

Source: Modified from ARA 1987 revised criteria.[1] Reprinted with permission of Wiley-Liss, Inc, a subsidiary of John Wiley & Sons, Inc. Mnemonic for the ARA classification criteria: "TRASH RX" (Dr. Caplan).

on which to establish the clinical diagnosis of RA. There is no pathognomonic ("gold standard") histologic or serologic pattern for rheumatoid arthritis; the diagnosis derives from a physician's interpretation of the clinical evidence, and may become apparent only with time.

Antibodies with affinity for the Fc component of IgG are referred to as *rheumatoid factor* (RF). While any isotype may demonstrate this function, IgM represents the majority of RA-associated rheumatoid factor. Techniques for detecting its presence include nephelometry (the most common method), ELISA, and latex agglutination. Roughly 70% of patients are positive for RF at the time they are diagnosed with RA (sensitivity). RF positivity increases with time, in the RA population (85% positive by 2 years following their diagnosis) as well as the non-RA population (20% of persons over 70 years of age). The specificity of rheumatoid factor is *poor*, and it has been described in many inflammatory states, such as hepatitis C (40%), subacute bacterial endocarditis, tuberculosis, cryoglobulinemia, and Sjögren's syndrome (80%). In general, RF positivity portends more severe RA, although clinical predictors are probably more predictive than RF.

While rheumatoid factor has facilitated the diagnosis of rheumatoid arthritis for nearly six decades, anticyclic citrullinated peptide antibodies (anti-CCP) are a more recent development. These molecules recognize peptides containing the uncommon modified amino acid citrulline, which is generated by deamination of arginine. Anti-CCP antibody tests appear to have a much higher specificity (95–98%) than does rheumatoid factor, and their clinical use is rapidly gaining favor. Second- and third-generation anti-CCP tests have an increased sensitivity (estimated to be approximately 80% for rheumatologist-diagnosed RA), when compared to the first-generation tests. In fact, anti-CCP antibody may precede the emergence of clinical symptoms. A variety of laboratory techniques have been employed to measure anti-CCP, including ELISA, latex agglutination, and other less common approaches.

Historically, physicians have relied on various laboratory tests as markers of disease activity in the inflammatory disorders. The most universally accepted indicators have been the erythrocyte sedimentation rate (ESR, SED rate) and C-reactive protein (CRP). ESR measurements provide an indirect assessment of acute-phase reactant and immunoglobulin levels by assessing their effect on the tendency of red blood cells to aggregate. In contrast, the pentameric protein CRP is itself an acute-phase reactant produced by the liver in response to a number of cytokines. It binds phospholipids and histones, activates complement, and modulates macrophage activation; thus, its purported teleological function is to mediate phagocytosis of encapsulated bacteria.

The initial degree of ESR and CRP elevation may correlate with rheumatoid arthritis disease activity. There is evidence, however, that ESR values tend to stay fairly stable during long-term follow-up and may remain elevated because of a persistent polyclonal gammopathy. CRP levels climb earlier and decline more rapidly than do ESR values. In addition, a high CRP prior to initiation of anti–tumor necrosis (anti-TNF) therapy may predict a patient's response. Very modest correlations have been described between patients' disease activity and their degree of anemia, thrombocytosis, and hypoalbuminemia. RF titer does not predict disease activity. It bears mentioning that in general, clinical and functional measures, such as hand grip and health assessment questionnaire disability index score (HAQ-DI), are more predictive of long-term prognosis (disability and mortality) than are current laboratory-based assessments.

While their roles have not been entirely elucidated, magnetic resonance imaging and musculoskeletal ultrasonography have been increasingly incorporated into many aspects of clinical practice and research trials. Recent studies have demonstrated that both imaging techniques may corroborate the presence of synovitis, as well as predict future erosions in patients with rheumatoid arthritis. Ultrasound has the potential added benefit of guiding joint aspirations and glucocorticoid injections.

Treatment

There is no known cure for rheumatoid arthritis. Fortunately, therapeutic options for patients have proliferated dramatically within the last few years (as of 2006). The goal of these therapies, generally speaking, is to suppress cellular activation and proliferation of inflammatory cells, thereby reducing the signs and symptoms of disease. Ideally, therapies should also prevent organ (articular and nonarticular) damage, as well as patient disability. Given that destructive changes may occur early in the disease process and that treatment regimens have become increasingly complex, rapid referral to a specialist is crucial.

Pharmacologic treatments achieve their immunomodulatory effects by targeting particular cell types (e.g., T cells, B cells) or their cytokine byproducts (tumor necrosis factor-α or interleukin-1). Some therapies likely bind a broad array of ligands, as is the case for glucocorticoids, or may be much more specific, as is the case for anti-B lymphocyte CD20 antibody (rituximab) and IL-1 receptor antagonist (anakinra).

Historically, treatment for RA involved the use of disease-modifying antirheumatic drugs (DMARDs) of a low molecular weight (methotrexate, gold, sulfasalazine, hydroxychloroquine, etc.). These drugs were administered as sequential monotherapy; that is, a treatment failure with a single medication would prompt transition to an alternative medication, with a gradual increase in the potency and toxicity of treatments. The use of specific combination therapies in clinical trials (e.g., methotrexate, hydroxychloroquine, and sulfasalazine or leflunomide with methotrexate) has produced clinical responses of greater magnitude than has monotherapy. Practicing physicians have been slow to adopt such complex regimen, however, often preferring a "step-up" approach (i.e., progressively adding agents to monotherapy treatment failures). Preliminary evidence suggests that the step-up approach is unfortunately suboptimal.

Until recently, only glucocorticoids alleviated patients symptoms rapidly (days to weeks), while more traditional disease-modifying antirheumatic drugs required longer to accomplish their effect. The introduction of biologics, such as anti-TNF therapy (etanercept, infliximab, and adalimumab), has shortened the interval between initiation of therapy and clinical response. Furthermore, the clinical response rates and ability to halt radiographic progression appear to be superior to that of traditional DMARDS, when evaluated in clinical trials. A vast array of newer biologic agents, including anti-CD20 antibody (riotuximab), CTLA4-Ig (abatacept), and anti-IL-6 [(MRA, tocilizumab) receptor antibody], are also being developed or gaining approval for use in rheumatoid arthritis. While the long-term role for these emerging therapies remains unclear, they indicate a vigorous effort under way to identify new treatments options for patients suffering with RA.

Reference

1. ARNETT, F. C., EDWORTHY, S. M., BLOCH, D. A., ET AL.: The American Rheumatism Association 1987 revised criteria for the classification of rheumatoid arthritis. *Arthritis Rheum. 31*:315–24, 1988.

Additional Reading

ATKINSON, J. P.: C-reactive protein: A rheumatologist's friend revisited. *Arthritis Rheum. 44*:995–6, 2001.

COLGLAZIER, C. L. AND SUTEJ, P. G.: Laboratory testing in the rheumatic diseases: A practical review. *South. Med. J. 98*:185–91, 2005.

ELLIOTT, J. R. AND O'DELL, J.: Rheumatoid arthritis. In *Rheumatology Secrets*, 2nd ed., S. WEST, ed., Hanley & Belfus, Philadelphia, 2002.

HOCHBERG, M., SILMAN, A., SMOLEN, J., WEINBLATT, M., AND WEISMAN, M., eds.: *Rheumatology*, 3rd ed., Mosby, Philadelphia, 2003.

KLIPPEL, J. H., CROFFORD, L. J., STONE, J. H., AND WEYAND, C. M., eds., *Primer on the Rheumatic Diseases*, Arthritis Foundation, Atlanta, 2001.

NAKAMURA, R. M.: Progress in the use of biochemical and biological markers for evaluation of rheumatoid arthritis. *J. Clin. Lab. Anal. 14*:305–13, 2000.

Case 84

Woman with a Rash and Lower Extremity Pain

Liron Caplan and Sterling G. West

A 25-year-old African-American female was in her usual state of health until she developed generalized fatigue, peripheral joint arthralgias, urinary frequency and urgency, and diffuse myalgias over the course of 2 weeks. After sun exposure, a flat nonpruritic erythematous rash appeared, consisting of nondistinct 1–2-cm lesions scattered about her arms, thighs, and face. After one month of symptoms, she reported to her family physician that the "sunburn" had not abated and that she now had difficulty urinating. In addition, her lower extremities ached with a "searing" pain. Urinalysis with microscopic analysis was performed, which revealed 4 WBCs/HPF, 2+ protein, and 7 RBCs/HPF. Her physician prescribed ciprofloxacin, amitriptyline, and a narcotic analgesic; however, she declined to fill the prescriptions.

The patient developed anorexia and lower extremity pain with weakness, nausea, and vomiting over the next week. On presentation to the emergency room, she also complained of fatigue, suprapubic pain, and fullness. The history was remarkable for frequent urinary tract infections over the prior 6 months, but no prior chronic health issues, surgeries, or pregnancies. Placement of a urinary catheter produced 1 L of clear output; she was thus admitted with urinary retention and severe pain of the lower extremities. Further questioning revealed that the patient was involved in a long-term monogamous relationship (which included unprotected intercourse), that she had a cousin with "lupus," that she smokes $\frac{1}{2}$ a pack per day, and that she had no known drug allergies.

On physical examination, the patient appeared to be a well-developed but ill-appearing woman. Vital signs consisted of a blood pressure of 110/58, a heart rate of 100, a temperature of 38.2°C and a room air oxygen saturation of 99%. Head and neck examination were normal. A grade 1/6 systolic murmur was noted on heart examination. Lungs were clear to auscultation. There was mild suprapubic tenderness on abdominal palpation, but no rebound or guarding was present. Rectal tone was diminished. Bowel sounds were active, and there was no costovertebral angle tenderness. The patient was unable to stand because of weakness (proximal strength 2+/5, distal strength 2−/5) and pain. The patellar deep tendon reflexes were diminished (0 − 1+) compared to biceps DTRs (2+), but all the cranial nerves were intact. Her skin examination was

Tietz's Applied Laboratory Medicine, Second Edition. Edited by Mitchell G. Scott, Ann M. Gronowski, and Charles S. Eby
Copyright © 2007 John Wiley & Sons, Inc.

significant for faint erythematous nonraised 1–2-cm lesions overlying the maxillae and distributed across the upper arms and thighs. The following laboratory results were obtained, including an anti–nuclear antigen (ANA) test:

Analyte	Value, Conventional Units	Reference Interval, Conventional Units	Value, SI Units	Reference Interval, SI Units
Sodium	137 mmol/L	135–145	Same	
Potassium	4.9 mmol/L	4.0–5.3	Same	
Chloride	101 mmol/L	98–107	Same	
CO_2, total	26 mmol/L	20–28	Same	
Calcium, total	9.7 mg/dL	8.5–10.5	2.42 mmol/L	2.12–2.62
Urea nitrogen	26 mg/dL	5–18	9.3 mmol/L	1.8–6.4
Creatinine	1.2 mg/dL	0.7–1.2	106 μmol/L	62–106
Glucose	93 mg/dL	70–110	5.2 mmol/L	3.9–6.1
Protein, total	8.1 g/dL	6.0–8.0	81 g/L	60–80
Albumin	3.0 g/dL	3.5–5.0	30 g/L	35–50
Bilirubin, total	0.1 mg/dL	0.2–1.2	2 μmol/L	3–21
ALP	51 U/L	35–120	μkat/L	0.6–2.0
ALT	15 U/L	8–47	μkat/L	0.1–0.8
AST	36 U/L	10–42	μkat/L	0.2–0.7
Hematocrit	34%	37–44	0.34 volume	0.37–0.44
Hemoglobin	11.5 g/dL	12–16	g/L	120–160
Platelets	$158 \times 10^3/\mu L$	150–400	$158 \times 10^9/L$	150–400
WBC	$3.8 \times 10^3/\mu L$	4–11	$3.8 \times 10^9/L$	4–11
Neutrophil count	$3.3 \times 10^3/\mu L$	1.8–6.6	$3.3 \times 10^9/L$	1.8–6.6
Lymphocyte count	$0.5 \times 10^3/\mu L$	1.2–3.3	$0.5 \times 10^9/L$	1.2–3.3
Qualitative ANA	Positive	Negative	Same	Same
ANA pattern	Speckled	None	Same	Same
ANA quantitative	1 : 5120	≤1 : 80	Same	Same
HIV-1/2 antibody	Negative	Negative	Same	Same

The admitting hospitalist consulted a rheumatologist for a possible diagnosis of systemic lupus erythematosus. Review of the patient's history and physical examination by the rheumatologist found that she had no evidence of current or prior oral ulcers, sicca symptoms (dry eyes and/or mouth), psychiatric symptoms, or alopecia; however, the patient did complain of positional chest pain for 2 weeks. The rheumatologist ordered complement C3 and C4 levels, extractable nuclear antigen (ENA) screen, dilute Russell viper venom time (dRVVT), lupus anticoagulant confirmation by phospholipid neutralization procedure (LAC-PNP), cardiolipin antibody screen, crithidia anti-dsDNA qualitative screen, anti-dsDNA antibody titers, and a 24-hour urine collection for protein and creatinine clearance. Positive values on the screening tests triggered additional "reflex" tests by the laboratory:

Analyte	Value, Conventional Units	Reference Interval, Conventional Units	Value, SI Units	Reference Interval, SI Units
C3 quantitation	76 mg/dL	83–185	760 mg/L	830–1850
C4 quantitation	10 mg/dL	12–54	100 mg/L	120–540

Analyte	Value, Conventional Units	Reference Interval, Conventional Units	Value, SI Units	Reference Interval, SI Units
ENA antibody screen	Positive	Negative	Same	
Anti-Smith (Sm) antibody	Positive	Negative	Same	
Anti-RNP antibody	Positive	Negative	Same	
Anti-SSA antibody	Positive	Negative	Same	
Anti-SSB antibody	Negative	Negative	Same	
DRVVT	Absent	Absent	Same	
LAC-PNP	Negative	Negative	Same	
Cardiolipin antibody screen	Positive	Negative	Same	
Cardiolipin IgG antibody	15 GPL/mL	<11	Same	
Cardiolipin IgM antibody	<10 MPL/mL	<10	Same	
Cardiolipin IgA antibody	<13 APL/mL	<13	Same	
Crithidia anti-dsDNA	Positive	Negative	Same	
Anti-dsDNA titer	1313 IU/mL	<25	Same	
24-hour urine protein	3430 mg/day	<150	Same	
24-hour urine creatinine	1600 mg/day	600–1500	13.5 mmol/day	5–13
Creatinine clearance	123 mL/min	75–115	1.18 mL/s	0.72–1.11

A subsequent magnetic resonance imaging of the spine revealed T2-weighted signal hyperintensity in the conus medullaris. On the basis of the clinical presentation, laboratory values, and studies, the patient was assigned the diagnosis of systemic lupus erythematosus (SLE), with neuropsychiatric, hematologic, and renal organ involvement. She was scheduled for a renal biopsy and given pulse-dose intravenous steroids.

Definition of the Disease

Pathophysiology

Systemic lupus erythematosus is a chronic, inflammatory, often multisystem disorder characterized by humoral autoimmunity. Specific autoantibodies gradually accumulate for years prior to the onset of clinical disease,[2] which reinforces data showing an increase in the concentration of autoantibodies—as well as their epitope specificity—preceding the diagnosis of SLE. Indeed, while self-reactive antibodies may be relatively common in the population, the prevailing wisdom indicates that antibodies must mature in their affinity for self-antigens before assuming a pathogenic role.

The mechanisms responsible for systemic lupus erythematosus have not been well articulated, but likely represent a complex interplay of genetic and environmental factors that ultimately result in disease-causing autoantibodies. Recent studies report that lupus patients have elevated blood levels of interferon α (IFN-α), suggesting that this cytokine may be a component of the disease mechanism, and/or a response to it.[3] Investigators have proposed that lupus arises in the presence of provocative antigens (particularly nuclear antigens), abnormal polyclonal B-cell activation, impaired apoptotic pathways, idiotypic network dysregulation, or a combination of these phenomena.

Similarly, an extensive panoply of candidate genetic susceptibility loci exists; at least 15 human and 30 murine genes have been identified thus far.[7] Potential human genes include those encoding (1) polymorphisms in the major histocompatibility complex (especially HLA-DR2), (2) immunoglobin heavy-chain Fc receptors (notably FcγRIIA and FcγRIIIA), (3) complement deficiencies (C1q, C4, and C2), (4) mannose-binding lectin, (5) cytotoxic T-lymphocyte antigen 4 (CTLA-4), and (6) the surface cell marker programmed cell death 1 (PD-1).

These genetic polymorphisms ultimately result in a diverse array of immune-mediated insults, including the reaction of free antibody with fixed antigens and microvascular injury as a result of antigen/antibody immune complex deposition.

Clinical Features

Systemic lupus is an uncommon disease, with an overall incidence of approximately 4 cases per 100,000 patient-years. SLE exhibits a striking gender bias, with a female to male ratio of 9 : 1. Likewise, incidence rates for non-Caucasians are 2–3 times that of Caucasians.

The potential target organ involvement can be extremely varied. In a substantial minority (perhaps 30%) of SLE patients, the disease is limited to arthralgias, scarring rashes, and cytopenias. However, serious organ dysfunction can include hemolytic anemia, recalcitrant serositis, neuropsychiatric disease, glomerulonephritis, and vasculitis. The various presentations of systemic lupus are represented in condensed form by the American College of Rheumatology (ACR) Classification Criteria (Table 84.1).[9] These manifestations are not exhaustive, though they do represent some of the more easily objectified characteristics of the disease.

Other common features include constitutional symptoms (fatigue and fever), lymphadenopathy, Raynaud's phenomenon (vasospastic episodes characterized by changes in the color of the digits), alopecia, and a polyclonal gammopathy. In large cohorts, the most frequent manifestations of SLE occurring at any time during the course of disease consist of arthritis (65–90%), cutaneous symptoms (40–85%), constitutional symptoms (40–80%), renal disease (20–70%), and Raynaud's phenomenon (20–60%).[5] Thus, the extreme phenotypic diversity of SLE mirrors its pathophysiologically heterogeneous background.

Diagnosis

As is the case with the classification criteria for rheumatoid arthritis (Case 83), the ACR classification criteria for SLE were designed to allow for systematic and consistent inclusion criteria in clinical trials. While they do serve to underscore many of the salient clinical features of systemic lupus, they were not originally intended as a standardized diagnostic definition. Rather, the diagnosis of lupus is based on a physician's clinical assessment. Consultation by a rheumatologist is therefore often advisable. It is likely that the classification criteria, already modified, will undergo further refinement in time. For example, the ACR now recognizes 19 neurologic and psychiatric manifestations of lupus, rather than simply seizures and psychosis.[1]

The anti–nuclear antibody (ANA), markedly positive in this patient, serves as the archetypal autoantibody. It has been argued that ANA positivity is necessary, but not

Table 84.1 Adapted Version of the ACR Classification Criteria for SLE[9]

Criterion	Definition[a]
Malar rash	Fixed erythema, flat or raised, over the malar eminences, tending to spare the nasolabial folds
Discoid rash	Erythematous raised patches with adherent keratotic scaling and follicular plugging; atrophic scarring may occur in older lesions
Photosensitivity	Skin rash as a result of unusual reaction to sunlight, by patient history or physician observation
Oral ulcers	Oral or nasopharyngeal ulceration, usually painless, observed by physician
Arthritis	Nonerosive arthritis involving 2 or more peripheral joints, characterized by tenderness, swelling, or effusion
Serositis	*Pleuritis*—convincing history of pleuritic pain or rubbing heard by a physician or evidence of pleural effusion, *or pericarditis* documented by ECG or rub or evidence of pericardial effusion
Renal disorder	*Persistent proteinuria* >0.5 g/day or $>3+$ if quantitation not performed, *or cellular casts*—may be red cell, hemoglobin, granular, tubular, or mixed
Neurologic disorder	*Seizures or psychosis*: occurring in the absence of either offending drugs or known metabolic derangements; e.g., uremia, ketoacidosis, or electrolyte imbalance
Hematologic disorder	*Hemolytic anemia* with reticulocytosis, *leukopenia*, $<4000/\mu L$ total on 2 or more occasions, *lymphopenia*, $<1500/\mu L$ on 2 or more occasions, *or thrombocytopenia*, $<100,000/\mu L$ in absence of offending drugs
Immunologic disorder	*Anti-DNA*—antibody to native DNA in abnormal titer, *anti-Sm*—presence of antibody to Smith nuclear antigen, *or* positive finding of *antiphospholipid antibodies* based on (1) an abnormal serum level of IgG or IgM anticardiolipin antibodies, (2) a positive test result for lupus anticoagulant using a standard method, or (3) a false-positive serologic test (VDRL), for syphilis known to be positive for at least 6 months and confirmed by negative *Treponema pallidum* immobilization or fluorescent treponemal antibody absorption test
Antinuclear antibody	An abnormal titer of antinuclear antibody by immunofluorescence or an equivalent assay at any point in time and in absence of drugs known to be associated with "drug-induced lupus" syndrome

[a]Only one from each row satisfies the criterion. For the purpose of identifying patients in clinical studies, a person shall be said to have systemic lupus erythematosus if any 4 or more of the 11 criteria are present, serially or simultaneously, during any interval of observation.
Source: Adopted from ARA 1982 revised criteria.[9] Reprinted with permission of Wiley-Liss, Inc., a subsidiary of John Wiley & Sons, Inc.

sufficient, for the diagnosis of SLE. This observation reflects the extraordinary false-positive rate of low-titer ANAs in the general population (as high as 30%), combined with the low prevalence of systemic lupus. Consequentially, even with a sensitivity approaching 99%, the positive predictive value of ANAs is only approximately 33%. Clearly, this laboratory test alone cannot serve as the basis for the diagnosis of lupus.

However, the negative predictive value of the ANA is calculated to be 99%. In summary, the ANA (when negative) is an excellent test to rule out systemic lupus, as it is virtually required for the diagnosis, but when assessed in a patient without the appropriate clinical features of SLE, false-positive results are common.

Indeed, autoantibody production remains one of the hallmarks of systemic lupus. Although over 100 self-reactive antibodies have been identified, only 10–15 have achieved routine clinical use.[8] The titer of anti-double-stranded DNA (anti-dsDNA) antibodies, for example, predict subsequent nephritis. Interestingly, while the classification criteria refer only to anti-Smith (Sm) antibodies, there are a number of commonly recognized antibodies to extractable nuclear antigens (ENA). Anti-SSA (anti-Ro) antibodies have been associated with a higher frequency of nephritis, as is the case with this patient. It has also been linked to photosensitivity, interstitial lung disease, cytopenias, and neonatal lupus. Anti-SSB (anti-La) antibodies, which are detected less frequently, have also been associated with neonatal lupus. Anti-Sm and anti-RNP antibodies target spliceosomes—proteins crucial to the processing of pre–messenger RNA. Anti-Sm antibodies are purportedly extremely specific for SLE, while anti-RNP antibodies have been associated with Raynaud's phenomenon, myositis, and pulmonary hypertension.

Active systemic lupus, especially within the setting of renal disease, is associated with low levels of serum C3 and C4. The C3 tends to be more sensitive than C4. Although the patient's urine dipstick analysis identified proteinuria in this case, preliminary evidence suggests that a urine protein : creatinine ratio is a much more reliable method of quantifying urinary protein loss. Additionally, while many clinicians do not pursue renal biopsy or initiate aggressive immunosuppressive therapy until after the serum creatinine becomes elevated, recent studies suggest that proteinuria itself may be an independent risk factor for mortality.

Treatment

Many complicated factors influence the choice of therapy in systemic lupus erythematosus. Because the data from studies are fairly limited, clinicians are largely forced to exercise judgment in balancing the need for therapeutic intervention with potentially severe adverse effects, rather than operating from fairly well-validated treatment protocols.

As the name implies, SLE is a prototypic systemic disease. Given all the phenotypic permutations of this malady, the physician must be rigorous in clearly defining (1) which organs are involved (preferably by relying on tissue/biopsy-proven results), (2) the extent/severity of involvement, (3) the patient's comorbidities, and (4) the likely efficacy and toxicities associated with each specific intervention. Once the health care professional has marshaled this information, an informed decision may be made with regard to therapy.

Potential interventions currently include immunosuppressives (azathioprine, cyclophosphamide, mycophenolate mofetil, corticosteroids, and antimalarials, among others), intravenous immunoglobulin, and plasmapharesis, which ostensibly remove the offending antibodies.[4] Biologic therapies, such as rituximab (anti-CD20 antibody), are being actively investigated as potential treatments for SLE. Adjunctive therapy attempts to control those factors that may precipitate worse disease. This may consist of the use of an angiotensin-converting enzyme inhibitor or angiotensin receptor blockade to reduce proteinuria and renovascular hypertension in lupus patients with glomerulonephritis. Similarly, anticoagulation may be indicated for patients with concomitant antiphospholipid syndrome.

References

1. ACR Ad Hoc Committee on Neuropsychic Lupus Nomenclature: The American College of Rheumatology nomenclature and case definitions for neuropsychiatric lupus syndromes. *Arthritis Rheum. 42*:599–608, 1999.

2. ARBUCKLE, M. R., McCLAIN, M. T., RUBERTONE, M. V. ET AL.: Development of autoantibodies before the clinical onset of systemic lupus erythematosus. *N. Engl. J. Med. 349*:1526–33, 2003.

3. HARDIN, J. A.: Directing autoimmunity to nucleoprotein particles: The impact of dendritic cells and interferon alpha in lupus. *J. Exp. Med. 197*:681–5, 2003.

4. HEJAILI, F. F., MOIST, L. M., AND CLARK, W. F.: Treatment of lupus nephritis. *Drugs 63*:257–74, 2003.

5. HOCHBERG, M., SILMAN, A., SMOLEN, J., AND WEINBLATT, M., eds.: *Rheumatology*, Mosby, Philadelphia, 2003.

6. KOTZIN, B. L.: Systemic lupus erythematosus. In *Rheumatology Secrets*, 2nd ed., S. WEST, ed., Hanley & Belfus, Philadelphia, 2002.

7. NATH, S. K., KILPATRICK, J., AND HARLEY, J. B.: Genetics of human systemic lupus erythematosus: The emerging picture. *Curr. Opin. Immunol. 16*:794–800, 2004.

8. SHERER, Y., GORSTEIN, A., FRITZLER, M. J., AND SHOENFELD, Y.: Autoantibody explosion in systemic lupus erythematosus: More than 100 different antibodies found in SLE patients. *Semin. Arthritus Rheum. 34*:501–37, 2004.

9. TAN, E. M., COHEN, A. S., FRIES, J. F. ET AL.: The 1982 revised criteria for the classification of systemic lupus erythematosus. *Arthritis Rheum. 25*:1271–77, 1982 and HOCHBERG, M. C.: Updating the American College of Rheumatology revised criteria for the classification of systemic lupus erythematosus (letter). *Arthritis Rheum. 40*:1725, 1997.

References

Case 85

Woman with Diarrhea and Anemia

Nikola Baumann

A 48-year-old woman presented to her primary care physician with a one-week history of fatigue, weakness, and six to seven bowel movements per day, all of which were watery, greenish-brown, and foul-smelling without any evidence of bleeding. The patient states that the diarrhea was usually associated with abdominal pain and bloating and that the symptoms had been intermittent for over 6 months. The patient had lost 7 lb in the past 2 months. Abdominal exam revealed a soft, flat abdomen with mild diffuse tenderness but no rebound or guarding. A stool specimen tested negative for fecal occult blood and positive for fecal fat. The physician ordered routine laboratory tests and an anemia workup. The results are listed below:

Analyte	Value, Conventional Units	Reference Interval, Conventional units	Value, SI Units	Reference Interval, SI Units
WBC	$9.2 \times 10^3/L$	4–10	$9.2 \times 10^9/L$	4–10
Hemoglobin	10.4 g/dL	12.0–16.0	104 g/L	120–160
Hematocrit	33.2%	37.0–47.0	0.33 volume	0.37–0.47
MCV	82.2 fL	84.0–99.0	Same	Same
Ferritin	6.0 ng/mL	10–291	13.5 pmol/L	23–654
Iron	17 μg/dL	37–170	3.0 μmol/L	6.6–30.4
TIBC	422 μg/dL	250–450	75.5 μmol/L	44.8–80.6
Sodium	137 mmol/L	135–145	Same	Same
Potassium	4.8 mmol/L	3.5–5.3	Same	Same
Chloride	102 mmol/L	98–108	Same	Same
CO_2, total	26 mmol/L	24–32	Same	Same
Urea nitrogen	12 mg/dL	6–20	4.3 mmol/L	2.1–7.1
Glucose	88 mg/dL	65–110	4.8 mmol/L	3.6–6.1
Protein, total	6.7 g/dL	6.3–8.2	67 g/L	63–82
Albumin	4.2 g/dL	3.4–5.0	42 g/L	34–50
AST	38 U/L	10–40	0.65 μkat/L	0.17–0.68
Alkaline phosphatase	76 U/L	40–125	1.3 μkat/L	0.68–2.13

The laboratory results were consistent with iron deficiency anemia and were otherwise normal. The physician then ordered serological testing for celiac disease and gastroenterology (GI) consultation:

Analyte	Value, Conventional Units	Reference Interval, Conventional Units	Value, SI Units	Reference Interval, SI Units
Antigliadin antibodies, IgA	17.0 EU	Negative <20	Same	Same
Antigliadin antibodies, IgG	19.0 EU	Negative <20	Same	Same
Antiendomysial antibodies, IgA screen	Positive	Negative	Same	Same
Antiendomysial antibodies, IgA titer	1 : 160	<1 : 10	Same	Same
Antitissue transglutaminase, IgG	50.0 EU	Neg <20 EU	Same	Same

A GI workup consisted of an upper endoscopy, sigmoidoscopy, and colonoscopy. Results of the flexible sigmoidoscopy and colonoscopy were negative. The esophagogastroduodenoscopy (EGD) revealed minimal esophagitis and gastric and duodenal inflammation. Gastric mucosal biopsies showed normal histology. Random biopsies of the duodenum were reported as "gastric-appearing mucosa with loss of normal villous architecture."

The diagnosis of celiac disease was made on the basis of the biopsy and serology findings, and the patient was placed on a gluten-free diet. She reported alleviation of symptoms and gained weight. Three months later, a follow-up biopsy of the small bowel was performed and histology appeared normal.

Definition of the Disease

Celiac disease (CD), also known as *gluten-sensitive enteropathy*, is an autoimmune disease of the small intestine that is triggered by the ingestion of gluten-containing grains such as wheat, rye, and barley in genetically susceptible individuals.[1-5] In patients with CD, T-cell infiltration into the intestinal epithelium leads to immunity-mediated destruction of the microscopic villi of the small intestine and subsequent malabsorption of nutrients. The major known disease contributors include the environmental factor gluten, as well as a genetic susceptibility in people with HLA-DQ2 or HLA-DQ8 alleles. Other unknown environmental factors may contribute to disease occurrence. Chronic inflammation and immunity-mediated tissue damage in the small intestine, including villous atrophy of the small intestinal mucosa, are characteristic of CD.

Epidemiological studies in the United States and Europe have shown the prevalence of CD to approach 1%.[1,7] The widespread occurrence of the disease has been documented in North and South America, Europe, North Africa, southern and western Asia, and Australia. The clinical presentation of the disease varies greatly, ranging from asymptomatic or "silent" to severe malnutrition. Celiac disease can present anywhere between infancy and adulthood to very old age. In children, the disease typically presents between 6 and 24 months with impaired growth, abnormal stools, abdominal distention, muscle wasting, hypotonia, poor appetite, and irritability.[4] In the long term, pediatric patients may exhibit permanent growth stunting. Adults may present with chronic ill health and GI symptoms, including episodic, nocturnal, or early morning diarrhea, flatulence, vague abdominal discomfort, and weight loss. Steatorrhea can be present in patients with severe CD. However, approximately 50% of adults with CD have no history of diarrhea, and the only diagnostic clue may be the presence of isolated nutritional deficiencies in conjunction with other extraintestinal manifestations. Iron, folate, or vitamin B_{12} deficiency may manifest as anemia, vitamin K deficiency may lead to prolonged prothrombin time, and vitamin D deficiency may be associated with bone diseases.

Extraintestinal Manifestations

CD has been shown to be closely associated with a number of other disorders. Dermatitis herpetiformis, a skin disease characterized by symmetric pruritic papulovesicular lesions and the presence of granular deposits of IgA in the skin, affects 10–20% of patients with CD and responds to withdrawal of gluten from the diet. CD is also strongly associated with type I diabetes and autoimmune thyroid disease, especially hypothyroidism. The prevalence of CD in type I diabetes patients is 3–8%.[2] Patients with untreated CD have an increased risk of certain types of cancer, specifically non-Hodgkin lymphoma, enteropathy-associated T-cell lymphoma, small intestinal adenocarcinoma, and esophageal or oropharyngeal squamous carcinoma. Neurological disorders, including peripheral neuropathy, cerebellar ataxia, epilepsy, and migraine, have also been shown to be associated with CD. Women with untreated CD may present with infertility, and infertility secondary to impotence or abnormally low sperm count is often found in men. A gluten-free diet resolves the CD-associated infertility in both men and women.

Because of the large percentage of CD patients who lack GI symptoms, it is important for the clinician to consider CD in the differential diagnosis in patients who present with those disorders that have been shown to be closely associated with CD.

Differential Diagnosis

In the classic presentation of CD, the differential diagnosis of malabsorption includes distinguishing between the following diseases: tropical sprue, celiac disease, Whipple's disease, irritable bowel syndrome, and inflammatory bowel disease (Crohn's disease and ulcerative colitis). Steatorrhea is often present in malabsorption syndromes and seldom assists in the differential diagnosis.

The "gold standard" for diagnosis is a small bowel biopsy showing histological findings consistent with CD followed by favorable clinical and histological response to gluten-free diet.[2,7] The characteristic, although not specific, pathology of CD is villous atrophy of the small intestinal mucosa. Resolution of the pathology on adherence to a gluten-free diet establishes the diagnosis of CD. Serological tests lend support but are not essential in the diagnosis.

Serological Markers of Celiac Disease

Serological testing for autoantibodies relevant to CD includes measurement of antigliadin antibodies (AGA), serum endomysial antibodies (EMA), tissue transglutaminase antibodies (tTG), and total serum IgA. Antigliadin antibodies are antibodies against the proteins present in the ethanol-soluble fraction of wheat gluten and can be measured using IgA- or IgG-specific AGA ELISA assays. The AGA test is the least sensitive (IgA AGA 75–90%; IgG AGA 69–85%) and least specific (IgA AGA 82–95%; IgG AGA 73–90%) serological test for the diagnosis of CD.[2] The lower sensitivity of AGA is illustrated in this patient's lab results, where AGA IgA and IgG were both negative, even though the other serological tests for CD were positive and the diagnosis of CD was confirmed by biopsy and response to a gluten-free diet.

IgA EMA are detected by indirect immunofluorescence using monkey esophagus or human umbilical cord frozen sections as substrate, and results are expressed as titers. Traditionally EMA was the preferred serological test for CD with the highest sensitivity (85–98%) and specificity (97–100%);[2] however, indirect IF is considered a labor-intensive, observer-dependent method. In 1997, it was shown that tTG is the autoantigen of endomysial antibodies, and ELISA assays for anti-tTG antibodies were developed.[6] IgA tTG antibodies are more sensitive (90–98%) than EMA and have similar specificity (94–97%).[2] Sensitivity and specificity variation are due to differences in methodology and the source of tTG (guinea pig or human recombinant). Approximately 2% of patients with the diagnosis of CD are IgA-deficient, which is a 10–16-fold higher occurrence than observed in the general population.[7] IgA deficiency in patients with CD often leads to negative serological test results in assays using anti-IgA antibodies. It is often useful to measure total serum IgA as part of the diagnostic workup for celiac disease, especially when IgA-based serology assays are being utilized.

The role of serological testing in the diagnosis of CD includes identification of patients for whom biopsy might be warranted because of the presence of characteristic symptoms, or because they are at increased risk for CD due to the presence of associated disorders. Once CD is biopsy-confirmed, serological tests may be used to monitor dietary compliance since they are seldom detectable 6–12 months after the introduction of a gluten-free diet. Further studies and improvements in methodology may allow serological testing to be used for screening of the general population and/or may eliminate the need for biopsy.

Pathogenesis

More than 98% of people with CD carry the HLA-class II molecules HLA-DQ2 and HLA-DQ8.[2] On ingestion of gluten, gluten peptides may preferentially bind to HLA-DQ2 or HLA-DQ8 on antigen-presenting cells leading to proliferation and production of proinflammatory cytokines by T cells in the lamina propria.[1] This inflammatory response induces the release of the intracellular enzyme, tissue transglutaminase (tTG), which is also an autoantigen of the disease. In susceptible individuals exposed to gluten, the production of autoantibodies directed against the proteins tTG and gliadin result in the characteristic inflammation and immunity-mediated tissue damage and collapse of the intestinal villi found in CD.

Treatment

The current treatment for CD is adherence to a strict gluten-free diet in which all products containing wheat, barley, and rye are eliminated. Oats are not toxic to patients with CD; however, it is often difficult to guarantee that commercially available oats are free from contamination by other grains. On a gluten-free diet, patients with CD generally respond quickly, including alleviation of clinical symptoms, normalization of intestinal changes on histology, and disappearance of the associated autoantibodies usually occurring within 6 months.

References

1. GREEN, P. H. R. AND JABRI, B.: Celiac disease. *Lancet.* *362*:383–91, 2003.
2. FARREL, R. J. AND KELLY, C. P.: Diagnosis of celiac sprue. *Am. J. Gastroenterol.* *96*:3237–46, 2001.
3. WONG, R. C. W., STEELE, R. H., REEVES, G. E. M., WILSON, R. J., PINK, A., AND ADELSTEIN, S.: Antibody and genetic testing in celiac disease. *Pathology.* *35*:285–304, 2003.
4. HILL, I. D., BHATNAGAR, S., CAMERON, D. J. S. ET AL.: Celiac Disease: Working Group Report of the First World Congress of Pediatric Gastroenterology, Hepatology, and Nutrition. *J. Ped. Gastroenterol Nutrit.* *35*:S78–88, 2002.
5. CERF–BENSUSSAN, N., CELLIER, C., HEYMAN, M., BROUSSE, N., AND SCHMITZ, J.: Celiac disease: An update on facts and questions based on the 10th International Symposium on Celiac Disease. *J. Ped. Gastroent. Nutrit.* *37*:412–21, 2003.
6. DIETRICH, W., LAAG, E., SCHOPPER, H. ET AL.: Identification of tissue transglutaminase as the autoantigen of celiac disease. *Nat. Med.* *3*:797–801, 1997.
7. ALAEDINI, A. AND GREENE, P. H. R.: Narrative review: Celiac disease: Understanding a complex autoimmune disorder. *Ann. Intern. Med.* *142*:289–98, 2005.

Part Twenty

Analytical Errors

Cases of analytical errors involving heterophile antibody are reported and discussed in Cases 86 and 87 (both edited by AMG); involving the urinary tract and prostate, in Case 88 (edited by MGS); and involving calcium values, in Case 89 (edited by MGS).

Tietz's Applied Laboratory Medicine, Second Edition. Edited by Mitchell G. Scott, Ann M. Gronowski, and Charles S. Eby
Copyright © 2007 John Wiley & Sons, Inc.

Case 86

Where's My Baby?

Jennifer A. Egan and David G. Grenache

A 25-year-old previously healthy woman presented to her physician with 2 weeks of intermittent, mild, abdominal pain. The pain was "crampy," rating 2–3 on a 10-point scale, and located in the midportion of her lower abdomen. It would come and go and was not related to eating. She had tried Pepto-Bismol and ibuprofen, but neither medication provided relief.

There were no significant issues in the patient's medical history. Her only other complaint was irregular menses since menarche at age 13. She was sexually active and reported inconsistent use of condoms. She denied any history of sexually transmitted diseases or pregnancy. The patient was a doctoral student and was nervous about an upcoming presentation to her graduate advisor and felt that her "stomach pain" made it difficult to concentrate.

She also said she had been worried she was pregnant, since her last menses was almost 6 weeks earlier—a time interval even more "irregular" than was usual. However, a urine home pregnancy test was negative just a few days prior to her visit, and she denied any vaginal bleeding, nausea, or breast tenderness. She reported no travel history; no new exposures to foods, chemicals, or drugs; no sick-people contacts; and—with the exception of her upcoming presentation—no new stressors.

Her vital signs including body mass index were normal, and she had no orthostatic hypotension. On exam, her abdomen was soft, nontender, without guarding or rebound. Bowel sounds were present and normoactive. The remainder of the physical was unremarkable.

Laboratory studies were performed and showed her serum electrolytes, renal and liver function tests, and a complete blood count to be within reference ranges. Her serum human chorionic gonadotropin (hCG) was elevated at 49 IU/L (nonpregnant <5 IU/L). No intrauterine or ectopic pregnancy could be identified by transvaginal and abdominal ultrasounds. She was urged to return to the clinic 2 days later for repeat measurement of serum hCG.

Two days later, the serum hCG concentration was unchanged at 55 IU/L. Clinical suspicion was of an abnormal pregnancy, and repeat ultrasound evaluations showed continued indeterminate findings.

She returned 2 days later. At this time, the hCG concentration was 50 IU/L. She had not experienced any further episodes of abdominal pain. Based on the lack of appropriate doubling of hCG concentrations, her physician diagnosed an ectopic pregnancy. Given her

---

Tietz's Applied Laboratory Medicine, Second Edition. Edited by Mitchell G. Scott, Ann M. Gronowski, Charles S. Eby, and Norbert W. Tietz
Copyright © 2007 John Wiley & Sons, Inc.

asymptomatic status and low hCG ($<$5000 IU/L), the patient was given a single intramuscular dose of methotrexate.

She returned to the clinic 7 days later. Her serum hCG concentration was 47 IU/L, and because it had not adequately dropped (a $>$25% decline from pretreatment level is expected), a second dose of methotrexate was administered.

The patient returned to the clinic a week later. Again, her hCG concentration was measured and found to be 58 IU/L, and imaging studies showed no evidence of intrauterine or ectopic pregnancy. She had experienced no further episodes of discomfort and no side effects.

Believing that she "just couldn't be pregnant," the patient stated that she had performed a home pregnancy test the night before and that the result was negative. Her physician decided to repeat the *urine* assay for hCG in the clinic, and that also produced a negative result.

He inquired with the clinical laboratory that performed the serum hCG test and was told that the immunoassay utilized mouse monoclonal antibodies for the quantification of hCG. As the test results were inconsistent with the clinical presentation of the patient, the laboratory technologist indicated that the results might be falsely positive because of the presence of heterophile antibodies in the patient's blood. After treatment of the patient's serum with a heterophile blocking reagent, repeat testing for hCG produced a result of $<$5 IU/L. The physician informed the patient that she had not experienced an ectopic or any other type of pregnancy.

Definition of the Problem

Immunoassay interference by endogenous antibodies reactive against reagent antibodies can be a serious problem. These interfering antibodies are variably referred to as human anti-animal antibodies, human anti-mouse antibodies, or heterophile antibodies. Heterophile (meaning "different affinity") antibodies are classically recognized as antibodies that have broad but weak reactivity for many different antigens. It is believed that they originate from the early stages of antibody production before the high-rate somatic mutations in the antigenically stimulated B cells produce antibodies with higher affinity for their antigens.[1]

It has been argued that heterophile antibodies should be distinguished from the human anti-animal antibodies (HAAAs) produced against specific animal immunoglobulins.[2] Unlike heterophile antibodies, HAAA typically result from exposure to a defined antigen such as treatment with a therapeutic animal immunoglobulin or to pharmaceutical agents derived from animal sources. Other potential sources of immunogens that can produce HAAA include vaccinations, animal husbandry, and even blood transfusions, although in many instances the source of the immunogen is not known.[3] The most commonly encountered HAAA is the human anti–mouse antibody (HAMA). This is most likely due to the use of mouse monoclonal antibodies in therapeutics, which stimulate the formation of HAMA and their common use as reagents in immunoassay systems.

Antibodies demonstrating interference in immunoassays that are not HAAA have also been described. In one report, serum from a patient with an IgM λ-paraprotein due to an *Escherichia coli* septicemia produced inappropriately elevated concentrations of troponin I, thyroid-stimulating hormone, α-fetoprotein, CA-125, and human chorionic gonadotropin.[4]

Mechanism of the Interference

Whether the interfering antibody is truly a heterophile immunoglobulin or a HAAA, the mechanisms by which they interfere with immunoassays remains the same. Figure 86.1 illustrates these different mechanisms. In two-site immunometric assays [panel (a)], two reagent antibodies are used that recognize distinct epitopes on the target antigen. One of these antibodies is bound to a solid phase and is used to capture the target antigen in the specimen, while the other antibody is labeled with a molecule that generates a signal that can be detected (such as a fluorophore). In this type of immunoassay, often called a "sandwich" immunoassay, the final immune complex consists of the target antigen bound between two antibodies. The intensity of the signal is proportional to the concentration of target antigen. The most common interference observed is a positive interference caused by heterophile antibodies crosslinking the capture and label antibodies in the absence of target antigen [panel (a)]. Negative interference producing falsely decreased results, while less common, has been documented.[5,6] Negative interference is

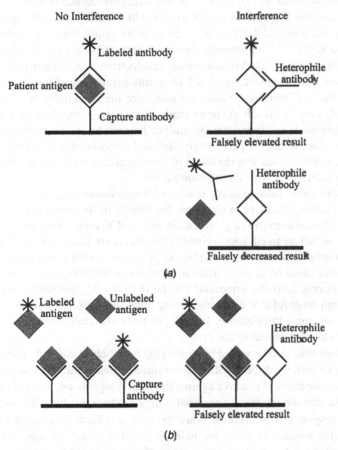

Figure 86.1 Immunoassay formats and potential mechanisms of interference from heterophile antibodies: (a) "sandwich" immunoassay, illustrating how interfering antibodies can cause either false increases or decreases in immunoassays; (b) "competitive" immunoassay, illustrating the mechanism of interference in immunoassays. See the text for an explanation of the mechanism.

caused by the heterophile antibody binding to only one of the two reagent antibodies, thereby preventing reaction with the target antigen [panel (a)].

In a competitive immunoassay, patient antigen and labeled reagent antigen compete for binding to a limited amount of capture reagent antibody [panel (b)]. In this immunoassay format, the concentration of patient antigen is inversely proportional to the intensity of the signal from bound reagent antigen. The presence of heterophile antibodies can cause interference if they bind to the capture antibody and prevent antigen binding. The effect would be a decreased signal intensity resulting in a falsely increased result. Heterophile antibody interference in competitive immunoassays is uncommon because the affinity of the capture antibody to the antigen is considerably stronger than the affinity of the heterophile antibody to the capture antibody. It is presumed that interference is only encountered when the heterophile antibody is present at unusually high concentrations.[7] The rheumatoid factor has also been implicated as a source of interference in a competitive immunoassay.[8]

Prevalence, Detection, and Prevention

Because there is no standard assay to test for them, the actual prevalence of heterophile antibodies and HAAA in clinical specimens is not known, although it is probably quite high.[9] For example, the prevalence of HAMA in three separate populations of blood donors ranged from 9% to 80%.[10–12] Fortunately, few of these antibodies cause interference. One study reported that 8.7% of 3445 immunoassay results from 10 specimens with heterophile antibodies were falsely positive, with 6% of results being clinically misleading.[13]

The low frequency of interference does not minimize the potentially disastrous consequences of a falsely elevated result. As an example, there are reports of women receiving inappropriate therapy such as chemotherapy and/or hysterectomy for presumed gestational trophoblastic disease due to persistently elevated concentrations of hCG.[14] Only after these invasive interventions was the cause of the elevated hCG discovered to be heterophile antibodies interfering with the immunoassay.

Because they can cause false-positive results with immunoassays, clinical suspicion of heterophile antibodies should be high when the results of an immunoassay are not consistent with the clinical scenario (e.g., when the serum hCG concentrations are persistently low positive or fail to trend appropriately). In situations where the analyte being measured is also normally present in the urine, as is the case with hCG, an initial step should be to perform a urine hCG test.[15] Human chorionic gonadotropin CG and its fragments are readily filtered into the urine and can be detected by qualitative urine tests. Because of their high molecular weight, interfering antibodies are not excreted into the urine and thus do not cause interference. In cases of truly elevated serum hCG, filtered hCG molecules would be detected in the urine.

Dilutional studies may also be useful in identifying heterophile antibody interference. Serum samples can be serially diluted with an appropriate diluent and the assay repeated. As the heterophile antibodies are reactive against the assay reagents and not the measured analyte, samples that contain interfering antibodies may produce results that deviate from the expected linear response.[3] For instance, when the sample is diluted by a factor of 2, the analyte concentration should decrease by half its original value. If this appropriate decrease is not observed, a heterophile antibody interference should be suspected.

The use of blocking agents is widely used for detecting and diminishing heterophile antibody interference. These agents may be nonimmune globulin from the same species of animal used to produce the assay antibodies or antibodies with specificity toward human immunoglobulins.[7] Blocking agents bind to heterophile antibodies and prevent their interference in immunoassays, although their effectiveness depends on numerous variables, including the heterophile antibody class, specificity, and concentration. Manufacturers of immunoassays now frequently include blocking agents in assay reagents to reduce interference from heterophile antibodies. Commercial blocking agents are also available. After incubation with blocking reagent, specimens suspected of containing interfering antibodies are reassayed, and results that are significantly lower suggest the presence of heterophile antibodies.

If a patient has a heterophile or a HAAA that produces a false result with one immunoassay, it may be helpful to repeat the test using a different immunoassay that employs antibodies produced from a different animal species. This method is not foolproof, however, as some patients may have broad heterophilic antibodies that are not species-specific. These antibodies may cross-react with multiple animal species and interfere with multiple assays.[16]

Special laboratory techniques are also available to remove interfering antibodies from serum prior to testing. Chromatographic methods such as affinity, cation exchange, and gel filtration chromatography have been used to successfully eliminate interference,[17] as have precipitation methods utilizing polyethylene glycol.[18] Protein A and protein G have also been used to absorb interfering antibodies from human serum.[5,17,6]

If desired, direct testing can be performed to confirm the presence of HAAA in suspected cases, although, as mentioned previously, there is no standard assay for detection. Multiple assay kits are currently available that are primarily sandwich immunoassays utilizing mouse IgG or IgM as capture and label antibodies for the detection of HAMA. Unfortunately, surveys of testing laboratories in the United States and Europe have shown significant intermethod and interlaboratory variability in the use of these assays to detect HAMA.[19]

In addition to the above mentioned steps to detect and eliminate heterophile antibody effects on immunoassay testing, multiple strategies have been attempted to prevent the formation of HAAA in susceptible persons (such as those receiving animal-derived therapies). One of these strategies is to treat patients who are receiving mouse antibody agents with a variety of immunosuppressant drugs. For example, studies have shown that giving patients cyclosporin A may prevent HAMA response.[20] Additionally, modifying the mouse antibody agents before they are administered may reduce HAMA formation. Such modifications include using the less immunogenic portions of the antibody molecule by removing the Fc fragments, using humanized or chimeric antibodies instead of pure mouse antibodies to avoid provoking an immune response, and coating the molecules with water-soluble polyethylene glycol (PEG)—a "stealth" technique—to reduce immunogenicity.[3] These modifications have shown variable success in reducing HAMA formation.

In conclusion, the presence of heterophile antibodies can lead to erroneous results generated by immunoassay techniques. Clinicians who do not recognize this as a possible cause of false-positive tests such as hCG may unnecessarily subject their patients to surgical procedures or chemotherapeutic agents for presumed disease. In order to prevent this inappropriate treatment, clinicians must be aware of the existence of interfering antibodies and have a high suspicion of them in patients who may be at risk.

Importantly, physicians must be strongly advised to contact the clinical laboratory in situations where the clinical picture is not consistent with immunoassay test results. When alerted to such discrepancies, the laboratory can investigate the possibility that heterophile antibodies are present and provide alternative methods of testing.

References

1. LEVINSON, S. S.: Antibody multi-specificity in immunoassay interference. *Clin. Biochem.* 25:77–87, 1992.
2. KAPLAN, I. V. AND LEVINSON, S. S.: When is a heterophile antibody not a heterophile antibody? When it is an antibody against a specific immunogen. *Clin. Chem.* 45:616–8, 1999.
3. KRICKA, L. J.: Human anti-animal antibody interferences in immunological assays. *Clin. Chem.* 45:942–56, 1999.
4. COVINSKY, M., LATERZA, O., PFEIFER, J. D. ET AL.: An IgM lambda antibody to Escherichia coli produces false-positive results in multiple immunometric assays. *Clin. Chem.* 46:1157–61, 2000.
5. HOWANITZ, P. J., LAMBERSON, H. V., HOWANITZ, J. H. ET AL.: Circulating human antibodies as a cause of falsely depressed ferritin values. *Clin. Biochem.* 16:341–3, 1983.
6. LUZZI, V. I., SCOTT, M. G., AND GRONOWSKI, A. M.: Negative thyrotropin assay interference associated with an IgG kappa paraprotein. *Clin. Chem.* 49:709–10, 2003.
7. LEVINSON, S. S. AND MILLER, J. J.: Towards a better understanding of heterophile (and the like) antibody interference with modern immunoassays. *Clin. Chim. Acta* 325:1–15, 2002.
8. NORDEN, A. G., JACKSON, R. A., NORDEN, L. E. ET AL.: Misleading results from immunoassays of serum free thyroxine in the presence of rheumatoid factor. *Clin. Chem.* 43:957–62, 1997.
9. KLEE, G. G.: Interferences in hormone immunoassays. *Clin. Lab. Med.* 24:1–18, 2004.
10. LIPP, R. W., PASSATH, A., AND LEB, G.: The incidence of non-iatrogenic human anti-mouse antibodies and their possible clinical relevance. *Eur. J. Nucl. Med.* 18:996–7, 1991.
11. THOMPSON, R. J., JACKSON, A. P., AND LANGLOIS, N.: Circulating antibodies to mouse monoclonal immunoglobulins in normal subjects—incidence, species specificity, and effects on a two-site assay for creatine kinase-MB isoenzyme. *Clin. Chem.* 32:476–81, 1986.
12. BOSCATO, L. M. AND STUART, M. C.: Incidence and specificity of interference in two-site immunoassays. *Clin. Chem.* 32:1491–5, 1986.
13. MARKS, V.: False-positive immunoassay results: A multicenter survey of erroneous immunoassay results from assays of 74 analytes in 10 donors from 66 laboratories in seven countries. *Clin. Chem.* 48:2008–16, 2002.
14. ROTMENSCH, S. AND COLE, L. A.: False diagnosis and needless therapy of presumed malignant disease in women with false-positive human chorionic gonadotropin concentrations. *Lancet* 355:712–15, 2000.
15. ACOG: Committee opinion: number 278, Nov. 2002. Avoiding inappropriate clinical decisions based on false-positive human chorionic gonadotropin test results. *Obstet. Gynecol.* 100:1057–9, 2002.
16. BRAUNSTEIN, G. D.: False-positive serum human chorionic gonadotropin results: Causes, characteristics, and recognition. *Am. J. Obstet. Gynecol.* 187:217–24, 2002.
17. TURPEINEN, U., LEHTOVIRTA, P., ALFTHAN, H. ET AL.: Interference by human anti-mouse antibodies in CA 125 assay after immunoscintigraphy: Anti-idiotypic antibodies not neutralized by mouse IgG but removed by chromatography. *Clin. Chem.* 36:1333–8, 1990.
18. FIAD, T. M., DUFFY, J., AND MCKENNA, T. J.: Multiple spuriously abnormal thyroid function indices due to heterophilic antibodies. *Clin. Endocrinol.* (Oxford). 41:391–5, 1994.
19. HAMA Survey Group: Survey of methods for measuring human anti-mouse antibodies. *Clin. Chim. Acta* 215:153–63, 1993.
20. WEIDEN, P. L., WOLF, S. B., BREITZ, H. B. ET AL.: Human anti-mouse antibody suppression with cyclosporin A. *Cancer* 73:1093–7, 1994.

Case 87

Elevated Concentrations, but Not Elevated Enough

Ann M. Gronowski

A 45-year-old male schoolteacher presented to his physician because of dizziness, vomiting, and recent vision problems. The patient had spoken to the physician several months prior complaining of recurrent headaches and irritability. The physician had urged him to come in for an examination, but the patient refused, indicating that he was "too busy" and would see if acetaminophen would relieve the headaches. A careful patient history also revealed a several-year decrease in libido and erectile dysfunction.

A blood sample was collected for endocrine testing, and the patient was scheduled for magnetic resonance imaging (MRI). Laboratory results are shown below:

Analyte	Value, Conventional Units	Reference Interval, Conventional Units	Value, SI Units	Reference Interval, SI Units
Prolactin	135 ng/mL	3–20	135 μg/L	3–20
Testosterone	98 ng/dL	280–1100	3.4 nmol/L	0.52–38.2
TSH	1.5 μU/mL	0.6–4.5	1.5 mU/L	0.6–4.5
FSH	1.1 mIU/mL	1.4–15.4	1.1 IU/L	1.4–15.4
LH	0.6 mIU/mL	1.24–7.8	0.6 IU/L	1.24–7.8

Imaging by MRI revealed a 54-mm-diameter, lobulated, locally invasive mass in the anterior skull base and anterior fossa. The diagnosis of a nonfunctioning macroadenoma was made, based on the observation that the serum prolactin concentration was less than 140 ng/mL, and surgical debulking was scheduled. By chance, the patient's sample was repeated by the laboratory as part of internal quality assurance testing. A series of dilutions revealed that the true prolactin concentration was 29,000 ng/mL. The original prolactin measurement was subject to the so-called high-dose "hook effect." The physician was notified immediately of this finding. The physician informed the laboratory that this was a very important finding and changed the patient's diagnosis to a macroprolactinoma. Because these tumors respond best to dopamine agonists, surgery

Tietz's Applied Laboratory Medicine, Second Edition. Edited by Mitchell G. Scott, Ann M. Gronowski, and Charles S. Eby
Copyright © 2007 John Wiley & Sons, Inc.

was canceled and the patient was placed on cabergoline. After several months, the serum prolactin concentration and size of the tumor decreased substantially.

Definition of the Disease

Prolactin-secreting tumors, or prolactinomas, are the most common form of pituitary tumors (~40%). Most prolactinomas are small microadenomas (<1 cm), but a few (<10%) are large macroadenomas (>1 cm). Prolactin's primary function is to stimulate lactation, but it also has effects on gonadal function. Elevated concentrations of serum prolactin in women typically cause infertility, oligo- or amenorrhea, and decreased libido. Galactorrhea occurs in up to 80% of women. In contrast, the most common symptoms of hyperprolactinemia in men include impotence, infertility, decreased libido, headaches, and visual disturbances. Galactorrhea and gynecomastia are rare in men.[2]

In general, serum prolactin concentrations parallel tumor size. Macroadenomas are typically associated with concentrations >375 ng/mL.[1,2] Some are associated with extremely high concentrations, >10000 ng/mL. However, up to 15–20% of macroadenomas are associated with serum prolactin concentrations <100 ng/mL. In such cases, compression of a non-prolactin-secreting tumor on the pituitary stalk, which thus interferes with the delivery of hypothalamic dopamine to the adenohypophysis, should be suspected. It can be difficult to distinguish between macroprolactinomas and nonfunctioning macroadenomas. Precise diagnosis is important because the methods for management of these two entities are quite different. While nonfunctioning macroadenomas respond best to surgical removal, macroprolactinomas respond best to dopamine agonists.

Differential Diagnosis

With a careful history, physical examination, thyroid function testing, and pregnancy test, most hypothalamic–pituitary disease can be excluded. A single serum prolactin concentration is usually adequate to demonstrate hyperprolactinemia. Normal concentrations are generally <20 mg/mL. However, because stress can stimulate prolactin, serum concentrations between 25 and 40 ng/mL should be repeated. The diagnosis of prolactinoma can be confirmed with gadolinium-enhanced MRI. Large pituitary tumors in patients with serum prolactin concentrations <140 ng/mL are considered nonfunctioning macroademnomas and generally respond well to surgical removal, while those found with serum prolactin concentrations of >375 ng/mL are associated with macroprolactinomas and should be treated with dopamine agonists.[1,3]

Serum prolactin is quantified by two-site "sandwich" immunoassays (Fig. 87.1a). In these tests, a capture antibody directed against one site on prolactin is immobilized to a tube, vial, well, or bead. Patient serum is added. The antibody binds, and immobilizes the prolactin in the serum sample (PRL + immobilized antibody). A second ("detection" or "tracer") antibody directed against a distant site on prolactin is linked to a tracer molecule (such as a radioisotope or an enzyme). This forms an immobilized "sandwich" complex (tracer–antibody + PRL + immobilized antibody. After washing, the amount of tracer is measured (in the case of enzyme assays, incubation with substrate is required). The amount of signal is directly proportional to the amount of prolactin in the sample. Quantitative prolactin tests are either "one-step" or "two-step." In a one-step assay, the serum is incubated with both immobilized and tracer antibodies simultaneously. In a two-step assay, the serum is first incubated with the immobilized antibody, and then washed before the addition of the

(a)

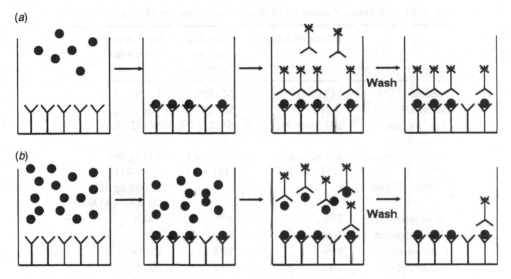

(b)

Figure 87.1   Assay format for (a) one-step sandwich assay with optimal amount of ligand and (b) ligand excess leading to the high-dose "hook effect."

tracer antibody. The one-step protocol is by far the most common protocol used because it is the fastest and the least complicated. The slower two-step protocol, however, avoids problems with hook effect and limits false-positive results due to heterophilic antibodies (see the Case 86, "Where's My Baby?").

The High-Dose "Hook Effect"

The "hook effect" is a major limitation of all one-step immunoassays. It occurs when extremely high concentrations of an analyte, such as prolactin, occupy all the sites on both the capture and detection antibodies, and thus prevent the formation of a "sandwich" immunoassay (Fig. 87.1b). The end result is that few or no tracer antibody + PRL + immobilized antibody complexes will be formed, yielding a false-negative result. The "hook effect" does not occur with two-step quantitative assays because excess analyte is washed away before the tracer antibody is added. Manufacturers of one-step sandwich assays have become more aware of this problem and have designed assays with more capture antibody, hence decreasing the chances of the hook effect. However, the hook effect still occurs and should always be a concern with one-step assays. This problem has been documented for numerous immunoassays, including prolactin, hCG, myoglobin, and PSA.[3–10] Physicians should be aware of these phenomena when evaluating large pituitary masses. As a rule, if a physician finds that the prolactin concentration is inconsistent with the clinical presentation or histological findings, the prolactin test should be repeated with 10- and 100-fold diluted samples.

Two reports, by St. Jean and Petakov, have described the clinical features of patients with pituitary macroadenomas who demonstrate the hook effect with serum prolactin.[3,6] These two studies reported that the hook effect occurs in 6–14% of patients with macroadenomas.[3,6] Both papers were very similar in their findings. In general, the patients who exhibit a hook effect tend to be younger, be male, and have very large (>20-mm) pituitary adenomas (Table 87.1).

Table 87.1 Clinical Features of 69 Patients with Pituitary Macroadenomas

	Macroprolactinomas	Nonfunctioning adenomas	Hook effect adenomas
Number	11 (16%)	54 (78%)	4 (6%)
Sex (M:F)	1:10	25:29	4:0
Age, median (range)	29 (20–70)	51 (21–79)	38 (32–52)
Prolactin, median (range)	428 ng/mL (72–3937)	72 ng/mL (81–151)	100 ng/mL (69–211)
After dilution	—	—	18,062 ng/mL (14,907–44,600)
Giant tumor[a]	27%	30%	100%
Hypogonadism	100%	60%	50%
Galactorrhea	89%	28%	25%
Visual failure	10%	70%	100%
ACTH deficiency	50%	71%	25%
FSH/LH deficiency	18%	52%	25%
TSH deficiency	9%	24%	0%

[a]Tumors with superior margin >20 mm above jugum sphenoidal.

Source: Adapted from St. Jean et al.[3]

It should be noted that this false-negative effect is also observed in qualitative serological agglutination assays used to detect serum antibodies.[11] This phenomenon is referred to as the *prozone effect*. In agglutination assays the reaction will be positive when the optimal ratio of antigen to antibody results in an insoluble precipitate that is visible to the eye. This optimal ratio of antibody to antigen (two to three antibody molecules for each antigen molecule) is referred to as the zone of equivalence. In the zone of antibody excess, or prozone, false-negative test results occur because excess antibodies prevent antibody/antigen lattice formation and hence prevent precipitation (Fig. 87.2).

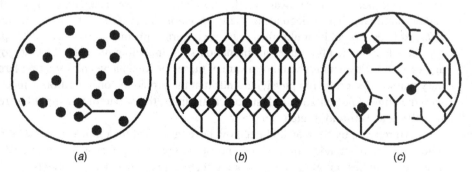

(a) (b) (c)

Figure 87.2 Assay format for agglutination assay and various ratios of antibody and ligand including (a) postzone due to antigen excess, (b) the optimal ratio resulting in a positive result, (zone of equivalence), and (c) prozone due to antibody excess.

Treatment

Treatments for pituitary tumors include either surgery or therapeutic treatment with a dopamine agonist. Although radiation therapy is still an option, it is rarely used in patients with prolactinomas, particularly those with microadenomas. If the tumor is large but non-functional, surgery is indicated. Surgery on functioning prolactin-secreting tumors does not reliably result in a long-term cure, and recurrence of hyperprolactinemia is common. If the tumor secretes prolactin, the treatment of choice is a dopamine agonist. In the United States, two drugs are approved for the treatment of hyperprolactinemia: bromocriptine, an ergot derivative; and cabergoline, a nonergot agonist. Bromocriptine has been the most commonly used agent for many years. Recently, cabergoline was introduced. It is better tolerated by patients and has an extremely long half-life, requiring only a single weekly dose compared to the 1–3 times daily administration of bromocriptine.

References

1. BEVAN, J. S., BURKE, C. W., ESSIRI, M. M., AND ADAMS, C. B.: Misinterpretation of prolactin levels leading to management errors in patients with sellar enlargement. *Am J. Med.* 82:29–32, 1987.
2. SCHLECHTE, J. A.: Prolactinoma. *N. Eng. J. Med.* 349:2035–41, 2003.
3. ST.-JEAN, E., BLAIN, F., AND COMTOIS, R.: High prolactin may be missed by immunoradiometric assay in patients with macroprolactinomas. *Clin. Endocrinol.* 44:305–9, 1996.
4. SCHOFL, C., SCHOFL-SIEGERT, B., KARSTENS, J. H. ET AL.: Falsely low serum prolactin in two cases of invasive macroprolactinoma. *Pituitary* 5:261–5, 2002.
5. FRIEZE, T. W., MONG, D. P., AND KOOPS, M. K.: "Hook effect" in prolactinomas: case report and review of literature. *Endocrine Pract.* 8:296–303, 2002.
6. PETAKOV, M. S., DAMJANOVIC, S. S., NIKOLIC-DUROVIC, M. M. ET AL.: Pituitary adenomas secreting large amounts of prolactin may give false low values in immunoradiometric assays. The hook effect. *J. Endocrinol. Invest.* 21:184–8, 1998.
7. FLAM, F., HAMBRAEUS-JONZON, K., HANSSON, L. O. ET AL.: Hydatidiform mole with non-metastatic pulmonary complications and a false low level of hCG. *Eur. J. Obstet. Gynecol. Reprod. Biol.* 77:235–7, 1998.
8. FIGNON, A., GUILLOTEAU, D., LANSAC, J., AND BESNARD, J. C.: Hook effect in immunoradiometric assay for human chorionic gonadotropine as a marker for trophoblastic disease. *Eur. J. Obstet. Gynecol. Reprod. Biol.* 61:183–4, 1995.
9. KIKUCHI, H., OHTA, A., TAKAHASHI, Y. ET AL.: High-dose hook effect in an immunochromatography-optical quantitative reader method for myoglobin. *Clin. Chem.* 49:1709–10, 2003.
10. FURUYA, Y., CHO, S., OHTA, S. ET AL.: High dose hook effect in serum total and free prostate specific antigen in a patient with metastatic prostate cancer. *J. Urol.* 166:213, 2001.
11. JURADO, R. L., CAMPBELL, J., AND MARTIN, P. D.: Prozone Phenomenon in secondary syphilis. *Arch. Intern. Med.* 153:2496–8, 1993.

Case 88

I Want To Go Home!

Mitchell G. Scott, Ph.D.

The patient is a 56-year-old white male who presented to the emergency department with a history of benign prostatic hypertrophy and now had fever, chills, and painful urination. The patient was diagnosed as likely having a urinary tract infection attributable to urethral obstruction. Blood and urine cultures were obtained, and the patient was discharged with oral levofloxacin antibiotic therapy. Two days later *Escherichia coli* was isolated from the blood and urine cultures, and the patient was called back to the hospital for admission. The patient was started on IV ampicillin/sulbactam and later switched to intravenous cefipime and oral ciprofloxacin following antibiotic sensitivity reports. On the third day of hospitalization, the patient complained of jaw pain but, in general, was beginning to feel better. Because of the jaw pain, tests for cardiac markers were requested. The ECG showed only nonspecific isolated Q wave in lead III and the patient did not complain of any specific chest pain. Other routine chemistry tests performed on this and subsequent days were unremarkable. Cardiac marker tests for the next 5 days were as follows:

Reference Interval	Cardiac Troponin I (<0.1 µg/L)	Creatine Kinase (<200 IU/L)	Creatine Kinase MB (<7 µg/L)
Hospitalizaiton Day			
Day 3 13 : 45	8.7	40	<2
19 : 00	12.7	35	<2
Day 4 06 : 00	17.3		
14 : 40	40.8		
Day 5 06 : 30	58.3	36	<2
20 : 00	106.2		
Day 6 05 : 00	115.0		
12 : 00	153.0	25	<2
Day 7 08 : 45	220.0	26	<2

On the basis of the cardiac troponin I (cTnI) results, he was transferred to the cardiac care unit with a diagnosis of non-Q-wave myocardial infarction. He was started on intravenous heparin, nitroglycerin, lopressor, and aspirin. However, a subsequent full cardiac workup failed to show any signs of ischemia, blockage, or other indications that the patient had suffered an infarct. On day 5 the laboratory noticed the discrepancy between the cTnI

Tietz's Applied Laboratory Medicine, Second Edition. Edited by Mitchell G. Scott, Ann M. Gronowski, and Charles S. Eby
Copyright © 2007 John Wiley & Sons, Inc.

results and CK-MB values and notified the patient's physician and began investigating the unusual results. By day 6 of hospitalization the patient was feeling fine, eating well while sitting up in bed, and insisting on going home. By day 7 studies were completed demonstrating that the patient's antibody response to his *E. coli* infection exhibited heterophilic, anti–mouse immunoglobulin activity and that the cTnI values were a result of interfering antibodies.[1]

Studies performed using samples from this patient also showed abnormally increased immunoassay results for thyrotropin, human chorionic gonadotropin, α-fetoprotein, and CA-125 that were consistent with hyperthyroidism and pregnancy, and suggestive of an occult neoplasm such as hepatic or ovarian cancer. None of these diagnoses were consistent with the rest of his medical examination and were also the result of an endogenous interfering antibody. In addition, the patient had what appeared to be a restricted IgM,λ paraprotein by immunofixation. When samples from the patient were incubated with either irrelevant murine monoclonal antibodies or formalin-killed *E. coli* organisms from his own blood culture, normal immunoassay values were obtained and the IgM,λ paraprotein disappeared from immunofixation.

Follow-up of Patient

One year following this hospitalization the patient still exhibited a cTnI value of 2.5 ng/mL using the same cTnI assay. In the interim, the manufacturer had modified the assay to minimize HAMA interference, and when the patient's samples that had produced cTnI values >100 ng/mL in the old version of the assay, were reanalyzed in the modified assay, all samples produced values <0.1 mg/mL. Three years after this admission there were no longer any detectable interfering antibodies in the patient's serum.

Endogenous Interfering Antibodies

Clinical laboratories strive to provide accurate and reproducible data to aid in the diagnosis and management of disease. However, erroneous values can be reported when the concentration of an analyte changes in a blood sample before it reaches the laboratory (due to improper drawing, storage, or handling of the sample) or when substances present in the sample interfere with the analytic process. The most common interferences are those caused by hemolyzed, icteric, or lipemic samples where the substance interferes with spectrophotometric measurements. Another, less appreciated, interferrant is the presence of endogenous antibodies with specificities that can cause erroneous results in immunoassays.

Immunoassays

Immunoassays are common tools in the clinical laboratory for determining the concentrations of proteins, hormones and drugs in blood or other body fluids. Most diagnostic immunoassays can be classified as either competitive inhibition assays or double antibody sandwich assays (Fig. 88.1). Inhibition assays are used to measure small molecules such as drugs, steroids, and thyroid hormones, while the sandwich assay format is generally used to measure larger protein molecules. In inhibition assays, antibodies are attached to a solid phase where they bind a labeled drug or hormone. Unlabeled drug or hormone in the patient sample competes with the labeled drug or hormone for binding to the antibodies.

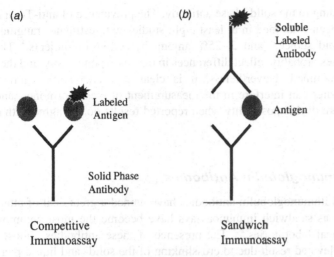

Figure 88.1 Typical assay configurations for competitive immunoassays (a), where endogenous antigen competes with labeled antigen for binding to a solid-phase antibody, and for two-site sandwich assays (b), where endogenous antigen is bound by a solid-phase antibody and a signal is generated when labeled antibody in solution binds another epitope on the antigen.

The amount of labeled drug or hormone bound by the antibody is inversely proportional to the amount of the substance in the patient sample. Sandwich assays are configured so that one set of antibodies is attached to a solid phase and a second set of labeled antibodies is in solution. After the protein of interest is bound to the solid-phase antibody, the soluble, labeled antibody forms a "sandwich" by binding to a second epitope on the protein. In this format the signal generated by the labeled antibody is directly proportional to the concentration of the protein in the patient sample.

Since the first competitive immunoassay was described in the 1950s by Berson and Yalow, the analytic specificity and sensitivities of immunoassays have improved tremendously so that clinical laboratories now routinely measure picomolar concentrations of a protein in blood in as little as 10 minutes. While these assays are robust and very accurate, clinicians need to be aware that there is a low incidence of patients who have endogenous antibodies that may interfere in these assays and lead to erroneous results.[2,3] The types of interfering antibodies can be classified into two general categories: endogenous autoantibodies and human anti–animal immunoglobulin (Ig) antibodies.

Autoantibodies

Endogenous autoantibodies to the analyte of interest can cause a falsely positive value in competitive immunoassays by binding the labeled hormone or drug and preventing it from being bound by the immobilized antibody. Examples of this have been described in assays that measure thyroxine (T4), tri-iodothyronine (T3), and testosterone.[4] Falsely decreased results due to endogenous autoantibodies have been described in competitive immunoassays for T3 and in sandwich assays for cardiac troponin I (cTnI).[5] The prevalence of interfering autoantibodies to most endogenous protein or hormone antigens is believed to be extremely low with only case reports described for most analytes. Autoantibodies to T3 and T4 have been examined more systematically; the most common finding is a falsely increased value.[4] This is due to the autoantibodies binding the labeled T3 or T4 and preventing their binding to the solid-phase antibody. The prevalence of anti-T4 or anti-T3 autoantibodies has been examined in at least eight studies with estimates ranging within 0–1.8% for euthyroid subjects and 2–25% among hyperthyroid subjects.[4] The wide ranges of the estimates probably reflect differences in the study populations and the immunoassay formats examined. Nevertheless, it is clear that endogenous anti–thyroid hormone autoantibodies can interfere in the measurement of these hormones, and clinicians should be aware of this possibility when reported results do not agree with clinical impression.

Anti-Animal Immunoglobulin Antibodies

Human anti–animal immunoglobulin antibodies have gained a great deal of attention in the recent literature as sandwich immunoassays have become the most common assay format used in clinical laboratories.[2,3] The presence of these antibodies almost always results in a falsely elevated result due to crosslinking of the solid- and liquid-phase antibodies even in the absence of the analyte (Fig. 88.2). Because murine monoclonal antibodies are used in most commercial diagnostic immunoassays, the anti–animal Ig antibody of most concern is human anti–mouse Ig antibodies (HAMA). The literature is replete with descriptions of patients with circulating HAMA that cause positive interferences in two-site "sandwich" immunometric assays. Falsely elevated results due to HAMA antibodies have been described for CEA, CA-125, TSH, AFP, cardiac troponin I, and hCG.[2,3] HAMA interference in HCG assays has gained particular attention due to the mistreatment of several patients believed to have trophoblastic disease as a result of falsely elevated hCG values[6] (see also Case 86). In the patient described here a HAMA antibody interfered and caused the markedly elevated cTnI even when he felt well, wished to go home, and had no other signs of myocardial infarction.[1]

The prevalence of interfering HAMA in the general population has been estimated to be as low as 0.7% and as high as 10%.[2] With a few exceptions the etiology of HAMA or other human anti–animal immunoglobulin antibodies is unclear. The use of murine

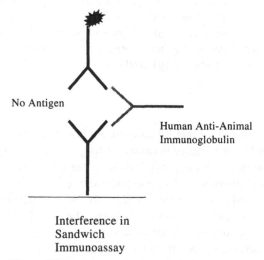

Figure 88.2   False-positive interference in a sandwich assay due to a human anti–animal immunoglobulin antibody crosslinking the solid phase and soluble antibodies in the absence of antigen.

monoclonal antibody–derived products for therapeutic purposes, or as diagnostic imaging tools, is an easily understood cause of HAMA antibodies.[2] However, even the lowest estimate of the prevalence of interfering antibodies is too high to be accounted for by individuals receiving parenteral administration of murine monoclonal antibody products. Beyond this, the etiology has been speculated to be a result of exposure to animal proteins in foods or from farm and other animal handling areas.[2]

More common than "true" anti–animal immunoglobulin antibodies, and of particular interest to clinical laboratories, are heterophilic antibodies that cross-react with animal immunoglobulins and crosslink the solid-phase capture antibody to the soluble detection antibody. When this occurs in two-site sandwich immunoassays, it almost always results in a false-positive signal. Heterophilic antibodies are those that bind multiple antigens as best represented by the IgM antibody against the Paul–Bunnell antigen on sheep, horse, and bovine RBC that develop in immune responses to the Epstein–Barr virus and form the basis for the "monospot" test. What induces heterophilic antibodies with HAMA activity is also a matter of speculation. Among antibodies that bind multiple antigens are those that are the products of germline VH and VL genes, some of which react with self-Ig and play an important role in the development of the mature immune system.[7] Related to these are rheumatoid factors, which are IgM anti-Ig antibodies. Recently, rheumatoid factor antibodies were clearly demonstrated to interfere in assays for free T4 and cTnI.[8,9] Because rheumatoid factor antibodies are relatively common in the elderly and patients with autoimmune disease, it is possible that these heterophilic antibodies may account for many instances of interference in immunometric assays. Finally, microbial antigens can induce broadly reactive heterophilic antibodies that also bind immunoglobulins.[10] In this patient it was demonstrated that the interfering antibody was an anti–E. coli antibody induced by an E. coli urinary tract infection that also avidly bound murine immunoglobulin.[1]

Prevalence of Interfering HAMA Antibodies

As mentioned above, estimates of the prevalence of interfering antibodies vary tremendously in the literature. One study using a cardiac troponin I assay known to be sensitive to HAMA interference examined the prevalence of interfering antibodies in 14,309 patients.[11] Twenty-five patients were found to have falsely elevated cTnI values due to HAMA antibodies. This prevalence of 0.17% is near the lower estimates in the literature. Half of the interfering antibodies were IgG and half were IgM. Interestingly, 8 of 13 patients for whom medical records were available had recent histories of bacterial infection, strengthening the theory that interfering heterophilic antibodies can be induced by microbial infection.

Detecting and Minimizing the Effect of Interfering Antibodies

Unfortunately, there are few methods available to the laboratory to detect the presence of endogenous interfering antibodies before reporting of results. One approach is rapid detection of inconsistent results between two related immunoassays. For instance, a high TSH value and a simultaneous high free T4 might suggest an interference in one of the assays. Another approach to detect these interferences in real time is to perform simultaneous analysis of an undiluted serum sample and a sample diluted 1 : 5. When HAMA interference is present, values from an immunoassay seldom exhibit a linear dilution pattern. Thus, when nonlinear results are observed, the laboratory can investigate for the presence of HAMA interference. However, this approach is costly and time-consuming considering the low prevalence of these interfering antibodies and is reserved only for those immunoassays that we have found to be particularly susceptible to HAMA interference. Taken together, it continues to be very important that clinicians be aware of this possibility and contact the laboratory for further investigations when the result of an immunoassay is inconsistent with a patient's clinical presentation.

Knowledge of heterophilic antibody interferences in immunoassays has led the FDA to require manufacturers to include the following statement in their package inserts: "As with any assay employing mouse antibodies, the possibility exists for interference by human anti-mouse (HAMA) in the sample." Manufacturers of diagnostic assays are also taking steps to minimize the impact of interfering anti–animal immunoglobulin antibodies. One approach has been to add "blocking" agents to immunoassay formulations. These agents generally consist of normal serum or irrelevant immunoglobulins of the same species used in the assay reagents. The goal of this approach is to saturate HAMA or heterophilic antibody activity in the patient sample so that the HAMA antibodies do not crosslink the analyte-specific antibodies of the assay.

References

1. COVINSKY, M., LATERZA, O., PFEIFER, J. D., FARKAS-SZALLASI, T., AND SCOTT, M. G.: An IgMλ antibody to Eschericia coli produces false-positive results in multiple immunometric assays. *Clin. Chem.* 46:1157–61, 2000.
2. KRICKA, L. J.: Human anti-animal antibody interferences in immunological assays. *Clin. Chem.* 45:942–56, 1999.
3. ISMAIL, A. A. A. AND BARTH, J. H.: Wrong biochemistry results (editorial). *Brit. Med. J.* 323:705–6, 2001.
4. DESPRÉS, N. AND GRANT, A. M.: Antibody interference in thyroid assays: A potential for clinical misinformation. *Clin. Chem.* 44:440–54, 1998.
5. BOHNER, J., VON PAPE, K. W., HANNES, W., AND STEGMANN, T: False-negative immunoassay results for cardiac troponin I probably due to circulating troponin I autoantibodies (letter). *Clin. Chem.* 42:2046, 1996.
6. COLE, L. A., RINNE, K. M., SHAHABI, S., AND OMRANI, A.: False-positive hCG assay results leading to unnecessary surgery and chemotherapy and needless

occurrences of diabetes and coma (letter). *Clin. Chem.* 45:313–4, 1999.
7. CASALI, P. AND NOTKINS, A. L.: CD5$^+$ B lymphocytes, polyreactive antibodies and the human B cell repertoire. *Immunol. Today 10*:364–70, 1989.
8. NORDEN, A. G. W., JACKSON, R. A., NORDEN, L. E., ET AL.: Misleading results from immunoassays of serum free thyroxine in the presence of rheumatoid factor. *Clin. Chem.* 43:957–62, 1997.
9. DASGUPTA, A. ET AL.: False positive troponin I in the MEIA due to the presence of rheumatoid factors in serum. *Am. J. Clin. Pathol. 112*:753–6, 1999.
10. POSNET, D. N. AND EDINGER, J.: When do microbes stimulate rheumatoid factor? *J. Exp. Med. 185*:1721–3, 1997.
11. KIM, W. J., LATERZA, O. F., HOCK, K. G. ET AL.: Performance of a revised cardiac troponin method that minimizes interferences from heterophilic antibodies. *Clin. Chem. 48*:1028–34, 2002.

Case 89

Is That Really the Calcium Value?

Mitchell G. Scott

A 72-year-old male was transferred from an outside hospital after concerns that a previously repaired abdominal aneurysm might be leaking. The patient had an open repair of an abdominal aneurysm 8 years prior to this presentation. He had presented to the outside hospital for evaluation of an enlarged prostate, weakness, and vague complaints of lower back pain. An abdominal computed tomography (CT) scan was performed, and an incidental finding of a large, possibly leaking abdominal aneurysm was observed in the same area as the previous graft. He was immediately transferred to a tertiary care hospital. On admission the patient was in no acute distress and denied any fevers, chills, abdominal pain, shortness of breath, nausea, vomiting, or diarrhea. Magnetic resonance imaging (MRI) studies with and without contrast agents were ordered. Laboratory values on admission were as follows:

Analyte	Value, Conventional Units	Reference Interval, Conventional Units	Value, SI Units	Reference Interval, SI Units
Sodium	141 mmol/L	135–145	Same	Same
Potassium	4.3 mmol/L	3.3–4.9	Same	Same
Chloride	107 mmol/L	97–110	Same	Same
Total CO$_2$	21 mmol/L	22–32	Same	Same
Glucose (random)	102 mg/dL	65–199	5.7 mmol/L	3.6–11.1
Creatinine	1.9 mg/dL	0.7–1.5	168 μmol/L	62–133
Urea nitrogen	26 mg/dL	8–25	9.3 mmol/L	2.8–8.9
Calcium	8.7 mg/dL	8.6–10.3	2.17 mmol/L	2.15–2.58
RBC	3.86 × 10/μL	4.5–5.7	3.86 × 10^{12}/L	4.5–5.7
Hemoglobin	11.4 g/dL	13.8–17.2	114 g/L	138–172
WBC	8.0 × 10^3/μL	3.8–9.8	8 × 10^9/L	3.8–9.8
Platelets	257 × 10^3/μL	140–440	257 × 10^9/L	140–440

The contrast agent for the MRI studies was the gadolinium, chelate, gadodiamide, and the MRI studies revealed a large, 8-cm abdominal aneurysm surrounding the previous graft with evidence of contrast agent leaking into the aneurysm sac. The aneurysm and

Tietz's Applied Laboratory Medicine, Second Edition. Edited by Mitchell G. Scott, Ann M. Gronowski, and Charles S. Eby
Copyright © 2007 John Wiley & Sons, Inc.

surrounding swollen soft tissue were impinging the right renal artery and ureter, leading to marked right kidney atrophy. Following these findings, surgery was scheduled the next day. Presurgery laboratory values were as follows:

Analyte	Value, Conventional Units	Reference Interval, Conventional Units	Value, SI Units	Reference Interval, SI Units
Sodium	137 mmol/L	135–145	Same	Same
Potassium	3.9 mmol/L	3.3–4.9	Same	Same
Chloride	104 mmol/L	97–110	Same	Same
Total CO_2	25 mmol/L	22–32	Same	Same
Glucose (random)	99 mg/dL	65–199	5.5 mmol/L	3.6–11.1
Creatinine	1.7 mg/dL	0.7–1.5	151 mmol/L	62–133
Urea nitrogen	18 mg/dL	8–25	6.4 mmol/L	2.8–8.9
Calcium	6.4 mg/dL	8.6–10.3	1.6 mmol/L	2.15–2.58
RBC	$4.0 \times 10^6/\mu L$	4.5–5.7	$4.0 \times 10^{12}/L$	4.5–5.7
Hemoglobin	12.0 g/dL	13.8–17.2	120 g/L	138–172
WBC	$7.8 \times 10^3/\mu L$	3.8–9.8	$7.8 \times 10^{9/}/L$	3.8–9.8
Platelets	$277 \times 10^3/\mu L$	140–440	$277 \times 10^{9/}/L$	140–440

After verifying the low calcium value, the laboratory phoned a nurse on the floor about the calcium value, which was a physician alert value. About one hour later the laboratory was contacted by the patient's physician asking if the low calcium value was "for real." The physician was considering administering calcium gluconate and postponing surgery. The calcium value was repeated by an alternative method and found to be 8.8 mg/dL. Once the physician was satisfied that the patient was not hypocalcemic, an open repair of the abdominal aneurysm was performed. Surgery was successful, and the patient was discharged in stable condition 5 days later.

Definition of Hypocalcemia

Calcium is the most tightly regulated of all electrolytes and has critical roles in many physiological functions, including muscle contraction, hormone secretion, cell division, and intracellular signaling pathways. It is also the most abundant cation in the body, with 99% of the total body calcium found in bone. Less than 1% of total body calcium is found in the blood, but this extracellular pool of calcium provides a pool for maintaining intracellular calcium, bone mineralization, and membrane potentials of cells. Intraindividual biologic variation is estimated to be only 2–3%. In the blood, calcium exists in three forms; 50% is the free (or ionized) form, 40% is bound to membrane proteins (mainly albumin), and 10% is complexed with anions such as bicarbonate, lactate, phosphate, and citrate. It is the free/ionized form of calcium in the blood that is biologically active, and it is this concentration that is tightly regulated by PTH and 1,25-hydroxy vitamin D (see also Case 31). Hypocalcemia is defined as a total blood calcium, concentration below 8.6 mg/dL which may represent a decrease in the free calcium, the bound calcium, or both. Symptoms of hypocalcemia include muscular excitability, tetany and seizures, and extreme hypocalcemia can lead to hypotension and ECG abnormalities.

Differential Diagnosis of Hypocalcemia

Probably the most common cause of hypocalcemia in hospitalized patients is due to hypo-albuminemia following surgery and fluid replacement. In this setting the total calcium will decrease by ~0.8 mg/dL for every 1-mg/dL decrease in albumin. Even though the total blood calcium in these patients is low, they will not show symptoms of hypocalcemia because the free/ionized calcium concentrations will be normal. In these patients the presence of a true hypocalcemia can be determined only by measuring ionized calcium using an ion-specific electrode. Chronic renal failure is another common cause of hypocalcemia and is a result of the hyperphosphatemia, low 1,25-hydroxy vitamin D, and skeletal resistance to PTH that occurs in renal failure (see also Case 29). In the present case, the elevated serum creatinine concentration and the right kidney atrophy both suggested that chronic renal failure was a possible cause of the observed hypocalcemia. Hypomagnesemia is another cause of hypocalcemia, as this decreases the secretion of PTH and also results in end-organ resistance to PTH. Other, rarer causes of hypocalcemia include hypoparathyroidism following parathyroidectomy and pseudohypoparathyroidism due to an inherited end-organ resistance to PTH. In the former, PTH concentrations will be low in a setting of hypocalcemia, while in the latter, the PTH concentrations will be elevated. Finally, patients undergoing plasma pheresis can exhibit classic symptoms of hypocalcemia, including muscle twitching and tetany, but will have normal total calcium concentrations in their blood. However, these patients will have a decreased ionized calcium, which is a result of increased complexed calcium due to citrate in the pheresis exchange fluid. While measurement of ionized calcium is readily available today and accurately assesses the biologically active calcium, it is not recommended for routine calcium measurements in chemistry panels. This is due to the change in pH that occurs with serum/plasma samples as they are processed in most laboratory labs. An increase of 0.1 pH units will increasase the ionized calcium value by ~0.2 mg/dL, due to increased albumin binding of calcium as the H+ ion concentration decreases. Thus, ionized calcium samples should be handled anearobically and tested as rapidly as possible.

One recently discovered but not widely recognized cause of pseudohypocalcemia is the presence of gadolinium-based contrast agents in the blood. This was the cause of the initial low calcium reading in this patient.

Gadolinium

Gadolinium, a lanthanide ion, is routinely administered intravenously as a contrast agent in magnetic resonance imaging examinations. Currently, there are four available gadolinium-based contrast agents on the U.S. market: gadodiamide (Omniscan; Amersham Health), gadopentetate dimeglumine (Magnevist; Schering), gadoversetamide (Opti-MARK; Mallinckrodt Medical), and gadoteridol (Prohance; Bracco). In April 2002, the manufacturers of Omniscan issued a change in product labeling to state that Omniscan interferes with colorimetric serum calcium determinations, producing falsely low calcium measurements. Almost simultaneously, an in vitro diagnostics company also issued a user bulletin at this time alerting clinical laboratories to the effect of this agent in their colorimetric calcium method. That method is one of the methods used by the clinical chemistry laboratory at this patient's hospital.

Characteristics of gadolinium that make it favorable as a contrast agent include its high paramagnetism and its exceptionally long electronic relaxation time. However, gadolinium ions interact with calcium-dependent biological systems and calcium channels[1] and also precipitate above pH 6, which can lead to gadolinium being trapped in the liver and other phagocytic tissues. These two characteristics of gadolinium make it necessary to chelate the ion with appropriate polyamino-polycarboxylic ligands for clinical use. These gadolinium chelates have favorable safety profiles—they are associated with no clinical incidence of nephrotoxicity[2] and with an extremely low incidence of allergic reactions.[3]

Gadolinium Interference with Calcium Measurement

Colorimetric methods for determining the concentration of total calcium in blood are based on the change of color when calcium binds to dyes such as o-cresolphthalein (OCP) or Arsenazo III. An interference in calcium values has been documented for gadodiamide and gadoversetamide in methods using OCP,[4–6] and for gadodiamide with Arsenazo III. In the OCP method used at this patient's hospital, calcium forms a purple complex with OCP that is measured with a spectrophotometer. The interference is due to the complete displacement of gadolinium[4,7] ion from gadodiamide by OCP, followed by the formation of a new gadolinium complex with OCP.[8] This complex has UV absorption characteristics different from those of the calcium–OCP complex, which causes the artifactually decreased calcium measurements observed in the presence of gadodiamide. Because this reaction occurs after OCP has been added, the observed calcium value does not reflect the true in vivo plasma calcium level. Gadolinium chelates do not affect ionized calcium measurements using ion-selective electrodes. Gadopentate dimeglumine and gadoteridol do not interfere with the OCP method.[7] The total displacement of Gd from its ligand by OCP is thought to be related to the weaker stability constants of gadodiamide and gadoversetamide (log $K_{eq} = 16.9$ and 16.6, respectively) when compared to other gadolinium chelates (gadopentate dimeglumine, 22.1; gadoteridol, 25.8).[5]

At one large medical center 20,000 MRI examinations were performed annually with approximately 14,000 patients/year receiving gadolinium chelate infusions. Calcium values were ordered for approximately 500 (3.6%) of these patients. In a study of 116 samples from 99 patients receiving gadolinium contrast medium, at least 28% of the samples had a clinically significant error (>0.7 mg/dL) when their plasma calcium was measured by the Roche OCP method.[7] Another study reported that a decrease >2 mg/dL in the plasma calcium measurement was noted in 4% of patients who had received gadodiamide infusions.[5] All of these patients were in the hypocalcemic range; 25 were in the alert range. However, none of these patients was noted to have symptoms characteristic of hypocalcemia. Thus, the decreased calcium values seen after administration of Omniscan are the result of an interference in the measurement and do not reflect the actual plasma calcium concentrations of the patients.

When interference due to gadodiamide is suspected, it may be helpful to measure ionized calcium or to use a method that is minimally affected by this interference.[7] The latter was done on this patient and assured the physician that the patient did not need an infusion of calcium gluconate and that he could be taken to surgery.

Gadolinium in Patients with Renal Insufficiency

In healthy subjects gadodiamide has a half-life of 78 minutes, and is cleared primarily by the kidney. However, observed periods of unexpectedly low calcium values persisting for

Table 89.1 Suggested Waiting Time between Administration of Gadodiamide and Collection of Sample for Calcium Determination[7]

Waiting time should be	If estimated GFR is
50 hours	20
18 hours	30
11 hours	40
8 hours	50
6 hours	60
5 hours	75
4 hours	90
3 hours	130

Source: Adapted from Ref. 7.

up to 2 days following contrast-enhanced MRI studies have been described. All of these occurred in patients with decreased renal function. Spuriously low calcium values have been reported in patients with severe renal insufficiency for up to 4.5 days after gadodiamide administration.[5]

Using calcium measurement data from 99 patients, a model was developed for the impact of this agent on plasma calcium values measured by an OCP method using the patient's GFR and the time elapsed since administration of gadodiamide.[7] This model can be used to calculate the minimum time after gadodiamide injection that is required to eliminate falsely decreased calcium values with a common OCP method (Table 89.1). During this period, or for a patient with unknown renal function, other calcium methods, such as ionized calcium measurement, should be used. The interference described above has been reported up to 188 hours after gadodiamide infusion in a patient with severely impaired renal function.[5]

References

1. BOURNE, G. W. AND TRIFARO, J. M.: The gadolinium ion: A potent blocker of calcium channels and catecholamine release from cultured chromaffin cells. *Neuroscience* 7:1615–22, 1982.
2. RUNGE, V. M.: Safety of magnetic resonance contrast media. *Top. Magn. Reson. Imaging* 12:309–14, 2001.
3. SHELLOCK, F. G. AND KANAL, E.: Safety of magnetic resonance imaging contrast agents. *J. Magn. Reson. Imaging* 10:477–84, 1999.
4. LIN, J. ET AL.: Interference of magnetic resonance imaging contrast agents with the serum calcium measurement technique using colorimetric reagents. *J. Pharm. Biomed. Anal.* 21:931–43, 1999.
5. PRINCE, M. R. ET AL.: Gadodiamide administration causes spurious hypocalcemia. *Radiology* 227:639–46, 2003.
6. DOORENBOS, C. J., OZYILMAZ, A., AND VAN WIJNEN, M.: Severe pseudohypocalcemia after gadolinium-enhanced magnetic resonance angiography. *N. Engl. J. Med.* 349:817–8, 2003.
7. KANG, H. P., ET AL.: Model for predicting the impact of gadolinium on plasma calcium measured by the o-cresolphthalein method. *Clin. Chem.* 50:741–6, 2004.

Part Twenty-One

Miscellaneous

Three cases in this section present and discuss gout in Case 90 (edited by
CSE), alcoholic liver disease (edited by MGS) in Case 91, and autoimmune
hemolytic anemia in Case 92 (edited by CSE), the final case in this volume.

Tietz's Applied Laboratory Medicine, Second Edition. Edited by Mitchell G. Scott, Ann M. Gronowski, and
Charles S. Eby
Copyright © 2007 John Wiley & Sons, Inc.

Case 90

A Man with Fever and Acute Polyarthritis

William Eugene Davis

A 51-year-old Caucasian male was hospitalized in a local hospital after presenting to the emergency room with a 2-day history of pain in the hands and shoulders and upper extremity weakness. He was febrile and reported a sore throat. Creatine kinase (CK) level and electromyography (EMG) were normal. Antinuclear antibodies and rheumatoid factor were absent. A throat culture grew group A streptococcus, and penicillin was given. On the third hospital day he developed difficulty walking due to pain in the knees and left ankle, and he was then transferred to the university hospital with fever and polyarthritis.

The patient gave a history of occasional sore throats that were rarely treated with antibiotics and a history of intermittent knee pain for several years. He complained of dysuria of one-week duration. He had no regular sexual partner and reported a new sexual contact one month previously. Social history revealed a seventh-grade education and employment as a parking lot attendant. His father died of cirrhosis and his mother, of suicide. He did not smoke but drank approximately 10 beers per week.

The temperature was 101.4°F (38.6°C), and other vital signs were normal. On physical examination he was mildly obese. The pharynx was not inflamed. A nonradiating systolic murmur was noted at the left sternal border. The physical examination was otherwise normal except for the musculoskeletal findings. Swelling, tenderness, and warmth were noted in the left second distal and third proximal interphalangeal joints, both wrists, the left elbow, both knees, and the left ankle and the shoulders were tender. Joint pain precluded assessment of motor strength.

On admission, blood, urine, and throat cultures were obtained. Admission laboratory data included the following:

Analyte	Value, Conventional Units	Reference Range, Conventional Units	Value, SI Units	Reference Range, SI Units
WBC	$10.8 \times 10^3/\mu L$	4.8–10.8	$10.8 \times 10^9/L$	4.8–10.8
Hemoglobin	15 g/dL	13–16	150 g/L	130–160
Neutrophils	55%	40–76	0.55	0.40–0.76

Tietz's Applied Laboratory Medicine, Second Edition. Edited by Mitchell G. Scott, Ann M. Gronowski, and Charles S. Eby

Analyte	Value, Conventional Units	Reference Range, Conventional Units	Value, SI Units	Reference Range, SI Units
Bands	9%	0–10	0.09	0.00–0.10
Lymphocytes	23%	20–52	0.23	0.20–0.52
Monocytes	12%	1–10	0.12	0.01–0.10
Hemoglobin	14 g/dL	12–16	140 g/L	120–160
Erythrocyte sedimentation rate	125 mm/h	0–15	Same	
C-reactive protein	20 mg/dL	0.0–1.4	200 mg/L	0.0–14
Urea nitrogen	12 mg/dL	7–18	4.3 mmol/L	2.5–6.4
Creatinine	1.2 mg/dL	0.5–1.4	106 μmol/L	44–124
Glucose	111 mg/dL	75–105	6.2 mmol/L	4.2–5.8
Urate	6.4 mg/dL	2.4–7.5	381 mmol/L	0.14–0.45

Aspiration of synovial fluid from the right knee and left ankle revealed the following:

Analyte	Right Knee	Left Ankle	Reference Interval
Appearance	Straw-colored	Cloudy	Clear, straw
Leukocytes	8750/μL $(8.75 \times 10^9/L)$	62,200/μL $(62.20 \times 10^9/L)$	63/μL $< 0.15 \times 10^9/L$
Polymorphonuclear cells	85% (0.85)	91% (0.91)	≤25% (≤.25)

Both specimens were Gram-stain-negative for bacteria. Compensated polarized light microscopy disclosed intracellular, negatively birefringent crystals characteristic of monosodium urate.

Blood and synovial fluid cultures were negative. Antistreptolysin O (ASO) and streptozyme titers were within normal limits. Hepatitis B surface antigen (HBsAg) was negative.

The patient was treated with indomethacin and bed rest, and his symptoms resolved completely over the next 5 days. X-rays of his feet, prior to discharge, showed erosions at the right first metatarsal head. On discharge, he was continued on indomethacin.

On return to clinic one month later, his serum urate level was 10.0 mg/dL, and urine uric acid excretion was 1037 mg/day (6.12 mmol/day), reference range 250–600 (1.48–3.54). He was subsequently treated with colchicine and allopurinol, and the serum urate level decreased to 6 mg/dL.

Differential Diagnosis

The differential diagnosis of fever and polyarthritis can be complex, including infectious disease, collagen vascular disorders, and a variety of miscellaneous conditions. In this patient, infectious causes had to be considered and excluded. Disseminated gonococcal infection was sought with appropriate cultures and acute rheumatic fever with throat cultures and serological tests. Empiric antibiotics were considered until synovial fluid analysis led to his diagnosis.

New onset of inflammatory arthritis is difficult to exclude in the acute setting. Some period of clinical observation is generally required. The absence of rheumatoid factor or antinuclear antibodies does not rule out rheumatoid arthritis or other systemic inflammatory disorders such as systemic lupus or systemic vasculitis. Additional studies that may help include complement levels, tests for cryoglobulin, and antineutrophil cytoplasmic antibody.

Crystal-mediated arthropathies include pseudogout and gout. In pseudogout, acute arthritis is limited to one or two joints, chondrocalcinosis (calcium deposits along the surface of articular cartilage) is evident on radiographs, and crystals characteristic of calcium pyrophosphate dihydrate (CPPD) are seen in synovial fluid. Pseudogout occurs in older patients and is associated with metabolic disorders of calcium metabolism, including hyperparathyroidism. This patient's diagnosis of gout was established when synovial fluid analysis revealed intracellular crystals characteristic of monosodium urate, in the absence of bacterial infection.

Definition and Classification

Gout represents a group of diseases in which prolonged hyperuricemia leads to deposition of urate salts in and around joints and other tissues. At physiological pH, most uric acid exists as monosodium urate. Saturation of serum occurs at a urate concentration of $\sim$7 mg/dL. Above this value the potential for precipitation of monosodium urate crystals exists, although plasma proteins allow stable supersaturated solutions in which the serum urate value may rise considerably higher.

The epidemiological definition of normouricemia (mean serum urate value plus or minus two standard deviations in a healthy population) varies depending on the analytic method and the population. Most laboratories now use a uricase assay in which uric acid is cleaved to produce allantoin and hydrogen peroxide. Oxygen consumption is directly proportional to uric acid in the sample. More commonly, the hydrogen peroxide produced reacts with a second reagent of known optical density that is then quantitated by differential spectrophotometry. The uricase method is very specific and gives upper limits of 7.0 mg/dL in men and 6.0 mg/dL in women in most population studies.

Hyperuricemia (serum urate $>$ 7.0 mg/dL) is a common laboratory finding, occurring in over 5% of adults on at least one occasion. Risk factors for hyperuricemia include increased body weight or mass index, elevated serum creatinine or urea nitrogen, alcohol intake, and male gender. Hyperuricemia leads to gout in a minority of instances. The majority of patients with asymptomatic hyperuricemia remain gout-free, but the greater the degree or duration of hyperuricemia, the more likely that gout will develop. The prevalence of clinical gout was estimated to be 13.6 per 1000 men and 6.4 per 1000 women in a 1986 study, but evidence suggests that the prevalence of disease is rising. The peak incidence occurs in middle-aged males.

When gout is present, hyperuricemia is classified as *primary*, if an inborn disorder of purine metabolism is present, or *secondary*, if another disease causes either overproduction or underexcretion of uric acid.

Overproduction of uric acid can be shown in 10–20% of patients with *primary hyperuricemia*. In these patients renal excretion of uric acid is $>$600 mg/dL (36 mmol/L) on a purine-restricted diet. Although the metabolic basis of overproduction is unidentified, and presumably multigenetic, in most patients, two enzymatic defects have been defined— overactivity of 5-phosphoribosyl-1-pyrophosphate (PRPP) synthetase and partial deficiency of hypoxanthine guanine phosphoribosyltransferase (HPRT).

In humans, uric acid is the degradation end product of purine metabolism. Inosinic acid, the parent purine compound, is synthesized de novo by a series of reactions, including the condensation of PRPP and L-glutamine in the presence of the enzyme amidophosphoribosyltransferase. High concentrations of PRPP accelerate this reaction and increase purine synthesis.

Purine nucleotides are degraded to hypoxanthine and xanthine and ultimately oxidized to uric acid in reactions catalyzed by the enzyme xanthine oxidase. Normally a salvage pathway allows conversion of hypoxanthine to inosine monophosphate (IMP) in the presence of PRPP and HPRT. Deficiency of HPRT leads to increased degradation of hypoxanthine and to underutilization of PRPP (which fuels de novo purine synthesis), resulting in increased uric acid formation.

Both HPRT deficiency and PRPP synthetase over activity are X-linked disorders. Affected males develop gout at an early age (15–30 years) and may be mentally retarded. The patient in this case was found to have normal HPRT and PRPP synthetase activities.

In the majority of patients with primary gout, hyperuricemia results from reduced renal uric acid clearance, so that urinary uric acid is normal or low in the presence of increased serum urate. Specific renal defects are under investigation to ascertain how urate transporter proteins, including the urate transporter 1 (URAT1) molecule, control the reabsorption and secretion of filtered urate.

Secondary hyperuricemia occurs when another primary disorder leads to either overproduction of uric acid or underexcretion. In myeloproliferative disorders, increased nucleic acid turnover raises uric acid production. Renal failure, diuretic therapy, and lead intoxication reduce uric acid excretion. Comorbidities that are independently associated with gout include hypertension, obesity, diabetes, and hyperlipidemia.

Clinical Features

Persistent hyperuricemia may lead to deposition of monosodium urate crystals in and around articular tissues. Clinical attacks of gout occur when crystals incite an acute inflammatory response in the synovial tissues. Physical trauma or rapid changes in the serum urate concentration may trigger attacks. The first attack is usually monoarticular and involves a lower extremity. Inflammation of the joint and periarticular tissues occurs rapidly, and joint effusions are extensive. Synovial fluid leukocyte counts are elevated (15,000–100,000/μL), and neutrophils predominate.

Acute attacks are self-limited and separated by asymptomatic, intercritical periods. Although the initial attack may be polyarticular, polyarthritis usually occurs later in the disease course. Fever may accompany acute attacks, along with elevations of the erythrocyte sedimentation rate (ESR) and acute-phase reactants such as the C-reactive protein. Eventually, uric acid deposition leads to grossly evident tophi around the joints or in subcutaneous tissue. Erosions may be visible on radiographs of the involved joints. Tophaceous gout is marked by chronic joint inflammation and deforming arthritis.

Diagnosis

The diagnosis of gout is made when intracellular crystals, typical of monosodium urate, are identified in the synovial fluid of an inflamed joint. Such crystals are needle-shaped and strongly negatively birefringent when examined by compensated polarized light microscopy. They appear yellow when oriented parallel to the axis of the compensator and blue when oriented perpendicular to it. The CPPD crystals of pseudogout are rhomboidal and weakly positively birefringent. They appear blue when oriented parallel to the axis of the compensator and yellow when perpendicular. CPPD disease and gout may coexist. "False negative" results on synovial fluid may be due to an inadequate specimen or to inadequate microscopic examination. Demonstration of uric acid crystals in material aspirated from a suspected tophus also confirms the diagnosis of gout.

Although hyperuricemia is a prerequisite for uric acid deposition, the serum urate level during an acute attack of gout may be normal. Baseline serum and urine levels should, therefore, be obtained during intercritical periods.

Treatment

Therapy of gout includes treatment of the acute gouty arthritis and treatment of the underlying hyperuricemia. Acute attacks of gout are treated with nonsteroidal antiinflammatory drugs (NSAIDs), colchicine, or glucocorticoids. NSAIDs inhibit the formation of proinflammatory prostaglandins by directly inhibiting the cyclooxygenase enzyme. The complex and profound antiinflammatory effects of glucocorticoids result from the regulation of transcription of a variety of target genes involved in inflammation. Colchicine inhibits the influx of neutrophils to the inflammatory site by interfering with microtubular processes involved in endothelial adhesion molecule expression and neutrophil chemotaxis. When attacks become recurrent and frequent, colchicine or NSAIDs may be given as prophylactic therapy. Although NSAIDs may be preferred for acute therapy because of the gastrointestinal toxicity of large doses of colchicine, they may be less favored for chronic prophylaxis owing to the risk of NSAID-induced gastropathy and renal insufficiency. Small doses of colchicine as given for prophylaxis are usually well-tolerated.

Lifestyle changes that should be advised at the initial diagnosis of gout include weight loss, reduced consumption of red meat and fish, and increased consumption of low-fat dairy products and vegetables. Definitive hypouricemic therapy is indicated in recurrent gout or tophaceous gout. Probenecid increases urinary uric acid excretion by inhibiting URAT1 in the proximal tubule and can be used in patients who are not "overproducers." Allopurinol and febuxostat are xanthine oxidase inhibitors that inhibit uric acid formation. Fungus-derived rasburicase is available for acute intravenous therapy of hyperuricemia associated with the tumor lysis syndrome, but no suitable uricase is available for chronic therapy at this time. Lowering the serum urate level below its saturation point (7.0 mg/dL) can allow dissolution of tissue deposits of monosodium urate to prevent further structural damage. Although initiation of hypouricemic drugs may trigger an acute attack of gout, appropriate long-term use of these agents can prevent chronic tophaceous gouty arthritis.

Additional Reading

BECKER, M. A. AND JOLLY, M.: Clinical gout and the pathogenesis of hyperuricemia. In *Arthritis and Allied Conditions, a Textbook of Rheumatology*, 15th ed., W. J. KOOPMAN AND L. W. MORELAND, eds., Lippincott, Williams and Wilkins, Philadelphia, 2004.

CHOI, H. K., ATKINSON, K., KARLSON, E. W., WILLETT, W. AND CURHAN, G.: Purine-rich foods, dairy and protein intake, and the risk of gout in men. *N. Engl. J. Med. 350*:1093–103, 2004.

CHOI, H. K., MOUNT, D. B., AND REGINATO, A. M.: Pathogenesis of gout. *Ann. Intern. Med. 143*:499–516, 2005.

TERKELTAUB, R. A.: Clinical practice. Gout. *N. Engl. J. Med. 349*:1647–55, 2003.

WORTMAN, R. L. AND KELLEY, W. N.: Gout and hyperuricemia. In *Harris: Kelley's Textbook of Rheumatology*. E. HARRIS, R. BUDD, AND G. FIRESTEIN, ET AL., eds., Saunders, St. Louis, 2005.

Case 91

Middle-Aged Alcoholic with Jaundice and Ascites

Luis R. Peña and Alvaro Koch

A 51-year-old white male came to the Emergency Department complaining of weakness, lack of appetite, shortness of breath, and abdominal distension. He was a known alcoholic who had failed detoxification programs several times in the past and continued to drink approximately one pint of vodka or gin per day. Eight months before presentation he had been admitted to another hospital with alcoholic hepatitis and at that time had suffered severe withdrawal symptoms. Soon after discharge, however, he resumed drinking. Two weeks prior to the current presentation, he developed a "cold" and lost his appetite. He began taking over-the-counter ibuprofen for non-specific pains and continued to drink. When he experienced profound weakness, shortness of breath, and abdominal bloating, he asked his girlfriend to take him to the hospital.

Physical examination revealed his wasted appearance, alcohol on his breath, icterus, and a protuberant abdomen. Vital signs included temperature, 98°F (36.8°C); respiratory rate, 24/min; pulse, 70 BPM; and blood pressure, 140/70 mm Hg without orthostasis. He had bilateral gynecomastia and sparse axillary hair; spider angiomata were present on his anterior chest. Cardiac examination revealed a hyperdynamic precordium with normal heart sounds; the lungs were normal to percussion and auscultation. The abdomen was tense with a fluid wave and shifting dullness. Liver and spleen were neither palpable nor ballotable, and the abdominal venous pattern, although prominent, drained normally. The testes were atrophic, and the legs showed petechial hemorrhages and 3+ edema. Palmar erythema was noted. Rectal examination provided a soft, brown stool that was positive for occult blood. Neurological examination disclosed poor concentration, but the patient was not disoriented. No asterixis was observed, but pain and light touch perception and proprioception were diminished in both lower extremities.

The patient's mother had died of a heart attack, and his father was an alcoholic. The patient had no history of previous operations or blood transfusion. He was divorced and childless.

Tietz's Applied Laboratory Medicine, Second Edition. Edited by Mitchell G. Scott, Ann M. Gronowski, and Charles S. Eby
Copyright © 2007 John Wiley & Sons, Inc.

On admission, laboratory values from blood and urine were as follows:

Analyte	Value, Conventional Units	Reference Range, Conventional Units	Value, SI Units	Reference Range SI units
Blood alcohol	97 mg/dL	0	21 mmol/L	0
Hemoglobin	9.5 g/dL	14–18	5.90 mmol/L	8.69–11.17
Hematocrit	30%	40–54	0.30	0.40–0.54
Leukocyte count	$11.5 \times 10^3/\mu L$	4.8–10.8	$11.5 \times 10^9/L$	4.8–10.8
MCV	106 fL	80–94	Same	
Platelet count	$97 \times 10^3/\mu L$	150–450	$97 \times 10^9/L$	150–450
Prothrombin time	16.2 s	11–15	Same	
Sodium	131 mmol/L	136–145	Same	
Potassium	4.0 mmol/L	3.8–5.1	Same	
Chloride	108 mmol/L	98–107	Same	
CO_2, total	13.8 mmol/L	23–31	Same	
Urea nitrogen	7 mg/dL	8–21	2.5 mmol urea/L	2.9–7.5
Creatinine	0.9 mg/dL	0.7–1.3	80 μmol/L	62–115
Glucose	110 mg/dL	70–105	6.1 mmol/L	3.9–5.8
Calcium	9.2 mg/dL	8.4–10.2	2.30 mmol/L	2.10–2.54
Phosphorus	4.5 mg/dL	2.7–4.5	1.45 mmol/L	0.87–1.45
Protein, total	5.6 g/dL	6.2–7.8	56 g/L	62–78
Albumin	2.3 g/dL	3.2–4.6	23 g/L	32–46
Cholesterol	126 mg/dL	140–220	3.25 mmol/L	3.62–5.69
Urate	6.1 mg/dL	2.6–7.2	363 μmol/L	155–428
Bilirubin, total	6.5 mg/dL	0.2–1.0	111 μmol/L	3–17
AST	210 U/L	10–42	3.50 μkat/L	0.17–0.70
ALT	56 U/L	10–60	0.93 μkat/L	0.17–1.00
ALP	180 U/L	42–121	3.0 μkat/L	0.7–2.0
GGT	320 U/L	7–64	5.33 μkat/L	0.12–1.07
Urinalysis	Specific gravity, 1.005; pH, 5.0; negative for glucose, protein, blood, and cells; bilirubin, 2+			

Ultrasonographic scan of the abdomen and right upper quadrant showed an intact gallbladder without gallstones; marked ascites was present with a slightly enlarged, inhomogeneous liver. Intrahepatic ducts were not dilated, and the common bile duct was normal size. The scan therefore did not suggest biliary obstruction.

The patient was treated with thiamine, folate, multivitamins, and vitamin K and was placed on a diet restricted to sodium <2 g/d and fluid <1.5 L/d. An intravenous line was placed to infuse 5% dextrose. Six liters of peritoneal fluid were removed by paracentesis, and the patient received 50 g of albumin immediately after paracentesis.

Laboratory results on the peritoneal fluid were as follows:

Analyte	Value, Conventional Units	Noninfected Ascites, Reference Range	Value, SI Units	Reference Range SI units
Leukocyte count, total	$105 \times 10^3/\mu L$	<350	$105 \times 10^9/L$	<350
Protein, total	1.5 g/dL	0.5–2.8	15 g/L	5–28
Albumin	0.3 g/dL	0.1–1.8	3 g/L	1–18
Glucose	95 mg/dL	70–105	5.3 mmol/L	3.9–5.8
Amylase	22 U/L	20–170	0.37 μkat/L	0.33–2.83
Gram stain	Negative			
Cytological examination	No malignant cells			

On the second hospital day, the patient began hallucinating, became violent, and had to be physically restrained. These withdrawal symptoms were successfully treated with oral oxazepam. On the fourth hospital day, spironolactone for treatment of his ascites was added to his drug regimen. A week after admission, his pedal edema and abdominal girth were improved; the liver became palpable 3 cm below the right costal margin and the spleen as well under the left costal margin. Serum electrolytes became normal. However, AST remained elevated (275 U/L; 4.58 μkat/L), and bilirubin had increased (9.7 mg/dL; 166 μmol/L). Despite three doses of vitamin K, his prothrombin time was still prolonged (15.6 s). Other serum liver function tests were performed:

Analyte	Value, Conventional Units	Reference Range, Conventional Units	Value, SI units	Reference Range, SI Units
HBsAg	Negative	Negative	Same	
Anti-hepatitis C Ab	Negative	Negative	Same	
α-Fetoprotein	<5.0 ng/mL	<8.5	<5.0 μg/L	<8.5
α₁-Antitrypsin	194 mg/dL	78–200	1.9 g/L	0.8–2.0
Ceruloplasmin	39 mg/dL	18–45	390 mg/L	180–450
Iron, total	27 μg/dL	65–170	5 μmol/L	12–30
Transferrin	123 mg/dL	220–400	1.23 g/L	2.20–4.00
% transferrin saturation	22%	20–50	0.22	0.20–0.50
Ferritin	117 ng/mL	30–270	117 μg/L	30–270

The patient remained mildly confused even after oxazepam was stopped. Plasma ammonia of 88 μmol/L (reference range, 11–35 μmol/L) suggested portosystemic encephalopathy. The patient responded to lactulose therapy. Presence of anemia and blood in the stool led to esophagogastroduodenoscopy (EGD); the examination showed large esophageal varices without evidence of a recent bleeding site. Colonoscopy showed no abnormality.

After two weeks, the patient was stable with minimal ascites, mild encephalopathy, and persistent jaundice. He was discharged after being scheduled for an outpatient clinic visit the next week. He failed to keep the appointment but returned two weeks later after an alcoholic binge. He was readmitted with a temperature of 100.2°F (39°C), massive ascites, a serum bilirubin of 22 mg/dL (376 μmol/L), and a hematocrit of 32% (0.32). Repeat paracentesis showed spontaneous bacterial peritonitis; the leukocyte count was $2.3 \times 10^3/\mu L$ ($2.3 \times 10^9/L$), and 95% of cells were granulocytes. Intravenous antibiotics were started, but the patient had a massive hematemesis and his hematocrit dropped to 17% (0.17). Intravenous octreotide was initiated at 50 mcg/hour and emergency EGD showed bleeding esophageal varices. Despite successful banding with bleeding control and supportive transfusions, the patient lapsed into a coma and died two days later.

Definition of Alcoholic Liver Disease

This case is classic for alcohol-induced cirrhosis with its three major complications: ascites, portosystemic encephalopathy, and bleeding from esophageal varices. This patient suffered also from many of the other complications of persistent alcohol abuse: acute alcoholic hepatitis, peripheral neuropathy, withdrawal syndrome, and spontaneous bacterial peritonitis. These manifestations in any patient further complicate management of the cirrhosis and darken the prognosis.

Alcoholic liver disease (ALD) includes three conditions: hepatic steatosis or fatty liver, alcoholic hepatitis, and cirrhosis.[1,2] Heavy alcohol abuse, even for as little as few days can lead to hepatic steatosis, the earliest stage of ALD and the most common alcohol induced liver disorder. This condition can be reversed when alcohol consumption stops. Heavy use of alcohol for longer periods of time may lead to the development of the more severe and potentially lethal alcoholic hepatitis.[3] Only 10–15% of abusers actually progress to acute alcoholic hepatitis; however, up to 70 percent of all alcoholic hepatitis patients eventually may go on to develop cirrhosis.[4] In 2000, ALD was the fourth most common cause of death in males between the ages of 45 and 54.[5]

Three theories of the mechanism by which ethanol causes damage in the liver and other tissues are:

1. Oxidation of ethanol in the liver by the enzyme alcohol dehydrogenase produces acetaldehyde, which is rapidly dehydrogenated with the reduction of NAD to NADH. Excess aldehyde may accumulate and act as a hepatotoxin. The highly reduced environment of cytoplasm and mitochondria inhibits fatty acid oxidation and the citric acid cycle so that lipogenesis is stimulated (leading to steatosis). Hyperuricemia and hyper-lactic acidemia may also develop, which stimulates collagen synthesis in myofibroblasts. Ethanol induces the hepatic cytochrome P-450 2E1 (CYP2E1) which generates release of free radicals, causing oxidative stress, with peroxidation of lipids, membrane damage, and altered enzyme activities. Products of lipid peroxidation such as 4-hydroxynonenal stimulate collagen generation and fibrosis. Oxidative stress and associated cellular injury promote inflammation, which is aggravated by increased production of tumor necrosis factor-alpha (TNF-α) in the Kupfer cells, thereby contributing to necrosis, and progression to fibrosis and cirrhosis.[6]

2. Damage may be mediated by immune mechanisms involving antibodies or sensitized T cells with specificities directed against hepatic antigens or both. One lesion often seen in hepatocytes in ALD is the "Mallory body,"[2,7] a perinuclear mass of dense, eosinophilic material. Mallory bodies and other proteins altered in response to ethanol toxicity might represent neoantigens that stimulate an autoimmune response.

3. The cell responsible for the synthesis of matrix proteins in all the types of fibrotic liver disease is the hepatic stellate cell (HSC). In pathological conditions such as chronic alcohol abuse, HSC lose retinoids, and synthesize a large amount of extracellular matrix (ECM) components including collagen, proteoglycan, and adhesive glycoproteins. There are some specific factor(s) that alcohol generates which converts this cells from the quiescent fat storing cells to myofibroblast. Ethanol, or the damage it causes, may activate collagen synthesis and may serve as an initiator for perivenular fibrosis and eventually for bridging fibrosis and cirrhosis.

Alcoholic Hepatitis: The diagnosis of alcoholic hepatitis (AH) is usually based on a history of prolonged alcohol intake and clinical findings of abdominal pain, anorexia, nausea, vomiting, fever, leukocytosis, and tender hepatomegaly.[2] Serum AST is characteristically elevated but <300 U/L (<5.00 μkat/L) and usually much higher than ALT. Low transaminase values may to be due to pyridoxine (vitamin B_6) deficiency in these patients that causes diminished activity to be measured in serum assays that are not supplemented with pyridoxal-5-phosphate.[8]

Liver biopsy can provide a histological diagnosis based on steatosis, lobular granulocyte infiltrates, and degenerating hepatocytes with or without Mallory bodies. However, liver biopsy is generally performed only in patients who seem to have a protracted course and fail to respond to alcohol abstinence, rehydration, and nutritional replacement of thiamine, folate, and protein. Alcoholic hepatitis is a serious lesion, and mortality rates of 17%, 23%, and 44% for mild, moderate, and severe cases, respectively, have been observed.[9] Often, as in this patient, alcoholic hepatitis is accompanied by an underlying alcoholic cirrhosis.

Alcoholic Cirrhosis: Micronodular cirrhosis can develop in ALD because of repeated episodes of alcoholic hepatitis with necrosis followed by fibrosis and regeneration. It is characterized by small (<3 mm in diameter), uniform nodules. In quiescent cirrhosis without active hepatitis, the liver shrinks and hardens. Patients can develop one or more of the manifestations of portal hypertension (ascites, esophageal varices, hypersplenism) or of liver failure (jaundice, prolonged prothrombin time, hypoalbuminemia, portosystemic encephalopathy, sensitivity to hepatically cleared medications). Only a few of these manifestations can be discussed here.

Symptoms of Alcoholic Liver Disease

Ascites: Ascites in alcoholic cirrhotics is due both to obstruction of hepatic lymphatic flow and to avid renal retention of sodium. Sodium retention arises because of marked peripheral vasodilation with a hyperdynamic circulation, high cardiac output, and low peripheral vascular resistance; this situation leads to contraction of the central plasma volume.[10] Spider angiomata and palmar erythema are probably manifestations of the peripheral arterial vasodilation. Reduced renal blood flow stimulates renin and aldosterone production, and despite total body sodium overload, very little sodium is excreted. Because renal cortical blood flow is maintained by prostaglandins, nonsteroidal anti-inflammatory drugs (such as ibuprofen), which inhibit cyclo-oxygenase, can lead to functional renal failure (the so-called hepatorenal syndrome) and exacerbation of sodium retention, and thus cause or worsen ascites.

Evaluation of ascites by paracentesis is very important in alcoholic cirrhotics in order to rule out spontaneous bacterial (or secondary) peritonitis and to differentiate cirrhotic ascites from malignant ascites.[11,12] In alcoholic cirrhosis, levels of protein and albumin in the fluid are very low. With spontaneous bacterial peritonitis, the absolute PMN count is, >250 cells/μL. Antibiotic treatment of the infection is imperative.

Treatment of ascites decreases the likelihood of spontaneous bacterial peritonitis, improves patient comfort and respiration, and permits percutaneous liver biopsy if the procedure is needed. More than 90% of compliant patients will respond to dietary sodium restriction and K^+-sparing diuretics such as spironolactone. However, diuretics take several weeks to eliminate ascites, and large-volume paracentesis (6–8 L/d until "dry") with intravenous administration of 40–50 g of albumin is now routine prior to starting a diuretic regimen. In patients with refractory ascites, placement of transjugular intrahepatic portosystemic shunt (TIPS) is significantly better than paracentesis for control of the ascites. Although it increases encephalopathy, it also is associated with a trend toward improved survival.[13]

Esophageal Varices: Increased portal pressures with a gradient of >12 mm Hg between the portal and hepatic venous systems lead to varices in the stomach and lower esophagus. These varices may bleed massively. Despite various approaches to prevention of variceal bleeding (prophylactic propranolol, portosystemic shunts of various types) and different ways to staunch bleeding (endoscopic banding, sclerotherapy, Sengstaken-Blakemore tubes, shunts, administration of octreotide or nitrates), patients with bleeding varices have a very poor prognosis. When an alcoholic patient presents with hematemesis or melena, orthostasis, and a falling hematocrit, variceal rupture should not be immediately assumed. Endoscopy should be routinely performed to rule out other causes such as ulcers or portal hypertensive gastropathy. If bleeding varices are found, endoscopic banding is the usual treatment.

Hypersplenism: With portal hypertension, the spleen enlarges and sequesters both platelets and leukocytes. Peripheral thrombocytopenia contributes to coagulopathy, and leukopenia to susceptibility to infection.

Anemia: Causes of anemia in ALD are complex; they include ethanol or acetaldehyde suppression of bone marrow function, vitamin deficiencies (e.g., folate), inflammation causing an "anemia of chronic disease," and acute and chronic blood loss leading eventually to iron deficiency. In most cases, the anemia that appears is macrocytic.

Liver Function Tests in ALD: Causes of jaundice in adults are numerous, among them, viral hepatitis, drug-induced hepatitis or cholestasis, biliary obstruction, or hemolytic anemia. With problems unrelated to the hepatobiliary systems, serum bilirubin is rarely >7 mg/dL (>120 μmol/L), and determination of conjugated (direct) bilirubin is unnecessary. Alcoholics presenting with jaundice should be promptly examined with ultrasonography of the right upper quadrant; if biliary obstruction is present, aggressive therapy to decompress the biliary tract is necessary.

In alcoholic hepatitis, AST and ALT are mildly elevated, and AST more so than ALT. Because these enzyme assays evaluate hepatocellular necrosis, levels may actually be normal in quiescent cirrhosis. Alkaline phosphatase (ALP) and γ-glutamyltransferase (GGT) are synthesized in excess by biliary ductular cells reacting to irritation or inflammation of the intra- or extrahepatic biliary system; levels are commonly increased in many liver and biliary diseases, including ALD, biliary obstruction, and metastatic tumor. GGT is also present in microsomes and thus is especially sensitive to alcohol-induced liver disease and may be increased when ALP is still normal. On the other hand, increased ALP with normal GGT is reason to look for a nonhepatobiliary cause for ALP elevation, e.g., bone disease.

Coagulation Tests: There are several reasons for disturbances of coagulation in ALD. Thrombocytopenia and prolonged prothrombin and partial thromboplastin times (PT and PTT) are the most commonly seen. Hypersplenism causes most cases of thrombocytopenia, but platelet consumption in a diffuse intravascular coagulopathy (DIC-like) syndrome can also occur. PT and PTT are prolonged owing to impaired hepatic production of factors II, VII, IX, X, protein C, and protein S, all of which require vitamin K for γ-carboxylation and activity. Liver failure alone may account for abnormal PT and PTT, but inadequate nutritional intake of vitamin K is also a possibility. A good test for residual reserve liver function in ALD patients is to see whether PT is corrected by administration of parenteral vitamin K (10 mg subcutaneously each day for three days).

Hypoalbuminemia: Low albumin contributes to ascites and edema in ALD patients. Liver failure, poor nutrition, inflammatory conditions and infections, and protein loss from the gut or kidneys are all factors that can cause or intensify hypoalbuminemia.

Encephalopathy: The encephalopathy of liver failure has been termed portosystemic encephalopathy (PSE). Current theories explain PSE as an inability of the compromised liver to convert ammonia into urea, coupled with accumulation in plasma of aromatic amino acids (AAA) and depletion of branched-chain amino acids (BCAA). BCAA depletion is the result of their preferential utilization instead of AAA by muscle. The postulate is that the combination of increased plasma ammonia and an altered ratio of BCAA to AAA leads to generation of false neurotransmitters responsible for encephalopathy. The measurement of plasma ammonia (collected on ice and assayed immediately) has often been used to determine whether a patient has PSE. However, plasma ammonia concentrations are often unreliable, and it is not recommended that such measurements be used to follow a patient's course. To treat PSE, the removal of ammonia with oral lactulose therapy is usually effective. Lactulose is a nonabsorbable sugar that is fermented by colonic bacteria. This process acidifies the colon and sequesters the ammonia in the colon lumen as NH_4^+. The use of dietary supplements or parenteral infusions of BCAA have not been shown to be beneficial.[14] In general, restriction of protein intake is contraindicated for patients with ALD since it may enhance existing nutritional deficiency. It may, however, be invoked should sensitivity to protein loads develop.

Drug Sensitivity and Feminization in Men: Patients with cirrhosis often have decreased activity of hepatic cytochromes P-450 and can be very sensitive to medications that require hepatic metabolism. This is especially true for certain sedatives, hypnotics, and psychoactive drugs. A good principle to follow is to avoid medication whenever possible; when medication cannot be avoided, use discretion in choosing the drugs and dosages. Male alcoholics often manifest feminization because estrogenic steroids, normally cleared by hepatic oxidative systems, accumulate. In addition, acute alcohol ingestion suppresses testosterone formation by the gonads, and this mechanism can be more important than estrogen accumulation in causing feminization.

Treatment

Treatment strategies for ALD include lifestyle changes to reduce alcohol consumption, nutritional support, pharmacological therapy, and possible liver transplantation (in selected patients with decompensated cirrhosis and documented abstinence).

Lifestyle Changes: Abstinence from alcohol is essential to prevent further liver damage and cirrhosis formation if not present. Smoking cessation and obesity control may influence the development of further liver injury and must be addressed.

Nutritional Support: Efforts should be made to treat malnutrition and specific nutritional deficiencies (balanced diet, dietary supplements of vitamins and minerals in particular folate, thiamine, calcium, and iron).

Pharmacological Therapy: Several investigators have given priority to the treatment of AH, given the fact that this form of ALD is associated with significant early mortality. There is no FDA-approved therapy for ALD; however, a few drugs have been use with some success, mainly in the treatment of severe acute alcoholic hepatitis:

Corticosteroids: Of the thirteen randomized clinical trials evaluating corticosteroids in patients with AH, five observed a survival benefit; however, Individual data from the three most recent randomized controlled trials and prospective studies have constantly shown that the use of corticosteroids improved 2-month survival (up to 80%) in patients with severe acute alcoholic hepatitis with a discriminant function) ≥ 32.[15] This survival advantage does not extend much longer than a year; therefore, corticosteroid usefulness may be only short-term.

Pentoxifylline: A large, randomized, double blind, placebo-controlled study by Akriviadis and colleagues in patients with severe acute alcoholic hepatitis showed improved survival during a 4-week period. The benefit appears to be related to a significant decrease in the risk of developing hepatorenal syndrome.[16]

Liver transplantation: Because of the shortage of donated organs and, since the liver damage is considered by many to be self-inflicted, transplantation to patients with ALD remains controversial. Patients must undergo a thorough evaluation to determine whether they are suitable candidates by remaining abstinent. A total of 41,734 liver transplants using organs from cadavers were performed in the United States between 1992 and 2001. Of these, 12.5% were performed in patients with ALD and 5.8% were performed in patients with ALD and concurrent infection with hepatitis C, making ALD the second most frequent reason for transplantation.[17]

References

1. LIEBER, C. S.: Biochemical and molecular basis of alcohol-induced injury of liver and other tissues. *N. Engl. J. Med. 319*:1639–1650, 1988.

2. ZAKIM, D., BOYER, T. D., AND MONTGOMERY, C.: Alcoholic liver disease. In: *Hepatology, A Textbook of Liver Disease*, 2nd ed., D. ZAKIM AND T. D. BOYER, eds., Saunders, Philadelphia, 1990.

3. U.S. Department of Health and Human Services, Alcohol Alert, NIAAA Publications Distribution Center, Number 64, January 2005.

4. BIRD, G. L., AND WILLIAMS, R.: Factors determining cirrhosis in alcoholic liver disease. *Mol. Aspects Med., 10*:97–105, 1988.

5. MANN, R. E., SMART, R. G., AND GOVONI, R.: The epidemiology of alcoholic liver disease. *Alcohol Res. Health 27*:209–219, 2003.

6. LIEBER, C. S.: Alcoholic fatty liver: its pathogenesis and mechanism of progression to inflammation and fibrosis. *Alcohol 34*:9–19, 2004.

7. FRENCH, S. W.: The Mallory body: Structure, composition, and pathogenesis. *Hepatology 1*:76–83, 1981.

8. LUDWIG, S., AND KAPLOWITZ, N.: Effect of pyridoxine deficiency on serum and liver transaminases in experimental liver injury in the rat. *Gastroenterology 79*:545–549, 1980.

9. MENDENHALL, C. L., AND the VA COOPERATIVE STUDY GROUP ON Alcoholic Hepatitis: Alcoholic Hepatitis. *Clin. Gastroenterol. 10*:417–441, 1981.

10. SCHRIER, R. W., ARROYO, V., AND BERNARDI, M., ET AL.: Peripheral vasodilation hypothesis. A proposal for the initiation of renal sodium and water retention in cirrhosis. *Hepatology 8*:1151–1157, 1988.

11. HOEFS, J. C.: Diagnostic paracentesis, a potent clinical tool. *Gastroenterology 98*:230–236, 1990.

12. RUNYON, B. A.: Spontaneous bacterial peritonitis: An explosion of information. *Hepatology 8*:171–175, 1988.

13. D'AMIGO, G., LUCA, A., AND MORABITO, A., ET AL.: Uncovered transjugular intrahepatic portosystemic shunt for refractory ascites: a meta-analysis. *Gastroenterology 129*:1282–1293, 2005.

14. ERIKSSON, L. S., AND CONN, H. O.: Branched-chain amino acids in the management of hepatic encephalopathy: An analysis of variants. *Hepatology 10*:228–246, 1989.

15. MATHURIN, P.: Corticosteroids for alcoholic hepatitis—what's next? J Hepatol. 43:526–533, 2005.

16. AKRIVIADIS, E., BOTLA, R., BRIGGS, W., ET AL.: Pentoxifylline improves short-term survival in severe acute alcoholic hepatitis: A double blind, placebo-controlled trial. *Gastroenterology 119*:1787–1791, 2000.

17. ANANTHARAJU, A., AND VAN THIEL, D. H.: Liver transplantation for alcoholic liver disease. *Alcohol Res. Health 27*:257–269, 2003.

Case 92

Where Did the Red Cells Go?

Arnel Urbiztondo

A 60-year-old man complained of progressive dyspnea over two weeks. Review of systems was negative for productive cough, chest pain, fever, myalgias, arthralgias, weight loss, change in bowel habits, or signs of gastrointestinal or genitourinary tract bleeding. He smoked two packs of cigarettes a day, and had stopped drinking alcohol five years ago on the advice of his physician. He was not taking any prescribed medicines, over-the-counter drugs, or natural health aids. No abnormalities were noted on physical exam other than a resting tachycardia (pulse 96/bpm), pale conjunctiva, and a 2/6 systolic ejection murmur. The following tests were performed in his doctor's office: urine dip stick, negative; stool occult blood test, negative; spun hematocrit, 25%. A CBC performed three months ago as part of a routine evaluation was normal. The patient was admitted to the hospital. Upper endoscopy and colonoscopy were immediately performed, and both studies were normal.

A hematologist/oncologist was consulted, and the following tests were obtained:

Analyte	Value, Conventional Units	Reference Interval, Conventional Units	Value, SI Units	Reference Interval, SI Units
WBC	$9.8 \times 10^3/\mu L$	4.0–10.0	$9.8 \times 10^9/L$	4.0–10.0
RBC	$2.1 \times 10^6/\mu L$	4.4–6.0	$2.06 \times 10^{12}/L$	4.4–6.0
Hemoglobin	6.9 g/dL	14–17	69 g/L	140–170
Hematocrit	21%	40–50	0.21 volume	0.40–0.50
MCV	102 fL	80–98	Same	—
Reticulocyte (%)	21%	0.5–1.5%	0.21 fraction	0.005–0.015
Absolute retic count	$432 \times 10^3/\mu L$	20–90	$432 \times 10^9/L$	20–90
Bilirubin total	1.0 mg/dL	0.2–1.3	17 μmol/L	3.4–22.2
AST	26 U/L	11–47	0.44 μkat/L	0.19–0.80
ALT	35 U/L	7–53	0.60 μkat/L	0.12–0.90
LDH	206 U/L	110–210	3.5 μkat/L	1.9–3.6
Haptoglobin	35 mg/dL	27–220	350 mg/L	270–2200

Notable findings on peripheral smear were marked polychromasia and 1–3 spherocytes per high powered field. A bone marrow biopsy was performed. The marrow was

Tietz's Applied Laboratory Medicine, Second Edition. Edited by Mitchell G. Scott, Ann M. Gronowski, and Charles S. Eby

hypercellular with increased erythropoiesis. Flow cytometry analysis of the bone marrow aspirate did not detect a clonal disorder.

Additional information was obtained from the blood bank when a sample was sent to type and screen the patient for possible transfusion: blood type, O+; antibody screen, positive; direct antiglobulin test (DAT) +2 polyspecific, +2 anti-IgG, negative anti-complement. Red cell bound IgG was eluted and tested against a panel of commercial red cells of known antigen phenotypes. The patient's eluate reacted specifically with Rh group antigen C positive red cells. Using red cell typing antisera, the patient's red cell phenotype was C positive. The patient was diagnosed with warm autoimmune hemolytic anemia displaying specificity for C antigen.

Diagnosis

Autoimmune hemolytic anemia (AIHA) is a group of disorders characterized by the presence of antibodies that are directed against antigenic targets on the patient's own red cells leading to hemolysis. Autoantibodies can recognize protein, polysaccharide, or glycoprotein epitopes. AIHA is classified based on the characteristics of the autoantibody (Table 92.1). This chapter will focus on warm autoimmune hemolytic anemias (WAIHA) and drug-induced hemolytic anemias. See Case 67 for a discussion of cold autoimmune hemolytic anemia and related disorders.

WAIHA is the most common form of immune hemolytic anemia, accounting for 50–70% of cases. Symptoms include shortness of breath, dizziness, and low grade fever, and may be accompanied by pallor and jaundice. The development of anemia is usually subacute, as in the patient described in this case, but can occur suddenly with rapid decompensation. Peak incidence of WAIHA is usually the seventh decade of life, although this disease has been reported in patients of all age groups. The antibody class is predominantly IgG with occasional cases of IgA, and rarely, IgM autoantibodies. Warm autoantibodies possess a high binding capacity for red cells at 37°C. Primary, or idiopathic, WAIHA accounts for half of the cases of WAIHA. Secondary WAIHA is usually associated with lymphoproliferative disorders, particularly low grade lymphomas, Hodgkin's disease, and chronic lymphocytic leukemia, autoimmune diseases such as systemic lupus erythematosis (SLE), primary agammaglobulinemia, pregnancy, and viral illnesses. Drug-induced WAIHA is the least common, but should always be considered, especially when initiation of a new medication is temporally related to the onset of symptoms. The patient in this case study was not taking any medications and a drug-induced mechanism was dismissed. An aggressive search for occult malignancy, including bone marrow exam, and chest, abdomen, and pelvic computerized axial tomography (CAT) scans was negative indicating that this was a case of primary WAIHA.

Specificity of Warm Autoimmune Antibodies

Warm autoimmune antibody specificity is complex. The autoantibodies found in the serum and those eluted from cells usually react with all commercial red cells tested, thus appearing to be non-specific. Almost 50%, however, have specificity for epitopes located on the Rh protein, as in our patient, whose antibody specificity appeared to be specific for Rh C antigen. However, the autoantibody could be absorbed from the patient's serum using C negative red cells, confirming that it recognized an epitope common to the Rh protein. There are reports of specificity against other blood group antigens, including

Kell, Kidd, Duffy, and Diego systems. Confirmation that the patient's red cell phenotype is identical to the 'specificity' of the autoantibody, as was done in this case, rules out the possibility of an alloantibody due to previous transfusion.

If the hemolytic anemia produces symptoms severe enough to require transfusion, it is critically important to ensure that an autoantibody with non-specific affinity is not obscuring detection of an underlying alloantibody that could further accelerate destruction of transfused red cells that express the target antigen. There are several ways to absorb the autoantibody in a patient's serum in order to uncover coexisting alloantibodies by using the patient's own red cells, if not recently transfused, or by using selected commercial red cells if the patient has been transfused.

Table 92.1 Classification of Autoimmune Hemolytic Anemia

I. **Warm Autoantibody**
    Antibody Class: IgG
    Thermal Amplitude: 37°C
A. Primary–etiology unknown/idiopathic
B. Secondary
    a. Lymphomas and chronic lymphocytic leukemia
    b. Other neoplastic conditions
    c. Autoimmune disorder (particularly systemic lupus erythematosus)
    d. Chronic inflammatory diseases (e.g., ulcerative colitis)
    e. Immunodeficiency disorders, congenital or acquired
C. Drug-induced hemolytic anemia

II. **Cold Autoantibody**
    Antibody Class: IgM
    Thermal Amplitude: 0–4°C
A. Acute
    a. Mycoplasma infection
    b. Infectious mononucleosis
    c. Other infectious conditions
B. Chronic
    a. Primary/idiopathic
    b. Secondary
        i. Chronic lymphocytic leukemia
        ii. Lymphomas

III. **Paroxysmal Cold Hemoglobinuria**
    Antibody Class: IgG
    Biphasic Hemolysin
A. Primary – idiopathic
B. Secondary
    a. Syphilis
    b. Viral infection

IV. **Mixed Cold and Warm Autoantibodies**
A. Primary
B. Secondary
    a. Associated with rheumatic disorders, particularly SLE

Differential Diagnosis

WAIHA must be distinguished from other causes hemolytic anemia. Elevated reticulocyte count, presence of spherocytes on peripheral smear, and increased osmotic fragility are non-specific findings, and may be observed in both inherited (hereditary spherocytosis) and acquired (DIC, TTP) non-immune causes of hemolysis. Detection of immunoglobin and/or complement bound to red cells confirms the diagnosis of WAIHA. The DAT is performed by incubating (at 37°C) a patient's rinsed red cells with a polyspecific antiserum that recognizes both human IgG and complement proteins. If red cells are coated with IgG and/or complement 3d, cross-linking of red cells by the antiserum will cause visible agglutination (scored +1 to +4). Subsequent testing with specific antisera to IgG and complement will complete the characterization of the AIHA process. About 20% of DATs are due to IgG alone (as seen in this patient), 70% IgG + complement, and 10% complement alone.

While the DAT is a sensitive test for AIHA, there will be patients (~10%) with DAT negative immune mediated hemolytic anemia. Explanations include a low density of bound antibody/complement, such that IgG molecules in the antisera are unable to crosslink red cells and produce agglutination, and non-IgG autoantibodies (IgA, IgM). In addition, a positive DAT can be non-specific and harmless, and is encountered in both healthy blood donors (~0.1%) and seriously ill patients (~8%) who show no evidence of hemolysis. Patients with WAIHA may also have unbound autoantibodies that can be detected by performing an indirect antiglobulin test (IAT). First incubate their serum with control red cells, rinsing them to remove unbound antibody, then incubate the red cells with IgG antisera, and observe for agglutination. The IAT is frequently negative due to absorption of all antibody to red cells. However, autoantibody can be 'recovered' by chemical or thermal elution of red cell bound immunoglobin to permit further characterization.

Pathogenesis of Hemolysis

Extravascular phagocytosis is the primary mechanism responsible for red cell destruction in WAIHA. As red cells pass through the spleen, the Fc region of bound IgG autoantibodies bind to Fc receptors on splenic macrophages leading to partial or complete phagocytosis. Similar to hereditary spherocytosis, partially phagocytized red cells are converted into rigid spherocytes, which are sequestered in splenic sinusoids and eventually destroyed. Fc receptors are also present on hepatic Kuppfer cells, but most of the extravascular hemolysis occurs in the spleen. Splenic and hepatic macrophages also have receptors for complement fragment C3b, and the presence of both IgG and complement fragments enhances the rate of phagocytosis. Autoantibody isotypes IgG1 and IgG3 are more efficient at binding complement and produce more avid phagocytosis than isotypes IgG2 and IgG4. Complement mediated intravascular hemolysis is uncommon in WAIHA, but if extravascular hemolysis is extremely brisk, elevated indirect bilirubin and LDH, and undetectable haptoglobin may occur.

Several mechanisms have been proposed or confirmed for drug-induced autoimmune hemolytic anemia. One classic, but uncommon, example is absorption of penicillin onto the red cell membrane and subsequent binding of penicillin-specific antibodies to the red cell causing increased destruction. To be clinically significant, the penicillin dose must be massive. When a penicillin specific IgG antibody is produced, it will only react with red cells that have absorbed the antibiotic in vitro.

Deposition of immune complexes, composed of a drug or its metabolite and a drug-specific antibody, on the surface of red cells may be the mechanism of some drug induced hemolytic anemias. Alternatively, a drug may bind to the red cell membrane and create neoantigens that stimulate autoantibodies that target the red cell and may activate complement. Finally, some medications, most frequently associated with the no longer popular antihypertension drug Aldomet, promote an IgG WAIHA that is independent of the presence of the drug. In this case, an eluate from IgG coated red cells will bind non-specifically to test red cells in the absence of the drug. When a drug responsible for AIHA is discontinued, recovery is typically rapid, except for the Aldomet-type autoantibody which may take months to resolve.

While many drugs can infrequently cause AIHA, second and third generation cephalosporin antibiotics deserve a special mention due to reports of severe, life-threatening hemolytic anemia linked to their use.

Treatment

The decision to transfuse red cells should be based on a clinical assessment of the patient's signs and symptoms of organ dysfunction rather than any particular hemoglobin trigger. Assuming there are no undetected alloantibodies, transfused red cells will be subject to hemolysis at the same rate as autologous red cells. However, a temporary increase in hemoglobin, while waiting for a response to treatment, can produce dramatic improvement in some patients.

Most WAIHA that are not drug-induced respond to immunosuppression with prednisone. The patient in this case was treated with prednisone, 1.0 mg/kg/day. Red cell transfusions were not necessary, hemoglobin rose rapidly, reticulocyte count decreased, and symptoms resolved. Prednisone was slowly tapered and discontinued at the end of three months, at which time his DAT was negative. Monitoring for clinical and laboratory signs of relapse will be necessary. In the event of a late relapse, a second course of prednisone would be administered. If a second remission is not obtained, or if control of hemolysis requires chronic prednisone doses of >15–20 mg/day, splenectomy is usually successful by removing the primary site of red cell destruction as well as a major site of antibody production. Patients that fail or cannot tolerate splenectomy are candidates for salvage therapies including; intravenous immune globulin (IVIg), which probably contains anti-idiotype antibodies that neutralize the pathologic autoantibody, anti-CD 20 rituximab to deplete immunoglobin producing B cells, azothioprine, cyclophosphamide, and other immunosuppressive drugs.

References

1. BRECHER, M. E. (ed.) *Technical Manual*, 15th ed. Bethesda, MD: American Association of Blood Banks, 461–464, 2005.
2. HARMENING, D., ET AL.: *Modern Blood Banking and Transfusion Practices*, 5th ed. Philadelphia PA: FA Davis Company, 436–456, 2005.
3. HILLYER, C. ET AL.: *Blood Banking and Transfusion Medicine, Basic Principles and Practice*, New York: Churchill Livingstone Publications, 378–382, 2003.
4. KUMAR, V., ABBAS, A., AND FAUSTO, N. (eds) *Pathologic Basis of Disease*, 7th ed. Philadelphia PA; Elsevier Saunders Publications, 637, 2005.
5. LICHTMAN, M. ET AL.: *Williams Hematology*, 7th ed. New York: McGraw-Hill Medical, 729–750, 2006.

Index

Abdominal pain, acute intermittent porphyria, 513–522. *See also* Acute intermittent porphyria

Abetalipoproteinemia, 585–588
  case presentation, 585–586
  defined, 586–587
  differential diagnosis, 587
  treatment, 587

Acidosis, chronic renal failure, 69

Acute coronary syndrome, acute myocardial infarction, 6. *See also* Coronary heart disease (CHD)

Acute intermittent porphyria, 513–522
  case presentation, 513–516
  definitions, 516–520
  diagnosis, 520–521

Acute myocardial infarction, 3–15
  anatomy, 7–8
  case presentation, 3–4, 11–12
  defined, 4, 12
  diagnostic criteria, 5–6
  differential diagnosis, 12–13
  pathogenesis, 6–7, 13–14
  precipitating factors, 7
  presenting symptoms, 4–5
  prognosis, 8–9
  treatment, 14

Acute promyelocytic leukemia (APL) with disseminated intravascular coagulation (DIC), 379–385
  acute leukemia forms, 381
  case presentation, 379–381
  diagnosis, 382
  disseminated intravascular coagulation complications, 383–385
  pathology, 381–382
  treatment, 382–383

Acute renal failure, 31–39. *See also* Chronic renal failure
  case presentation, 31–36
  differential diagnosis, 37–39
  treatment, 39

Addison disease, 167–173
  case presentation, 167–169
  defined, 170
  diagnosis, 172
  differential diagnosis, 170–172
  treatment, 172

Adrenocortical disease, 147–195
  Addison disease, 167–173
    case presentation, 167–169
    defined, 170
    diagnosis, 172
    differential diagnosis, 170–172
    treatment, 172
  congenital adrenal hyperplasia (CAH), 149–154
    case presentation, 149–150
    clinical features, 151–152
    commentary, 154
    defined, 150–151
    diagnosis, 152–154
    treatment, 154
  Cushing syndrome, 155–165
    case presentation, 155–159
    defined, 159–161
    diagnosis, 162–163
    diagnostic testing, 163–164
    differential diagnosis, 161–162
    treatment, 165
  multiple endocrine neoplasia (MEN) syndrome, 183–188
    case presentation, 183–184
    defined, 184–185
    diagnosis, 185
    differential diagnosis, 185
  pheochromocytoma, 189–195
    case presentation, 189–191
    defined, 191–192
    differential diagnosis, 192–195
  primary hyperaldosteronism (Conn's syndrome), 175–182
    case presentation, 175–177
    defined, 177–178

Tietz's Applied Laboratory Medicine, Second Edition. Edited by Mitchell G. Scott, Ann M. Gronowski, Charles S. Eby, and Norbert W. Tietz
Copyright © 2007 John Wiley & Sons, Inc.

Adrenocortical disease (*Continued*)
  primary hyperaldosteronism (*Continued*)
    diagnosis confirmation and subtype
      differentiation, 180–181
    differential diagnosis and screening, 178–180
    treatment, 181
Adrenocortical dysplasia, Cushing syndrome, 161
Adrenocorticotrophic hormone (ACTH):
  Addison disease, 170, 171, 172
  congenital adrenal hyperplasia (CAH), 150,
    152, 154
  Cushing syndrome, 157, 158, 160, 163, 164
Allergic bronchopulmonary aspergillosis
  (ABPA), 315–318
  case presentation, 315–316
  defined, 316–317
  differential diagnosis, 317
  treatment, 317–318
Allograft rejection, renal transplant cyclosporin
  toxicity, 44–45
Analytical error, 615–639
  calcium values, 635–639
    case presentation, 635–636
    defined, 636
    gadolinium, 637–639
    hypocalcemia differential diagnosis, 637
  heterophile antibodies:
    HAA antibodies, 617–622
      case presentation, 617–618
      interference mechanism, 619–620
      prevalence, detection, and prevention,
        620–621
      problem definition, 618
    prolactinomas, 623–627
      case presentation, 623–624
      defined, 624
      differential diagnosis, 624–625
      "hook effect," 625–626
      treatment, 627
  urinary tract and prostate, 629–634
    case presentation, 629–630
    endogenous interfering antibodies, 630–633
      anti-animal immunoglobulin antibodies,
        632–633
      autoantibodies, 631–632
      immunoassays, 630–631
    follow-up, 630
    interference detection and minimization,
      633–634
Anemia, chronic renal failure, 69, 419–423. *See also*
  Celiac disease (CD); Chronic lymphocytic
  leukemia (CLL) with autoimmune hemolytic
  anemia (AHA); Pernicious anemia (PA)

Anemia with chronic disease, 419–423
  case presentation, 419–420
  differential diagnosis, 420–421
  treatment, 421–422
Angelman syndrome (AS), 287–291
  case presentation, 287–288
  defined, 288
  diagnosis, 289–291
  pathogenesis, 288–289
  prognosis, 291
Anti-animal immunoglobulin antibodies:
  heterophile antibodies, 617–622
  urinary tract and prostate, 632–633
Antidiuretic hormone (ADH). *See* Syndrome
  of inappropriate secretion of antiduretic
  hormone (SIADH)
Antioxidants, nonalcoholic fatty liver disease
  (NAFLD), 127–128
Antiphospholipid syndrome (venous
  thromboembolism):
  clinical presentation, 463–464
  defined, 461
  diagnosis, 461–462
  pathophysiology, 462–463
  thrombosis and, 462
  treatment, 464
Arginine vasopressin. *See* Syndrome of
  inappropriate secretion of antiduretic
  hormone (SIADH)
Arthritis, sitosterolemia, 589–592. *See also*
  Rheumatoid arthritis
Ascites, 99–102
  case presentation, 99–101
  evaluation and management, 101–102
Aspergillus, allergic bronchopulmonary
  aspergillosis (ABPA), 315–318
Atherosclerosis, acute coronary syndrome, 6–7
ATP7B gene, Wilson's disease, 94
Autoimmune disease, 593–613
  celiac disease (CD), 609–613
    case presentation, 609–610
    defined, 610–611
    differential diagnosis, 611
    extraintestinal manifestations, 611
    pathogenesis, 612
    serological markers, 611–612
    treatment, 612
  rheumatoid arthritis, 595–600
    case presentation, 595–596
    clinical features, 595
    diagnosis, 595–599
    pathophysiology, 595
    treatment, 599–600

systemic lupus erythematosus (SLE), 601–607
  case presentation, 601–603
  clinical features, 604
  diagnosis, 604–606
  pathophysiology, 603–604
  treatment, 606
Autoimmune hemolytic anemia (AHA). *See*
    Chronic lymphocytic leukemia (CLL) with
    autoimmune hemolytic anemia (AHA)
Azathioprine. *See* Thiopurine
Azotemia, chronic renal failure, 68

Back pain, renal osteodystrophy, 75–78
Bilateral micronodular hyperplasia, Cushing
    syndrome, 161
Bilirubin metabolism, Gilbert's
    syndrome, 107–109
Bone alkaline phosphatase isoenzyme, bone
    markers, 230
Borrelia burgdorferi, Lyme disease, 311–314
Breast cancer, 337–341
  case presentation, 337
  defined, 337–338
  differential diagnosis, 338–339
  treatment, 339–340
Breath testing, *Helicobacter pylori* infection, 323

Calcineurin inhibitor effects and toxicity, renal
    transplant cyclosporin toxicity, 43–44
Calcium value error:
  case presentation, 635–636
  defined, 636
  gadolinium, 637–639
  hypocalcemia differential diagnosis, 637
Cancer. *See* Breast cancer; Hematologic disorders
    (malignant); Nonhematologic malignancies;
    Prostate cancer
Carcinoid syndrome, 249–253
  case presentation, 249–250
  defined, 250–251
  diagnosis, 251–252
  treatment and prognosis, 252–253
Cardiac disease. *See* Acute myocardial infarction
Catechol-*O*-methyl transferase (COMT),
    pheochromocytoma, 191
Celiac disease (CD), 609–613
  case presentation, 609–610
  defined, 610–611
  differential diagnosis, 611
  extraintestinal manifestations, 611
  pathogenesis, 612
  serological markers, 611–612
  treatment, 612

Cerebral venous thrombosis, venous
    thromboembolism (acquired), 459–464. *See
    also* Venous thromboembolism (acquired)
Chronic bronchitis, chronic obstructive pulmonary
    disease (COPD), 21, 22
Chronic hyponatremia, syndrome of inappropriate
    secretion of antidiuretic hormone (SIADH),
    79–87. *See also* Syndrome of inappropriate
    secretion of antidiuretic hormone (SIADH)
Chronic lymphocytic leukemia (CLL) with
    autoimmune hemolytic anemia (AHA),
    371–377
  case presentation, 371–372
  diagnosis, 372–374
  differential diagnosis, 374–376
  prognosis, 374
  treatment, 377
Chronic myelogenous leukemia (CML), 393–399
  case presentation, 393
  confirmation tests, 395–396
  cytogenics, 396–397
  defined, 396
  differential diagnosis, 394–395
  genetic diagnosis, 397–398
  prognosis, 398
  treatment, 398–399
Chronic obstructive pulmonary disease (COPD):
  case presentation, 19–21
  commentary, 21–23
  pulmonary disease, 19–23
  pulmonary function tests, 21
  treatment, 23
Chronic renal failure, 65–74. *See also* Acute renal
    failure
  case presentation, 65–66
  chemistry and hematology, 67–69
    acidosis, 69
    anemia, 69
    azotemia, 68
    electrolytes, 68–69
    proteinuria, 67–68
  creatinine assays, 73
  defined, 66–67
  diagnosis, 69
  glomerular filtration rate (GFR) estimation, 69–70
  Modification of Diet in Renal Disease Study
    (MDRD) equation for glomerular filtration
    rate (GFR), 71–72
  treatment, 73–74
Chronic sinusitis, pain management,
    pharmacogenomics, 539–542
Cirrhosis, ascites, 99–102. *See also* Ascites; Liver
    disease

"Club drug" abuse, 557–560

Coagulation factors, protein C and, venous thromboembolism (hereditary), 456

Coagulation factor V Leiden hypercoaguability, 551–554
  case presentation, 551–552
  defined, 552–553
  differential diagnosis, 553
  treatment, 553–554

Cocaine abuse. *See also* "Club drug" abuse; Drug abuse
  acute myocardial infarction, 11–15
  intravenous cocaine, Hepatitis C, 111

Cockcroft–Gault equation, glomerular filtration rate (GFR) estimation, 70

Cold agglutinin disease, 491–495
  case presentation, 491–492
  defined, 492–493
  differential diagnosis, 493
  paroxysmal cold hemoglobinuria, 494–495
  pathophysiology, 493–494
  treatment, 494

Colitis, thiopurine pharmacogenetics, 543–549

Collagen crosslinks, bone markers, 230

Colle's fracture. *See* Osteoporosis

Congenital adrenal hyperplasia (CAH), 149–154
  case presentation, 149–150
  clinical features, 151–152
  commentary, 154
  defined, 150–151
  diagnosis, 152–154
  treatment, 154

Conn's syndrome. *See* Primary hyperaldosteronism (Conn's syndrome)

Coronary heart disease (CHD), 575–579
  case presentation, 575–576
  defined, 576
  differential diagnosis, 576–577
  pathogenesis, 577
  treatment and prevention, 577–579

Cough, chronic obstructive pulmonary disease (COPD), 22

Creatinine assays, chronic renal failure, 73

Cryptococcus neoformans antigen, West Nile virus infection, 330

Cultures, *Helicobacter pylori* infection, 325

Cushing syndrome, 155–165
  case presentation, 155–159
  defined, 159–161
  diagnosis, 162–163
  diagnostic testing, 163–164
  differential diagnosis, 161–162
  treatment, 165

Cyclosporine A (CsA) metabolism, 533–537. *See also* End-stage renal disease (ESRD) osteodystrophy; Renal transplant cyclosporin toxicity
  case presentation, 533–535
  "personalized medicine" approach, 535–536

Cystic fibrosis, 25–30
  case presentations, 25–27
  defined, 27
  differential diagnosis, 27–28
  pathogenesis, 28–30
  treatment, 30

Depression, Wilson's disease, 91–97. *See also* Wilson's disease

Diabetes mellitus, 197–215
  case presentation, 199–200
  Cushing syndrome, 161
  defined, 200–201
  differential diagnosis, 201
  hypoglycemia, 211–215
    case presentation, 211–212
    defined, 212–213
    differential diagnosis, 213–214
    pathogenesis, 214
    treatment, 215
  ketoacidosis, 205–209
    case presentation, 205–206
    defined, 206
    differential diagnosis, 206–207
    pathogenesis, 207–208
    treatment, 208
  pathogenesis, 201–202
  treatment, 202–203

Diabetes mellitus type 1, defined, 200

Diabetes mellitus type 2:
  defined, 200–201
  nonalcoholic fatty liver disease (NAFLD), 124, 127

Disseminated intravascular coagulation (DIC), acute promyelocytic leukemia (APL) with, 383–385. *See also* Acute promyelocytic leukemia (APL) with disseminated intravascular coagulation (DIC)

Drug abuse:
  "club drug" abuse, 557–560
  cocaine abuse, acute myocardial infarction, 11–15
  intravenous cocaine, Hepatitis C, 111
  opioids, 561–565

Dyspnea, chronic obstructive pulmonary disease (COPD), 23

Ecchymoses, acute promyelocytic leukemia (APL) with DIC, 379–385

Edema:
chronic obstructive pulmonary disease (COPD), 23
nephrotic syndrome, 55–63 (*See also* Nephrotic syndrome)

Electrolytes, chronic renal failure, 68–69

Emphysema, chronic obstructive pulmonary disease (COPD), 21–22

Endoscopy, *Helicobacter pylori* infection, 324

End-stage renal disease (ESRD) osteodystrophy, 219–224. *See also* Cyclosporine A (CsA) metabolism
case presentation, 219–220
defined, 220–221
differential diagnosis, 222–223
pathogenesis, 221–222
treatment, 223

Epstein–Barr virus (EBV), 301–304
case presentation, 301–302
defined, 302–303
differential diagnosis, 303–304
treatment, 304

Erythrocytosis, thombocytosis and, polycythemia vera differential diagnosis, 402–404

Familial hypercholesterolemia, sitosterolemia differential diagnosis, 591

Focal segmental glomerulosclerosis (FSGC), nephrotic syndrome, 57–62. *See also* Nephrotic syndrome

Foot ulcer. *See* T-cell leukemia (lymphoma, peripheral)

Gadolinium, calcium values, 637–639

Genetically inherited disease, 255–298
Angelman syndrome (AS), 287–291
case presentation, 287–288
defined, 288
diagnosis, 289–291
pathogenesis, 288–289
prognosis, 291
hemochromatosis, 293–298
case presentation, 293–294
defined, 294–295
differential diagnosis, 295–296
iron overload diagnosis, 296–297
pathogenesis, 295
screening for, 298
treatment, 297
isovaleric acidemia (IVA), 281–286
case presentation, 281–283
defined, 283–284

differential diagnosis, 285–286
pathogenesis, 284–285
treatment, 286
maple syrup urine disease, 275–280
case presentation, 275–277
defined, 277
differential diagnosis, 278–279
pathogenesis, 278
treatment, 279
medium-chain acyl CoA dehydrogenase (MCAD), 255–261
case presentation, 255–258
defined, 258
differential diagnosis, 260
pathogenesis, 258–259
prognosis and treatment, 260–261
methylmalonic acidemia, 263–267
case presentation, 263–264
defined, 264–265
differential diagnosis, 266–267
pathogenesis, 265–266
prognosis and treatment, 267
ornithine transcarbamylase (OTC) deficiency, 269–273
case presentation, 269–270
defined, 271
differential diagnosis, 271–272
patient outcome, 270–271
treatment, 272

Germ cell tumor, 355–362
case presentation, 355
defined, 355–357
human chorionic gonadotropin (hCG), 357–358
human chorionic gonadotropin (hCG) assays, 358–359
laboratory investigation, 359–361

Gestational trophoblastic disease, 363–368
case presentation, 363–364
defined, 364–365
differential diagnosis, 365–366
pathogenesis, 366
treatment, 366–367

Gilbert's syndrome, 105–109
case presentation, 105–106
defined, 106
differential diagnosis, 107
pathogenesis, 107–109
treatment, 109

Glomerular filtration rate (GFR, chronic renal failure), 66–74. *See also* Chronic renal failure
estimation of, 69–70
Modification of Diet in Renal Disease Study (MDRD) equation, 71–72

Glomerular nephritis, 49–53
Gout, 643–647
  case presentation, 643–644
  clinical features, 646
  definition and classification, 645–646
  diagnosis, 646–647
  differential diagnosis, 644–645
  treatment, 647
Graves disease, 131–137
  case presentation, 131–132
  defined, 132–133
  diagnosis, 134–136
  differential diagnosis, 133–134
  treatment, 136

Haemophilus influenzae:
  chronic obstructive pulmonary disease (COPD), 21
  sinusitis, 539
Hashimoto's thyroiditis, 139–142
  case presentation, 139–140
  defined, 140
  diagnosis, 141–142
  etiology, 140–141
  treatment, 142
Helicobacter pylori infection, 319–327
  case presentation, 319–320
  defined, 321–322
  diagnosis, 323–326
  symptoms, 322
  treatment, 326
Hematologic disorders (benign), 409–509
  anemia with chronic disease, 419–423
    case presentation, 419–420
    differential diagnosis, 420–421
    treatment, 421–422
  cold agglutinin disease, 491–495
    case presentation, 491–492
    defined, 492–493
    differential diagnosis, 493
    paroxysmal cold hemoglobinuria, 494–495
    pathophysiology, 493–494
    treatment, 494
  hemolytic disease (Rh), 497–501
    case presentation, 497–498
    defined, 498
    laboratory testing, 500–501
    pathogenesis, 498–499
    prevention and diagnosis, 499–500
  hemophilia, 443–451
    bleeding disorders, 449–450
    case presentation, 443–444
    clinical aspects, 444–445
    complications, 446–447

    diagnosis, 447–448
    genetics, 445–446
    treatment, 448–449
  heparin-induced thrombocytopenia (HIT), 435–441
    case presentation, 435–437
    commentary, 441
    defined, 438
    differential diagnosis, 437
    laboratory detection of antibodies, 439–440
    management, 440–441
    pathophysiology, 438–439
  hereditary spherocytosis (HS), 503–509
    case presentation, 503–505
    defined, 505–506
    differential diagnosis, 506–507
    pathogenesis, 507–508
    spherocytosis diagnosis, 507
    treatment, 509
  pernicious anemia (PA), 425–433
    case presentation, 425–427
    clinical features, 431
    defined, 427–429
    diagnosis, 431–432
    pathophysiology, 429–430
    treatment, 432–433
  qualitative platelet disorder, 465–474
    case presentation, 465–466
    diagnosis, 469–473
    differential diagnosis, 466–469
    treatment, 473
  sickle cell disease, 411–417
    case presentation, 411–412
    differential diagnosis, 412–415
    pathophysiology, 415
    treatment, 415–416
  thrombotic thrombocytopenic purpura (TTP), 485–490
    case presentation, 485–486
    clinical presentation, 487–488
    differential diagnosis, 486–487
    pathophysiology, 488
    testing and management, 488
    treatment, 489
  venous thromboembolism
      (acquired), 459–464
    antiphospholipid syndrome, 461
      clinical presentation, 463–464
      diagnosis, 461–462
      pathophysiology, 462–463
      thrombosis and, 462
      treatment, 464
    case presentation, 459–461

venous thromboembolism (hereditary), 453–457
  case presentation, 453–454
  defined, 456
  diagnosis, 454–455
  hyperhomocysteinemia, 456–457
  protein C and coagulation factors, 456
  prothrombin gene mutation G20210A, 456
  testing for, 455
  treatment, 457
von Willebrand disease, 475–483
  case presentation, 475–476
  defined, 480
  diagnosis, 481–482
  differential diagnosis, 476–479
  management, 482–483
  molecular dynamics, 479
Hematologic disorders (malignant), 369–407
  acute promyelocytic leukemia (APL) with DIC,
    379–385
    acute leukemia forms, 381
    case presentation, 379–381
    diagnosis, 382
    disseminated intravascular coagulation
      complications, 383–385
    pathology, 381–382
    treatment, 382–383
  chronic lymphocytic leukemia (CLL) with
    autoimmune hemolytic anemia (AHA),
    371–377
    case presentation, 371–372
    diagnosis, 372–374
    differential diagnosis, 374–376
    prognosis, 374
    treatment, 377
  chronic myelogenous leukemia
    (CML), 393–399
    case presentation, 393
    confirmation tests, 395–396
    cytogenics, 396–397
    defined, 396
    differential diagnosis, 394–395
    genetic diagnosis, 397–398
    prognosis, 398
    treatment, 398–399
  polycythemia vera, 401–407
    case presentation, 401–402
    clinical follow-up, 402
    defined, 404
    diagnosis, 404–405
    differential diagnosis, 402–404
    pathogenesis, 405–406
    prognosis, 407
    treatment, 406–407

T-cell leukemia (lymphoma, peripheral), 387–391
  case presentation, 387–388
  differential diagnosis, 388–389
  incidence and characteristics, 389–390
  treatment, 390–391
Heme pathway, porphyrias and, 516–520
Hemochromatosis, 293–298
  case presentation, 293–294
  defined, 294–295
  differential diagnosis, 295–296
  iron overload diagnosis, 296–297
  pathogenesis, 295
  screening for, 298
  treatment, 297
Hemolytic disease (Rh), 497–501
  case presentation, 497–498
  defined, 498
  laboratory testing, 500–501
  pathogenesis, 498–499
  prevention and diagnosis, 499–500
Hemophilia, 443–451
  bleeding disorders, 449–450
  case presentation, 443–444
  clinical aspects, 444–445
  complications, 446–447
  diagnosis, 447–448
  genetics, 445–446
  treatment, 448–449
Hemophilus influenza, cystic fibrosis, 27
Hemoptysis, glomerular nephritis, 49–53
Hemostasis disorders, differential diagnosis,
  476–479. *See also* Von Willebrand disease
Heparin-induced thrombocytopenia
  (HIT), 435–441
  case presentation, 435–437
  commentary, 441
  defined, 438
  differential diagnosis, 437
  laboratory detection of antibodies, 439–440
  management, 440–441
  pathophysiology, 438–439
Hepatic porphyria, acute intermittent porphyria,
  520–521. *See also* Acute intermittent porphyria
Hepatitis, Wilson's disease, 91–97. *See also*
  Wilson's disease
Hepatitis A virus, 114–115
Hepatitis B virus, 115–116
Hepatitis C, 111–120
  case presentation, 111–114
  classification, 114–119
  treatment, 119
Hepatitis C virus, 116–119
Hepatolenticular degeneration. *See* Wilson's disease

Hereditary hemochromatosis (HH):
  pathophysiology, diagnosis, and management,
    102–104
  porphyria cutanea tarda (PCT), 528–529
  treatment, 529–530
Hereditary spherocytosis (HS), 503–509
  case presentation, 503–505
  defined, 505–506
  diagnosis, 507
  differential diagnosis, 506–507
  pathogenesis, 507–508
  treatment, 509
Hereditary venous thromboembolism. *See* Venous
  thromboembolism (hereditary)
Heterophile antibody errors:
  HAA antibodies, 617–622
    case presentation, 617–618
    interference mechanism, 619–620
    problem definition, 618
  prolactinomas, 623–627
    case presentation, 623–624
    defined, 624
    differential diagnosis, 624–625
    "hook effect," 625–626
    treatment, 627
Histology, *Helicobacter pylori* infection, 324
Human chorionic gonadotropin (hCG), germ cell
  tumor, 357–359
Human glandular kallikrein 2, prostate cancer
  diagnosis, 352
Human leukocyte antigen (HLA) matching, renal
  transplant cyclosporin toxicity, 43
Hyperhomocysteinemia, venous thromboembolism
  (hereditary), 456–457
Hyperlipidemia, nonalcoholic fatty liver disease
  (NAFLD), 124, 127
Hyperparathyroidism, 233–239
  case presentation, 233–234
  defined, 234–236
  differential diagnosis, 236–238
  treatment, 238
Hypertension, Cushing syndrome, 155–165. *See also*
  Cushing syndrome
Hyperthyroidism, Graves disease, 132
Hypoalbuminemia, nephrotic syndrome, differential
  diagnosis, 59
Hypoalphalipoproteinemia. *See* Tangier disease
Hypocalcemia, differential diagnosis, 637
Hypocholesterolemia, abetalipoproteinemia
  differential diagnosis, 587
Hypoglycemia, 211–215
  case presentation, 211–212
  defined, 212–213

  differential diagnosis, 213–214
  pathogenesis, 214
  treatment, 215
Hyponatremia, chronic, syndrome of inappropriate
  secretion of antiduretic hormone (SIADH),
  79–87. *See also* syndrome of inappropriate
  secretion of antiduretic hormone (SIADH)
Hypothyroidism, Hashimoto's thyroiditis, 139–142.
  See also Hashimoto's thyroiditis

Infectious disease, 299–333
  allergic bronchopulmonary aspergillosis (ABPA),
    315–318
    case presentation, 315–316
    defined, 316–317
    differential diagnosis, 317
    treatment, 317–318
  Epstein–Barr virus (EBV), 301–304
    case presentation, 301–302
    defined, 302–303
    differential diagnosis, 303–304
    treatment, 304
  Helicobacter pylori, 319–327
    case presentation, 319–320
    defined, 321–322
    diagnosis, 323–326
    symptoms, 322
    treatment, 326
  Lyme disease, 311–314
    case presentation, 311
    defined, 311–312
    differential diagnosis, 313–314
    treatment, 314
  neurosyphilis, 305–309
    case presentation, 305–306
    defined, 306–307
    differential diagnosis, 307–308
    treatment, 308–309
  pain management, pharmacogenomics, 539–542
  West Nile virus infection, 329–333
    case presentation, 329–330
    defined, 330
    differential diagnosis, 331–332
    pathogenesis, 332
    treatment, 332–333
Inferior petrosal venous sinus sampling (IPSS),
  Cushing syndrome, 164
Infertility, Cushing syndrome, 155–165. *See also*
  Cushing syndrome
Insulinlike growth factors (IGFs), prostate cancer
  diagnosis, 352–353
Insulin resistance (IR), nonalcoholic fatty liver
  disease (NAFLD), 125

Intravascular coagulation, disseminated (DIC). *See*
    Acute promyelocytic leukemia (APL) with
    disseminated intravascular coagulation (DIC)
Intravenous cocaine, Hepatitis C, 111
Iodine deficiency, Hashimoto's thyroiditis, 140–141
Iron overload, hemochromatosis, 296–297
Isovaleric acidemia (IVA), 281–286
    case presentation, 281–283
    defined, 283–284
    differential diagnosis, 285–286
    pathogenesis, 284–285
    treatment, 286
Jaundice. *See* Hereditary spherocytosis (HS)

Ketoacidosis, 205–209
    case presentation, 205–206
    defined, 206
    differential diagnosis, 206–207
    pathogenesis, 207–208
    treatment, 208

Leukemia. *See* Acute promyelocytic leukemia (APL)
    with disseminated intravascular coagulation
    (DIC); Chronic lymphocytic leukemia (CLL)
    with autoimmune hemolytic anemia (AHA);
    Chronic myelogenous leukemia (CML);
    Hematologic disorders (malignant); T-cell
    leukemia (lymphoma, peripheral)
Leukopenia:
    acute promyelocytic leukemia (APL) with DIC,
        379–385
    thiopurine pharmacogenetics, 543–549
Lipid disorders, 573–592
    abetalipoproteinemia, 585–588
        case presentation, 585–586
        defined, 586–587
        differential diagnosis, 587
        treatment, 587
    coronary heart disease, 575–579
    coronary heart disease (CHD):
        case presentation, 575–576
        defined, 576
        differential diagnosis, 576–577
        pathogenesis, 577
        treatment and prevention, 577–579
    sitosterolemia, 589–592
        case presentation, 589–590
        defined, 590
        differential diagnosis, 590–591
        treatment, 591
    Tangier disease, 581–584
        case presentation, 581–582
        defined, 582–583

differential diagnosis, 583–584
        treatment, 584
Liver disease, 89–128
    ascites, 99–102
        case presentation, 99–101
        evaluation and management, 101–102
    Gilbert's syndrome, 105–109
        case presentation, 105–106
        defined, 106
        differential diagnosis, 107
        pathogenesis, 107–109
        treatment, 109
    hepatitis C, 111–120
        case presentation, 111–114
        classification, 114–119
        treatment, 119
    hereditary hemochromatosis (HH), 102–104
    nonalcoholic fatty liver disease (NAFLD),
        121–128
        case presentation, 121–123
        clinical presentation, 126
        defined, 123
        epidemiology, 123–124
        natural history, 124
        pathogenesis, 125
        pathology, 124–125
        treatment, 126–128
    Wilson's disease, 91–97
        case presentation, 91–93
        commentary, 95–96
        manifestations of, 94–95
        pathophysiology, 94
        treatment, 96–97
Lung cancer, chronic hyponatremia with,
    syndrome of inappropriate secretion of
    antidiuretic hormone (SIADH), 79–87.
    See also Syndrome of inappropriate secretion
    of antidiuretic hormone (SIADH)
Lyme disease, 311–314
    case presentation, 311
    defined, 311–312
    differential diagnosis, 313–314
    treatment, 314
Lymphocytosis. *See* Chronic lymphocytic leukemia
    (CLL) with autoimmune hemolytic anemia
    (AHA)
Lymphoma. *See* T-cell leukemia (lymphoma,
    peripheral)

Macronodular adrenal dysplasia, Cushing
    syndrome, 161
Magentic resonance imaging (MRI), Cushing
    syndrome, 164

Malignancies. *See* Hematologic disorders
  (malignant); Nonhematologic malignancies
Maple syrup urine disease (MSLID), 275–280
  case presentation, 275–277
  defined, 277
  differential diagnosis, 278–279
  pathogenesis, 278
  treatment, 279
Medium-chain acyl CoA dehydrogenase
  (MCAD), 255–261
  case presentation, 255–258
  defined, 258
  differential diagnosis, 260
  pathogenesis, 258–259
  prognosis and treatment, 260–261
Medullary thyroid carcinoma
  (MTC), 143–146
  case presentation, 143–144
  defined, 144
  differential diagnosis, 145
  treatment, 145–146
Metabolic acidosis, 567–572
  case presentation, 567–568
  defined, 568–570
  differential diagnosis, 570–571
  with oliguria, renal transplant cyclosporin
      toxicity, 41–47 (*See also* Renal transplant
      cyclosporin toxicity)
  treatment, 571–572
Methylmalonic acidemia, 263–267
  case presentation, 263–264
  defined, 264–265
  differential diagnosis, 266–267
  pathogenesis, 265–266
  prognosis and treatment, 267
Microangiopathic hemolytic anemia (MAHA),
  thrombotic thrombocytopenic
  purpura (TTP), 486–487
Modification of Diet in Renal Disease Study
  (MDRD) equation, for glomerular
  filtration rate (GFR), chronic renal
  failure, 71–72
Moraxella catarrhalis, sinusitis, 539
Multiple endocrine neoplasia (MEN) syndrome,
  183–188. *See also* Pheochromocytoma
  case presentation, 183–184
  classification, 185–187
  defined, 184–185
  diagnosis, 185
  differential diagnosis, 185
  pheochromocytoma, 183–188
Myelogenous leukemia. *See* Chronic myelogenous
  leukemia (CML)

Nephritis, nephrosis and, nephrotic syndrome, 57–58
Nephrosis, nephritis and, nephrotic syndrome, 57–58
Nephrotic syndrome, 55–63
  case presentation, 55–57
  clinical findings, 57
  commentary, 62
  differential diagnosis, 59
  laboratory results, 59–61
  pathophysiology, 57–59
  treatment, 61–62
Neurosyphilis, 305–309
  case presentation, 305–306
  defined, 306–307
  differential diagnosis, 307–308
  treatment, 308–309
Nonalcoholic fatty liver disease
  (NAFLD), 121–128
  case presentation, 121–123
  clinical presentation, 126
  defined, 123
  epidemiology, 123–124
  natural history, 124
  pathogenesis, 125
  pathology, 124–125
  treatment, 126–128
Nonhematologic malignancies, 335–368
  breast cancer, 337–341
    case presentation, 337
    defined, 337–338
    differential diagnosis, 338–339
    treatment, 339–340
  germ cell tumor, 355–362
    case presentation, 355
    defined, 355–357
    human chorionic gonadotropin (hCG), 357–358
    human chorionic gonadotropin (hCG) assays,
        358–359
    laboratory investigation, 359–361
  gestational trophoblastic disease, 363–368
    case presentation, 363–364
    defined, 364–365
    differential diagnosis, 365–366
    pathogenesis, 366
    treatment, 366–367
  ovarian cancer, 343–347
    case presentation, 343–344
    defined, 344–345
    differential diagnosis, 345–346
    treatment, 346–347
  prostate cancer, 349–354
    case presentation, 349–350
    defined, 350
    differential diagnosis, 351–353

pathophysiology, 350–351
screening, 353
treatment, 353
Non-ST-segment elevation AMI (NSTEMI), acute
    myocardial infarction, 4, 6, 7, 8–9, 11

Obesity, nonalcoholic fatty liver disease (NAFLD),
    124, 127
Oliguria, with metabolic acidosis, renal transplant
    cyclosporin toxicity, 41–47. See also Renal
    transplant cyclosporin toxicity
Opioid drug abuse, 561–565
Ornithine transcarbamylase (OTC) deficiency,
    269–273
    case presentation, 269–270
    defined, 271
    differential diagnosis, 271–272
    patient outcome, 270–271
    treatment, 272
Osteocalcin, bone markers, 230
Osteodystrophy. See Renal osteodystrophy; Renal
    osteodystrophy (end-stage renal disease)
Osteoporosis, 225–231
    bone markers, 229–231
    case presentation, 225–226
    defined, 226–228
    diagnosis, 228
    treatment and monitoring, 229
Ovarian cancer, 343–347
    case presentation, 343–344
    defined, 344–345
    differential diagnosis, 345–346
    treatment, 346–347

Pain management, pharmacogenomics, 539–542
Pancytopenia, thiopurine pharmacogenetics,
    543–549
Papillary thyroid carcinoma. See Medullary thyroid
    carcinoma (MTC)
Parathyroid hormone (PTH):
    hyperparathyroidism, 233–239
        case presentation, 233–234
        defined, 234–236
        differential diagnosis, 236–238
        treatment, 238
    osteoporosis, 227–228
    renal osteodystrophy, 75–78, 220–223
Paroxysmal cold hemoglobinuria, cold agglutinin
    disease, 494–495
PCR amplification, Helicobacter pylori infection,
    325–326
Peripheral T-cell leukemia (lymphoma). See T-cell
    leukemia (lymphoma, peripheral)

Pernicious anemia (PA), 425–433
    case presentation, 425–427
    clinical features, 431
    defined, 427–429
    diagnosis, 431–432
    pathophysiology, 429–430
    treatment, 432–433
"Personalized medicine" approach, cyclosporine A
    (CsA) metabolism, 535–536
Pharmacogenomics, 531–554. See also Toxicology
    coagulation factor V Leiden hypercoaguability,
        551–554
        case presentation, 551–552
        defined, 552–553
        differential diagnosis, 553
        treatment, 553–554
    cyclosporine A (CsA) metabolism, 533–537
        case presentation, 533–535
        "personalized medicine" approach, 535–536
    opioid drug abuse, 564–565
    pain management, 539–542
    thiopurine, 543–549
        case presentation, 543–544
        diagnosis, 548
        differential diagnosis, 544
        dynamics of, 546–547
        metabolism and toxicity, 544–546
        treatment, 548
Pheochromocytoma, 189–195. See also Multiple
    endocrine neoplasia (MEN) syndrome
    case presentation, 189–191
    defined, 191–192
    differential diagnosis, 192–195
    multiple endocrine neoplasia (MEN)
        syndrome, 183–188
Platelet disorder. See Qualitative platelet disorder
Pneumonia:
    acute promyelocytic leukemia (APL) with DIC,
        379–385
    sickle cell disease, 411–417
Polycythemia vera, 401–407
    case presentation, 401–402
    clinical follow-up, 402
    defined, 404
    diagnosis, 404–405
    differential diagnosis, 402–404
    pathogenesis, 405–406
    prognosis, 407
    treatment, 406–407
Porphyria cutanea tarda (PCT), 523–530
    case presentation, 523–524
    clinical features, 526
    defined, 525–526

Porphyria cutanea tarda (*Continued*)
  diagnosis, 527–528
  generally, 524–525
  hereditary hemochromatosis (HH) and, 528–529
  pathophysiology, 526–527
  treatment, 529–530
Porphyrias, 511–530
  acute intermittent porphyria, 513–522
    case presentation, 513–516
    definitions, 516–520
    diagnosis, 520–521
  porphyria cutanea tarda (PCT), 523–530
    case presentation, 523–524
    clinical features, 526
    defined, 525–526
    diagnosis, 527–528
    generally, 524–525
    hereditary hemochromatosis (HH) and,
      528–529
    pathophysiology, 526–527
    treatment, 529–530
Prerenal azotermia, acute renal failure, differential
  diagnosis, 38–39
Primary hyperaldosteronism (Conn's syndrome),
  175–182
  case presentation, 175–177
  defined, 177–178
  diagnosis confirmation and subtype differentiation,
    180–181
  differential diagnosis and screening, 178–180
  treatment, 181
Primary micronodular hyperplasia, Cushing
  syndrome, 161
Prolactinomas (heterophile antibodies), 623–627
  case presentation, 623–624
  defined, 624
  differential diagnosis, 624–625
  "hook effect," 625–626
  treatment, 627
Prostate cancer, 349–354. *See also* Urinary
  tract and prostate errors
  case presentation, 349–350
  defined, 350
  differential diagnosis, 351–353
  pathophysiology, 350–351
  screening, 353
  treatment, 353
Prostate-specific antigen (PSA), prostate cancer
  diagnosis, 351–352
Prostatic acid phosphatase (PAP), prostate cancer
  diagnosis, 352
Protein C, coagulation factors and, venous
  thromboembolism (hereditary), 456

Proteinuria, chronic renal failure, 67–68
Prothrombin gene mutation G20210A, venous
  thromboembolism (hereditary), 456
Pseudohyponatremia, syndrome of
  inappropriate secretion of antiduretic hormone
  (SIADH), 84
Pseudomonas aeruginosa, cystic fibrosis, 27
Pulmonary disease, 17–30
  chronic obstructive pulmonary disease (COPD),
    19–23
    case presentation, 19–21
    commentary, 21–23
    pulmonary function tests, 21
    treatment, 23
  cystic fibrosis, 25–30
    case presentations, 25–27
    defined, 27
    differential diagnosis, 27–28
    pathogenesis, 28–30
    treatment, 30
Pulmonary function tests, chronic obstructive
  pulmonary disease (COPD), 21
Pulmonary infiltration, glomerular
  nephritis, 49–53

Qualitative platelet disorder:
  case presentation, 465–466
  diagnosis, 469–473
  differential diagnosis, 466–469
  hematologic disorders (benign), 465–474
  treatment, 473

Renal disease, 31–87. *See also* Cyclosporine A
  (CsA) metabolism
  acute renal failure, 31–39
    case presentation, 31–36
    differential diagnosis, 37–39
    treatment, 39
  anemia with chronic disease, 419–423
    case presentation, 419–420
    differential diagnosis, 420–421
    treatment, 421–422
  chronic renal failure, 65–74
    case presentation, 65–66
    chemistry and hematology, 67–69
      acidosis, 69
      anemia, 69
      azotemia, 68
      electrolytes, 68–69
      proteinuria, 67–68
    creatinine assays, 73
    defined, 66–67
    diagnosis, 69

glomerular filtration rate (GFR) estimation, 69–70
Modification of Diet in Renal Disease Study (MDRD) equation for glomerular filtration rate (GFR), 71–72
treatment, 73–74
glomerular nephritis, 49–53
nephrotic syndrome, 55–63
case presentation, 55–57
clinical findings, 57
commentary, 62
differential diagnosis, 59
laboratory results, 59–61
pathophysiology, 57–59
treatment, 61–62
osteodystrophy, 75–78
case presentation, 75
defined, 75–76
differential diagnosis, 76–77
treatment, 77–78
osteodystrophy (end-stage renal disease), 219–224
case presentation, 219–220
defined, 220–221
differential diagnosis, 222–223
pathogenesis, 221–222
treatment, 223
renal transplant cyclosporin toxicity, 41–47
allograft rejection, 44–45
calcineurin inhibitor effects and toxicity, 43–44
case presentation, 41–43
human leukocyte antigen (HLA) matching, 43
renal tubular acidosis (RTA), 45–47
uremic acidosis, 45
syndrome of inappropriate secretion of antidiuretic hormone (SIADH), 79–87
case presentation, 79–80
clinical features, 84
defined, 82
differential diagnosis, 80–82
laboratory findings, 84–86
ADH and renin measurements, 86
pseudohyponatremia, 84
serum osmolality, 84–86
water-loading test, 86
pathogenesis, 82–84
treatment, 86–87
Renal failure. See Acute renal failure; Chronic renal failure; Renal disease
Renal osteodystrophy, 75–78
case presentation, 75
defined, 75–76
differential diagnosis, 76–77
treatment, 77–78

Renal osteodystrophy (end-stage renal disease), 219–224
case presentation, 219–220
defined, 220–221
differential diagnosis, 222–223
pathogenesis, 221–222
treatment, 223
Renal transplant cyclosporin toxicity, 41–47. See also Cyclosporine A (CsA) metabolism; End-stage renal disease (ESRD) osteodystrophy
allograft rejection, 44–45
calcineurin inhibitor effects and toxicity, 43–44
case presentation, 41–43
human leukocyte antigen (HLA) matching, 43
renal tubular acidosis (RTA), 45–47
uremic acidosis, 45
Renal tubular acidosis (RTA), renal transplant cyclosporin toxicity, 45–47
Renin measurements, ADH and, syndrome of inappropriate secretion of antidiuretic hormone (SIADH), 86
Rheumatoid arthritis, 595–600
case presentation, 595–596
clinical features, 595
diagnosis, 595–599
pathophysiology, 595
treatment, 599–600
Rh hemolytic disease (Rh). See Hemolytic disease (Rh)

Seizures, hyperparathyroidism, 233–239
Serology, Helicobacter pylori infection, 324
Serum osmolality, syndrome of inappropriate secretion of antidiuretic hormone (SIADH), 84–86
Sickle cell disease, 411–417
case presentation, 411–412
differential diagnosis, 412–415
pathophysiology, 415
treatment, 415–416
Sinus pain, pain management, pharmacogenomics, 539–542
Sitosterolemia, 589–592
case presentation, 589–590
defined, 590
differential diagnosis, 590–591
treatment, 591
Spherocytosis. See Hereditary spherocytosis (HS)
Splenomegaly, chronic myelogenous leukemia (CML), 395
Sputnum production, chronic obstructive pulmonary disease (COPD), 22

Staphylococcus aureus:
    cystic fibrosis, 27
    sinusitis, 539
Stool antigen detection, *Helicobacter pylori*
    infection, 323
Streptococcus pneumoniae, sinusitis, 539
ST-segment elevation AMI (STEMI), acute
    myocardial infarction, 4, 6, 7, 8
Syndrome of inappropriate secretion of antidiuretic
    hormone (SIADH), 79–87
    case presentation, 79–80
    clinical features, 84
    defined, 82
    differential diagnosis, 80–82
    laboratory findings, 84–86
        ADH and renin measurements, 86
        pseudohyponatremia, 84
        serum osmolality, 84–86
        water-loading test, 86
    pathogenesis, 82–84
    treatment, 86–87
Syphilis. *See* Neurosyphilis
Systemic lupus erythematosus (SLE), 601–607
    case presentation, 601–603
    clinical features, 604
    diagnosis, 604–606
    pathophysiology, 603–604
    treatment, 606

Tangier disease, 581–584
    case presentation, 581–582
    defined, 582–583
    differential diagnosis, 583–584
    treatment, 584
Tartrate-resistant acid phosphatase (TRAP), bone
    markers, 230
T-cell leukemia (lymphoma, peripheral), 387–391
    case presentation, 387–388
    differential diagnosis, 388–389
    incidence and characteristics, 389–390
    treatment, 390–391
Thiopurine, 543–549
    case presentation, 543–544
    diagnosis, 548
    differential diagnosis, 544
    drug-metabolizing enzymes, 548–549
    metabolism and toxicity, 544–546
    pharmacogenetics, 546–547
    treatment, 548
Thrombocytopenia. *See* Heparin-induced
    thrombocytopenia (HIT)
Thrombocytosis:
    chronic myelogenous leukemia (CML), 394

erythrocytosis and, polycythemia vera differential
    diagnosis, 402–404
Thromboembolism. *See* Venous thromboembolism
    (acquired); Venous thromboembolism
    (hereditary)
Thrombotic thrombocytopenic purpura (TTP),
    485–490
    acute renal failure, differential diagnosis, 37–38
    case presentation, 485–486
    clinical presentation, 487–488
    differential diagnosis, 486–487
    pathophysiology, 488
    testing and management, 488
    treatment, 489
Thyroid disease, 129–146
    Graves disease, 131–137
        case presentation, 131–132
        defined, 132–133
        diagnosis, 134–136
        differential diagnosis, 133–134
        treatment, 136
    Hashimoto's thyroiditis, 139–142
        case presentation, 139–140
        defined, 140
        diagnosis, 141–142
        etiology, 140–141
        treatment, 142
    hyperparathyroidism, 233–239
        case presentation, 233–234
        defined, 234–236
        differential diagnosis, 236–238
        treatment, 238
    medullary thyroid carcinoma (MTC), 143–146
        case presentation, 143–144
        defined, 144
        differential diagnosis, 145
        treatment, 145–146
Thyrotoxicosis, Graves disease, 132
Thyrotropin-releasing hormone (TRH), Graves
    disease, 134
Toxicology, 555–572. *See also* Pharmacogenomics
    "club drug" use, 557–560
    metabolic acidosis, 567–572
        case presentation, 567–568
        defined, 568–570
        differential diagnosis, 570–571
        treatment, 571–572
    opioid drug abuse, 561–565

Urease testing, *Helicobacter pylori* infection, 325
Uremia, glomerular nephritis, 49–53
Uremic acidosis, renal transplant cyclosporin
    toxicity, 45

Urinary tract and prostate errors, 629–634. *See also*
    Prostate cancer
  case presentation, 629–630
  endogenous interfering antibodies, 630–633
    anti-animal immunoglobulin antibodies,
        632–633
    autoantibodies, 631–632
    immunoassays, 630–631
  follow-up, 630
  interference detection and
        minimization, 633–634
Urine production, nephrotic syndrome, 55–63. *See
    also* Nephrotic syndrome

Venous thromboembolism (acquired), 459–464
  antiphospholipid syndrome, 461
    clinical presentation, 463–464
    diagnosis, 461–462
    pathophysiology, 462–463
    thrombosis and, 462
    treatment, 464
  case presentation, 459–461
Venous thromboembolism (hereditary), 453–457
  case presentation, 453–454
  defined, 456
  diagnosis, 454–455
  hyperhomocysteinemia, 456–457
  protein C and coagulation factors, 456
  prothrombin gene mutation G20210A, 456
  testing for, 455
  treatment, 457
Venous thrombosis, coagulation factor V Leiden,
    551–554

von Willebrand disease, 475–483
  case presentation, 475–476
  defined, 480
  diagnosis, 481–482
  differential diagnosis, 476–479
  management, 482–483
  molecular dynamics, 479

Water-loading test, syndrome of inappropriate
        secretion of antidiuretic hormone (SIADH), 86
Weight gain, Cushing syndrome, 155–165. *See also*
    Cushing syndrome
West Nile virus infection, 329–333
  case presentation, 329–330
  defined, 330
  differential diagnosis, 331–332
  pathogenesis, 332
  treatment, 332–333
Wilson's disease, 91–97
  case presentation, 91–93
  commentary, 95–96
  manifestations of, 94–95
  pathophysiology, 94
  treatment, 96–97

Xanthomas, sitosterolemia, 589–592

Zollinger–Ellison syndrome (ZES), 243–248
  case presentation, 243–244
  defined, 245–246
  differential diagnosis, 246–247
  follow-up, 244
  treatment, 247